Basics of Blood Management

Basics of Blood Management

Petra Seeber

MD

Department of Anesthesiology
Critical Care Medicine
Pain Management, Emergency Medicine
HELIOS Klinik Blankenhain
Wirthstr. 5
99444 Blankenhain
Germany

Aryeh Shander

MD, FCCM, FCCP, Chief

Department of Anesthesiology, Critical Care Medicine
Pain Management and Hyperbaric Medicine
Englewood Hospital and Medical Center
350 Engle Street
Englewood, NJ 07631
and
Clinical Professor of Anesthesiology, Medicine and Surgery
Mount Sinai School of Medicine, Mount Sinai Hospital,
New York

FIRST EDITION

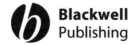
Blackwell
Publishing

Published by Blackwell Publishing
Blackwell Publishing, Inc., 350 Main Street, Malden, Massachusetts 02148-5020, USA
Blackwell Publishing Ltd, 9600 Garsington Road, Oxford OX4 2DQ, UK
Blackwell Publishing Asia Pty Ltd, 550 Swanston Street, Carlton, Victoria 3053, Australia

First published 2007

1   2007

Library of Congress Cataloging-in-Publication Data

Seeber, Petra.
    Basics of blood management / Petra Seeber, Aryeh Shander. – 1st ed.
        p. ; cm.
    Includes bibliographical references and index.
    ISBN: 978-1-4051-5131-3
  1. Transfusion-free surgery.   2. Blood–Transfusion.   3. Blood banks.
I. Shander, Aryeh.   II. Title.
    [DNLM: 1. Blood Substitutes–therapeutic use.   2. Blood Banks–organization & administration.   3. Blood Loss, Surgical–prevention & control.
4. Blood Transfusion. WH 450 S451b 2008]

    RD33.35.S44 2008 2007
    617–dc22

                                                                    2007005030

ISBN: 978-1-4051-5131-3

A catalogue record for this title is available from the British Library

Set in 9.25/11.5 Minion by Aptara Inc., New Delhi, India
Printed and bound in Singapore by Fabulous Printers Pte Ltd

Development Editor: Rebecca Huxley
Commissioning Editor: Maria Khan
Editorial Assistant: Jennifer Seward
Production Controller: Debbie Wyer

For further information on Blackwell Publishing, visit our website:
http://www.blackwellpublishing.com

The publisher's policy is to use permanent paper from mills that operate a sustainable forestry policy, and which has been manufactured from pulp processed using acid-free and elementary chlorine-free practices. Furthermore, the publisher ensures that the text paper and cover board used have met acceptable environmental accreditation standards.

Contents

Acknowledgments

We thank the following individuals for their review and valuable comments: Philip Battiade, Dr Charles and Nicole Beard, Prof. Dr Jochen Erhard, Shannon Farmer, David Grant, Renate Lange, Gregg Lobel, MD, FAAP, David Moskowitz, MD, Barbara Shackford, CRNA, MS, Mark Venditti, MD, and Prof. Max Woernhard.

Preface

The benefit-to-risk ratio of blood products needs constant evaluation. Blood products, as therapeutic agents, have had the test of time but lack the evidence we expect from other medicinals. Blood, an organ, is used as a pharmaceutical agent by the medical profession, due to the achievements in collection, processing, banking, and distribution. The fact that the most common risk of blood transfusion is blood delivery error supports the notion that blood is handled as a pharmaceutical agent. Over the last few decades, the risk of blood transfusion and associated complications has raised concerns about safety of blood by both the public and health-care providers. At the same time, experience with patients refusing blood and data on blood conservation brought to light the real possibility of other modalities to treat perisurgical anemia and to avoid it with blood conservation methods. In addition to risks and complications, data became available demonstrating the behavioural aspect of transfusion practice versus an evidence-based practice. In this book, the authors address many aspects of modern transfusion medicine, known blood conservation modalities, and new approaches to the treatment of perisurgical anemia, as well as special clinical considerations. This approach, now termed "blood management" by the Society for the Advancement of Blood Management (SABM, www.sabm.org), incorporates appropriate transfusion practice and blood conservation to deliver the lowest risk and highest benefit to the patient. In addition, it brings all these modalities to the patient's bedside and above all is a patient-centered approach. Blood management is a multidisciplinary, multimodality concept that focuses on the patient by improving patient outcome, making it one of the most intriguing and rewarding fields in medicine.

Blood management requires an understanding of all elements of blood and transfusions. It includes the philosophy, biology, physiology, and ethical considerations, as well as demonstrating the practical application of various techniques. This publication introduces the reader to blood management and explains how to improve medical outcomes by avoiding undue blood loss, enhancing the patient's own blood, and improving tolerance of anemia and coagulopathy until any of these underlying conditions are successfully remedied.

This introduction to blood management is intended for the training and early practicing clinicians. It is meant to be both informative and practical and spans many of the medical specialties that encounter blood and transfusions as part of their daily practice. It will aid in tailoring individual care plans for the different patients. Finally, it addresses the structure and function of a blood management program, a novel approach to blood conservation, and improved patient outcome.

In this book, blood management is considered from an international perspective, so attention is paid to conditions encountered in developing as well as industrial countries. Techniques such as cell salvage are performed differently in economically deprived countries; HIV, hepatitis, and malaria may or may not be a threat to the blood supply, depending on geographic location; oxygen, intravenous fluids, and erythropoiesis-stimulating proteins may be readily available in some countries or inaccessible in others. The book is intended to broaden the readers' horizons, discussing working conditions encountered by blood managers around the world. Many of the clinical scenarios and the exercise that follow are intended for the reader to adapt the information to the prevailing circumstances in their location.

This book is unique in the fact that it is the first dedicated in its entirety to the concept of blood management. The authors hope that this book will stimulate the readers to further advance blood management through shared experience and research. It is intended to be informative, practical, enjoyable and will stimulate debate and discussion as well as help patients in need.

Petra Seeber and Aryeh Shander
March 2007

1 History and organization of blood management

With this introductory chapter the reader will be given a glimpse into the organization of blood management and its history—a history that is still extremely active and changes day to day.

Objectives of this chapter

1 Identify historical developments that led to today's concept of blood management.
2 Demonstrate the benefits of blood management.
3 Identify blood management as "good clinical" practice.
4 Show that blood management and its techniques should be used in all cases that qualify.
5 Help understand how a blood management program works.

Definitions

Bloodless medicine and surgery: Bloodless medicine is a multimodality, multidisciplinary approach to safe and effective patient care *without* the use of allogeneic blood products. Bloodless medicine and surgery utilizes pharmacological and technological means as well as medical and surgical techniques to provide the best possible care without the use of donor blood.

Transfusion-free medicine and surgery: Since "bloodless medicine" is kind of a misnomer, the term "transfusion-free medicine" was coined and is used instead.

Blood conservation: "Blood conservation is a global concept engulfing all possible strategies aimed at *reducing* patient's exposure to allogeneic blood products" [1]. This concept does not exclude the use of allogeneic blood entirely.

Blood management: Blood management is the philosophy to improve patient outcomes by integrating all

available techniques to reduce or eliminate allogeneic blood transfusions. It is a patient-centered, multidisciplinary, multimodal, planned approach to patient care. Blood management is not an "alternative," it is the standard of care.

A brief look at history

History of bloodless medicine, transfusion-free medicine, blood conservation, and blood management

The term "bloodless medicine" is often associated with the belief of Jehovah's Witnesses to refrain from the use of blood, therefore ruling out the option of blood transfusion. The essence of bloodless medicine, and lately, blood management, however, is not restricted to the beliefs of a religious group. To get a better understanding as to what bloodless medicine and blood management means, let us go back to the roots of these disciplines.

One is not completely wrong to attribute the origin of the term "bloodless medicine" to the endeavor of Jehovah's Witnesses to receive treatment without resorting to donor blood transfusion. Their attitude toward the sanctity of blood greatly influences their view of blood transfusion. This was published as early as 1927 in their journal *The Watchtower* (December 15, 1927). Although the decision to refuse blood transfusion is a completely religious one, the Witnesses frequently used scientific information about the side effects of donor blood transfusion. The booklet entitled *Blood, Medicine and the Law of God* (published in 1961) addressed issues such as transfusion reactions, transfusion-related syphilis, malaria, and hepatitis.

Refusing blood transfusions on religious grounds was not easy. Repeatedly, patients were physically forced to take donor blood, using such high-handed methods as incapacitation by court order, strapping patients to the bed (even with the help of police officers), and secretly adding sedatives to a patient's infusion. In the early 1960s, representatives of Jehovah's Witnesses started visiting physicians to explain the reasons why transfusions were refused by the Witness population. Often, during the same visit, they offered literature which dealt with techniques that were acceptable to the Witness patients, informing physicians of the availability of the so-called transfusion alternatives. After a few years of work, the governing body of Jehovah's Witnesses announced the formation of Hospital Liaison Committees (1979). These continued to "support Jehovah's Witnesses in . . . *their* determination to prevent their being given blood transfusions, to clear away misunderstandings on the part of doctors and hospitals, . . . to establish a more cooperative spirit between medical institutions and Witness patients" and to "alert hospital staff to the fact that there are valid alternatives to the infusion of blood" (italics ours). Occasionally, the Witnesses even went to court to fight for their rights as patients. In a great number of cases, the Witnesses' position was upheld by the courts.

Although many physicians had difficulty with the concept of bloodless medicine, there were some physicians who took up the challenge to provide the best possible medical care without the use of blood transfusions. These were in fact the earliest blood managers. As their experience in performing "bloodless" surgery increased, more complex procedures such as open heart surgery, orthopedic surgery, and cancer surgery could be performed. Even children and newborns could successfully be treated without transfusing blood. Not before long, those pioneering physicians published their results with Witness patients, thereby encouraging other doctors to adopt the methods used in performing such surgical interventions.

Among the first ones who rose to the challenge was the heart surgeon Denton Cooley of Texas. In the early 1960s, his team devised methods to treat Witness patients. Reporting on his early experiences, he published an article in a 1964 issue of *The American Journal of Cardiology*. In the article "Open heart surgery in Jehovah's Witnesses" his team described the techniques used. In 1977, Cooley reported his experiences with more than 500 patients [2].

Cooley's example was followed by many other courageous physicians. For instance, in 1970 Dr Pearce performed bloodless open heart surgery in New Orleans. His efforts did not go unnoticed. Newspapers reported on these spectacular cases. Perhaps out of curiosity or out of the earnest desire to learn, many colleagues visited Dr Pearce's team in the operating room to learn how to do "bloodless hearts." Dr Jerome Kay, from Los Angeles, also performed bloodless heart surgery. In 1973 he reported that he is now performing bloodless heart surgery on the majority of his patients. The call for bloodless treatments spread around the whole world. Dr Sharad Pandey of the KEM hospital in Mumbai, India, adopted bloodless techniques from Canada and tailored them to fit Indian conditions. Centers in Europe and the rest of the world started adopting those advances as well.

It is understandable that Witness patients preferred the treatment of physicians who had already proven their willingness and ability to treat them without using donor blood. The good reputation of such physicians spread and so patients from far away were transferred to their facilities. This laid the foundation for organized "bloodless programs." One of the hospitals with such a program was the Esperanza Intercommunity Hospital in Yorba Linda, California, where a high percentage of patients were Witnesses. Dr Herk Hutchins, an experienced surgeon and a Witness himself, was known for his development of an iron-containing formula for blood-building. Among his team was the young surgeon Ron Lapin. Later, he was famed for his pioneering work in the area of bloodless therapies. Critics labeled him a quack. Nevertheless, he continued and was later honored for opening one of the first organized bloodless centers in the world, as well as for publishing the first journal on this topic, and for his efforts to teach his colleagues. During his career, he performed thousands of bloodless surgeries.

All of those pioneers of blood management had to rise to the challenge of using and refining available techniques, adjusting them to current needs, and individualizing patient care. They adopted new technologies as soon as this was reasonable. Much attention was paid to details of patient care, thus improving the quality of the whole therapy. They also fought for patients' rights and upheld those rights. Many involved in the field of blood management confirm the good feeling of being a physician in the truest sense. There is no need to force a particular treatment. Such an attitude is a precious heritage from the pioneers of blood management. Now, at the beginning of the twenty-first century, this pioneer spirit can still be felt at some meetings dedicated to blood management.

Military use of blood and blood management

Over the centuries, the armies of different nations contributed to what is now available for blood management, but not on religious grounds. It can actually be said that the military made many crucial contributions to blood management by taking care of the thousands of wounded operated on before transfusions became feasible. In fact, every surgery performed before the era of blood transfusion was, strictly speaking, a "bloodless surgery." Surgeons were confronted with blood loss, but had no way to replace blood. This meant it was imperative to stop hemorrhage promptly and effectively and to avoid further blood loss. During the centuries, battlegrounds were the places where surgeons were massively confronted with blood loss and it was on the battlefield that hemorrhage was recognized as a cause of death. Hemorrhaging victims needed surgery. It was then that techniques of bloodless medicine and blood management were invented. The experience of the early surgeons serving near the battlefield is applicable in today's blood management schemes. William Steward Halsted, a surgeon on the battlefield, described uncontrolled hemorrhage [3] and later taught his trainees at Johns Hopkins the technique of gentle tissue handling, surgery in anatomic ways, and meticulous hemostasis (Halstedian principles). His excellent work provides the basis of the surgical contribution to a blood management program.

As soon as transfusions became somewhat practical, the military used them for their purposes. Since war brought about a deluge of hemorrhaging victims, there was a need for a therapy. The First World War brought the advent of blood anticoagulation. This made it possible to transport blood to the wounded and reduced the use of living donors in the field. But there were other problems. Storage times and problems with logistics called for improvements in blood therapy. During the Second World War, the problem of storage of blood was partly overcome by the advent of blood banks. Another development was due to Cohn's fractionation of blood, which led to the production of plasma as a volume expander for war victims. The United States extensively used plasma for volume expansion in World War II.

Although the World Wars propelled the development of transfusion medicine, these simultaneously propelled the development of alternative treatments. Tremendous problems with availability and logistics as well as with compatibility of blood made transfusions near the battlefield dangerous, difficult, and expensive. Those problems, as well as inherent risks of transfusions, led to the search for other ways of treatment. Intravenous fluids had been described in earlier medical literature [4, 5], but the pressing need to replace lost blood and the difficulties involved in transfusions provided a strong impetus for military medicine to change practice. In this connection, note the following report appearing in the Providence *Sunday Journal* of May 17, 1953: "The Army will henceforth use dextran, a substance made from sugar, instead of blood plasma, for all requirements at home and overseas, it was learned last night. An authoritative Army medical source, who asked not to be quoted by name, said 'a complete switchover' to the plasma substitute has been put into effect, after 'utterly convincing' tests of dextran in continental and combat area hospitals during the last few months. This official said a major factor in the switchover to dextran was that use of plasma entails a 'high risk' of causing a disease known as serum hepatitis—a jaundice-like ailment. Not all plasma carries this hazard, he emphasized, but he added that dextran is entirely free of the hazard. 'We have begun to fill all orders from domestic and overseas theaters with dextran instead of plasma.'"

Efforts to develop another "blood substitute" were intensified by US military in 1985. Major investments supported research, either by contract laboratories or by military facilities themselves [6]. This time, not the search for a plasma expander but the search for an oxygen carrier was the driving force behind the army's efforts.

Promising products in the sector of blood management were readily introduced to the military. One example is a cell-saving device. The surgeon Gerald Klebanoff, who served in the Vietnam War, introduced a device for autotransfusion in the military hospitals. Another example is the recombinant clotting factor VIIa. Although officially declared to be a product for use in hemophiliacs, the Israeli army discovered its potential to stop life-threatening hemorrhage and therefore included it in their treatment of injured victims.

Also, in recent times, the military showed a keen interest in blood management. After the attack on the World Trade Center in New York on September 11, 2001, physicians of the US military approached the Society for the Advancement of Blood Management and asked about blood management. They were aware that a war in a country like Afghanistan would also require preparation on the part of the physicians. The high costs of transfusions in war times (up to US $9000 must be calculated for one unit of red blood cells when transfused in countries like Afghanistan) and logistic difficulties called for blood-conserving approaches. Consequently, specialists in the field of blood management met together with representatives of the US military, the result of which was an initiative named STORMACT® (strategies to reduce military and civilian transfusion). The consensus of this initiative was a blood management concept to be used to treat victims of war and disaster as well as patients in a preclinical setting.

Transfusion specialists support blood management

Interestingly, right from the beginning of transfusion medicine, the development of blood transfusion and transfusion alternatives were closely interwoven. "Alternatives" to transfusion are as old as transfusion itself.

The first historically proven transfusions in humans were performed in the seventeenth century. The physicians were aiming to cure mental disorders rather than the substitution of lost blood. But the very first transfusion specialists were in fact also the first people to try infusions that were later called transfusion alternatives. For instance, it was reported that Christopher Wren was involved in the first transfusion experiments. He was also the first to inject asanguinous fluids, such as wine and beer. After two of Jean Baptiste Denise's (a French transfusionist) transfused patients died, transfusion experiments were prohibited in many countries. Even the Pope condemned those early efforts. For a long time, transfusions came to a halt.

In the beginning of the nineteenth century, the physician James Blundell was looking for a method of prohibiting the death of female patients due to profuse hemorrhage related to childbirth. His amazing results with retransfusion of the women's shed blood rekindled the interest of the medical community in transfusion medicine. Due to his work with autotransfusion he was named in the list of the "fathers of modern transfusion medicine." This demonstrates again that transfusion medicine and alternatives to allogeneic transfusion are closely related.

After Blundell demonstrated that retransfusion of shed blood saved lives, other physicians followed his example. This gave new impetus to transfusion medicine, and in 1873 Jennings [7] published a report of about 243 transfusions in humans, of which almost half of the cases died. Allogeneic transfusions remained dangerous. Blood groups were not known at that time. Technical problems with the transfusion procedure itself resulted in complications and effective anticoagulants were still unknown. Frustration around this situation led some researchers to look for alternative treatments in the event of hemorrhage. Barnes and Little came up with normal saline as a blood substitute [8]. Hamlin tried milk infusions [9]. The use of gelatin was also experimented with. But soon, normal saline was introduced into medical practice. One of the advocates of normal saline, W.T. Bull, wrote in 1884 [10]: "The danger from loss of blood, even to two-thirds of its whole volume, lies in the disturbed relationship between the caliber of the vessels and the quantity of blood contained therein, and not in the diminished number of red blood corpuscles;

and ... this danger concerns the volume of the injected fluids also, it being a matter of indifference whether they be albuminous or containing blood corpuscles or not."

In the early 1900, Landsteiner's discovery of the blood groups was probably the event that propelled transfusion medicine to where it is today. Some 10–15 years later, when Reuben Ottenberg introduced routine typing of blood into clinical practice, the way was paved for blood transfusions. About that time, technical problems had been solved by new techniques and anticoagulation was in use. Russian physicians (Filatov, Depp, Yudin) stored cadaver blood. The groundwork for the first blood bank was laid in 1934 in Chicago by Seed and Fantus [11], and as already mentioned, the wars of the first half of the twentieth century brought about changes in transfusion medicine. After two World Wars the medical community had a seemingly endless and safe stream of blood at their disposal. Adams and Lundy published an article, suggesting a possible transfusion trigger of a hemoglobin level of 10 mg/dL and a hematocrit of 30. For nearly four decades thereafter, physicians transfused to their liking, convinced that the benefits of allogeneic transfusions outweigh their potential risks.

As time went by, reports about blood-borne diseases increased. In 1962, when the famous article of J.G. Allen [12] again demonstrated a connection between transfusion and hepatitis, an era of increased awareness about transfusion-transmissible diseases began. But the risk of hepatitis transmission did not concern the general medical community, and it became an acceptable complication of banked blood. It was not until the early 1980s that the medical community and the public became aware of the risks of transfusions. The discovery that an acquired immunodeficiency syndrome was spread by allogeneic transfusion heightened public awareness, and the demand for safer blood and bloodless medicine increased. Other problems with allogeneic transfusions such as immunosuppression added to the concerns. Again, as in the centuries before, it was the ones concerned most about transfusion issues who were looking for alternative approaches. Lessons learned from the work with the Jehovah's Witnesses community were ready to be applied on a wider scale. In the United States, the National Institute of Health launched a consensus conference on the proper use of blood. The Adams and Lundy's 10/30 rule was revised, and it was agreed upon that a hemoglobin level of 7 mg/dL would be sufficient in otherwise healthy patients.

With time, the incentives for better blood management and blood conservation change. The role of immunomodulation with allogeneic blood is controversial but, nonetheless, offers a reason for blood conservation;

the incremental increase of blood products is another and lastly, sporadic but serious blood shortages are all good reasons to consider effective blood management.

Blood management today and tomorrow

Currently, there are more than 100 organized bloodless programs in the United States. Many are transitioning to become blood management programs. This is not unique to the United States since many more programs have been established worldwide. Most of them were formed as a result of the initiatives of Jehovah's Witnesses. However, a growing number of those programs have now realized the benefits that all patients can receive from this care. The increasing number of patients asking for treatment without blood demonstrates a growing demand in this field. Concerns about the public health implications of transfusion-related hazards have led governmental institutions, around the globe, to encourage and support the establishment of these programs.

The growing interest in blood management is reflected by these activities described herein. Major medical organizations (e.g., the American Association of Blood Banks, AABB) are now including blood management issues on the agenda of their regular meetings. Many transfusion textbooks and regular medical journals have incorporated the subject of blood management in their publications. A growing body of literature invites further investigation (compare Appendix B). In addition, professional societies dedicated to furthering blood management were founded throughout the world. It is their common goal to provide a forum for the exchange of ideas and information among professionals engaged in the advancement and improvement of blood management in clinical practice. This is done by facilitating cooperation among existing and future programs for blood conservation, transfusion-free or bloodless medicine and blood management; also, by reinforcing the clinical and scientific aspects of appropriate transfusion practice, by encouraging and developing educational programs for health-care professionals and the public, and by contributing to the active continuing medical education of its members. Usually, interested persons from a variety of medical and nonmedical backgrounds are invited to participate.

Clearly, out of humble beginnings as an outsider specialty, blood management has evolved to be in the mainstream of medicine. It improves the outcome for the patient, reduces costs, and brings satisfaction for the physician—a clear win–win situation. Blood management is plainly good medical practice.

What are the future trends in blood management? As long as there is a need for medical treatment, blood management will develop. Many new drugs and techniques are on the horizon. To date, there are many techniques available to reduce or eliminate the use of donor blood that it is not necessary to wait for the future. A commitment to blood management is what will change the way blood is used. The authors of this book hope that the information provided by its pages will be another piece in the puzzle that will eventually define future blood management by a new generation of physicians.

Blood management as a program

The organized approach to blood management is a program. These programs are named according to the emphasis each one puts on different facets of blood management, such as bloodless programs, transfusion-free programs, blood conservation programs, or global blood management programs. No matter what a hospital calls its program, there are some basic features that good quality programs have in common.

The administration

The basis for establishing a program is not primarily a financial investment but rather a great deal of commitment on the part of the hospital. Administration, physicians, nurses, and other personnel need to be involved. Only the sincere cooperation of those involved will make a program successful.

The heart and soul of a program is its coordinator with his/her in-hospital office [13, 14]. As a historical prospective, coordinators are often members of Jehovah's Witnesses. However, as such programs are more widely accepted, there is an increasing number of coordinators with other backgrounds. Usually, coordinators are employed and paid by the hospital.

During the initial phases of development of the program, the coordinators may be burdened with significant workload. Together with involved physicians, the coordinator has to recruit additional physicians who are willing and able to participate in the program. Since successful blood management is a multidisciplinary endeavor, specialists from a variety of fields need to be involved. (What, for instance, is the use of a dedicated anesthesiologist if surgeons do not participate?) The coordinator meets with the heads of the clinical departments and works toward mutual understanding and cooperation. Each physician willing to participate needs to meet with the coordinator to affirm the physician's commitment to the program and to enhance his/her knowledge of basic ethical and medical principles involved. To ensure a lasting and dependable cooperation between physicians and the program, both parties sign a contract. This contract outlines the points that are crucial for blood management with its legal, ethical, and medical issues.

The coordinator is also instrumental for the initial and continuous education of participating and incoming staff. She/he may use in-service sessions, invite guest speakers, collect and distribute current literature, get information on national and international educational meetings, and help staff interested in hands-on experience in the field of blood management. Ideally, participating staff members take care of their education themselves and contribute to the success of the program.

From the beginning of the program, there needs to be a set of policies and procedures. Guidelines as to cooperation with other staff members need to be worked out. It is prudent to have the hospital lawyer review all such documents. Each individual hospital must find a way to educate patients, document their will, and make sure that patients are treated according to their will and they are clearly identifiable. Transfers of patients to and from the hospital need to be organized. A mode of emergency transferal needs to be established. Procedures already in existence such as storage and release of blood products and rarely used drugs for emergencies need to be reviewed. Most probably, there are many medical procedures already available in the hospital that just need to be adapted to the needs of the program. Additional blood management procedures and devices are to be introduced to the hospital staff. The use of hemodilution, cell salvage, platelet sequestration, autologous surgical glue, and other methods needs to be organized. Besides, departments not directly involved in patient care can contribute to the development of policies and procedures. This holds true for administrative offices, the blood bank, laboratory, technical department, pharmacy, and possibly the research department. There are also a variety of issues that need legal and ethical clarification. In keeping with national and international law, issues involved with pediatric and obstetric cases need to be clarified well before the first event arises. Forms need to be developed and a protocol for obtaining legal consent and/or advance directive must be instituted.

To assure continuing support on the part of the administration and the public, some measures of quality control and assurance need implementation. Statistical data from the time before the establishment of a certain procedure should be available for comparison with those obtained after its institution and during the course of its implementation. This is a valuable instrument to demonstrate the effectiveness of procedures and their associated costs. It also serves as an aid in decision making regarding possible and necessary changes. If records are kept up-to-date, developments and trends can be used as an effective tool for quality assurance and for the identification of strong and weak points in a program. Such records are also helpful for negotiations with sponsors and financial departments, discussions with incoming physicians, and for public relations.

The coordinators, and later their staff, need to be well informed about policies and procedures in their hospital and the level of care the facility can provide. There may be times when burden of cases or the severity of a patient's condition outsize the faculty's capacity or capability. In such cases, a list of alternative hospitals better suited to perform a certain procedure should be available.

Good communication skills are essential for the daily activities of the coordinator since he/she is the link between patients and physicians. The coordinator is in constant contact with the patient and his/her family and is involved in the development of the plan of care of every patient in the program. The coordinator informs the staff involved in the care of the patient about issues pertaining to blood management. In turn, staff members inform the coordinator about the progress of the patient. Planned procedures are discussed and any irregular development is reported. Thus, developing problems can be counteracted at an early stage, thereby avoiding major mishaps.

There is virtually no limit to the ingenuity of a coordinator. She/he is a pioneer, manager, nurse, teacher, host, helper, and friend. No successful program is possible without a coordinator. The last chapter in this book will further describe how the coordinator can work effectively for the development of a blood management program.

The physician's part

Several studies on transfusion practice in relation to certain procedures demonstrate a striking fact: A great institutional variability exists in transfusion practice, for no medical reason. For example, in a study on coronary bypass surgery the rate of transfusions varied between 27 and 92% [15]. What was the reason? Did physicians who transfused frequently care for sicker patients? No, the major differing variable was the institution—and with it were the physicians. This is in fact good news. If the physician's behavior can be modified to appropriately limit the transfusion rate, then a blood management program can effectively reduce transfusions.

Basic and continuous education is crucial for physicians participating in a blood management program. To start with, physicians should intercommunicate about currently available techniques of blood management which relate to their field of practice and compare their own knowledge and skills with others. The result of such an honest comparison identifies the strong and weak areas in their practice of blood management. Then, new approaches, techniques, and equipment should be added as needed. However, remember that not all techniques fit all physicians and not all physicians fit all techniques. After all, it is not a sophisticated set of equipment that makes good blood management—it is a group of skilled physicians. That is why it is desirable that all physicians in a blood management program be aware of the experiences and skills of their colleagues, in order to make these available to the patients.

Another group of professionals that is essential for the program to succeed are the nurses. Nurses play a vital role as they contribute much to patient identification, education, and care. Nursing staff must therefore also be included in the process of initial and continuing education.

Commitment, education, cooperation, and communication are key factors for a successful blood management program. To make each treatment a success, it requires the concerted effort by physicians, coordinators, nurses, administration, and auxiliary staff on the one side, and the patient with his/her family on the other.

Key points

- Blood management is a good clinical practice that should be applied for all patients.
- Blood management is best practiced in an organized program.
- Blood management improves outcomes, is patient centered, multidisciplinary, and multimodal.
- Respect for patients, commitment, education, cooperation, and communication are the cornerstones blood management builds on.

Questions for review

- What role did the following play in the development of modern blood management: Jehovah's Witnesses, physicians, the military, and transfusion specialists?

- What do the following terms mean: bloodless medicine, transfusion-free medicine, blood conservation, blood management?
- What are the important facets of a comprehensive blood management program?

Suggestions for further research

What medical, ethical, and legal obstacles had early blood managers to overcome? How did they do so? What can be learned from their experience?

Exercises and practice cases

Read the article of Adams and Lundy that builds the basis for the 10/30 rule.

Homework

Analyze your hospital and answer the following questions:
What measures are taken to identify patients?
What is done to comply with legal requirements when it comes to documentation of patients' preferences for treatment?
What steps are taken to ensure the patients' wishes are heeded?

References

1 Baele, P. and P. Van der Linden. Developing a blood conservation strategy in the surgical setting. *Acta Anaesthesiol Belg*, 2002. **53**(2): p. 129–136.

2 Ott, D.A. and D.A. Cooley. Cardiovascular surgery in Jehovah's witnesses. Report of 542 operations without blood transfusion. *JAMA*, 1977. **238**(12): p. 1256–1258.

3 Halsted, W.S. *Surgical Papers by William Steward Halsted*. John Hopkins Press, Baltimore, MD, 1924.

4 Mudd, S. and W. Thalhimer. *Blood Substitutes and Blood Transfusion*, Vol. 1. C.C. Thomas, Springfield, IL, 1942.

5 White, C. and J. Weinstein. *Blood Derivates and Substitutes. Preparation, Storage, Administration and Clinical Results Including Discussion of Shock. Etiology, Physiology, Pathology and Treatment*, Vol. 1. Williams and Wilkins, Baltimore, MD, 1947.

6 Winslow, R.M. New transfusion strategies: red cell substitutes. *Annu Rev Med*, 1999. **50**: p. 337–353.

7 Jennings, C. *Transfusion: It's History, Indications, and Mode of Application.* Leonard & Co., New York, 1883.

8 Diamond, L. A history of blood transfusion. In *Blood, Pure and Eloquent.* McGraw-Hill, New York, 1980.

9 Spence, R. Blood substitutes. In L.D., Petz, S., Kleinman, S.N., Swisher, and R.K., Spence (eds.) *Clinical Practice of Transfusion Medicine.* Churchill-Livingstone, New York, 1996. p. 967–984.

10 Bull, W. On the intravenous injection of saline solutions as a substitution for transfusion of blood. *Med Rec,* 1884. **25**: p. 6–8.

11 Fantus, B. Therapy of the Cook County Hospital (blood preservation). *JAMA,* 1937. **109**: p. 128–132.

12 Allen, J. Serum hepatitis from transfusion of blood. *JAMA,* 1962. **180**: p. 1079–1085.

13 Vernon, S. and G.M. Pfeifer. Are you ready for bloodless surgery? *Am J Nurs,* 1997. **97**(9): p. 40–46; quiz 47.

14 deCastro, R.M. Bloodless surgery: establishment of a program for the special medical needs of the Jehovah's Witness community—the gynecologic surgery experience at a community hospital. *Am J Obstet Gynecol,* 1999. **180**(6, Pt 1): p. 1491–1498.

15 Stover, E.P., *et al.* Institutional variability in red blood cell conservation practices for coronary artery bypass graft surgery. Institutions of the MultiCenter Study of Perioperative Ischemia Research Group. *J Cardiothorac Vasc Anesth,* 2000. **14**(2): p. 171–176.

2 Physiology of anemia and oxygen transport

Tolerance of anemia while it is being treated is one of the cornerstones of blood management. This chapter explains the physiological and pathophysiological mechanisms underlying the body's oxygen transport and use of oxygen. This will help to understand how the body deals with states of reduced oxygen delivery and efforts to increase delivery. Furthermore, it enables the reader to reflect critically on current and future therapeutic measures to increase oxygen availability to tissue.

Objectives of this chapter

1 Review factors that influence oxygen delivery.
2 Learn how to calculate oxygen delivery and consumption.
3 Identify mechanisms the body uses to adapt to acute and chronic anemia.
4 Define the vital role of the microcirculation.
5 Describe tissue oxygenation and tissue oxygen utilization.

Definitions

Anemia: Anemia is a reduction in the total circulating red blood cell mass, usually diagnosed by a decrease in hemoglobin concentration. Thresholds for anemia depend on the age and gender of the patient. Typically, anemia is said to exist in an adult male when hemoglobin is below 13.5 g/dL. In adult females, anemia is diagnosed when the hemoglobin is below 12 g/dL.

Regular physiology

A single equation describes the whole concept...

Let us jump right into the subject, using the well-known equation where oxygen delivery is simply calculated by multiplying the cardiac output by arterial oxygen content.

$$DO_2 = Q \times (Hgb \times 1.34 \times SaO_2 + 0.003 \times PaO_2) \times 10 \tag{1}$$

where DO_2, oxygen delivery; Q, flow in L/min; Hgb, hemoglobin in g/dL; 1.34, Hufner's number; SaO_2, oxygen saturation of hemoglobin in %; 0.003, oxygen solubility in plasma; PaO_2, partial pressure of oxygen in arterial blood in mm Hg.

The equation describes the concept of systemic oxygen transport (macrocirculation), the knowledge of which constitutes a sound basis for understanding therapeutic interventions that enhance oxygen delivery.

One of the crucial factors of oxygen transport is the flow (Q) or cardiac output (CO), which is determined by the stroke volume (SV) and the heart rate (HR) (CO = SV × HR). Flow is permanent for oxygen delivery since neither red cells nor any other blood constituent would reach their target if sufficient flow were lacking.

Another crucial player in oxygen transport is hemoglobin. In healthy individuals, most of the oxygen in blood is bound to hemoglobin. One molecule of hemoglobin can hold a maximum of four oxygen molecules. In vivo, 1 g hemoglobin has the potential to bind approximately 1.34 mL oxygen (Hufner's number). In order to know exactly how much oxygen is bound to hemoglobin, another variable must be known. This is the oxygen saturation (SaO_2), the percentage of hemoglobin molecules that actually have bound oxygen.

Besides the oxygen bound by hemoglobin, a small amount of oxygen is physically dissolved in plasma. This amount is linearly dependent on the partial pressure of oxygen "above" the plasma, namely the inspiratory oxygen fraction (FiO_2). The higher the FiO_2, the more oxygen is dissolved. The amount of oxygen physically dissolved in plasma also depends on the specific Bunsen solubility coefficient α of oxygen. A Bunsen solubility coefficient of 0.024 means that there is 0.024 mL oxygen dissolved in 1 mL blood at normal body temperature (37°C) at a pressure of 1 atm. Using the Henry Dalton equation, it can be calculated that 0.003 mL O_2/mL blood is physically dissolved in normal arterial blood ($PO_2 = 95$ mm Hg, $PCO_2 = 40$ mm Hg). Thus, the number 0.003 in eqn. (1) is the amount of physically dissolved oxygen in the blood under "normal" conditions. Although the amount of physically dissolved oxygen might appear insignificant compared to the amount of oxygen transported by hemoglobin, it should be borne in mind that every single molecule of oxygen bound to hemoglobin had to be physically dissolved in blood before it entered the red cell. Later it will be shown that the amount of physically dissolved oxygen is crucial for patients with severe anemia.

A single equation describes the whole concept . . . does it?

Imagine a patient with a very low serum calcium level. What treatment should be used? Substituting the body's calcium stores sounds reasonable, but a doctor could also prescribe the patient pebbles and ask him/her to swallow them. The body's content of calcium would certainly increase dramatically. Most would object, "But that is complete nonsense," and they would be right, because it is obvious that the calcium contained in the pebbles does not reach the place where it is needed and cannot be used by the body. On the contrary, it may even cause harm to the patient.

The same holds true for patients suffering from a lack of oxygen carrying red cells. Initially the idea of filling the patient up may sound reasonable. However, the main point is easily overlooked if only macrocirculatory oxygen delivery is kept in mind; namely, Do I reach the goal of delivering oxygen to the tissue? And one step further: Do I succeed in maintaining aerobic metabolism? Just increasing the hemoglobin level by transfusing may,

at times, be similar to feeding a stone to a patient with low calcium level. A number is changed, but the condition is not improved. For this reason the second half of oxygen delivery needs to be taken into consideration: the microcirculation.

How do red cells take up oxygen?

How about accompanying red cells on their journey through the human body. The trip starts in the capillary bed of the lungs. Here is where the red cells deliver carbon dioxide and take up oxygen.

Pulmonary gas exchange is governed by Fick's law of diffusion, stating that the flux of diffusing particles (here oxygen and carbon dioxide) is proportional to their concentration gradient. Driven by this gradient, oxygen and carbon dioxide molecules move across membranes in the lung, in vessel walls and red cells, as well as through fluids in random walk. Due to the immense surface of the lung across which oxygen and carbon dioxide gradients develop, the exchange of oxygen and carbon dioxide is performed rapidly. Hemoglobin molecules further support the uptake of oxygen by red cells as hemoglobin molecules diffuse within the cell, also following a gradient. Once hemoglobin is oxygenated by means of oxygen diffusion across the red cell membrane, the oxygenated hemoglobin diffuses into the center of the red cell whereas deoxyhemoglobin diffuses toward the cell membrane, ready for oxygen uptake.

The processes of carbon dioxide release and oxygen uptake interact closely. As the partial pressure of carbon dioxide decreases, the affinity of hemoglobin for oxygen increases (Haldane effect). This effect supports the oxygenation of red cells in the lung.

The rate of oxygen uptake by human red cells is approximately 40 times slower than the corresponding rate of oxygen combination with free hemoglobin. The reason being that the hemoglobin in red cells is surrounded by several layers: cytoplasm, cell membrane, and a fluid layer adjacent to the red cell membrane. Oxygen therefore has to diffuse over a long distance before it can penetrate the cell. In particular the unstirred layers around the red cell pose a barrier to oxygen uptake. The impact of the red cell membrane to resist gas exchange is a subject of controversy and may in fact be negligible [1, 2]. The uptake of oxygen by red cells appears mainly to depend on the thickness of unstirred fluid layers [1] (and less on pH, 2,3-diphosphoglycerate (2,3-DPG) level, and membrane resistance).

How do red cells reach the microvasculature in the tissue?

Let us follow the red cells even further. As already described, they brought CO_2 for exhalation to the lung and have taken up oxygen. Now the red cells are ready for their next mission. They have to travel to the microcirculation to deliver the oxygen.

As the blood is impelled by the heart, it is urged from large vessels into the narrower areas of the human vasculature. The red cells then slow down. The resulting reduction in red cell velocity leads to a reduction in hematocrit in a determined segment of vessel relative to the hematocrit of blood entering or leaving the tube. This dynamic reduction of the intravascular hematocrit is called the Farhaeus effect [3]. The hematocrit in the microcirculation is about 30% of that in the systemic circulation and it remains constant until the systemic hematocrit is lowered to less than 15% [4].

As the red cells travel down the road toward the smallest capillaries, they tend to aggregate and build "rouleaux" formations, which look like stacks of coins [3]. This is due to macromolecular bridging and osmotic water exclusion from the gap between neighboring red cell membranes. Red cells line up in the center of the vessel where they have the maximum velocity. A plasma layer at the vessel wall works as kind of a lubricant to help the cells pass through the capillary. This arrangement of cells and plasma leads to a marked reduction in the viscosity so that blood viscosity in the microcirculation is close to that of plasma [3]. This effect was described by Farhaeus and Lindqvist when they wrote, "Below a critical point at a diameter of about 0.3 mm the viscosity decreases strongly with reduced diameter of the tube" [5].

The smallest capillaries have a diameter of less than 3 μm, and red cells a diameter of about 7–8 μm. Red cells are therefore much bigger than the roads they have to travel, but this poses no real problem since red cells are as soft as a sponge and are easily deformable. They virtually squeeze through the capillaries. It is obvious, then, that red cell deformability is essential for the perfusion of the microcirculation [6].

Now, the red cells have arrived in the microcirculation and are eager to give their oxygen to the tissues. But where exactly? Formerly, the Krogh model was used to explain tissue oxygenation. It described a single capillary with a surrounding cylinder of tissue. Oxygen gradients between the tissue and the vasculature were thought to be the driving forces of tissue oxygenation. Capillaries were the only structures thought to participate in the oxygen exchange with the tissue. Tissue sites farthest away from the capillary got the least oxygen. More recent research, however, has revealed that tissue oxygen distribution is even in all parts of tissue between vessels. The capillary–tissue oxygen gradient is very low, namely only about 5 mm Hg. Capillaries are nearly at equilibrium with the tissue and deliver oxygen to pericapillary regions only [7]. Thus, capillaries do not contribute significantly to tissue oxygenation. Most of the oxygen is delivered to the tissues via arterioles. Oxygen gradients were found to be greatest between arterioles and the tissue. Significant amounts of oxygen (30%) leave the vessels already at the arteriolar level. This is surprising since the tissue surrounding the arterioles does not have a metabolic demand high enough to justify an uptake of great oxygen amounts. In fact, only 10–15% of the losses can be explained by the oxygen consumption of the tissue surrounding the arterioles. There is no good explanation of where the other 85–90% of the oxygen remains. Probably, this oxygen serves the high metabolic demand of the endothelium [7]. Such demand may be explained by the enormous amount of endothelial synthesis (e.g., nitric oxide (NO), renin, interleukin, prostaglandins, and prostacyclin, etc.), transformation (of bradykinin, angiotensin, etc.), and constant work to adjust vascular tone.

Before continuing the trip with the red cells, let us step back and have a look at the whole microcirculation. Tissue as a whole depends on a network of capillaries (microvasculature), not only for delivery of oxygen but also for removal of metabolites. According to Fick's law, the size of the area of diffusion is one main component in the exchange of oxygen and metabolites. In the microcirculation, the area of diffusion depends on the number of vessels available for exchange. The term "functional capillary density" (FCD) has been coined to describe the "size" of the microvasculature. This term refers to the number of functional, that is, perfused, capillaries per unit tissue volume [8]. Decreased FCD lowers tissue oxygenation uniformly (without causing oxygenation inhomogeneity) [7] and is associated with poor outcome.

To maintain tissue survival, adequate FCD is essential. Several factors modify FCD. The diameter of the capillaries depends on the surrounding tissue and internal pressure. This means that capillaries embedded in tissue cannot increase their diameter but they can collapse if they are not properly perfused. Sufficient arterial pressure and an adequate volume status are therefore needed for capillary perfusion. Another factor that modifies FCD and capillary blood flow is the metabolic requirement of the

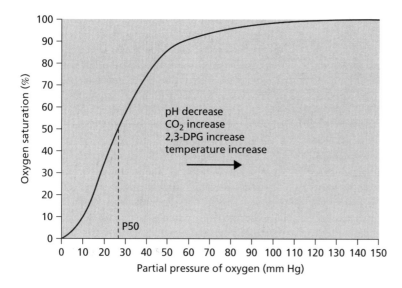

Fig 2.1 Oxygen dissociation curve.

tissue. Demand increases blood flow and excess of oxygen decreases blood flow. This mechanism is partially mediated by NO. Hemoglobin is able to scavenge NO and, therefore, constrict vessels. Hence, it seems red cells counteract their own work of delivering oxygen by blocking (constricting) their own road (vessels). This is not the case, however. The explanation for this phenomenon lies in the fact that hemoglobin comes in two different forms: R (relaxed, with high oxygen affinity) and T (tense, with low oxygen affinity). In the R form, hemoglobin not only transports oxygen but can also take up an NO compound (= S-nitrosylation). When the hemoglobin arrives at precapillary resistance vessels, it loses some oxygen and starts its transition from R to T. This change liberates the NO and causes dilatation of the arterioles [9]. With this mechanism, oxygen-loaded red cells open their doors to the tissue in order to deliver oxygen.

How do red cells give oxygen and how is it taken up by tissue?

The quantity of oxygen released by red cells depends much on the oxygen affinity of hemoglobin molecules. It is this affinity that translates oxygen flow into available oxygen. A common method to depict the behavior of hemoglobin is the oxygen dissociation curve (Fig. 2.1). The oxygen dissociation curve is sigmoid-shaped. This is due to conformational changes in the hemoglobin molecule that occur when it loads or releases oxygen. The uptake of each oxygen molecule alters the hemoglobin

conformation and so it enhances the uptake of the next oxygen molecule. A change in the hemoglobin's oxygen affinity profoundly affects oxygen release to the tissue, whereas the oxygen uptake by hemoglobin is scarcely affected.

There are several factors that per se can influence the hemoglobin's affinity for oxygen (Fig. 2.1). Those factors include temperature, CO_2, H^+, and 2,3-DPG [10]. Red blood cells deliver oxygen to metabolically active tissues. Such tissues release CO_2 that diffuses into the red cells. By carbonic anhydrase, CO_2 and H_2O react to H^+ and HCO_3^-. The resulting HCO_3^- is exchanged with extracellular Cl^-, which leads to an intracellular acidification. The resulting decrease in pH facilitates oxygen dissociation from hemoglobin. Also, 2,3-DPG, a glycolytic intermediate, binds to deoxyhemoglobin and stabilizes hemoglobin in the deoxy form, thus reducing hemoglobin's oxygen affinity and supporting oxygen release. In fact, this 2,3-DPG is so important that no oxygen can be unloaded by the red cells if it is completely lacking.

After being released from the hemoglobin molecule, oxygen has to pass several layers until it reaches the tissue. In contrast to oxygen uptake by red cells, release of oxygen depends mainly on the affinity of hemoglobin in the red cell and not so much on the thickness of surrounding unstirred fluid layers [1]. Deoxygenation therefore depends on pH and 2,3-DPG (lowered pH and increased 2,3-DPG levels facilitate release of oxygen) [1]. Only at very low hemoglobin concentrations chemical reactions limit release of oxygen from hemoglobin.

After the oxygen is released by the hemoglobin and has passed all barriers on its way to the tissue, the mitochondria accept the delivered oxygen molecules. Oxygen may have traveled via free flow or by means of a "coach" to a myoglobin molecule. The latter is called myoglobin-facilitated oxygen diffusion. "Deoxymyoglobin captures oxygen immediately as it crosses the interface: the newly formed oxymyoglobin diffuses away . . . . The effect is to make the oxygen pressure gradient from capillary lumen to the sarcoplasma more steep, thereby enhancing the oxygen flux" [11]. This effect maintains oxygen flow to the mitochondria under conditions of low extracellular oxygen pressure.

Does the tissue use oxygen?

The human body depends on oxygen for adenosine triphosphate (ATP) generation and maintenance of aerobic metabolism. ATP, the body's main energy source, is generated in the mitochondria using molecular oxygen. Only if the mitochondria actually use the oxygen, offered oxygen can do its job. This means that oxygen utilization is defined by the mitochondria.

Interestingly, there is a genetic component to the work of the mitochondria. Inherited or acquired changes in the enzyme supply determine how effectively oxygen can be used. Drugs such as propofol, which inhibit oxidative phosphorylation, can influence the mitochondria and thus the use of delivered oxygen [12]. Other factors influence tissues' (and mitochondria's) use of oxygen as well. The energy demand of the tissue influences how much oxygen is used. In turn, factors that influence the tissue's metabolism also influence the rate of its oxygen use. NO inhibits mitochondrial respiration, and thus oxygen consumption. On the other hand, lack of NO increases metabolism and tissue oxygen consumption [13]. The influence of the body temperature on oxygen extraction is well known: Higher body temperature increases oxygen demand, extraction [14], and utilization. There are many more factors that alter the body's energy requirement and thus the oxygen demand of the tissue: physical activity, hormones (catecholamines, thyroid hormones), infections, psychological stress, pain and anxiety, digestion and repair of tissues, just to name a few.

All organs and tissues, with the exception of the central nervous system, are able to use the delivered oxygen to the full, that is, 100%. This is also true for the myocardium [15]. In a healthy individual, however, there is a wide safety margin. Oxygen delivery in healthy resting humans exceeds the needs fourfold. The body as a whole uses only about one in four of the hemoglobin's oxygen molecules. The amount of oxygen used is called oxygen consumption (VO_2). Another way to express the use of oxygen is the oxygen extraction ratio O_2ER. It describes the percentage of oxygen extracted from the hemoglobin molecule. The total body's normal resting O_2ER equals about 20–25%. But the organ-specific oxygen extraction varies. Kidneys extract only 5–10%, and the heart at rest 55% [4]. It can be seen from such numbers that oxygen delivery is not the only determinant in the body's oxygen balance. Only the concerted efforts of all systems included in oxygen supply and use make aerobic life possible.

Pathophysiology of anemia

The human body is a marvel of creation. It is equipped with amazing mechanisms to maintain its function and to ensure that its tissue and organ systems tolerate a broad variety of conditions. This is also true for diminished levels of hemoglobin. Oxygen delivery remains sufficient over a wide range of hemoglobin levels, and even when hemoglobin levels have decreased markedly, the body can survive. All this is due to a variety of compensatory mechanisms, some of which are reviewed on the following pages.

The initial adaptation to blood loss is not mainly a reaction to a decrease in oxygen-carrying capacity but rather the body's reaction to hypovolemia. If left alone, the human body initiates a series of changes: first, to restore blood volume and second, to restore red cell mass. Within minutes, heart rate and stroke volume increase. The adrenergic system and the renin-angiotensin-aldosterone system are stimulated, releasing vasoactive hormones. This leads to the constriction of vascular sphincters in the skin, skeletal muscle, kidneys, and splanchnic viscera. The blood flow is redistributed to high-demand organs, namely the heart and brain [16]. To restore intravascular volume, fluids are first shifted from the interstitial space to the vessels, and later from the intracellular to the extracellular space. Due to adaptations in renal function, water and electrolytes are conserved. The liver is stimulated to produce osmotic active agents (glucose, lactate, urea, phosphate, etc.), which results in a net shift of fluid into the vasculature [16] and thus preload increases. Unless compensatory mechanisms fail, cardiac output is restored within 1–2 minutes [17].

However, if the body's compensatory mechanisms fail, cardiac output and oxygen delivery decrease. At that point, restoration of blood volume (not red cell volume) is mandatory. If fluids are infused, cardiac output can be increased and the untoward effects of hypovolemia averted.

Blood flow is restored and the body is able to repair damage and replenish the loss of red cell mass.

In the following paragraphs, the trip through the human body is repeated—this time under anemic, yet normovolemic, conditions. The assumption is that the patient is already volume-resuscitated and that adaptive mechanisms are mainly due to reduced red cell mass rather than reduced intravascular volume.

Adaptation of the body: acute is not the same as chronic

It is not uncommon to meet persons with a hemoglobin value of less than 4 g/dL doing their normal job—the only clinically observable effect being reduced exercise tolerance. On the other hand, some patients with the same hemoglobin level are hardly capable of lifting their head. Responses to blood loss and anemia are obviously not uniform. How the body responds to anemia depends on the rapidity of blood loss, the underlying condition of the patient, drugs taken, preexisting hemoglobin level, etc. [18]. Some adaptive mechanisms are more pronounced in acute anemia while others are more common in chronic anemia.

Adaptive mechanisms to anemia: macrocirculation

Leonardo da Vinci said: "Movement is the cause of all life." This also holds true for blood loss and anemia. In anemia, increased flow, that is, cardiac output, compensates for the losses in hemoglobin. In the acute setting, cardiac output increases with increasing levels of volume-resuscitated anemia. This is mainly due to increases in stroke volume. The influence of the heart rate in increasing the cardiac output is a subject of debate. Results conflict depending on the animal species studied and the patients and their conditions (anesthetized versus awake, influence of drugs taken). It seems, however, that an increase in the heart rate is not the main determinant in increasing the cardiac output of acutely anemic, volume-resuscitated individuals [18, 19].

Two major mechanisms are responsible for increased cardiac output. The most important is a reduction in blood viscosity. This results in increased venous flow with increased flow to the right heart. Preload increases, resulting in an enhanced cardiac output. Afterload is reduced by the decrease in blood viscosity. The other important cause for the increase in cardiac output is stimulation of the sympathetic nerve system. Via the sympathetic nerve system

and a catecholamine release, myocardial contractility (and heart rate) increases, and again, the cardiac output increases.

Both, in acute and chronic anemia cardiac output is increased by means of viscosity reduction and sympathetic nerve stimulation. And if anemia is becoming chronic, the heart adapts to the increased workload with left ventricular hypertrophy.

In the discussion of macrocirculatory adaptations to anemia, special consideration must be given to the heart. The myocardium requires more oxygen than any other organ and has a high O_2ER even at rest. When the heart's oxygen demand increases, e.g., by increased cardiac workload, the heart can slightly increase its oxygen extraction. The major increase in oxygen delivery to the heart, however, is due to vasodilatation of the coronary arteries. Normally, there is a great reserve in myocardial blood flow [20]. However, if myocardial blood flow cannot be increased, the heart may not be able to receive the oxygen it needs for its vital work. On the one hand, increased myocardial work is beneficial to compensate anemia. But then, increased myocardial work increases the heart's oxygen demand. Since an increase in the cardiac output is a crucial factor in compensating for the loss of oxygen-carrying capacity, it is vital for the heart to be able to increase its output on demand. Several factors can impair the heart's ability to increase output. Coronary stenosis, myocardial insufficiency, sepsis, anesthetics, and other drugs may compromise the work of the heart [21]. In such situations, the increase in cardiac output may not be sufficient to compensate for the lost red cell mass. Studies show that patients with different pathologies of the heart are more susceptible to ischemia than other patient populations and tolerate anemia less than the same patients without cardiac pathology.

Closely related to anemia-induced changes in cardiac output is the alteration of vascular tone. Again, the sympathetic nerve system plays an important role in this [18]. Increased activity of aortic chemoreceptors has been postulated to change vasomotor tone, and thus afterload [4]. Part of the reduction in afterload may also be due to hypoxic vasodilatation.

An increase in cardiac output and a reduction in vascular tone lead to an increased blood flow. The flow is directed to high-demand organs, with the brain and heart first in line to get a major portion of the blood [22]. Even under normal conditions they extract most of the oxygen offered by the hemoglobin [4] and are therefore supply dependent. Redistribution of the blood flow takes place at the expense of noncritical organs [23], e.g., the skin.

Volume-resuscitated anemic patients have a greater plasma volume than healthy, nonanemic humans. This volume serves to transport physically dissolved oxygen. While the portion of physically dissolved oxygen is almost insignificant in nonanemic patients, it must not be underestimated in severely anemic patients. At times, it may constitute a major portion of the total oxygen delivered by the blood [24].

Another adaptive mechanism of anemia tolerance is increased oxygen extraction. As shown above, given normal conditions, on average only one out of four oxygen molecules carried by a hemoglobin molecule is extracted by the body. Most tissues would be able to extract much more oxygen from the hemoglobin. In fact, in severe states of anemia, most tissues can extract nearly 100% of the oxygen offered. The increase in O_2ER is thus a valuable tool to compensate for decreased oxygen carriers.

The extent to which the above-mentioned adaptive mechanisms are being used by the body differs from patient to patient: The degree of anemia as well as the condition of the patient, the comorbidities, and the rapidity of the development of anemia play a role. If anemia becomes a chronic state, systemic vascular resistance returns to normal. Cardiac output is not increased to the same high degree as in acute anemia. Redistribution of blood flow from organs, with excess flow to other organs, takes place [4]. A combination of adaptive mechanisms enable a chronically anemic body to meet oxygen demand, even at times when hemoglobin levels are extremely low.

As a combined effect of reduction of blood viscosity, increase in cardiac output, etc., delivery of oxygen increases as the hematocrit starts to decrease. Oxygen delivery reaches its maximum at a hematocrit of 25–33% [4]. At hematocrits above 45 and below 25, oxygen delivery decreases. Adaptation in cardiac output compensates for decreased oxygen-carrying capacity. This results in an almost constant delivery of oxygen to the capillaries, as long as red cell losses do not exceed about 50% in healthy persons [13].

Adaptive mechanisms to anemia: microcirculation

As shown above, the microcirculation plays a crucial role in oxygen delivery to the tissue. It does not come as a surprise, then, that on the microcirculatory level there are also many mechanisms that compensate for decreased red cell mass. In fact the microcirculation is where the advantages of hemodilution matter most [19].

How do red cells take up oxygen?

Adaptive mechanisms begin again in the lung, the place where red cells exchange gases. Despite a reduction of the blood's capacity for carrying O_2 and CO_2, even severe anemia is associated with remarkable stability of the pulmonary gas exchange [25]. Compensatory mechanisms kick in, ensuring that O_2 transport and CO_2 elimination are not impaired [26].

In anemia, lung perfusion is altered. Less hemoglobin molecules are available for interaction with NO, which preserves the vasodilatatory effect of NO. Resistance to pulmonary blood flow is thus decreased [27]. This leads to an increased flow of blood through the pulmonary vasculature. This flow increases the shear stress in the endothelium, thus further increasing the production of vasodilatating NO. Those vasodilatatory effects counteract hypoxic pulmonary vasoconstriction [25]. In anemia there is a tendency toward reduced heterogenicity of pulmonary blood flow. Selective constriction of pulmonary vessels diverts blood to better ventilated alveoli [28]. NO may also alter airway tone, leading to a redistribution of ventilation. All this results in improved gas exchange in the lung. Several studies showed that arterial partial pressure of oxygen in anemic patients may even be greater than in nonanemic patients.

How do red cells reach their goal, the microvasculature in the tissue?

There is a clear relationship between hematocrit and viscosity. As the hematocrit decreases, blood viscosity decreases and red cells travel at a higher speed. When traveling at this high speed, they do not have sufficient time to lose oxygen on the way to the tissue. Therefore, in anemic conditions red cells arrive in the microcirculation with more oxygen than that in nonanemic conditions [4].

Since FCD is important for tissue survival, several mechanisms are employed in anemia to recruit capillaries. The blood flow in the capillaries of anemic patients is more homogenous than in nonanemic ones [19]. Several mechanisms account for this. Hemoglobin has a very high affinity for NO. This property is a crucial factor for regulating the interaction of red cells and the endothelium. Red cells have the ability to constrict the vascular bed by scavenging the vasodilatator NO. This effect is concentration dependent; that is, the lower the hematocrit, the more the vasodilatation and the better tissue perfusion. A better flow of blood in anemic states results. "Physical stimuli such as fluid shear stress, pulsatile stretching of the vessel wall, or a low arterial PO_2, also stimulate the release of NO above the basal level" [29]. Furthermore, in anemia, red cells do not aggregate readily and are able to pass through the narrowest capillary. Arterial/venular diffusional shunting is diminished because of the increased blood velocity and the decreased red cell residence time in the vessels [13]. While in the acute anemic setting the body is only able to recruit available capillaries, in the chronic anemic setting new vessels develop (neoangiogenesis).

Capillary vessels need arterial pressure to remain open. As blood viscosity decreases in anemia, flow increases because less arterial pressure is lost struggling with high blood viscosity. Thus, the lowered blood viscosity improves capillary perfusion. For this reason hemodilution is used therapeutically to improve tissue oxygenation. However, the beneficial effect of reducing the blood viscosity is only apparent as long as the heart can compensate for lost hemoglobin by improving flow. At the point where the heart can no longer compensate for the red cell loss, this beneficial effect ceases to exist. Hemodilution beyond this point reduces viscosity still further, inducing vasoconstriction and thus reducing FCD. At that point, a therapeutic maneuver may be employed to improve tissue perfusion again. Vessels are dependent on shear stress to open. By artificially increasing blood viscosity, shear stress to the vessels can be exerted, eliciting a vasodilatatory response. This may result in recovery of FCD [8, 13, 30].

In a summary of some interesting findings about the relationship of blood viscosity and transfusions the author stated: "Microcirculatory studies show that the organism compensates for reduced blood viscosity only up to reductions coincident with the conventional transfusion trigger and that reductions beyond this point lower functional capillary density. These studies show that the critical limit for tissue survival at the transfusion trigger is functional capillary density. Functional capillary density is important, primarily, for the extraction of tissue metabolism byproducts and, secondly, for tissue oxygenation. Thus, the transfusion trigger signals a condition where the circulation no longer compensates for significantly lowered viscosity due to hemodilution. Continued hemodilution with high-viscosity plasma expanders beyond the transfusion trigger is shown to maintain functional capillary density and improve tissue perfusion, suggesting that the conventional transfusion trigger is a viscosity trigger . . ." [31]. And after a discussion of the benefits of higher blood viscosity after reaching the "transfusion trigger," the author concluded: "It is a corollary to these considerations that the level of oxygen carrying capacity required to safely oxygenate the tissue may be much lower than that dictated by medical experience if microvascular function is maintained" [13].

How do the red cells give oxygen and how does the tissue take up oxygen?

In states of anemia, the oxygen affinity of hemoglobin is lowered as is reflected in a right shift in the oxygen dissociation curve. This facilitates oxygen release to the tissue. The right shift in the oxyhemoglobin dissociation curve is the result of increases of 2,3-DPG in red cells [18]. In contrast to chronic anemia, however, facilitated O_2 dissociation does not play too big a role in acute anemia where 2,3-DPG levels do not change significantly [20]. Theoretically, in anemia also a shift in pH toward greater acidity may enhance oxygen release (Bohr effect). However, this effect is probably not clinically relevant since immense changes in pH are needed to release significant amounts of oxygen from red cells [18].

Reserves in oxygen delivery are used in anemia, and this is reflected in an increased oxygen extraction ratio. Normally, the tissue extracts only about 20–30% of the total oxygen delivered. In anemia, the tissue may extract much more so that body O_2ER as a whole increases to 50–60%. As a consequence, the mixed venous oxygen partial pressure decreases.

In extreme anemia, oxygen uptake by the tissue seems to be limited. This may be due to the increased flow and the decreased transit time of red cells in the microvasculature. Time available for oxygen diffusion may be insufficient [32]. Also, erythrocyte spacing (increased distance between adjacent red cells during anemia) and the diffusion distance may contribute to this phenomenon [33].

Does the tissue use oxygen?

The last stop on this trip through the anemic body is again the tissue with the mitochondria, the place where a decrease in oxygen delivery should matter most. Intracellular mechanisms sense the decrease of O_2 in the tissue. In response, hypoxia-dependent gene expression is stimulated. A key factor in this process is the hypoxia-inducible factor 1α (HIF1α). It "induces the expression of genes that influence angiogenesis and vasodilatation, erythropoiesis and increased breathing, as well as glycolytic enzyme genes for anaerobic metabolism" [34]. Interestingly, the basic mechanisms of hypoxia tolerance are shared by different species, including humans. The following model was described for animals.

So, what happens if a cell senses a decrease in oxygen supply? Does the cell die? Not right away. The cell needs oxygen mainly to produce energy (ATP). So it makes sense that in anticipation of reduced oxygen (that is, energy) supply, energy demand is reduced. What does a cell need energy from ATP for? Almost all energy is needed for protein synthesis and degradation, maintenance of ion gradients, and synthesis of glucose and urea. And, in fact, in an initial defense phase, cells greatly (>90%) and rapidly suppress their protein, glucose, and urea synthesis. Interestingly, ion gradients over membranes remain constant, although the pumping activity of ion pumps is reduced to save energy. The cells use different mechanisms to accomplish this miracle. For instance, liver cells reduce cell membrane permeability, a process called channel arrest. Nerve cells reduce the firing frequency (spike arrest). Employing such measures, many cells can attain an energy balance at a lower level (ATP demand = ATP supply). This may ensure long-term survival in hypoxia. Hypoxia-sensitive cells, however, do not attain a new balance.

After the defense phase, a second, "rescue" phase, follows. Cells are now aiming at long-term hypoxia survival. To that end, cells reactivate some protein biosynthesis to prepare the cell for survival with extremely low ATP turnover. Hypoxia-dependent expression of key factors (such as HIF 1) regulates this process. Housekeeping genes consolidate and stabilize the cell, and enzymes for anaerobic ATP production are upregulated [34, 35]. With changes like these, cells can function for a while with a very low oxygen delivery.

Relationship between oxygen delivery and oxygen consumption

As mentioned initially, the aim of anemia therapy is to match the tissue's demand for oxygen with supply. This demand is reflected by tissue oxygen consumption VO_2. There is a relationship between oxygen delivery and oxygen consumption (Fig. 2.2). Oxygen consumption remains constant over a wide range of delivery. At the point where oxygen consumption becomes supply dependent, tissue hypoxia may occur. This point is called "critical oxygen delivery," DO_{2crit}^*. This, however, is no fixed number, leaving room for therapeutic interventions.

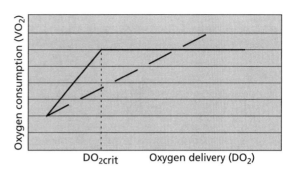

Fig 2.2 Relationship between oxygen delivery and oxygen consumption. Continuous line: healthy individuals; dashed line: pathologic as in severe illness (with a wider range of dependence of VO_2 on DO_2 and a higher DO_{2crit}).

Practical implications

The oxygen delivery equation $[DO_2 = CO \times (Hgb \times 1.34 \times SaO_2 + 0.003 \times PaO_2) \times 10]$ may serve as a mnemonic for available anemia treatments. Every variable in the equation can be considered, based on which therapeutic interventions can be evaluated to optimize oxygen delivery. The cardiac output can be optimized by administering balanced amounts of intravenous fluids and removing negative inotropic influences or increasing positive inotropics as tolerated. The hemoglobin level can be increased, not only by speeding up endogenous hematopoiesis, but also by avoiding undue hemoglobin losses. Arterial oxygen partial pressure and oxygen saturation can be increased, using supplemental oxygen and mechanical ventilation as indicated. In addition, the amount of oxygen dissolved in plasma can be increased further by increasing the atmospheric pressure (hyperbaric oxygen).

A more complete picture of anemia therapy, though, is achieved when not only an increase of oxygen delivery is aimed at, but also a reduction of oxygen demand is contemplated. Oxygen delivery and consumption are related, since $VO_2 = DO_2 \times O_2ER$. While not many interventions are available to increase oxygen extraction, there are quite a few things that can be done to reduce oxygen consumption. "The four pillars of anemia therapy" (Fig. 2.3) summarize how an understanding of physiology and pathophysiology translates into a plan of care. With the appropriate combination of factors that not only increase oxygen delivery but also reduce oxygen consumption, even hemoglobin levels way below the supposed

The four pillars of anemia therapy

Minimize bloodloss	Optimize O_2-delivery	Reduce oxygen need	Enhance hematopoiesis
Stop bleeding	Volume therapy	Manage pain	Prescribe vitamins B + C, folate, iron
Minimize phlebotomy	Increase inspired oxygen fraction	Sedate	Administer erythropoietin or anabolics
Provide ulcer prophylaxis	Treat thoracic injuries	Intubate, ventilate, relax	Avoid marrow depressants
Avoid hemolytic drugs	Optimize ventilation	Give antioxidants	Consider other growth factors (CSF)
Normalize clotting	Intubate	Maintain normothermia	Pay attention to appropriate nutrition
Give contraceptives	Give hyperbaric oxygen	Consider β-blockade	
Avoid hypertension and hypervolemia			

Fig 2.3 The four pillars of anemia therapy.

critical border can be tolerated for some time without lasting damage [36], and even severely anemic patients can be treated successfully.

Key points

• Many mechanisms are used by the body to survive even severe anemia; these include the following:
– increased cardiac output
– redistribution of blood flow to organs with high oxygen demand
– increased oxygen extraction by tissues
– improved FCD
– decreased oxygen affinity of hemoglobin
– metabolic adaptations to tolerate lower oxygen delivery.
• Therapeutic interventions are aimed at finding a new balance between oxygen delivery and oxygen consumption, either by increasing oxygen delivery or by reducing oxygen consumption or both at the same time.

Questions for review

• What mechanisms support red cell oxygen uptake and oxygen release?
• Where is oxygen release from the red cells to the tissue regulated?
• What does the term functional capillary density mean? How can it be influenced?
• How do cells prepare when decreasing oxygen levels are detected?
• How is blood flow altered in anemic states?
• How do adaptation methods for acute and chronic anemia differ?

Suggestions for further research

What different forms of hypoxia are there and how do they differ?

Exercises and practice cases

Work with the following case, which was reported in a journal [37].

A 37-year-old woman with a long history of Crohn's disease presented for bowel resection and drainage of an abdominal abscess. Her preoperative hematocrit was 30. She consented to surgery but asked for therapy without use of donor blood. The patient was taken to the operating room and surgery started. After the abdominal cavity was opened, she started hemorrhaging and in a period of 1 hour she lost 3 L of blood. Her hematocrit during surgery was 17. After surgery, her hematocrit dropped to 4 (hemoglobin approx. 1.3 g/dL). At that point, the patient was intubated and given morphine, muscle relaxants, oxygen ($FiO_2 = 1.0$), crystalloids, and colloids. Her body temperature was 30°C (blood pressure 130/70 mm Hg, heart rate 88, cardiac output 5.3 L/min).

Using the following questions, try to understand the pathophysiology of her condition.

1 How did the patient adapt to the chronic anemia with a hematocrit of 30?

2 Which pathophysiological mechanisms were activated in the patient when she had an intraoperative hematocrit of 17?

3 Calculate how much oxygen was delivered in the patient when she had a hematocrit of 4? How was the oxygen delivered?

References

1 Vandegriff, K.D. and J.S. Olson. Morphological and physiological factors affecting oxygen uptake and release by red blood cells. *J Biol Chem*, 1984. **259**(20): p. 12619–12627.

2 Coin, J.T. and J.S. Olson. The rate of oxygen uptake by human red blood cells. *J Biol Chem*, 1979. **254**: p. 1178–1190.

3 Pries, A.R., T.W. Secomb, and P. Gaehtgens. Biophysical aspects of blood flow in the microvasculature. *Cardiovasc Res*, 1996. **32**(4): p. 654–667.

4 Tuman, K.J. Tissue oxygen delivery: the physiology of anemia. *ACNA*, 1990. **8**: p. 451–469.

5 Farhaeus, R. and T. Lindqvist. The viscosity of the blood in narrow capillary tubes. *Am J Physiol*, 1931. **96**: p. 562–568.

6 Langenfeld, J.E., et al. Correlation between red blood cell deformability and changes in hemodynamic function. *Surgery*, 1994. **116**(5): p. 859–867.

7 Intaglietta, M., P.C. Johnson, and R.M. Winslow. Microvascular and tissue oxygen distribution. *Cardiovasc Res*, 1996. **32**(4): p. 632–643.

8 Mazzoni, M.C., A.G. Tsai, and M. Intaglietta. Blood and plasma viscosity and microvascular function in hemodilution. A perspective from La Jolla, California. *Eur Surg Res*, 2002. **34**(1–2): p. 101–105.

9 Stamler, J.S., et al. Blood flow regulation by S-nitrosohemoglobin in the physiological oxygen gradient. *Science*, 1997. **276**(5321): p. 2034–2037.

10 Longmuir, I.S. The effect of hypothermia on the affinity of tissues for oxygen. *Life Sci*, 1962. **1**: p. 297–300.

11 Wittenberg, B.A. and J.B. Wittenberg. Transport of oxygen in muscle. *Annu Rev Physiol*, 1989. **51**: p. 857–878.

12 Clay, A.S., M. Behnia, and K.K. Brown. Mitochondrial disease: a pulmonary and critical-care medicine perspective. *Chest*, 2001. **120**: p. 634–648.

13 Intaglietta, M. Microcirculatory basis for the design of artificial blood. *Microcirculation*, 1999. **6**(4): p. 247–258.

14 Schumacker, P.T., et al. Effects of hyperthermia and hypothermia on oxygen extraction by tissues during hypovolemia. *J Appl Physiol*, 1987. **63**(3): p. 1246–1252.

15 Zander, R. Oxygen supply and acid-base status in extreme anemia. *AINS*, 1996. **31**(8): p. 492–494.

16 Stehling, L. and H.L. Zauder. How low can we go? Is there a way to know? *Transfusion*, 1990. **30**(1): p. 1–3.

17 Zander, R. Pathophysiology of hypovolemic shock. *Anasthesiol Intensivmed Notfallmed Schmerzther*, 2001. **36**(Suppl 2): p. S137–S139.

18 Hebert, P.C. and S. Szick. The anemia patient in the ICU: how much does the heart tolerate? *AINS*, 2001. **26**: p. S94–S100.

19 Landrow, L. Perioperative hemodilution. *Can J Surg*, 1987. **30**: p. 321–325.

20 Wahr, J.A. Myocardial ischaemia in anaemic patients. *Br J Anaesth*, 1998. **81**(Suppl 1): p. 10–15.

21 Morgan, T.J., et al. Siggaard-Andersen algorithm-derived p50 parameters: perturbation by abnormal hemoglobin-oxygen affinity and acid-base disturbances. *J Lab Clin Med*, 1995. **126**(4): p. 365–372.

22 Borgstrom, L., H. Johannsson, and B.K. Siesjo. The influence of acute normovolemic anemia on cerebral blood flow and oxygen consumption of anesthetized rats. *Acta Physiol Scand*, 1975. **93**(4): p. 505–514.

23 Van der Linden, P., et al. Influence of hematocrit on tissue O2 extraction capabilities during acute hemorrhage. *Am J Physiol*, 1993. **264**(6, Pt 2): p. H1942–H1947.

24 Habler, O., et al. Hyperoxia in extreme hemodilution. *Eur Surg Res*, 2002. **34**(1–2): p. 181–187.

25 Deem, S., et al. Mechanisms of improvement in pulmonary gas exchange during isovolemic hemodilution. *J Appl Physiol*, 1999. **87**(1): p. 132–141.

26 Deem, S., et al. CO2 transport in normovolemic anemia: complete compensation and stability of blood CO2 tensions. *J Appl Physiol*, 1997. **83**(1): p. 240–246.

27 Agarwal, J.B., R. Paltoo, and W.H. Palmer. Relative viscosity of blood at varying hematocrits in pulmonary circulation. *J Appl Physiol*, 1970. **29**(6): p. 866–871.

28 Lopez-Barneo, J. Oxygen-sensing by ion channels and the regulation of cellular functions. *Trends Neurosci*, 1996. **19**(10): p. 435–440.

29 Motterlini, R., K.D. Vandegriff, and R.M. Winslow. Hemoglobin-nitric oxide interaction and its implications. *Transfus Med Rev*, 1996. **10**(2): p. 77–84.

30 Deem, S., *et al*. Effects of the RBC membrane and increased perfusate viscosity on hypoxic pulmonary vasoconstriction. *J Appl Physiol*, 2000. **88**(5): p. 1520–1528.

31 Tsai, A.G. and M. Intaglietta. Hemodilution and increased plasma viscosity for the design of new plasma expanders. *TATM*, 2001. **3**: p. 17–23.

32 Gutierrez, G., *et al*. Skeletal muscle PO_2 during hypoxemia and isovolemic anemia. *J Appl Physiol*, 1990. **68**(5): p. 2047–2053.

33 Hogan, M.C., D.E. Bebout, and P.D. Wagner. Effect of hemoglobin concentration on maximal O_2 uptake in canine gastrocnemius muscle in situ. *J Appl Physiol*, 1991. **70**(3): p. 1105–1112.

34 Csete, M. Respiration in anesthesia pathophysiology and clinical update: cellular response to hypoxia. *ACNA*, 1998. **16**: p. 201–210.

35 Hochachka, P.W., *et al*. Unifying theory of hypoxia tolerance: molecular/metabolic defense and rescue mechanisms for surviving oxygen lack. *Proc Natl Acad Sci U S A*, 1996. **93**(18): p. 9493–9498.

36 Welte, M. Is there a "critical hematocrit?". *Anaesthesist*, 2001. **50**(Suppl 1): p. S2–S8.

37 Lichtenstein, A., *et al*. Unplanned intraoperative and postoperative hemodilution: oxygen transport and consumption during severe anemia. *Anesthesiology*, 1988. **69**(1): p. 119–122.

3

Anemia therapy I: erythropoiesis-stimulating proteins

Untreated and progressive anemia increases both morbidity and mortality of patients. Anemia, therefore, must be detected, properly diagnosed, and treated. Ideally, the patient's own bone marrow should be able to produce the needed red blood cells. This chapter is one in a series of two that deal with anemia and anemia therapy. Here, we will consider hormone and cytokine therapy of anemia, and in the next chapter we will deal with the raw products of blood building.

Objectives of this chapter

1 Review the physiological role of hormones and cytokines in erythropoiesis.
2 Get to know more about recombinant human erythropoietin (rHuEPO) as a drug.
3 Define the settings in which erythropoietin (EPO) is beneficial.
4 Compare EPO with its analogies.

Definitions

Erythropoietin: EPO is a naturally occurring hormone that stimulates erythropoiesis, that is, the synthesis of blood. A recombinant equivalent (rHuEPO) is available for therapeutic use.
Novel erythropoiesis-stimulating protein: Novel erythropoiesis-stimulating protein (NESP) is an analogy of rHuEPO. It stimulates erythropoiesis by the same mechanisms as done by naturally occurring EPO.
Anabolic steroids: These are the hormones derived from androgens. They not only influence metabolism but also have effects on erythropoiesis.

A brief look at history

For decades, it has been known that there is a factor (an EPO) that stimulates the production of red blood cells. It was possible to transfer this factor from one individual to another. Transfusing plasma of anemic individuals into someone else caused acceleration of hematopoiesis [1]. It was not until 1977, however, when Miyake and colleagues [2] isolated that factor from the urine of patients with aplastic anemia. Early experiments used material extracted from urine. The cumbersome process of purification limited the use of this factor for research. Yet, it was possible to identify the gene for EPO. In 1985, Lin *et al.* and Jacobs *et al.* [1, 3] cloned that gene, and EPO became the first hematopoietic growth factor ever cloned [4]. This laid the foundation for mass production of human recombinant erythropoietin and accelerated research in this field. In 1987, Sawyer *et al.* described the receptor for EPO [5, 6] and shed further light on the interaction of the hormone and its target.

With record speed, rHuEPO found its way into clinical practice. Kidney failure as the cause of anemia due to a lack of EPO was the first condition that was successfully treated with rHuEPO. Recently, other potential clinical benefits of EPO have been discovered, suggesting an expanded use of these agents in other disease states.

Erythropoietin

Erythropoietin in normal erythropoiesis

EPO is a natural hormone. Prior to birth, it is produced in the liver. Within weeks, main production shifts to the kidneys. After total nephrectomy, residual EPO is

Table 3.1 Review: steps in erythropoiesis.

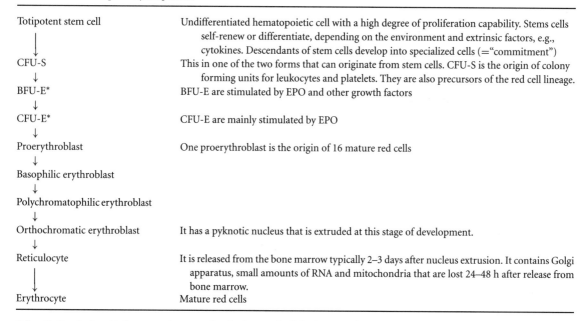

Totipotent stem cell	Undifferentiated hematopoietic cell with a high degree of proliferation capability. Stems cells self-renew or differentiate, depending on the environment and extrinsic factors, e.g., cytokines. Descendants of stem cells develop into specialized cells (="commitment")
↓	
CFU-S	This in one of the two forms that can originate from stem cells. CFU-S is the origin of colony forming units for leukocytes and platelets. They are also precursors of the red cell lineage.
↓	
BFU-E*	BFU-E are stimulated by EPO and other growth factors
↓	
CFU-E*	CFU-E are mainly stimulated by EPO
↓	
Proerythroblast	One proerythroblast is the origin of 16 mature red cells
↓	
Basophilic erythroblast	
↓	
Polychromatophilic erythroblast	
↓	
Orthochromatic erythroblast	It has a pyknotic nucleus that is extruded at this stage of development.
↓	
Reticulocyte	It is released from the bone marrow typically 2–3 days after nucleus extrusion. It contains Golgi apparatus, small amounts of RNA and mitochondria that are lost 24–48 h after release from bone marrow.
↓	
Erythrocyte	Mature red cells

Follow the lines in the table from top to bottom and review how a red cell develops out of a totipotent stem cell.

*The terms BFU-E and CFU-E describe the cell's growth patterns under laboratory conditions.

CFU-S, colony-forming units—spleen; BFU-E, burst-forming units—erythroid; CFU-E, colony-forming units—erythroid.

detectable. This remaining EPO is synthesized in the liver. In an adult, the liver constitutes less than 5% of the total EPO production.

Basal EPO secretion has a circadian cycle with levels higher in the evening than in the morning. There are no stores of preformed EPO [4]. EPO is produced as demand arises. Current thinking is that the main stimulus for secretion of EPO is hypoxia. This may be caused by anemia, lung disease, or high-altitude living. The EPO gene has an enhancer where hypoxic-inducing factor (HIF)-1α + β (a transcription factor that is induced by hypoxia) attaches and induces EPO gene transcription and subsequent EPO synthesis.

Normal EPO levels in nonanemic persons range between 6 and 32 U/L. The levels are similar in men and women. In severe hypoxia or anemia, EPO levels may rise 1000 times above normal. Provided there is enough EPO, basal erythropoiesis may increase by 6–8 times [7].

The target of EPO is the EPO receptor. This receptor consists of extracellular, transmembrane, and intracellular domains. EPO binds to its receptor on the cell surface. Afterward, it is ingested into the cell by receptor-mediated endocytosis. Tyrosines on the intracellular domain of the receptor are phosphorylated and an intracellular signaling process is initiated. As a result, gene expression in the nucleus is modulated. This affects the changes EPO mediates.

EPO acts as a "survival factor" in erythropoiesis (Table 3.1). It is not involved in the commitment of the erythroid lineage. EPO mainly promotes survival, proliferation, and differentiation of erythroid progenitors. Therefore, it saves cells from natural cell death (apoptosis). In hematopoiesis, the main EPO targets are progenitor cells: burst-forming units erythroid (BFU-E) and colony-forming units erythroid (CFU-E) [8]. BFU-E exhibit only a small number of EPO receptors and are relatively resistant to the influence of EPO. The main EPO receptors in the erythroid lineage are CFU-Es. They react even at low concentrations of EPO. Erythropoietin receptors are also found on proerythroblasts. In the late erythroid precursors, EPO receptors diminish. There are no receptors on reticulocytes and erythrocytes. Besides influencing the survival of erythroid progenitors, EPO accelerates the release of reticulocytes from the bone marrow. Therapy with rHuEPO also increases the amount of fetal hemoglobin by increasing the number of reticulocytes.

Recombinant human erythropoietin as a drug

rHuEPO is a sialylglycoprotein. It has three N-linked oligosaccharide chains. The carbohydrate part of rHuEPO with its sialic acid is used for biological activities in the body. If it were not for sialic acid residues, EPO would be removed from circulation within minutes.

Under laboratory conditions, it is possible to synthesize rHuEPO through different cell lines. Nowadays, Chinese hamster ovary cells are used for the pharmacological production of rHuEPO. Recombinant human erythropoietin is biologically active and reacts in a way similar to the natural hormone purified from urine. To date, several forms of rHuEPO are commercially available: EPO α, EPO β, and EPO ω. They have slightly different carbohydrate residues but are equally effective in stimulating erythropoiesis.

rHuEPO requires parenteral application (either intravenously or subcutaneously) to stimulate erythropoiesis. Intraperitoneal application is also possible. Patients on peritoneal dialysis may prefer this route of administration. The half-life of rHuEPO given intravenously is 3–16 hours and declines after multiple injections. If given subcutaneously, the half-life is about 12–28 hours. It takes 5–18 hours until maximum serum concentration is reached. Bioavailability of subcutaneously administered rHuEPO is approximately 30%.

The metabolic "fate" of rHuEPO is poorly understood. When used by erythrocyte precursors, it is removed from circulation by being taken up into these cells. Less than 5% of the administered rHuEPO is excreted unchanged through the kidneys. Parts of the remaining hormone are desialylated and metabolized by the liver.

Dose and response relationship: The onset of hematocrit recovery in normal postsurgical patients with severe anemia shows a 1-week lag if no rHuEPO is given. This is so because endogenous EPO has to be synthesized and iron stores need to be replenished. In contrast, the erythropoietic effect of rHuEPO starts almost immediately. It takes some time until the results can be detected by laboratory testing. The higher the initial doses of rHuEPO, the faster hematocrit recovery occurs [9]. Reticulocytosis can be detected within 2–3 days. Some laboratories are also able to count the immature reticulocyte fraction. This is a valuable tool in detecting early response to rHuEPO therapy.

rHuEPO dosage is calculated on an individual basis. Much depends on the patient's underlying medical condition and the response to therapy. Daily administration is warranted in patients with severe anemia and in those who need rapid increase in red cell mass. Other dosing schedules of rHuEPO include thrice or once a week. This may be the case with patients with sufficient time to prepare for elective surgery. It appears that rHuEPO therapy on a weekly schedule for some weeks prior to surgery is as effective as daily perioperative rHuEPO dosing [10]. Please refer to Table 3.2 for dosage recommendations to administer rHuEPO in different clinical settings [11–28].

Side effects

rHuEPO is remarkably safe and well tolerated by patients. Only about 10% of patients receiving rHuEPO experience self-limiting flu-like symptoms with bone pain. This is an expression of hemopoiesis activation. Other than with cases of renal disease, significant side effects were rarely reported.

A hypertensive response after rHuEPO administration was observed mainly in patients with chronic renal failure. This hypertension may be the result of the reversal of anemic vasodilatation and the increase in hematocrit. Hemodynamic adaptation to the reversal of anemia may be too slow in uremic patients and so hypertension may develop. Controlled slow increase of hematocrit levels in such patients reduces the risk of severe hypertension. Hypertension may resolve spontaneously by continuing EPO therapy. Regular blood pressure monitoring is advisable for patients receiving rHuEPO. If necessary, antihypertensive therapy can be started.

Seizures were also observed in dialysis patients receiving rHuEPO, especially during the initial treatment phase when the hematocrit can rise rapidly. Often, there is a combination of hypertension and seizures. The danger of provoking a seizure is reduced if rHuEPO is administered in a way that induces a gradual increase in hematocrit.

Slight allergic reactions after administration of rHuEPO were reported (such as urticaria). Another type of immune response is the development of antibodies to rHuEPO (and natural EPO), leading to pure red cell aplasia (PRCA). This was reported mainly in patients on long-term treatment and in those with uremia and myelodysplastic syndromes. While this is very rare, it is a serious side effect. After an increased incidence of rHuEPO-induced PRCA was reported, this phenomenon was investigated. It appeared that not all commercially available brands of rHuEPO were associated with PRCA. The most likely explanation is that compounds from the rubber plungers of prefilled rHuEPO syringes are responsible for the increased immunogenicity of rHuEPO. The packages of rHuEPO are no longer

Table 3.2 rHuEPO dose regimens in the literature.

Field	Setting	Dose
Hematology	Patients with sickle cell/β-thalassemia	200 U/kg daily
Hematology	Aplastic anemia	200 or 400 U/kg s.c. for 12 wk or longer
Immunology	Rheumatoid arthritis	40–300 U/kg twice weekly
Immunology	Inflammatory bowel disease	150 U/kg twice weekly for 12 wk
Intensive care	Critically ill patients	300 U/kg s.c. daily for 5 days, then every other day
Intensive care	Multiorgan dysfunction syndrome	600 U/kg i.v. thrice weekly
Nephrology	Anemic patients with chronic renal failure	50–100 U/kg in the correction phase and 25–100 U/kg in the maintenance phase, each thrice weekly; some patients require more
Obstetrics	Anemic pregnant women	300 U/kg twice weekly
Oncology	High-dose chemo-radiotherapy	10,000 U daily beginning 2 wk prior to chemotherapy
Orthopedics	Preoperative autologous donation	50–150 U/kg s.c. twice weekly
Pediatrics	Premature babies	300 U/kg twice weekly
Pediatrics	Children with congenital hypoplastic anemia	2000 U/kg per day
Surgery	Cancer patients undergoing gastrointestinal surgery	300 U/kg 12 days before surgery + 100 U/kg 4 and 8 days later
Surgery	Preoperatively for cardiac surgery	Five times 500U/kg i.v. over 14 days preoperatively
Surgery	Prior to cardiac surgery	100 U/kg, 4 days prior to surgery
Surgery	Prior and after pediatric cardiac surgery	300 U/kg, prior and after surgery
Surgery	If time permits to prepare the patient for general surgery	100–150 U/kg, s.c. six doses (e.g., twice weekly for 3 wk) prior to surgery plus i.v. iron or 150–300 U/kg s.c., 6–10 doses (e.g., twice weekly for 3 wk) plus iron p.o.
Surgery	If time permits to prepare the patient for cardiac surgery	600 U/kg 14 and 7 days prior to surgery plus i.v. iron or 150–300 U/kg s.c. daily for 7 days prior to surgery plus iron p.o.
Urology	Prior to radical prostatectomy	600 U/kg 14 and 7 days prior to surgery

s.c., subcutaneous; p.o., per os; i.v., intravenous.

shipped with the traditional rubber plungers. If PRCA should occur in any patient, rHuEPO needs to be stopped immediately. Switching to another brand of rHuEPO does not improve the situation. Actually, rHuEPO is contraindicated if antibodies develop. Immunosuppressive therapy with corticoids, cyclosporine, cyclophosphamide, immunoglobulins, or plasmapheresis should be initiated once the diagnosis is confirmed. Spontaneous reversal of the PRCA can occur, but it seems to be rare.

In addition to the above mentioned side effects, venous thrombosis, cancer progression and worsening of diabetic retinopathy have been discussed to be related to rHuEPO therapy. As yet, a cause-and-effect relationship has not been established.

While rHuEPO mainly influences the erythroid precursors, it has also some influence on megakaryocytes and on precursors of leukocytes. Increased platelet counts and monocyte counts were observed in patients with renal failure, although levels remained within normal limits.

On rare occasions, thrombocytosis, requiring low-dose aspirin therapy, has been reported.

Some of the side effects or rHuEPO are actually beneficial. Mild defects in hemostasis observed in uremic and severely anemic patients were corrected by using rHuEPO [17]. "Tests performed in small numbers of hemodialysis patients at baseline and following normalization of hematocrit with epoetin therapy have demonstrated improved cerebral blood flow, information processing, overall cognitive function, mood state, subjective health and physical activity, and decreased dialysis-related and general treatment-related stress, and fatigue, following correction of anemia." Anemia therapy using rHuEPO was shown to reverse insulin resistance as well as amino acid and lipid abnormalities in dialysis-dependent patients [29]. Also in dialysis patients, rHuEPO normalizes the decreased metabolic rate in muscles [30]. Reduced fatigue and improved well-being are also observed in patients with cancer-related anemia that is treated with rHuEPO [17].

Effects not directly related to erythropoiesis

In recent years, insight has been gained into the biological role of EPO. As mentioned above, EPO acts as a hormone. In this endocrine function, it originates mainly in the kidneys and is transported by the blood plasma to the target tissues. EPO receptors are distributed in the whole body and are found in the brain and other neural tissue. The heart, retina, vessels, lungs, liver, gastrointestinal tract, ovaries, and the uterus also carry EPO receptors. Apart from kidney and liver, other tissues are able to produce EPO and EPO-like molecules. It seems that these tissues do not release EPO into the circulation. The synthesized EPO is used by neighboring cells (paracrine) or by the producing cell itself (autocrine).

In the paracrine and autocrine process, EPO has a wide spectrum of actions. Such actions obviously can be mimicked by exogenously administered rHuEPO. It protects tissues by preventing vascular spasm, apoptosis, and inflammatory responses. rHuEPO is able to protect the brain, myocardium, and other tissues from hypoxia [31]. Its neuroprotective properties were demonstrated in patients with cerebral ischemia and spinal cord injury. Experimental evidence supports the assumption that EPO plays a role in the regeneration after brain and spinal injury [32–34]. rHuEPO also protects the heart from ischemia due to infarction or surgery. It activates multiple biochemical pathways and seems to mimic ischemic preconditioning. rHuEPO may therefore not only be beneficial therapy in increasing red cell mass but may also protect tissues until hypoxia is resolved. This effect has been shown to occur even if rHuEPO was given shortly prior to and immediately following the insult [35].

EPO also has an effect on muscles. Minutes after administration, muscle strength is detectably increased. EPO can even be found in human milk. Epithelial tissue in the mammary gland produces EPO and secretes it with the milk. The suckling baby may benefit from the oral intake of EPO [36].

Erythropoietin hyporesponsiveness

The term "erythropoietin hyporesponsiveness" (or erythropoietin resistance) refers to situations where—despite sufficiently high doses of rHuEPO—the erythropoietic response is undetectable or minimal. Several conditions cause EPO hyporesponsiveness. Many of them are treatable. Causes of EPO hyporesponsiveness that are not treatable do not necessarily constitute a contraindication for rHuEPO therapy, though. Patients who do not respond initially may respond to higher doses of rHuEPO.

Treating EPO hyporesponsiveness is imperative if the patient is to derive any benefit. Continuation of the rHuEPO therapy in cases of obvious EPO hyporesponsiveness may be a wastage. Often, the reason for EPO hyporesponsiveness can be elucidated and treated.

Erythropoiesis can be increased above the basal level. This potential increase, however, is limited by iron availability. Healthy humans can provide sufficient iron to triple their basal erythropoiesis level. If erythropoiesis is increased more than threefold, a functional iron deficiency develops. This happens even in the presence of full iron reserves (= relative iron deficiency). Patients who require rHuEPO may also exhibit absolute iron deficiency. Dialysis patients, for instance, lose blood from frequent testing and the process of dialysis itself. Occult gastrointestinal hemorrhage may further increase blood loss and subsequently lead to depletion of iron stores. No matter whether a patient has a measurable iron deficiency or not, patients who receive rHuEPO therapy require iron supplementation.

Iron may also cause an EPO hyporesponsiveness if iron overload is present. Even in this case, functional iron deficiency can occur. Treatment with supplemental iron may resolve this problem, but it may also contribute to further iron overload. To circumvent this effect, ascorbic acid infusions (e.g., 200–500 mg, i.v.; three times a wk) were proposed instead of iron infusions [37]. Ascorbic acid is able to mobilize iron from the stores and increases iron utilization in the erythroid progenitor cells. Ascorbic acid infusions in iron overload may not only increase the hematocrit when given with rHuEPO but may also reduce rHuEPO requirements.

Closely related to the iron metabolism is aluminum metabolism. Both metals are bound to transferrin. Aluminum inhibits iron uptake in the gastrointestinal tract, decreases iron utilization, and interferes with heme biosynthesis. Therefore, it can cause EPO hyporesponsiveness. Especially, patients on dialysis are prone to aluminum overload. Monitoring aluminum serum levels is warranted in such patients. If indicated, chelation therapy with desferrioxamine may be prescribed.

Infection and inflammation in chronic diseases can also cause EPO hyporesponsiveness. Cytokines involved in the inflammatory process act on different stages of erythropoiesis. Interferon-γ downregulates the EPO receptor at the surface of erythroid precursors [4]. Tumor necrosis factor suppresses EPO production in the kidneys. Optimizing the treatment of infection and inflammation reduces certain cytokine levels and may recover EPO responsiveness. In some cases, however, it may be necessary to treat inflammation-related anemia with high doses of rHuEPO since this can overcome the inhibitory effects of cytokines [38].

Hyperparathyroidism may diminish the body's response to rHuEPO. High serum levels of parathyroid hormone exert toxic effects on EPO synthesis and erythropoiesis. Furthermore, it can cause marrow fibrosis, interfering with red cell production. Surgical or medical (therapy with vitamin D analogues) correction of hyperparathyroidism improves the response to rHuEPO [38].

Logically, the lack of raw materials for erythropoiesis also causes EPO hyporesponsiveness. Deficiency of any of the hematinics (as discussed in the next chapter) can be the culprit. This is true not only for iron but also for folate, vitamins B_6 and B_{12}, and L-carnitine. Substitution of deficient vitamins and their derivatives may resolve EPO hyporesponsiveness and may even decrease rHuEPO requirements and costs.

Several other factors can cause EPO hyporesponsiveness. Among them are uremia, severe metabolic acidosis, and oxalosis [39]. Patients with hemoglobinopathies, red cell enzyme deficiencies, and other red cell abnormalities may not respond to the usual doses of rHuEPO [40].

Various drugs may interfere with rHuEPO therapy. Theophylline, an adenosine antagonist, lowers plasma levels of EPO in normal humans. The rate of EPO secretion is related to the activity of the renin-angiotensin-aldosteron system [39].

Flow charts like the one shown in Fig. 3.1 are helpful for the efficient work-up of patients with EPO hyporesponsiveness.

Adjuvant therapy

The therapy with rHuEPO is relatively costly. Adjuvant therapies are available to increase the effectiveness of rHuEPO therapy and reduce total costs. While studies on adjuvant therapies usually deal with patients on dialysis, basic principles apply to other patient groups as well. Consider some supplements that are valuable as adjuvants to rHuEPO therapy.

Iron: As long as there is no contraindication to iron therapy, it should be given to all patients on rHuEPO. The next chapter will deal with the details of iron therapy.

Ascorbic acid: It can resolve functional iron deficiency even in patients with iron overload. It facilitates the uptake of iron in the gastrointestinal tract and supports hemopoiesis.

Vitamin D: The erythropoiesis in patients with secondary hyperparathyroidism can be improved with vitamin D therapy and its analogues, since the unwanted

effects of high parathyroid hormone levels are alleviated. It is still a matter of discussion whether therapy with vitamin D analogues is also beneficial for patients without hyperparathyroidism. Some patients experience an improvement of their anemia by taking calcitriol even if they do not have hyperparathyroidism. Currently, vitamin D analogues are not officially recommended for anemia therapy [39].

Vitamins of the B group: Vitamins of the B group, such as B_{12}, B_6, and folic acid were shown to be deficient in patients with rHuEPO therapy. Since the turnover of those vitamins is increased in accelerated erythropoiesis, patients should receive sufficient amounts of those vitamins [39].

L-Carnitine: L-Carnitine is able to increase the reticulocyte count and hematocrit even if no rHuEPO is given. If given together with rHuEPO, it can increase the effectiveness of rHuEPO. L-Carnitine may also increase erythrocyte membrane stability and has a beneficial effect on erythrocyte survival. Several studies demonstrate a reduced need of rHuEPO if L-carnitine is given concomitantly [41]. Because of a lack of hard scientific data, official recommendations for the routine use of L-carnitine have not been published. However, a trial of L-carnitine may be indicated in patients with suspected deficiency [39, 41].

Cytokines: Certain cytokines participate in the regulation of erythropoiesis. Insulin-like growth factor 1 is one of them. Its receptors are found on erythrocyte precursors and on mature red cells. Insulin-like growth factor is able to decrease the apoptosis of CFU-E's and enhances the maturation and proliferation of the erythron. In a similar manner, interleukin-3 can enhance erythropoiesis. Those cytokines are candidates for future use in concert with rHuEPO [39].

Who benefits from recombinant human erythropoietin therapy?

rHuEPO is one of those drugs used by athletes to improve their performance. The participants of the Olympic Games and other official sports events are not permitted to use rHuEPO since it would not be considered fair play. This vividly demonstrates that rHuEPO is a potent drug that works in healthy people as well. In the medical setting, rHuEPO can be used in healthy, nonanemic patients. It also helps in accelerating recovery from anemia due to a variety of sources. The indications of rHuEPO therapy can be classified as follows:

– Stimulation of normal erythropoiesis with appropriate levels of EPO to prevent either initiation or progression of anemia.

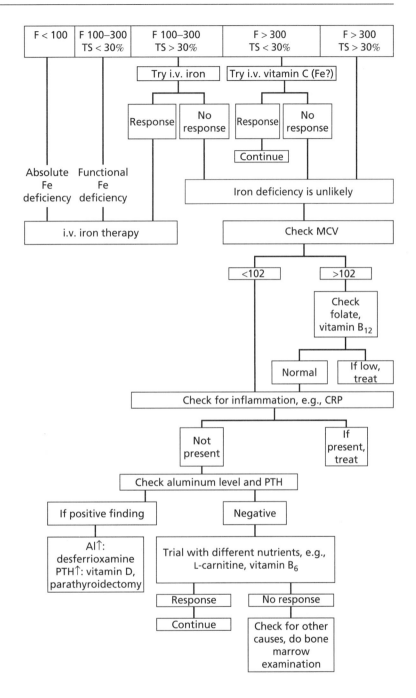

Fig 3.1 Erythropoietin hyporesponsiveness. A1, aluminium; CRP, C-reactive protein; PTH, parathyroid hormone; F, ferritin; MCV, mean corpuscular volume; TS, transferrin saturation.

– Stimulation of normal erythropoiesis with low levels of EPO.

– Stimulation of impaired erythropoiesis with low, normal, or high levels of EPO.

Prevention is better than cure

Patients who are expected to develop anemia in the course of their treatment are candidates for preventive measures.

Patients scheduled for chemotherapy were shown to benefit from preventive rHuEPO therapy and also those who are anemic at the onset of their chemotherapy. Patients who develop anemia during the first therapy cycle also benefit from rHuEPO application. rHuEPO helps such patients to keep an acceptable hemoglobin level by boosting their own erythropoiesis. Transfusions are reduced [42].

rHuEPO also prevents anemia in the *surgical setting*. If given prior to and during *preoperative autologous blood donation*, more autologous units can be donated [43]. *Acute normovolemic hemodilution* is facilitated by an increased preoperative hematocrit. More units can be drawn before the patient reaches the lowest acceptable hemoglobin level. The more units are drawn before reaching this level, the lower the likelihood of allogeneic transfusion exposure.

Patients who do not donate their blood before surgery benefit as well [43–45]. The hemoglobin level is a key predictor for the use of perioperative allogeneic transfusions. Increasing the preoperative hematocrit to high-normal values increases the tolerable blood loss [24] and decreases the use of allogeneic transfusions. Perioperative hematocrit values of 45–50% are usually tolerated.

Practice tip

Prescribing rHuEPO before surgery
Here is a proposal of a therapeutic regimen for a slightly anemic average adult patient who will undergo hip replacement in 14 days.
Rp:
rHuEPO 20,000 U subcutaneously on
Monday–Wednesday–Friday for 2 wk
Plus daily:
Iron tablets 200 mg—1–1–1
Vitamin B_{12} tablets 500 mcg—1–0–0
Folate tablets 20 mg—1–1–1
Vitamin C tablets 100 mg 1–1–1
Monitoring:
Finger stick hemoglobin every Friday and blood pressure measurement with every injection

---

Boosting normal erythropoiesis

There are situations where erythropoiesis is already stimulated by endogenous EPO but, for some reason, a more rapid recovery of the blood count is needed. Since the speed of hemoglobin recovery depends on the serum levels of EPO, giving additional rHuEPO accelerates the replenishment of the red blood cells. Usually, mid to high doses of rHuEPO are given to expedite recovery.

Blood loss is a normal feature of surgery and childbirth. If this blood loss exceeds a certain amount, patients are left anemic. Here is where rHuEPO comes into play. It is used to improve postoperative and postpartum red cell mass recovery [46]. Patients reach an acceptable hemoglobin level earlier and are able to leave the hospital sooner. rHuEPO given after surgery with major blood loss is the ideal treatment for patients who cannot receive allogeneic transfusion. rHuEPO therapy must be considered in virtually every surgical procedure leading to considerable anemia.

rHuEPO also plays a role in pregnancy complicated with anemia. Anemia during pregnancy and gestation may endanger mother and child. It increases the risk of miscarriage, infections, and periportal hemorrhage. If iron and vitamin therapy alone are not sufficient, rHuEPO can be added [18].

When erythropoietin is missing

Some forms of anemia are due to low levels of endogenous EPO. One example of this kind of anemia is the anemia due to kidney failure. Often, there is ongoing blood loss, and additional factors complicate anemia and weaken the response to rHuEPO. For this reason usually higher doses of rHuEPO are given. rHuEPO is effective treatment for anemia in patients with renal failure. Regardless of their dialysis dependency, rHuEPO therapy usually abolishes transfusions.

Premature babies have a relative EPO deficiency. The immature kidneys are not able to produce sufficient amounts of EPO. This is especially true during the phase when erythropoietin is switched from the hepatic to the renal production. During this time, babies benefit from rHuEPO therapy and transfusions may be decreased or eliminated [47, 48].

When erythropoiesis is impaired

A great variety of hematologic disorders are accompanied by anemia. In such settings, the use of rHuEPO is often very effective. Here are two examples:

Sickle cell disease: Patients with sickle cell disease were shown to benefit from rHuEPO therapy. In the course of their disease, they suffer hemolysis and painful crisis. The underlying defect is the presence of the abnormal sickle hemoglobin. If patients are given rHuEPO, the level of normally present fetal hemoglobin increases and the amount of sickle hemoglobin decreases. This leads to improvement in the condition of the patients [11].

Aplastic anemia: rHuEPO alone, or in combination with other hematopoietic growth factors, has been successfully used in the treatment of patients with aplastic anemia [12].

Erythropoiesis is also impaired in patients with chronic inflammatory disease. Inflammatory cytokines hinder EPO's ability to attach to its receptor and to stimulate erythropoiesis. They decrease the sensitivity of erythrogenic progenitor cells to EPO [13]. As a means of compensation, higher levels of endogenous EPO circulate in the serum. Anemia may exist despite high levels of endogenous EPO. Nevertheless, rHuEPO may be beneficial. Very high doses of rHuEPO partially counteract the effects of inflammatory cytokines and abolish anemia.

Some relatively common chronic disorders were studied in order to evaluate potential benefits of rHuEPO therapy. The following represent some of them:

Rheumatoid arthritis: Inflammatory cytokines may affect hematopoiesis. If an optimal anti-inflammatory therapy cannot improve anemia, rHuEPO is available to increase hematocrit levels [49, 50].

Inflammatory bowel disease: Plasma concentration of EPO is raised in patients with inflammatory bowel disease. Despite these raised levels, concentrations are inadequate to reverse anemia. rHuEPO is effective in increasing the hemoglobin level [14].

Anemia associated with acquired immunodeficiency syndrome: Anemia is common among patients with acquired immunodeficiency syndrome. This is not only due to the presence of the disease but also due to administered therapies (e.g., zidovudine). rHuEPO can be used to reverse the anemia developing in acquired immunodeficiency syndrome patients [51].

Malignancy: rHuEPO is useful when dealing with malignancy in cancer patients [52]. Such patients may be anemic due to an inhibition of their erythropoiesis by cytokines, blood loss, and/or hemolysis. In addition, their therapy induces anemia due to myelosuppression or nephrotoxic drugs such as cisplatin. rHuEPO either increases the hematocrit levels or prevents it from falling. It also allows for a more intensive therapy regimen [19]. Stem cell and bone marrow harvesting as well as bone marrow transplantation are facilitated by rHuEPO therapy. Mild anemia associated with cancer, which is typically not considered an indication for allogeneic transfusion, has an impact on the patient's well-being since patients feel tired frequently. Fatigue caused by anemia is another setting where rHuEPO is used [53]. This dramatically improves the patient's quality of life.

Patients in an intensive care unit are often anemic. Approximately 85% of patients admitted to the intensive care unit for more than 1 week receive donated red blood cells. Most of the transfusions administered there are not due to acute blood loss. Rather, patients develop anemia over the course of time. This multifactor process includes a reduced erythropoietic response due to inflammation and iatrogenic blood loss. rHuEPO is able to alleviate the anemia of critical illness [16].

Recombinant human erythropoietin and transfusions

In many studies and reviews, rHuEPO therapy was shown to reduce the use of red blood cell transfusions [10, 54]. The most impressive reductions of allogeneic transfusion were achieved in patients with kidney failure. The transfusion rate of patients on dialysis dropped drastically since the introduction of rHuEPO into clinical practice. More than 95% of all renal patients treated with rHuEPO respond favorably and do not receive transfusions any more [55].

Increasing the hemoglobin level prior to surgery can reduce patient's exposure to donor blood. Patients with perioperative rHuEPO application are transfused less than patients not receiving rHuEPO. This was shown to be the case in a variety of surgical interventions including cardiac and urologic procedures in adults and children [23–26, 28].

Patients with a variety of medical conditions respond to rHuEPO therapy and are transfused less than patients not on rHuEPO. This is true for anemia due to rheumatoid arthritis [13], anemia in critically ill patients [15], patients with sickle cell disease and thalassemia [11], as well as many cancer patients [56].

The number of patients who do not accept blood transfusions is growing. The use of rHuEPO may now allow for treatments that traditionally would call for frequent transfusions. Complicated surgical procedures such as liver transplantation and open-heart surgery were safely performed in combination with the perioperative application of rHuEPO. High-dose chemotherapy without allogeneic transfusion is possible with the use of certain growth factors, including rHuEPO [19]. With the use of rHuEPO, stem cell and bone marrow transplantation without exposure to allogeneic blood were performed.

Future developments

The therapy of chronic, EPO-dependent anemia requires regular injections of rHuEPO. To make EPO substitution more convenient, different methods of replacement are under investigation. Some success was reported when viral vectors for encoding EPO were injected into animals. Repeated injections were useless, since the animals developed

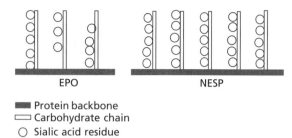

EPO NESP

■ Protein backbone
▭ Carbohydrate chain
○ Sialic acid residue

Fig 3.2 Structure of erythropoietin and novel erythropoietin-stimulating protein (engineered to contain five N-linked carbohydrate chains carrying sialic acid residues).

antibodies against the virus [57]. Another way to introduce EPO into an organism is by means of cell implantation. Cells are genetically engineered to release EPO. After encapsulation of the cells, antigenicity is reduced, and the cells can be implanted into patients. Implantation of such cell-capsule combinations provides the body with a source of human EPO [58].

Novel erythropoiesis-stimulating protein (darbepoetin)

EPO depends on its sialic acid molecules for a prolonged plasma half-life. If these molecules are lost, EPO is rapidly cleared from the blood. In turn, the half-life of EPO is increased when it contains more sialic acid molecules. Based on this fact, it was hypothesized that increasing the amount of sialic acid would increase serum half-life, and indeed it did. An analogue of EPO, a novel erythropoiesis stimulating protein (NESP) was engineered by adding two additional N-linked oligosaccharide chains (with sialic acid residues) to the EPO molecule (Fig. 3.2). This prolonged the half-life of the new drug considerably. The NESP remains in the blood stream approximately three times longer than does rHuEPO [59].

NESP is a molecule that is somewhat larger than EPO (38,000 compared to 30,400 Da). It stimulates erythropoiesis in the same way as EPO [60], by attaching to the EPO receptor and initiating the biochemical cascade that induces changes in the nucleus of cells.

Side effects of NESP are similar to those found with rHuEPO therapy. One area of concern was neutralizing antibodies. Since NESP is a new molecule that has no endogenous equivalent, it may be immunogenic. However, so far, antibodies do not seem to be a cause for concern.

The greatest advantage of NESP is its prolonged half-life. This allows for less frequent administration. A single

shot once a week or even once every 2–3 weeks is sufficient to maintain the required erythropoiesis. Especially patients dependent on long-term EPO substitution benefit from this. Several studies conducted in dialysis patients demonstrated the clinical value of NESP [61]. The same is true of cancer patients [62, 63]. NESP is useful for initiating of anemia therapy as well as for maintenance therapy [60].

Anabolic steroids

The average hematocrit of men is higher than that of women. This is the result of the natural androgen testosterone, stimulating formation of EPO. It increases the endogenous EPO production and enhances the sensitivity of erythroid progenitors to available EPO. Persons with bilateral nephrectomy do not benefit much from androgen therapy, since the presence of at least one kidney is needed for a favorable response to androgen therapy in anemia.

Anabolic steroids are derivatives of androgens. Among them are 19-nortestosteron derivates and 17-alkylated androgens. Examples of androgens used for anemia therapy are nandrolone (e.g., 200 mg/wk i.m.) [64–67] and danazol [68–70].

Androgen therapy has been tried for a variety of anemia types, such as in bone marrow failure and myelofibrosis. About half of the patients with anemia, particularly in cases with bone marrow involvement, respond with an increase in red cell mass. Aplastic anemia may also respond well to androgens. Before the advent of rHuEPO, androgens, with their anabolic effect, were also used in the management of anemia in dialysis patients [71]. When used in elderly males (>50 yr) on dialysis, it increases hemoglobin levels to a similar degree as equivalent doses of rHuEPO would [64].

The cost of anabolics is considerably lower than that of equivalent doses of rHuEPO. This finding led to a renaissance of androgen therapy. Androgen therapy alone or a combination of rHuEPO and androgens may lower the costs of anemia therapy.

Androgen therapy is coupled with significant side effects. A consistent effect of androgens is the retention of water and sodium chloride, which causes edema. This responds to the use of diuretics. Androgens have a virilizing effect (deep voice, hirsutism), which is especially disturbing when the drug is used in women. Only if the prescribed androgens are withdrawn as soon as the first outward effects appear, a complete recovery can be expected. If androgens are given to females for a prolonged time, the virilizing effects remain even after the discontinuation of the drug. Androgens also have virilizing effects in both male and female children and cause premature closure of epiphyses. Some drugs have a feminizing effect, which may cause gynecomastia. Anabolic effects increase albumin and body weight, an effect not considered disturbing. In addition, triglycerides are increased by administration of androgens. This is reversible after discontinuation of the therapy. Liver dysfunction and liver cancer were also reported in patients receiving androgens, particularly of the group of 17-alkylated androgens [64]. Therapy with androgens generally is contraindicated in pregnancy since it can pass the placenta barrier, causing fetal virilization. Carcinoma of the prostate and disturbed liver function are contraindications to the use of androgens as well.

Prolactin

Prolactin is a hormone with anabolic properties. It was shown to act on hematopoietic precursors as these have a prolactin receptor. This receptor is similar to the EPO receptor.

Recombinant human prolactin has been used successfully to reduce anemia in animals treated with the myelosuppressive agent azidothymidine [72] and in humans with bone marrow failure [73].

Indirectly increasing endogenous prolactin by means of metoclopramide therapy has proven effective therapy for anemia as well. Patients with Diamond–Blackfan anemia can be treated with metoclopramide for extended periods. This may eliminate their being transfused [74, 75].

Key points

• rHuEPO is a safe and effective tool in the therapy of anemia. The response to rHuEPO therapy depends on the dose given. To prevent or treat functional iron deficiency, iron therapy should accompany rHuEPO therapy. If EPO hyporesponsiveness is present, adjuvant therapies are warranted. Adjuvant therapy may overcome EPO hyporesponsiveness and may decrease the need for rHuEPO. rHuEPO therapy reduces allogeneic transfusions in a great variety of cases. Combining rHuEPO therapy with other techniques of blood management further reduces the patient's exposure to donor blood.
• The NESP is a synthetic analogue to rHuEPO. Its half-life is prolonged. This may allow for less frequent applications.

• Anabolic steroids exert some influence on erythropoiesis by releasing endogenous EPO. They may be used as an adjuvant or alternative to rHuEPO in selected cases.
• Recombinant human prolactin and metoclopramide may provide effective hematopoietic therapy for selected patients.

Questions for review

• How does human erythropoiesis take place?
• What is the role of EPO in human erythropoiesis?
• Which recombinant erythropoietic agents are available? What are their properties?
• How is rHuEPO used for blood management?
• How is EPO hyporesponsiveness overcome?
• What is the role of androgens, recombinant human prolactin, and metoclopramide in blood management?

Suggestions for further research

Characterize the following erythropoietic agents: endogenous EPO, EPO α, EPO β, EPO ω, and darbepoetin. What differences are clinically relevant and why?

Homework

Get a package insert of rHuEPO and NESP, read it, and file it.

Ask a sales representative to provide you with current articles on EPO/NESP.

Inquire about the contact details of the providers of the following drugs and note their prices: rHuEPO, NESP, danazol, nandrolone, recombinant human prolactin, metoclopramide. Note the information in your address book (Appendix E).

Exercises and practice cases

A 39-year-old patient with placenta previa who has heavy vaginal hemorrhage is taken to your emergency room. She does not give consent to blood transfusion. Her hematocrit is 37% at admission. You take her to the operating room immediately and her problem is solved surgically. After surgery, she has a hematocrit of 22%. The next day, her hematocrit is 5.6%. She is no longer hemorrhaging. Your colleagues already gave her oxygen and 6% hetastarch. The patient is sedated and has sufficient analgesia [76].

What do you prescribe for her today? Please, give also exact dosing.

How do you follow up?

Do you expect side effects of your treatment? If so, which? How would you treat them?

Read the original case report in the literature [76] to find out how the mentioned patient was actually treated. Would you have done something different?

References

1 Tabbara, I.A. Erythropoietin. Biology and clinical applications. *Arch Intern Med*, 1993. **153**(3): p. 298–304.

2 Miyake, T., C.K. Kung, and E. Goldwasser. Purification of human erythropoietin. *J Biol Chem*, 1977. **252**(15): p. 5558–5564.

3 Jacobs, K., *et al.* Isolation and characterization of genomic and cDNA clones of human erythropoietin. *Nature*, 1985. **313**(6005): p. 806–810.

4 Lacombe, C. and P. Mayeux. The molecular biology of erythropoietin. *Nephrol Dial Transplant*, 1999. **14**(Suppl 2): p. 22–28.

5 Sawyer, S.T., S.B. Krantz, and J. Luna. Identification of the receptor for erythropoietin by cross-linking to Friend virus-infected erythroid cells. *Proc Natl Acad Sci U S A*, 1987. **84**(11): p. 3690–3694.

6 Sawyer, S.T., S.B. Krantz, and E. Goldwasser. Binding and receptor-mediated endocytosis of erythropoietin in Friend virus-infected erythroid cells. *J Biol Chem*, 1987. **262**(12): p. 5554–5562.

7 Goodnough, L.T., B. Skikne, and C. Brugnara. Erythropoietin, iron, and erythropoiesis. *Blood*, 2000. **96**(3): p. 823–833.

8 van Iperen, C.E., *et al.* Erythropoietic response to acute and chronic anaemia: focus on postoperative anaemia. *Br J Anaesth*, 1998. **81**(Suppl 1): p. 2–5.

9 Atabek, U., *et al.* Erythropoetin accelerates hematocrit recovery in post-surgical anemia. *Am Surg*, 1995. **61**(1): p. 74–77.

10 Goldberg, M.A. Perioperative epoetin alfa increases red blood cell mass and reduces exposure to transfusions: results of randomized clinical trials. *Semin Hematol*, 1997. **34**(3, Suppl 2): p. 41–47.

11 Bourantas, K., *et al.* Preliminary results with administration of recombinant human erythropoietin in sickle cell/beta-thalassemia patients during pregnancy. *Eur J Haematol*, 1996. **56**(5): p. 326–328.

12 Bessho, M., *et al.* Treatment of the anemia of aplastic anemia patients with recombinant human erythropoietin in combination with granulocyte colony-stimulating factor: a multicenter randomized controlled study. Multicenter Study Group. *Eur J Haematol*, 1997. **58**(4): p. 265–272.

13 Murphy, E.A., *et al.* Study of erythropoietin in treatment of anaemia in patients with rheumatoid arthritis. *BMJ*, 1994. **309**(6965): p. 1337–1338.

14 Schreiber, S., *et al.* Recombinant erythropoietin for the treatment of anemia in inflammatory bowel disease. *N Engl J Med*, 1996. **334**(10): p. 619–623.

15 Corwin, H.L., *et al.* Efficacy of recombinant human erythropoietin in the critically ill patient: a randomized, double-blind, placebo-controlled trial. *Crit Care Med*, 1999. **27**(11): p. 2346–2350.

16 Gabriel, A., High-dose recombinant human erythropoietin stimulates reticulocyte production in patients with multiple organ dysfunction syndrome. *J Trauma*, 1998. **44**(2): p. 361–367.

17 Faulds, D. and E.M. Sorkin. Epoetin (recombinant human erythropoietin). A review of its pharmacodynamic and pharmacokinetic properties and therapeutic potential in anaemia and the stimulation of erythropoiesis. *Drugs*, 1989. **38**(6): p. 863–899.

18 Breymann, C., *et al.* Recombinant human erythropoietin and parenteral iron in the treatment of pregnancy anemia: a pilot study. *J Perinat Med*, 1995. **23**(1–2): p. 89–98.

19 Estrin, J.T., *et al.* Erythropoietin permits high-dose chemotherapy with peripheral blood stem-cell transplant for a Jehovah's Witness. *Am J Hematol*, 1997. **55**(1): p. 51–52.

20 Tryba, M. Epoetin alfa plus autologous blood donation in patients with a low hematocrit scheduled to undergo orthopedic surgery. *Semin Hematol*, 1996. **33**(2, Suppl 2): p. 22–24; discussion 25–26.

21 Braga, J., *et al.* Maternal and perinatal implications of the use of human recombinant erythropoietin. *Acta Obstet Gynecol Scand*, 1996. **75**(5): p. 449–453.

22 Niemeyer, C.M., *et al.* Treatment trial with recombinant human erythropoietin in children with congenital hypoplastic anemia. *Contrib Nephrol*, 1991. **88**: p. 276–280; discussion 281.

23 Braga, M., *et al.* Erythropoietic response induced by recombinant human erythropoietin in anemic cancer patients candidate to major abdominal surgery. *Hepatogastroenterology*, 1997. **44**(15): p. 685–690.

24 Sowade, O., *et al.* Avoidance of allogeneic blood transfusions by treatment with epoetin beta (recombinant human erythropoietin) in patients undergoing open-heart surgery. *Blood*, 1997. **89**(2): p. 411–418.

25 Yazicioglu, L., *et al.* Recombinant human erythropoietin administration in cardiac surgery. *J Thorac Cardiovasc Surg*, 2001. **122**(4): p. 741–745.

26 Shimpo, H., *et al.* Erythropoietin in pediatric cardiac surgery: clinical efficacy and effective dose. *Chest*, 1997. **111**(6): p. 1565–1570.

27 Messmer, K. Consensus statement: using epoetin alfa to decrease the risk of allogeneic blood transfusion in the surgical

setting. Roundtable of Experts in Surgery Blood Management. *Semin Hematol*, 1996. **33**(2, Suppl 2): p. 78–80.

28 Chun, T.Y., S. Martin, and H. Lepor. Preoperative recombinant human erythropoietin injection versus preoperative autologous blood donation in patients undergoing radical retropubic prostatectomy. *Urology*, 1997. **50**(5): p. 727–732.

29 Mak, R.H. Effect of recombinant human erythropoietin on insulin, amino acid, and lipid metabolism in uremia. *J Pediatr*, 1996. **129**(1): p. 97–104.

30 Fagher, B., H. Thysell, and M. Monti. Effect of erythropoietin on muscle metabolic rate, as measured by direct microcalorimetry, and ATP in hemodialysis patients. *Nephron*, 1994. **67**(2): p. 167–171.

31 Lewis, L.D. Preclinical and clinical studies: a preview of potential future applications of erythropoietic agents. *Semin Hematol*, 2004. **41**(4, Suppl 7): p. 17–25.

32 Erbayraktar, S., *et al.* Asialoerythropoietin is a nonerythropoietic cytokine with broad neuroprotective activity in vivo. *Proc Natl Acad Sci U S A*, 2003. **100**(11): p. 6741–6746.

33 Ehrenreich, H., *et al.* Erythropoietin therapy for acute stroke is both safe and beneficial. *Mol Med*, 2002. **8**(8): p. 495–505.

34 Calvillo, L., *et al.* Recombinant human erythropoietin protects the myocardium from ischemia-reperfusion injury and promotes beneficial remodeling. *Proc Natl Acad Sci U S A*, 2003. **100**(8): p. 4802–4806.

35 Baker, J.E. Erythropoietin mimics ischemic preconditioning. *Vascul Pharmacol*, 2005. **42**(5–6): p. 233–241.

36 Semba, R.D. and S.E. Juul. Erythropoietin in human milk: physiology and role in infant health. *J Hum Lact*, 2002. **18**(3): p. 252–261.

37 Tarng, D.C. and T.P. Huang. A parallel, comparative study of intravenous iron versus intravenous ascorbic acid for erythropoietin-hyporesponsive anaemia in haemodialysis patients with iron overload. *Nephrol Dial Transplant*, 1998. **13**(11): p. 2867–2872.

38 Danielson, B. R-HuEPO hyporesponsiveness—who and why? *Nephrol Dial Transplant*, 1995. **10**(Suppl 2): p. 69–73.

39 Horl, W.H. Is there a role for adjuvant therapy in patients being treated with epoetin? *Nephrol Dial Transplant*, 1999. **14**(Suppl 2): p. 50–60.

40 Kuhn, K., *et al.* Analysis of initial resistance of erythropoiesis to treatment with recombinant human erythropoietin. Results of a multicenter trial in patients with end-stage renal disease. *Contrib Nephrol*, 1988. 66: p. 94–103.

41 Bommer, J. Saving erythropoietin by administering l-carnitine? *Nephrol Dial Transplant*, 1999. **14**(12): p. 2819–2821.

42 Wolchok, J.D., *et al.* Prophylactic recombinant epoetin alfa markedly reduces the need for blood transfusion in patients with metastatic melanoma treated with biochemotherapy. *Cytokines Cell Mol Ther*, 1999. **5**(4): p. 205–206.

43 Colomina, M.J., *et al.* Preoperative erythropoietin in spine surgery. *Eur Spine J*, 2004. **13**(Suppl 1): p. S40–S49.

44 Christodoulakis, M. and D.D. Tsiftsis. Preoperative epoetin alfa in colorectal surgery: a randomized, controlled study. *Ann Surg Oncol*, 2005. **12**(9): p. 718–725.

45 Weber, E.W., *et al.* Effects of epoetin alfa on blood transfusions and postoperative recovery in orthopaedic surgery: the European Epoetin Alfa Surgery Trial (EEST). *Eur J Anaesthesiol*, 2005. **22**(4): p. 249–257.

46 Breymann, C., R. Zimmermann, R. Huch, and A. Huch. Erythropoietin zur Behandlung der postpartalen Anämie. In *Hämatologie, München Sympomed*, 1993. 2: p. 49–55.

47 Kumar, P., S. Shankaran, and R.G. Krishnan. Recombinant human erythropoietin therapy for treatment of anemia of prematurity in very low birth weight infants: a randomized, double-blind, placebo-controlled trial. *J Perinatol*, 1998. **18**(3): p. 173–177.

48 Ohls, R.K. Erythropoietin to prevent and treat the anemia of prematurity. *Curr Opin Pediatr*, 1999. **11**(2): p. 108–114.

49 Goodnough, L.T. and R.E. Marcus. The erythropoietic response to erythropoietin in patients with rheumatoid arthritis. *J Lab Clin Med*, 1997. **130**(4): p. 381–386.

50 Wilson, A., *et al.* Prevalence and outcomes of anemia in rheumatoid arthritis: a systematic review of the literature. *Am J Med*, 2004. **116**(Suppl 7A): p. 50S–57S.

51 Fischl, M., *et al.* Recombinant human erythropoietin for patients with AIDS treated with zidovudine. *N Engl J Med*, 1990. **322**(21): p. 1488–1493.

52 Stasi, R., *et al.* Management of cancer-related anemia with erythropoietic agents: doubts, certainties, and concerns. *Oncologist*, 2005. **10**(7): p. 539–554.

53 Jilani, S.M. and J.A. Glaspy. Impact of epoetin alfa in chemotherapy-associated anemia. *Semin Oncol*, 1998. **25**(5): p. 571–576.

54 Laupacis, A. and D. Fergusson. Erythropoietin to minimize perioperative blood transfusion: a systematic review of randomized trials. The International Study of Peri-operative Transfusion (ISPOT) Investigators. *Transfus Med*, 1998. **8**(4): p. 309–317.

55 Cazzola, M., F. Mercuriali, and C. Brugnara. Use of recombinant human erythropoietin outside the setting of uremia. *Blood*, 1997. **89**(12): p. 4248–4267.

56 Seidenfeld, J., *et al.* Epoetin treatment of anemia associated with cancer therapy: a systematic review and meta-analysis of controlled clinical trials. *J Natl Cancer Inst*, 2001. **93**(16): p. 1204–1214.

57 Svensson, E.C., *et al.* Long-term erythropoietin expression in rodents and non-human primates following intramuscular injection of a replication-defective adenoviral vector. *Hum Gene Ther*, 1997. **8**(15): p. 1797–1806.

58 Rinsch, C., *et al.* A gene therapy approach to regulated delivery of erythropoietin as a function of oxygen tension. *Hum Gene Ther*, 1997. **8**(16): p. 1881–1889.

59 Glaspy, J. Phase III clinical trials with darbepoetin: implications for clinicians. *Best Pract Res Clin Haematol*, 2005. **18**(3): p. 407–416.

60 Macdougall, I.C. Novel erythropoiesis stimulating protein. *Semin Nephrol*, 2000. **20**(4): p. 375–381.

61 Brunkhorst, R., *et al.* Darbepoetin alfa effectively maintains haemoglobin concentrations at extended dose intervals relative to intravenous or subcutaneous recombinant human erythropoietin in dialysis patients. *Nephrol Dial Transplant*, 2004. **19**(5): p. 1224–1230.

62 Schwartzberg, L.S., *et al.* A randomized comparison of every-2-week darbepoetin alfa and weekly epoetin alfa for the treatment of chemotherapy-induced anemia in patients with breast, lung, or gynecologic cancer. *Oncologist*, 2004. **9**(6): p. 696–707.

63 Cvetkovic, R.S. and K.L. Goa. Darbepoetin alfa: in patients with chemotherapy-related anaemia. *Drugs*, 2003. **63**(11): p. 1067–1074; discussion 1075–1077.

64 Teruel, J.L., *et al.* Androgen versus erythropoietin for the treatment of anemia in hemodialyzed patients: a prospective study. *J Am Soc Nephrol*, 1996. **7**(1): p. 140–144.

65 Gascon, A., *et al.* Nandrolone decanoate is a good alternative for the treatment of anemia in elderly male patients on hemodialysis. *Geriatr Nephrol Urol*, 1999. **9**(2): p. 67–72.

66 Teruel, J.L., *et al.* Androgen therapy for anaemia of chronic renal failure. Indications in the erythropoietin era. *Scand J Urol Nephrol*, 1996. **30**(5): p. 403–408.

67 Teruel, J.L., *et al.* Evolution of serum erythropoietin after androgen administration to hemodialysis patients: a prospective study. *Nephron*, 1995. **70**(3): p. 282–286.

68 Cervantes, F., *et al.* Efficacy and tolerability of danazol as a treatment for the anaemia of myelofibrosis with myeloid metaplasia: long-term results in 30 patients. *Br J Haematol*, 2005. **129**(6): p. 771–775.

69 Cervantes, F., *et al.* Danazol treatment of idiopathic myelofibrosis with severe anemia. *Haematologica*, 2000. **85**(6): p. 595–599.

70 Harrington, W.J., Sr., *et al.* Danazol for paroxysmal nocturnal hemoglobinuria. *Am J Hematol*, 1997. **54**(2): p. 149–154.

71 Hardman, J. *Goodman and Gilman's The Pharmacological Basis of Therapeutics*. McGraw-Hill, New York, 1995. p. 1441ff.

72 Woody, M.A., *et al.* Prolactin exerts hematopoietic growth-promoting effects in vivo and partially counteracts myelosuppression by azidothymidine. *Exp Hematol*, 1999. **27**(5): p. 811–816.

73 Jepson J.H. and E.E. McGarry. Effect of the anabolic protein hormone prolactin on human erythropoiesis. *J Clin Pharmacol*, 1974(May–June): p. 296–300.

74 Akiyama, M., *et al.* Successful treatment of Diamond-Blackfan anemia with metoclopramide. *Am J Hematol*, 2005. **78**(4): p. 295–298.

75 Abkowitz, J.L., *et al.* Response of Diamond-Blackfan anemia to metoclopramide: evidence for a role for prolactin in erythropoiesis. *Blood*, 2002. **100**(8): p. 2687–2691.

76 Koenig, H.M., *et al.* Use of recombinant human erythropoietin in a Jehovah's Witness. *J Clin Anesth*, 1993. **5**(3): p. 244–247.

4 Anemia therapy II (hematinics)

Erythropoiesis depends on three prerequisites to function properly: a site for erythropoiesis, that is, the bone marrow; a regulatory system, that is, cytokines acting as erythropoietins; and raw materials for erythropoiesis, among them hematinics. This second chapter on anemia therapy will introduce the latter, their role in erythropoiesis, and their therapeutic value.

Objectives of this chapter

1 Review the physiological basis for the use of hematinics.
2 Relate the indications for the therapeutic use of hematinics.
3 Define the role of hematinics in blood management.

Definitions

Hematinics: Hematinics are vitamins and minerals essential for normal erythropoiesis. Among them are iron, copper, cobalt, and vitamins A, B_6, B_{12}, C, E, folic acid, riboflavin, and nicotinic acid.

Iron: Iron is a trace element that is vital for oxidative processes in the human body. Its ability to switch easily from the ferrous form to the ferric state makes it an important player in oxygen binding and release.

Physiology of erythropoiesis and hemoglobin synthesis

Hematinics are the fuel for erythropoiesis. When treating a patient with anemia, it is necessary to administer hematinics in order to support the patient's own erythropoiesis in restoring a normal red blood cell mass. A review of erythropoiesis and hemoglobin synthesis will provide the necessary background information to prescribe hematinics effectively.

Erythropoiesis starts with the division and differentiation of stem cells in the bone marrow. In the course of erythropoiesis, DNA needs to be synthesized, new nuclei need to be formed, and cells need to divide. For all these processes, hematinics are needed. Folates and vitamin B_{12} are important cofactors in the synthesis of the DNA. They are necessary for purine and pyrimidine synthesis. Folates provide the methyl groups for thymidylate, a precursor of DNA synthesis.

Erythropoiesis continues while the newly made red cell precursors synthesize hemoglobin. This synthesis consists of two distinct, yet interwoven processes: the synthesis of heme and the synthesis of globins. The heme synthesis, a ring-like porphyrin with a central iron atom, starts with the production of δ-aminolevulinic acid (ALA) in the mitochondria (Table 4.1). ALA then travels to the cytoplasm. There, coproporphyrinogen III is synthesized out of several ALA molecules. The latter molecule travels back to the mitochondria where it reacts with protoporphyrin IX. With the help of the enzyme ferrochelatase, iron is introduced into the ring structure and the resulting molecule is heme.

Parallel to the synthesis of heme, the synthesis of globin chains takes place. Physiologically, it matches the needs of erythropoiesis. After the globins are synthesized, the pathway of globin synthesis and heme synthesis comes together. This final pathway, the assembly of the hemoglobin molecule, occurs in the cytoplasm of the red cell precursor. In the process of folding the primary amino acid sequence, each globin molecule binds a heme molecule. After this process, dimers of an alpha-chain and a non-alpha-chain form. Later, the dimers are assembled into the functional hemoglobin molecule.

During life, the human body synthesizes different kinds of hemoglobins. The differences between those hemoglobins are the result of the type of globin chains produced (Table 4.2). Apart from a short period in embryogenesis, healthy humans always have hemoglobins that consist of two alpha-chains and two non-alpha-chains. During fetal life and 7–8 months thereafter, considerable

Table 4.1 Hemoglobin synthesis.

Step	Enzyme	Place	Cofactor
Succinyl CoA + glycine forms ALA	ALA synthase, pyridoxal phosphatase	Mitochondria	Pyridoxal phosphate
2× ALA form porphobilinogen	ALA dehydratase	Cytoplasm	
4× porphobilinogen form uroporphyrinogen III	Two-step process: hydroxymethylbilane synthase (= porphobilinogen deaminase), uroporphyrinogen III cosynthase	Cytoplasm	
Uroporphyrinogen converted to coproporphyrinogen III	Uroporphyrinogen decarboxylase, converting four acetates to methyl residues	Cytoplasm	
Coproporphyrinogen III converted to protoporphyrin IX	Two-step process: coproporphyrinogen III oxidase for decarboxylation of propionate to vinyl residues, protoporphyrin oxidase for oxidation of the methylene bridges between pyrrole groups	Mitochondria	
Insertion of iron in protoporphyrin IX	Ferrochelatase	Mitochondria	

ALA, δ-aminolevulinic acid; CoA, coenzyme A.

amounts of hemoglobin F are present. After this period, hemoglobin A is the major hemoglobin present, with trace amounts (less than 3%) of hemoglobin A2. Alpha-chains are encoded for on chromosome 16, whereas the non-alpha-chains are encoded for on chromosome 11. A set sequence of non-alpha-globins is found on chromosome 11, beginning from the 5′ to the 3′ end of the DNA molecule in the sequence epsilon, gamma, delta, and beta. The genes are activated in this sequence during human development. Based on the molecular pattern given by the genes that encode the globins, RNA and globin chains are synthesized.

Table 4.2 Human hemoglobin types.

Type of hemoglobin	Globin chains
Embryonic hemoglobins	Gower1: zeta × 2 plus epsilon × 2
	Gower2: alpha × 2 plus epsilon × 2
	Portland: zeta × 2 plus gamma × 2
Fetal hemoglobin	HgbF: alpha × 2 plus gamma × 2
Adult hemoglobin	HgbA: alpha × 2 plus beta × 2 HgbA2: alpha × 2 plus delta × 2

Hgb, hemoglobin.

Iron therapy in blood management

Physiology of iron

Iron plays a key role in the production and function of hemoglobin. It is able to accept and donate electrons, thereby easily converting from the ferrous (Fe^{2+}) to the ferric form (Fe^{3+}) and vice versa. This property makes iron a valuable commodity for oxygen-binding molecules. On the other hand, iron molecules may be detrimental. Too much iron stored in the body likely inhibits erythropoiesis. Besides, iron can also damage tissues by promoting the formation of free radicals. If the storage capacity of ferritin is superseded (in conditions when body iron stores are in excess of 5–10 times normal), iron remains free in the body and may cause organ damage. The same happens if iron is rapidly released from macrophages. Another interesting feature of iron is that its metabolism is tightly interwoven with immune functions. Since iron promotes the growth of bacteria and possibly of cancer, iron metabolism is modified when patients have infections or cancer. In these conditions, the body employs several mechanisms to reduce the availability of iron.

The body iron stores of normal humans contain about 35–45 mg/kg body weight of iron in the adult male and somewhat less in the adult female. More than two-third of this iron is found in the red cell lining. Most of the remaining iron is stored in the liver and the reticuloendothelial macrophages. Storage occurs as iron bound to ferritin, and mobilization of iron from ferritin occurs by a reducing process using riboflavin-dependent enzymes.

The turnover of iron mainly takes place within the body. Old red cells are taken up by macrophages that process the iron contained in them and load it to transferrin for reuse. By this recycling process, more than 90% of the iron needed for erythropoiesis is gained. Only a small amount of new iron (1–2 mg) enters the body each day. There are no mechanisms to actively excrete iron. The loss of iron takes place by shedding endothelial cells containing iron and by blood loss.

Since the maintenance of adequate iron stores is of vital importance, many mechanisms help in the regulation of iron uptake and recycling. Dietary iron is taken up by enterocytes in the duodenum. These enterocytes are programmed, during their development, to "know" the iron requirements of the body. The low gastric pH in conjunction with a brush border enzyme called ferrireductase helps the iron to be converted from its ferrous form (Fe^{2+}) to ferric iron (Fe^{3+}). The divalent metal transporter 1 (DMT1) is located close to the ferrireductase in the membrane of the enterocytes. This transports iron through the apical membrane of the enterocyte after it was reduced by the ferrireductase. The absorption of iron in the gut is regulated by several mechanisms. After a diet rich in iron, enterocytes stop taking up iron for a few hours ("mucosal block"), probably believing that there is sufficient iron in the body (although this may not be the case). Iron deficiency can cause a two- to threefold increase in iron uptake by the enterocytes. Furthermore, erythropoietic activity is able to increase iron absorption, a process that is independent of the iron stores in the body. Acute hypoxia is also able to stimulate iron absorption [1].

The absorbed iron is either stored in the enterocyte, bound to ferritin (up to about 4500 iron atoms per ferritin molecule), or it is transported through the basolateral membrane into the plasma. The transporter in the basolateral membrane is known to need hephaestin (which is similar to the copper-transporter ceruloplasmin) to carry the iron into the plasma. After being transported into plasma, iron is converted back to the Fe^{3+} form. Probably, hephaestin aids in this conversion [2]. Transferrin in the plasma accepts a maximum of two incoming Fe^{3+} ions.

Iron-loaded transferrin attaches to transferrin receptors on the cell surface of various cells, among them red cell precursors. The receptors are located near clarithrin-coated pits. The clarithrin-coated pits hold the transferrin receptor and the transferrin–iron complex together. In addition, a DMT1, which is close to the membrane that contains the clarithrin-coated pit, is incorporated. As a result, the pits are ingested by the cell by endocytosis and form endosomes. A proton pump in the membrane of the endosomes lowers the pH in the endosome. This leads to changes in the protein structure of the transferrin and triggers the release of free iron into the endosome. The DMT1 pumps the free iron out of the endosome and the endosome membrane fuses with the cell membrane again to release the transferrin receptor and the unloaded transferrin for further use. In erythroid cells, the free iron in the cytoplasm is absorbed by mitochondria. This process is facilitated by a copper-dependent cytochrome oxidase. The iron in the mitochondria is used to transform protoporphyrin into heme. In nonerythroid cells, iron is stored as ferritin and hemosiderin [1].

An interesting mechanism for the regulation of iron metabolism was recently found. This suggests that the liver is not only a storage place of iron but also acts as the command center. While searching for antimicrobial principles in body fluids, Park and his colleagues [2] found a new peptide in the urine that had antimicrobial properties. The same peptide was found in plasma. Due to the peptide's synthesis in the liver (hep-) and its antimicrobial properties (-cidin), the peptide was called hepcidin. Hepcidin is a small, hair-needle-shaped molecule with 20–25 amino acids (hepcidin-20, −22, −25) and four disulfide bonds that link the two arms of the hair-needle to form a ladder-like molecule.

From the early experiments with hepcidin, it was concluded that hepcidin is the long-looked-for regulator of iron metabolism. It seems to regulate the transmembrane iron transport. Hepcidin binds to its receptor ferroportin. Ferroportin is a channel through which iron is transported. When hepcidin binds to ferroportin, ferroportin is degraded and iron is locked inside the cell [3]. By this mechanism, hepcidin locks iron in cells and blocks the availability of iron in the blood. Conversely, when hepcidin levels are reduced, more iron is available.

A closer look at hepcidin revealed its unique properties in the regulation of iron metabolism. In the initial studies about hepcidin in the urine, one urine donor developed an infection and hepcidin levels in the urine increased by about 100 times. This finding led to more research, the results of which are summarized in Table 4.3 [4, 5].

Table 4.3 Regulation of hepcidin.

Hepcidin decreases	Hepcidin increases
– in anemia and hypoxia – by non-transferrin-bound iron (as in thalassemias, some hemolytic anemias, hereditary hemochromatosis, hypo-/a-transferrinemia)	– in inflammation – in iron ingestion and parenteral iron application – after transfusion
A lack of hepcidin causes • iron accumulation • hyperabsorption of iron • increased release of storage iron • release of iron from macrophages with resulting decrease of iron in the spleen	Superfluous hepcidin causes • decreased iron stores • microcytic hypochromic anemia • reduced iron uptake in the small intestine • inhibition of release of iron from macrophages • inhibition of iron transport through the placenta to the fetus

It is evident from Table 4.3 that anemia causes a decrease in hepcidin, making iron available for erythropoiesis. In contrast, inflammation and infection increase hepcidin levels and reduce the availability of iron. This may act as a protection when bacteria or tumor tissue is present since the growth of both of these relies on iron. However, under such circumstances, increased hepcidin may also induce anemia due to iron deficiency. Overproduction of hepcidin during inflammation may be responsible for anemia during inflammation [6].

The concept of hepcidin as a key regulator of iron metabolism offers potential for diagnostic and therapeutic use. Patients with hemochromatosis, who are deficient in hepcidin, could be treated with hepcidin or similar peptides, once they become available. In chronic anemia due to inflammation, detection of hepcidin provides a new diagnostic tool in the differential diagnosis of anemia.

Therapeutic use of iron

Iron deficiency anemia is the most common form of treatable anemia. Absolute iron deficiency develops if the iron intake is inadequate or if blood loss causes loss of iron. Iron uptake is impaired if the amount of iron in food is insufficient, if the pH of the gastric fluids is too high (antacids), and if there are other divalent metals that compete with the iron on the DMT1 protein. After bowel resection, the surface area available for iron absorption is reduced, also limiting the iron uptake. This can also occur in bowel inflammation and in other diseases causing malabsorption. Iron loss is increased in all forms of blood loss, such as gastrointestinal hemorrhage, parasitosis, menorrhagia, pulmonary siderosis, trauma, phlebotomy, etc.

Relative or functional iron deficiency develops as a result of inflammation and malignancy. The term "functional iron deficiency" refers to patients with iron needs despite sufficient or even supranormal iron levels in the body stores. Iron is stored in the macrophages, but it is not recycled. The stored iron is trapped and cannot be mobilized easily for erythropoiesis. Anemia develops despite these normal or supranormal iron stores. Iron therapy may also be warranted under such circumstances. This may be true for patients with anemia due to infection or chronic inflammation being treated with recombinant human erythropoietin (rHuEPO).

Iron therapy is indicated in states of absolute or functional iron deficiency. If patients are eligible for oral iron therapy, this is the treatment of choice. There are many oral iron preparations available. Ferrous salts (ferrous sulfate, gluconate, fumarate) are equally tolerable. Controlled release of iron causes less nausea and epigastric pains than conventional ferrous sulfate. Most cases of absolute iron deficiency can be managed by oral iron administration. Iron absorption is best when the medication is taken between meals. Occasional abdominal upset, after taking the iron, can be reduced if iron is taken with meals. For iron stores to be replenished, the treatment with iron supplements must be continued over several months.

Several additional factors increase or interfere with the iron absorption from the intestine. Ascorbic acid (vitamin C) prevents the formation of less-soluble ferric iron and increases iron uptake. Meat, fish, poultry, and alcohol enhance iron uptake as well, while phytates (inositol phosphates, soy), calcium (in calcium salts, milk, cheese), polyphenols (tea, coffee, red wine (with tannin)), and eggs inhibit iron absorption [7].

Unlike patients with light to moderate iron deficiency anemia, some groups of patients neither respond to nor tolerate oral iron medication. Others need a rapid replenishment of their iron reserves. For some patients, oral iron may be contraindicated when it adds to the damage already caused by chronic inflammatory bowel diseases. In these cases, parenteral iron therapy is warranted. The classical intravenous iron preparation is iron dextran. It is generally well tolerated. However, some concerns arose to its use. Side effects of iron dextrane include flushing, dizziness, backache, anxiety, hypotension, and occasionally respiratory failure and even cardiac arrest. Such symptoms remind us of anaphylactic reactions. Anaphylaxis is probably due to the dextrane in the product. Also a specific effect of free iron contributes to the symptoms. Since dextrane is partially responsible for the adverse effects of iron dextrane, it was proposed that iron preparations free of dextrane might be safer. Other iron preparations are now available to avoid the use of dextrane. Sodium ferric gluconate, a high-molecular-weight complex, contains iron hydroxide, as iron dextrane does. However, it is stabilized in sucrose and gluconate and not in dextrane. Another iron preparation, iron sucrose (iron saccharate), is also available. The dextrane-free products cause similar side effects, such as nausea and vomiting, malaise, heat, back and epigastric pain, and hypotension. In contrast to iron dextrane, the reactions are short-lived and lighter. It is recommended that, due to their safety, the dextrane-free products should be favored when they are available [8]. Even patients who had allergic reactions to iron dextrane can safely be managed with other products.

When intravenous iron therapy is warranted, the amount of iron to be given can be infused in a single dose or in divided doses. It is recommended that iron be diluted in normal saline (not in dextrose, since administration hurts more). The amount of iron can be calculated using the following equations:

Dose in mg Fe = $0.0442 \times (13.5 - \text{hemoglobin current})$ $\times$ lean body weight $\times 50 + (0.26 \times$ lean body weight) $\times 50$

Or

Dose in mg Fe = $(3.4 \times$ hemoglobin deficit $\times$ body weight in kg $\times$ blood volume in mL/kg body weight)/100.

A male has a blood volume of 66 mL/kg and a female about 60 mL/kg.

In addition to the amount of iron calculated by this formula, an additional 1000 mg should be given to fill iron stores.

For example, a 70-kg female has a hemoglobin level of 8 g/dL and is scheduled for parenteral iron therapy. How much iron does she need?

If we consider a hemoglobin level of 14 g/dL to be normal for this woman, she has a deficit of 6 g/dL.

Therefore, calculate:

$(3.4 \times 6 \text{ g/dL} \times 70 \text{ kg} \times 60 \text{ mL/kg} = 856{,}800)/100 = 856.8$ mg.

Meaning the woman has an iron deficit of about 857 mg. In addition, a further 1000 mg should be given to replenish the stores.

> **Practice tip**
>
> A simpler way to estimate the iron needs of an adult is to multiply the hemoglobin deficit by 200 mg. Additional 500 mg should be given to replenish iron stores.

The above-mentioned patient would receive approximately 1700 mg of iron ($6 \times 200 + 500$) using this calculation method.

There are different iron products available for parenteral use. Table 4.4 gives vital information [9] for their practical use.

Markers of iron deficiency

It is usually simple to recognize and diagnose iron deficiency anemia. Microcytic anemia and hypochromic anemia together with low body iron (as measured by transferrin saturation, serum iron, and ferritin) are the classical findings. However, there is an increasing number of patients whose iron needs are not easily monitored by the classical iron markers. Among them are patients with the so-called functional iron deficiency. Since iron status and immunity are closely related, most biochemical markers of the iron status are affected by inflammation and/or infection. Table 4.5 describes commonly used and newer markers of the iron reserves [10–13].

Most hospitals do not offer all methods to monitor iron status mentioned in Table 4.5. Nevertheless, a reliable differential diagnosis (Table 4.6) is possible using commonly available tests. For instance, in addition to the red cell count and the red cell indices (MCV, MCHC), the three following parameters should be sufficient for an exact diagnosis of iron deficiency:

- *Ferritin concentration:* If it is below 12–15 mcg/L, there is a sure indication for iron therapy. If ferritin is above 800–1000 mcg/L, there seems to be too much iron stored in the body and iron therapy needs to be adapted.
- *Transferrin saturation:* It indicates the amount of iron in circulation. If it is below 20%, there seems to be an iron deficit and if it is below 15%, this is a certain indication for iron therapy. If it is above 50%, enough iron should be available.
- *Percentage of hypochromic red cells:* The percentage of hypochromic red cells indicates if red cell synthesis is iron deficient. If the value is above 2.5%, then it

Table 4.4 Commonly used parenteral iron formulas.

Iron preparation	Iron dextrane	Iron sucrose	Iron gluconate
Allergic reactions	Relatively common	Rare	?
Anaphylactoid reactions, e.g., due to free iron	Rare	Rare	Occasionally (iron complex instable)
Availability of iron	Takes 4–7 days until iron available	Immediately	Immediately
Stability	Very stable	Stable	Instable 250 mg safely possible
Recommended dose given in one session (during at least which time)	Do not exceed 20 mg/kg body weight (4–6 h); it has been reported that up to 3–4 g have been given over several hours	500 mg, do not exceed 7 mg/kg body weight (3.5 h)	
Test dose required	Yes, 10 mg, (no guarantee that patient will not react allergically)		
Remarks	There are different types of iron dextrane with slightly different properties		Contains preservatives that may be dangerous for newborns

Other available parenteral iron preparations include iron polymaltose (= iron dextrin), chondroitin sulfate iron colloid, iron saccharate, and iron sorbitol.

is abnormal. Values above 10% indicate absolute iron deficiency.

Copper therapy in blood management

Copper deficiency can cause anemia. In early experiments in anemia therapy of animals on iron feed, it was shown that iron-deficient anemic animals did not improve if copper was lacking in their feed. Adding copper to their feed cured the anemia [14]. This was an interesting result, because hemoglobin does not contain copper. It was found out later that a lack of copper influences hematopoiesis by interfering with iron metabolism due to impaired iron absorption, iron transfer from the reticuloendothelial cells to the plasma, and inadequate ceruloplasmin activity mobilizing iron from the reticuloendothelial system to the plasma. Additionally, copper is a component of cytochrome-c oxidase, an enzyme that is required for iron uptake by mitochondria to form heme. Defective mitochondrial iron uptake, due to copper deficiency, may lead to iron accumulation within the cytoplasm, forming sideroblasts. Copper deficiency may also shorten red cell survival [15].

The average daily Western diet contains 0.6–1.6 mg of copper. Meats, nuts, and shellfish are the richest sources of dietary copper. Because of the ubiquitous distribution of copper and the low daily requirement, acquired copper deficiency is rare. However, it has been reported in premature and severely malnourished infants, in patients with malabsorption, in parenteral nutrition without copper supplementation, and with ingestion of massive quantities of zinc or ascorbic acid. Copper and zinc are absorbed primarily in the proximal small intestine. Zinc interferes directly with intestinal copper absorption.

When copper deficiency anemia is present, the patient presents with macrocytic or microcytic anemia, occasionally accompanied by neutropenia or thrombocytopenia [16–19]. Erythroblasts in the bone marrow are vacuolized. The serum copper level is lower than the normal serum copper level of 70–155 µg/dL. The ceruloplasmin level may also be lower than normal. Treatment of copper deficiency is administered by copper sulfate solution (80 mg/(kg day)) per os or by intravenous bolus injection of copper chlorite [20].

Vitamin therapy in blood management

Vitamins play an important role in blood management. They not only influence hematopoiesis, but also have an impact on other aspects of blood management such as

Table 4.5 Available essays for the monitoring of iron therapy.

Essay	Reference values	Description	Use and limitations
Bone marrow aspirate	Normal: stainable iron present	"Gold standard"; if stainable iron is missing, iron deficiency is present	Too invasive for routine use in the diagnosis of iron deficiency
Classic biochemical markers			
Serum iron	50–170 μg/dL or female: 10–26 μmol/L; male: 14–28 μmol/L (μmol/L × 5.58 = μg/dL)	Iron bound to transferrin	Diurnal variations (higher concentrations late in the day); diet-dependent; infection and inflammation lower serum iron
Transferrin	2.0–4.0 g/L in adults; higher in children	Iron-binding transport protein in plasma and extracellular fluid	Increased by oral contraceptives; decreased in infection or inflammation
Total iron-binding capacity (TIBC)	Normal: 240–450 μg/dL	Measures indirectly the transferrin level (TBIC in μmol/L = transferrin in d/L × 22.5)	High in iron deficiency anemia, late pregnancy, polycythemia vera; low in cirrhosis, sickle cell anemia, hypoproteinemia, hemolytic, and pernicious anemia
Transferrin saturation (TS)	20–50%	Ratio of the serum iron to the TIBC	Oral contraceptives cause inappropriately low TS
Ferritin (F)	<100 μg/L in healthy predicts functional Fe deficiency; <12–20 μg/L is highly specific for iron deficiency	Storage protein of iron; currently accepted laboratory test for iron deficiency; however, disagreement on the lower reference value that indicates iron deficiency	Acute-phase protein; increased in infection/ inflammation, hyperthyroidism, liver disease, malignancy, alcohol use, oral contraceptives; does not reflect iron stores in anemia of chronic disease
Newer biochemical markers			
Serum transferrin receptor (sTfR)	Male: 2.16–4.54 mg/dL; female: 1.79–4.63 mg/dL (extremely dependent on method)	Truncated form of the tissue transferrin receptor; reflects total body mass of cellular transferrin; concentration of circulating sTfR is determined by erythroid marrow activity: estimate of red cell precursor mass which is inversely related to erythropoietin concentrations	Not an acute-phase reactant; higher in patients with iron deficiency than in noniron deficiency, but not sufficient to discriminate between both; decreased in hypoplastic anemia, increased in hyperplastic anemia and iron deficiency
R/F-ratio	>1.5–4.0: absolute iron deficiency; <0.8–1.0 for iron deficiency in inflammation	= sTfR/F most sensitive method to distinguish between anemia of iron deficiency and anemia of chronic disease	Estimates body iron stores; value limited in liver disease and inflammation/infection (C-reactive protein (CRP) screening recommended to identify patients with infection)

(*cont.*)

Table 4.5 *Continued.*

Essay	Reference values	Description	Use and limitations
Erythrocyte zinc protoporphyrin (ZPP)	ZPP < 40 mmol/mol Hgb may exclude iron deficiency	In case of iron deficiency, zinc instead of iron is incorporated into protoporphyrin, and ZPP accumulates in the red cells	ZPP reflects intracellular iron deficiency/supply of iron to red cells; ZPP is also increased in hemolytic anemia, anemia of chronic disease, lead intoxication
Red cell and reticulocyte indices			
% of hypochromic red cells (%HYPO)	Pathologic: >2.5–6.0%; highly pathologic is >10%	Cells with a mean corpuscular Hgb concentration <280 g/L	It takes prolonged iron deficiency to develop pathological %HYPO; also increased with reticulocytosis
Reticulocyte count	0.5–2.0%	Seen as response to red cell synthesis: it takes 18–36 h for reticulocytes to be seen in circulation	Estimate of response to anemia therapy, e.g., with rHuEPO; increases in reticulocyte count after iron therapy indicates iron deficiency
Hemoglobin content of reticulocytes ((CHr) in pg/cell)	Pathologic if ≤29 pg in some patients, e.g., children; pathologic if <20–24 pg		Not useful in thalassemias since reticulocytes have already a low CHr; not useful in chemotherapy since megaloblastic/macrocytic erythropoiesis causes increased CHr
Immature reticulocyte fraction		Reticulocytes with medium to high fluorescence based on fluorescence intensity (of RNA residues)	

TfR, transferrin receptor; R/F, serum transferrin receptor/ferritin; pg, picogram; RNA, ribonucleic acid; Hgb, hemoglobin.

Table 4.6 Differential diagnosis of absolute and functional iron deficiency.

	Absolute iron deficiency	Functional iron deficiency
Serum iron	Low	Low (or normal)
Transferrin	High	Low (or normal)
Transferrin saturation	low	Low (or normal)
Ferritin	low	(Normal or) high
TfR in serum	Increased	Normal
Serum iron-binding capacity		Low
R/F-ratio	High	Low

TfR, transferrin receptor; R/F, serum transferrin receptor/ferritin.

the prevention of hemorrhage. The following paragraphs shed light on the background and use of vitamins.

Vitamin B$_{12}$

The term vitamin B$_{12}$ stands for a group of chemical compounds called cobalamins. They have a common corrin ring with a central cobalt ion and differ with regard to the chemical groups added to this atom.

Cobalamins are found in food. The highest levels are found in animal products such as meat. The ingested vitamin is freed from the food by acid in the stomach and by enzymatic activity. Most of the vitamin B$_{12}$ is bound to the so-called R protein and transported to the duodenum where the protein is degraded by pancreatic proteases. The free vitamin now binds to the intrinsic factor, a protein produced by parietal cells of the gastric mucosa. The complex of the intrinsic factor and the vitamin is resistant to further enzymatic degradation and continues its journey down to the ileum where the complex binds to receptors for the intrinsic factor. These facilitate the uptake of vitamin B_{12}. A small amount of the ingested vitamin B_{12} (about 1%) is taken up without the use of intrinsic factor. Vitamin B_{12} is transported by a plasma protein called transcobalamin II and is absorbed by the liver where it is stored, bound to transcobalamin I.

The normal requirement of vitamin B_{12} is 1–2 μg/day. The human body stores the vitamin, and it may take 2–4 years until the stores are depleted. Only after that do the typical clinical symptoms of vitamin B_{12} deficiency appear. A lack of vitamin B_{12} occurs if the dietary intake is too low, if intrinsic factor is lacking (after gastrectomy or due to autoimmune processes), in pancreatic insufficiency (with a lack of proteases for the degradation of R protein), or if malabsorption is present (in cases of colonization of the small intestine with bacteria, Crohn's disease, Celiac's disease).

A lack of B_{12} stops the function of folate coenzymes, necessary for DNA synthesis. Since vitamin B_{12} is a cofactor for enzymes that aid in the conversion of folate, a lack of vitamin B_{12} causes "folate trapping," a condition of functional deficiency of folate. Folate is available but cannot be changed into the form the body typically uses, namely, tetrahydrofolate (THF) (see below). DNA synthesis is impaired. Cell division and formation of the nucleus in red cell precursors are hindered. Therefore, megaloblasts accumulate in the bone marrow and immature red cells are found in the blood. The lack of vitamin B_{12} affects the blood count. If a vitamin B_{12} deficiency is manifest, megaloblastic anemia results. In addition, neurological sequelae develop. Sometimes, bleeding diathesis with thrombocytopenia may be present.

When clinical signs and basic laboratory results suggest a deficiency in vitamin B_{12}, specific tests are warranted. The measurement of serum vitamin B_{12} (normal level of about 160–960 ng/L) is a step in the right direction. Homocysteine and methylmalonic acid levels are raised early in vitamin B_{12} deficiency. These are more sensitive markers for vitamin B_{12} deficiency than serum B_{12} levels, but they are less specific.

Vitamins B_{12}, for pharmaceutical use, contain cyano, methyl, and hydroxyl groups (cyanocobalamin, methylcobalamin, and hydroxycobalamin). Traditionally, vitamin B_{12} is applied as an intramuscular or subcutaneous shot to circumvent gastroenteral passage and the need for intrinsic factor, etc., for uptake. However, since about 1% of the ingested vitamin is taken up passively, daily high-dose vitamin B_{12} (500–1000 μg), given sublingually or orally, meets the needs of patients with a lack of vitamin B_{12}, even if the intrinsic factor is lacking [21]. If vitamin B_{12} needs to be administered to patients where oral application is not possible, injections are recommended. Shots with 500–1200 μg are commonly given. Alternatively, nasal spray containing hydroxycobalamin is available.

Absolute vitamin B_{12} deficiency is clearly an indication for vitamin B_{12} therapy. Transfusions are contraindicated in patients who suffer from anemia that can be corrected by replenishment of B_{12} stores. In patients undergoing rHuEPO therapy or in those recovering from other kinds of anemia, B_{12} supplementation is sometimes recommended to meet the increased vitamin needs of erythropoiesis and to prevent neurological sequelae resulting from vitamin B_{12} deficiency. Patients with sickle cell disease should be monitored closely for vitamin B_{12} deficiency since the hyperhomocysteinemia associated with this condition may worsen sickle cell disease [22]. (Hyperhomocysteinemia is a risk factor for endothelial damage contributing to sickle cell vasoocclusive disease.)

Folates

Folates are derived from folic acid by the addition of glutamic acid or carbon units or by their reduction to dihydrofolates and tetrahydrofolates (DHF, THF). Folates are used by the body to accomplish the transfer of carbon groups. The synthesis of purines, pyrimidines, and thymidylates for DNA synthesis depends on such carbon group transfers.

Folates in the food (that is, polyglutamates, when food is derived from plants) are hydrolyzed in the bowel to monoglutamates and are absorbed in the small intestine. In the mucosa, they are transformed to methyltetrahydrofolate and enter the plasma and cells as such.

Hematological changes based on a lack of folate include a megaloblastic blood smear, and later, anemia. In addition, thrombocytopenia and a bleeding diathesis can develop. The clinical differentiation between anemia due to vitamin B_{12} or folate cannot be made without vitamin essays. It is possible to monitor folate levels in serum or in red cells. While the serum folate is affected by immediate changes of folate, such as folate ingestion or acute loss in hospitalized patients, red cell folate may be a better indicator for the folate reserves of a patient. However, a low vitamin B_{12} level also causes low red cell folate without an actual lack of folate.

Folates are readily available in fresh vegetables, but are destroyed by cooking. Patients with a poor diet are at risk for folate deficiency. Also, patients with disorders in the gastrointestinal tract that lead to malabsorption may suffer from folate deficiency (such as Celiac's disease). Alcohol and some drugs (sulfasalazine, cholestyramine) impair the absorption of folates as well. A lack of folate can occur in states of increased requirement, such as pregnancy, lactation, and conditions of rapid cell turnover. In general, folate may be required for all patients with a rapid cell turnover. The increased need of folate in hematological disorders such as hemolytic anemia and myelofibrosis is of special interest. Folic acid may also be lacking in patients with erythropoietin hyporesponsiveness. Even if folate serum levels are within the normal range, the mean corpuscular volume increases during rHuEPO therapy, suggesting an increased folate demand in patients undergoing rHuEPO therapy [23]. Folate serum levels may also be within normal or near-normal range in critically ill patients who suddenly develop a syndrome consisting of hemorrhage, severe thrombocytopenia, and a megaloblastic bone marrow. When this occurs, even if no megaloblastic anemia may be present, folate therapy may be considered, since it has been shown to rapidly reverse this condition. It was even recommended as a prophylactic treatment for critically ill patients as the described condition is common among this group [24].

Riboflavin

Riboflavin, as a vitamin, was isolated from milk in 1879. It is a heterocyclic isoalloxazine ring with ribitol. Its biologically active forms are FAD (flavin adenine dinucleotide) and FMN (flavin mononucleotide). Small amounts of free riboflavin are present in food, but FAD and FMN are the most common forms. In order to be absorbed by the small intestine, FAD and FMN are hydrolyzed to riboflavin. Absorption is facilitated by a saturable active transporter. In the enterocytes, riboflavin undergoes changes and enters the plasma either as riboflavin or as FMN. Riboflavin is also found in the colon, most probably as the result of the biological activity of the bacterial flora in the colon. This microbial source may be more important than previously thought. In the blood, riboflavin is bound to albumin and immunoglobulins.

Riboflavin deficiency is endemic in many regions of the world, especially those feeding on products other than milk and meat and those who do not have a balanced vegetable diet. In industrial nations, riboflavin is often present in fortified products. Elderly persons are prone to a lack of riboflavin. Since riboflavin is sensitive to light,

hyperbilirubinemic newborns treated with phototherapy may also have riboflavin deficiency.

Anemia may be the result of riboflavin deficiency. Patients with this pathology develop erythroid hypoplasia and reticulocytopenia (pure red cell aplasia). Also, iron metabolism is impaired. A lack of riboflavin impairs iron absorption and iron mobilization from reserves [25]. Since riboflavin is required for the activation of red cell glutathione reductase, the activity of this enzyme is reduced in riboflavin deficiency.

Therapeutic doses of riboflavin were shown to cause a raise in hemoglobin when given to young adults [26].

Vitamin C

Ascorbic acid is derived from glucose, using L-gulonolactone oxidase. Humans do not have this enzyme and cannot perform this metabolic step. Therefore, the intake of ascorbic acid is essential for humans.

Vitamin C is required for folic acid reductase, the enzyme synthesizing the active form of folate, THF. Ascorbic acid is also used in the uptake of iron and its mobilization from its stores.

A lack of vitamin C is rare in patients with a reasonable nutrition. If it occurs, scurvy results—a condition that leads to hemorrhage due to impaired vessel integrity and hemostasis. About 80% of patients with scurvy are also anemic.

Intravenous vitamin C application was shown to increase hemoglobin in iron-overloaded patients. The vitamin facilitates iron release from iron stores and increases the iron utilization [27]. Furthermore, it enhances iron uptake from oral iron preparations. Ascorbic acid was also shown to reverse the adverse effects of certain psychopharmaceuticals on coagulation.

L-Carnitine

L-Carnitine is a derivative of butyrate. It is ingested with food and synthesized in the body itself. States of L-carnitine deficiency may develop when its biosynthesis is impaired, such as in cirrhosis and renal failure, or it is lost during hemodialysis. Other conditions may also decrease carnitine levels, such as catabolism in critically ill patients, preterm infants, or in patients on drugs as valproate and zidovudine.

Typically, L-carnitine is needed for the β-oxidation of fatty acids in the mitochondria. L-Carnitine also exerts pharmacological effects. It seems to reduce apoptosis in erythroid precursors. Besides this, it stabilizes the membrane of the red cells and increases their osmotic resistance [28].

L-Carnitine therapy may be indicated in patients with anemia due to renal failure. It may alleviate erythropoietin hyporesponsiveness and may increase the blood count by other unknown mechanisms. L-Carnitine is also beneficial in patients with thalassemia major. In this case, it increases the hemoglobin level and reduces allogeneic transfusions [29]. The recommended dose for thalassemia patients is 50 mg/kg body weight/day, given for at least 6 months.

Vitamin B$_6$

Vitamin B$_6$ comes in different forms: pyridoxine, pyridoxal, pyridoxamine, and their phosphates. The different forms seem to have equal vitamin activity since they are interconvertible in the body. The active form of vitamin B$_6$ is pyridoxal phosphate, the major form transported in the plasma.

Pyridoxine is essential for heme synthesis. The very first step of heme synthesis depends on pyridoxal phosphate as a cofactor. A lack of vitamin B$_6$ leads to sideroblastic anemia. Sideroblastic anemia is characterized by ring sideroblasts in the bone marrow, impaired heme synthesis, and storage of iron in the mitochondria. Sideroblastic anemia is a heterogenous group of disorders. Genetic disorders, toxins (ethanol), and drugs (isoniacid, chloramphenicol) can trigger sideroblastic anemia. Vitamin B$_6$ effectively treats various kinds of sideroblastic anemia. Presumably, high doses of pyridoxine can counteract the resulting defect in the heme synthesis.

A trial of pyridoxine should be given in patients with sideroblastic anemia. Beginning with 100 mg/day orally, and thereafter a maintenance dose of 50 mg daily, seems to be a reasonable regimen [30]. Short-term intravenous regimen are also applicable, e.g., 180–500 mg pyridoxal phosphate daily [31].

Other vitamins

Several other vitamins also seem to influence hematopoiesis and are suitable for certain blood-related disorders.

Vitamin A: There is a strong relationship between serum vitamin A levels and the hemoglobin concentration. Vitamin A deficiency results in anemia that is similar to that of iron deficiency. Serum iron levels are low but the iron stores in the liver and bone marrow are increased. Iron therapy, in such cases, does not correct the anemia. When vitamin A is given, iron is mobilized from stores and increases red cell production. An increase in erythropoietin levels was demonstrated in vitro after administration of vitamin A. However, this does not seem to play an important role in certain anemic patients. On the contrary, anemic patients when given vitamin A may reduce their erythropoietin level despite their increase of red cell mass after vitamin A therapy [32].

Vitamin-B group: Pantothenic acid deficiency is not associated with anemia, while niacin deficiency (pellagra) is.

Vitamin E: Low-birth-weight babies are born with low vitamin E levels and they may develop hemolytic anemia if a diet with polyunsaturated fatty acids and iron is given. In such babies, vitamin E therapy corrects the anemia quickly. Patients with cystic fibrosis may develop severe anemia due to a lack of vitamin E. In this case, water-soluble vitamin E preparations are recommended.

Vitamin K: Vitamin K is not considered a hematinic vitamin since it does not contribute directly or indirectly to red cell production. It is used in the therapy of coagulation disorders.

Interactions of hematinics

Niacin deficiency is increased by iron deficiency [33]. Superfluous zinc intake reduces copper and iron availability, leading to anemia. Riboflavin deficiency interferes with the metabolism of other B vitamins by enzymatic activity. The list of interactions of hematinics is very long. A thorough knowledge of the interactions of hematinics is vital in improving response to therapy and to treat anemia effectively as well as to avoid side effects of hematinic therapy. You are encouraged to dig a little deeper into this matter. The source material at the end of the chapter will help you find more information.

Implications for blood management

Hematinics are vital for blood management. Their shrewd use is usually a cost-effective way to reduce the patient's exposure to donor blood. The following is a list of settings where hematinics can be used to potentially prevent allogeneic transfusions [34].

Primary prevention of anemia

The primary prevention of anemia includes providing patients, and prospective patients, with all the hematinics they need under the special circumstances they find themselves in. In fact, anemia caused by nutritional deficiencies is rarely due to the lack of a single nutrient. Rather, multiple components of hematopoiesis are usually missing in nutritional anemia. In different regions of the world, there are different hematinics that are typically lacking in the population. Certain patient groups also have specific needs. In order to be effective, primary prophylaxis of anemia has to consider these differences.

Among the nutritional anemia, iron deficiency is number 1 in the world. In addition, deficiency of vitamins A, B_{12}, C, E, folic acid, riboflavin, and zinc is also attributed to anemia. Many different nutritional supplements are now available for the primary prevention of anemia prevalent in different regions of the world.

Certain groups of patients are prone to develop nutritional anemia, and primary prevention means supplying them with what they need. Multiple hematinic deficiency anemia is common in pregnant women. Twenty percent of pregnant women in industrialized countries and up to 75% of pregnant women in developing countries are anemic [35]. Areas with chronic food shortages, as well as frequent pregnancies and prolonged lactation, may leave pregnant women deprived of vital hematinics and leave them anemic [35]. Efforts to prevent anemia in populations with a high prevalence of hematinic deficiency include using micronutrient-fortified foods or medical preparations.

Patients with anemia due to a lack of hematinics are prone to receive blood transfusions. Primary prevention of anemia by the consumption of hematinics may lower the risk of receiving allogeneic transfusions. This is especially true for malnourished women of childbearing age who receive hematinics when they become pregnant and give birth. Elderly, malnourished individuals also receive lesser transfusions when receiving hematinics to replenish their blood—prior to a possible blood loss. The same may be true for children and patients with certain medical conditions such as renal failure, Crohn's disease, and cystic fibrosis.

Prevention and therapy of iatrogenically induced hematinic deficiency

Medical interventions can cause a need for hematinics. The therapy of anemia aims at normalizing the red cell count. Ideally, the body itself does this. Medication is used to treat the underlying condition leading to anemia or by increasing erythropoiesis. In either case, if the therapy is successful and the body starts recovery of the red cell mass, hematinics are needed as fuel. If such are not available, the physician's intervention induces vitamin deficiency.

An example of this is the therapy of sickle cell anemia. If therapy is successful, erythropoiesis increases and supplies the needed red cell mass. Concurrently, hematinics need to be given. Giving one hematinic may increase the demand of another. If this vitamin is not available in sufficient amounts to meet the needs of the increased erythropoiesis, a deficiency state develops, which, in the case of vitamin B_{12}, may lead to neurological sequelae.

If hematinics are lacking, a physician's therapy may not be successful. rHuEPO therapy may serve as an example. rHuEPO spurs on erythropoiesis. However, if hematinics are lacking, erythropoietin hyporesponsiveness develops and rHuEPO therapy is ineffective, since the red cell mass cannot be restored.

Other iatrogenic influences: Some drugs impair the erythropoiesis, while hematinics may abolish the negative effects of the medication. Isoniacid, an antibiotic, often leads to anemia. If pyridoxine is given, anemia can be prevented.

Therapy of anemia due to hematinic deficiency

The main indication for the application of hematinics is their absolute deficiency. Anemia, developing due to a lack of hematinics, is easily treated with the missing hematinic. Iron deficiency ranks number 1 on the list of hematinic deficiencies. Other commonly encountered deficiencies are those of B_{12}, folate, and riboflavin. Blood transfusions are contraindicated if hematinic therapy can effectively resolve anemia. Two examples may illustrate this:

Induced iron deficiency: Patients receiving surgery after hip fracture are often elderly and, typically, have, or develop, iron deficiency anemia during hospitalization. Parenteral iron application may speed up recovery after surgery. It reduces the patients' exposure to allogeneic blood products and seems to reduce the length of hospital stay and reduces mortality [36].

> **Practice tip**
>
> For example, to treat anemia of elderly patients with hip fracture, the following regimen may be used:
> 100 mg iron sucrose i.v. upon admission and just before surgery and another 100 mg dose between admission and surgery if the hemoglobin level is below 12 g/dL (= 200–300 mg preoperatively) [36].

Combined vitamin deficiency: Patients with sickle cell disease have a greater need for vitamins. Regular treatment with an appropriate combination of hematinics in combination with a comprehensive prophylactic and treatment schedule reduces their exposure to transfusions. An impressive example is a Nigerian Sickle Cell Clinic and Club using, among others, therapy with hematinics. They were able to reduce the transfusion rate of their patients from 90 to 2% and their mortality rate from 20.7 to 0.6% [37].

Practice tip

Patients with sickle cell anemia should receive a combination of hematinics. Here is an example of what can be prescribed for them:
Folate, 5 mg: once daily
Vitamin B compound: 3× daily
Vitamin C, 100–200 mg: 3× daily
Vitamins A and E: 1–3× daily, according to individual need

Treatment of anemia not related to an absolute deficiency of hematinics

Hematinics can also be used to treat anemia if there is no absolute deficiency of a specific hematinic. Vitamin B_6, for example, is recommended in patients with certain kinds of sideroblastic anemia. High-dose vitamin E may compensate for genetic defects (glutathione synthetase, G-6-P dehydrogenase deficiency), which limit the red cells' defense against oxidative injury, and it often increases the life span of erythrocytes. Vitamin E also reduces the number of irreversibly sickled erythrocytes in sickle cell disease [20]. While still controversial, certain kinds of myelodysplastic syndromes and leukemia benefit from vitamin substitution, and transfusion reduction or elimination has been reported [38].

Patients with thalassemia and other forms of anemia not due to vitamin deficiency, often lack substantial amounts of vitamins, especially of those associated with oxidative stress. When vitamins are lacking, some enzyme system functions are drastically reduced in red cells (catalase, glutathione peroxidase, and reductase), while others are increased (superoxide dismutase). In addition, the red cell membrane is changed. These patients seem to benefit from substituting the missing vitamins to achieve supranormal levels [39–42].

Hematinics as an adjunctive to rHuEPO therapy

Hematinics are generally low-cost drugs. If given to resolve erythropoietin hyporesponsiveness, or to optimize the erythropoietic response to rHuEPO, costs can be saved by lowering the required rHuEPO dosage.

Hematinics as an adjunctive to other medical therapies in blood management

Some hematinics are not used to directly influence erythropoiesis. Vitamin C, for instance, is primarily given to enhance iron uptake in the gastrointestinal tract. The increased availability of iron is the factor that influences erythropoiesis. Riboflavin, vitamin A, and copper act similarly—by also increasing the availability of iron.

Hematinics as therapy of other blood management related issues

Sometimes, minerals and vitamins are given to treat a condition leading to increased blood loss rather than to increase erythropoiesis. Vitamin C is a good example. Certain psychotherapeutic drugs impair coagulation. Vitamin C seems to antidote this effect. Another example is vitamin K that contributes to the coagulation process as well and sometimes prevents the use of allogeneic blood products.

Key points

• Hematinics fuel hematopoiesis. Without hematinics, hematopoiesis is not possible.
• Anemia, due to hematinic deficiency, is a contraindication for transfusions and warrants supplementation of the deficient nutrient.
• Absolute and functional iron deficiency warrant iron therapy.

Do you remember?

• What happens when hepcidin increases and how does this take place?
• Which vitamins play a role in erythropoiesis and how do they do so?
• Do hematinics influence use of allogeneic transfusions? Do they reduce morbidity and mortality?

Suggestions for further research

What is the relationship between transferrin and lactoferrin? How do they interact with iron, and what role does this play in the defense against bacteria?

Exercises and practice cases

How much iron is needed for a previously healthy male who lost so much blood during a car accident that his hemoglobin level dropped to 6 mg/dL?

Homework

Go to your hospital laboratory and find out what parameters can be determined to detect (a) a lack of iron and (b) a lack of vitamins.

Ask your hospital pharmacy which oral and parenteral iron preparations are available and what vitamins are on stock. Make some notes about the dose per tablet, vial, etc. and about the price.

Ask for the availability of all other hematinics mentioned in this chapter and note prices and dosages as above. Note the producers of the hematinics in your address book in the Appendix E.

Find out where hematinics are routinely used in your hospital. Check, for instance, the birth clinic, the general practitioners, the hematologists and oncologists, the pediatricians, and the surgeons. Make a note of current standards that are applicable in your hospital with regard to hematinic use.

References

1 Andrews, N.C. Disorders of iron metabolism. *N Engl J Med*, 1999. **341**(26): p. 1986–1995.

2 Park, C.H., *et al.* Hepcidin, a urinary antimicrobial peptide synthesized in the liver. *J Biol Chem*, 2001. **276**(11): p. 7806–7810.

3 Vyoral, D. and J. Petrak. Hepcidin: a direct link between iron metabolism and immunity. *Int J Biochem Cell Biol*, 2005. **37**(9): p. 1768–1773.

4 Ganz, T. Hepcidin, a key regulator of iron metabolism and mediator of anemia of inflammation. *Blood*, 2003. **102**(3): p. 783–788.

5 Kearney, S.L., *et al.* Urinary hepcidin in congenital chronic anemias. *Pediatr Blood Cancer*, Oct. 11, 2005.

6 Roy, C.N. and N.C. Andrews. Anemia of inflammation: the hepcidin link. *Curr Opin Hematol*, 2005. **12**(2): p. 107–111.

7 Hallberg, L. and L. Hulthen. Prediction of dietary iron absorption: an algorithm for calculating absorption and bioavailability of dietary iron. *Am J Clin Nutr*, 2000. **71**(5): p. 1147–1160.

8 Fishbane, S. and E.A. Kowalski. The comparative safety of intravenous iron dextran, iron saccharate, and sodium ferric gluconate. *Semin Dial*, 2000. **13**(6): p. 381–384.

9 Danielson, B.G. Structure, chemistry, and pharmacokinetics of intravenous iron agents. *J Am Soc Nephrol*, 2004. **15**: p. S93–S98.

10 Brugnara, C. Iron deficiency and erythropoiesis: new diagnostic approaches. *Clin Chem*, 2003. **49**(10): p. 1573–1578.

11 van Tellingen, A., *et al.* Iron deficiency anaemia in hospitalised patients: value of various laboratory parameters. Differentiation between IDA and ACD. *Neth J Med*, 2001. **59**(6): p. 270–279.

12 Joosten, E., *et al.* Serum transferrin receptor in the evaluation of the iron status in elderly hospitalized patients with anemia. *Am J Hematol*, 2002. **69**(1): p. 1–6.

13 Brittenham, G.M., *et al.* Clinical consequences of new insights in the pathophysiology of disorders of iron and heme metabolism. *Hematology (Am Soc Hematol Educ Program)*, 2000: p. 39–50.

14 Hart, E.B. *Iron in Nutrition: VII. Copper as a Supplement to Iron for Hemoglobin Building in the Rat.* Department of Agricultural Chemistry, University of Wisconsin, Madison, 1928.

15 Hassan, H.A., C. Netchvolodoff, and J.P. Raufman. Zinc-induced copper deficiency in a coin swallower. *Am J Gastroenterol*, 2000. **95**(10): p. 2975–2977.

16 Gregg, X.T., V. Reddy, and J.T. Prchal. Copper deficiency masquerading as myelodysplastic syndrome. *Blood*, 2002. **100**(4): p. 1493–1495.

17 Fuhrman, M.P., *et al.* Pancytopenia after removal of copper from total parenteral nutrition. *JPEN J Parenter Enteral Nutr*, 2000. **24**(6): p. 361–366.

18 Manser, J.I., *et al.* Serum copper concentrations in sick and well preterm infants. *J Pediatr*, 1980. **97**(5): p. 795–799.

19 Masugi, J., M. Amano, and T. Fukuda. Letter: copper deficiency anemia and prolonged enteral feeding. *Ann Intern Med*, 1994. **121**(5): p. 386.

20 Beutler, E., *et al. Williams Hematology*, 6th edn. McGraw-Hill, New York, 2001. p. 417ff.

21 Nyholm, E., *et al.* Oral vitamin B_{12} can change our practice. *Postgrad Med J*, 2003. **79**: p. 218–220.

22 Dhar, M., R. Bellevue, and R. Carmel. Pernicious anemia with neuropsychiatric dysfunction in a patient with sickle cell anemia treated with folate supplementation. *N Engl J Med*, 2003. **348**: p. 2204–2208.

23 Pronai, W., *et al.* Folic acid supplementation improves erythropoietin response. *Nephron*, 1995. **71**(4): p. 395–400.

24 Mant, M.J., *et al.* Severe thrombocytopenia probably due to acute folic acid deficiency. *Crit Care Med*, 1979. **7**(7): p. 297–300.

25 Powers, H.J. Riboflavin (vitamin B-2) and health. *Am J Clin Nutr*, 2003. **77**: p. 1352–1360.

26 Ajayi, O.A., *et al.* Haematological response to supplements of riboflavin and ascorbic acid in Nigerian young adults. *Eur J Haematol*, 1990. **44**(4): p. 209–212.

27 Lin, C.L., *et al.* Low dose intravenous ascorbic acid for erythropoietin-hyporesponsive anemia in diabetic hemodialysis patients with iron overload. *Ren Fail*, 2003. **25**(3): p. 445–453.

28 Evangeliou, A., *et al.* Carnitine metabolism and deficit—when supplementation is necessary? *Curr Pharm Biotechnol*, 2003. **4**(3): p. 211–219.

29 El-Beshlawy, A., *et al.* Apoptosis in thalassemia major reduced by a butyrate derivative. *Acta Haematol*, 2005. **114**: p. 155–159.

30 Alcindor, T., *et al.* Sideroblastic anaemias. *Br J Haematol*, 2002. **116**: p. 733–743.

31 Murakami, R., *et al.* Sideroblastic anemia showing unique response to pyridoxine. *Am J Pediatr Hematol Oncol*, 1991. **13**(3): p. 345–350.

32 Cusick, S.E., *et al.* Short-term effects of vitamin A and antimalarial treatment on erythropoiesis in severely anemic Zanzibari preschool children. *Am J Clin Nutr*, 2005. **82**(2): p. 406–412.

33 Oduho, G.W., *et al.* Iron deficiency reduces the efficacy of tryptophan as a niacin precursor. *J Nutr*, 1994. **124**(3): p. 444–450.

34 Hallak, M., *et al.* Supplementing iron intravenously in pregnancy. A way to avoid blood transfusions. *J Reprod Med*, 1997. **42**(2): p. 99–103.

35 Makola, D., *et al.* A micronutrient-fortified beverage prevents iron deficiency, reduces anemia and improves the hemoglobin concentration of pregnant Tanzanian women. *J Nutr*, 2003. **133**: p. 1339–1346.

36 Cuenca, J., *et al.* Role of parenteral iron in the management of anaemia in the elderly patient undergoing displaced subcapital hip fracture repair: preliminary data. *Arch Orthop Trauma Surg*, 2005. **125**(5): p. 342–347.

37 Akinyanju, O.O., A.I. Otaigbe, and M.O. Ibidapo. Outcome of holistic care in Nigerian patients with sickle cell anaemia. *Clin Lab Haematol*, 2005. **27**(3): p. 195–199.

38 Giagounidis, A.A., *et al.* Treatment of myelodysplastic syndrome with isolated del(5q) including bands q31–q33 with a combination of all-trans-retinoic acid and tocopherol-alpha: a phase II study. *Ann Hematol*, 2005. **84**(6): p. 389–394.

39 Dhawan, V., *et al.* Antioxidant status in children with homozygous thalassemia. *Indian Pediatr*, 2005. **42**(11): p. 1141–1145.

40 Das, N., *et al.* Attenuation of oxidative stress-induced changes in thalassemic erythrocytes by vitamin E. *Pol J Pharmacol*, 2004. **56**(1): p. 85–96.

41 Rachmilewitz, E.A., A. Shifter, and I. Kahane. Vitamin E deficiency in beta-thalassemia major: changes in hematological and biochemical parameters after a therapeutic trial with alpha-tocopherol. *Am J Clin Nutr*, 1979. **32**(9): p. 1850–1858.

42 Rachmilewitz, E.A., A. Kornberg, and M. Acker. Vitamin E deficiency due to increased consumption in beta-thalassemia and in Gaucher's disease. *Ann N Y Acad Sci*, 1982. **393**: p. 336–347.

5 Growth factors

Human hematopoiesis is regulated by an intricate system of factors that regulate growth, maturation, and death of hematopoietic cells. In health, this enables the hematopoietic system to adapt to the needs of the organism. The idea of modulating such systems to promote health is intriguing. In fact, it has been possible to modulate certain conditions with the use of growth factors. This chapter gives a short abstract of the current quest for agents to modify hematopoiesis. It shows what efforts led to success and where further work is needed.

Objectives of this chapter

1 Summarize what is known about the role of growth factors in hematopoiesis.
2 Become familiar with a variety of hematological growth factors currently used.
3 Understand the role of available growth factors and their current and potential use in blood management.

Definitions

Hormones: Hormones are substances that have a specific regulatory effect on the organs. Classically, they are secreted by endocrine glands and are transported by the blood to their target tissues.
Cytokines: Cytokines are proteins that are secreted by leukocytes and some nonleukocytic cells, which act as intercellular mediators. In contrast to hormones, they are produced by a certain cell type rather than by specialized glands and act locally in a paracrine or autocrine fashion.
Interleukins: Interleukins are factors that stimulate the growth of hematopoietic and other cells and regulate their function.
Colony-stimulating factors: Colony-stimulating factors (in hematology) are glycoproteins that regulate proliferation, differentiation, maturation, and function at different levels of hematopoiesis.
Hematopoietic cell growth factors: Hematopoietic cell growth factors comprise a family of hematopoietic regulators with biological specificities defined by their ability to support proliferation and differentiation of different lines of blood cells.

Hematopoiesis and the role of growth factors

Hematopoiesis is a sequential development of the final blood cells, or corpuscles, out of a pluripotent stem cell. A series of developments cause the stem cell to develop different lines of cells. The result is the production of red cells (compare Chapter 3), platelets, or white cells. The cell's division, maturation, and function are regulated by the activities of a variety of cytokines (growth factors). Some cytokines develop multiple cell lines, others are specific for one cell line. Some cytokines contribute only in the initial phase of hematopoiesis, while others act later on in the development of blood corpuscles. Refer to Fig. 5.1 to get an impression of the maturation process of platelets and white cells.

Megakaryopoiesis

Originating from their stem cells, megakaryocytes develop. These undergo endomitosis (that is, they undergo several mitoses without dividing their cytoplasm), thereby growing to become the largest cell in the bone marrow. Megakaryocytes carry receptors for growth factors, permitting these factors to influence their development. After reaching a certain growth and maturation level, megakaryocytes shed platelets. This happens when the cytoplasm breaks along demarcation membranes. It takes about 5 days for the stem cell to mature and finally shed platelets.

The final platelet is made up of three distinct zones. The outer zone consists of the glycocalyx and the plasma

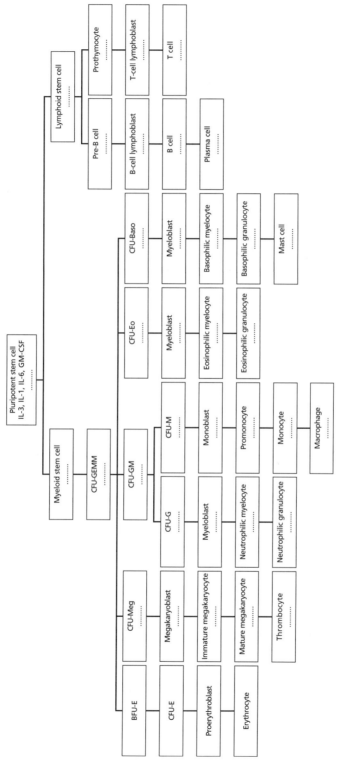

Fig 5.1 Human hematopoiesis. Baso, basophil; BFU, bust-forming units, CFU, colony-forming units; E, erythrocyte; Eo, eosinophil; G, granulocyte; GEMM, granulocyte erythrocyte megakaryocyte; GM, granulocyte macrophage; M, monocyte/macrophage; Meg, megakaryocyte; MM, monocyte macrophage.

membrane with the platelet receptors. These receptors facilitate the adherence of platelets to collagen and support the aggregation and activation of platelets. They also bind growth factors. Another platelet zone is the sol-gel zone with tubular systems, microfilaments, and thrombosthenin. The central zone of the platelet is the metabolic (organelle) zone with organelles and granules. The granules contain a variety of substances needed for the function of the platelets. There are dense granules (ATP, ADP, calcium, magnesium, serotonin, epinephrine), alpha granules (platelet-derived growth factor, platelet factor 4, plasminogen activator inhibitor 1, albumin, and fibrinogen), and lysosomes (hydrolytic enzymes).

Leukopoiesis

Leukopoiesis starts with the stem cell. Early during development, two distinct lines of white cells divide: the lymphoid line (lymphopoiesis) and the myeloid line (myelopoiesis). Lymphopoiesis results in the synthesis of T cells and B cells. This area is rarely the target of therapeutic intervention with growth factors. Myelopoiesis, which results in the development of monocytes and granulocytes, is more often the target of therapeutic intervention with growth factors.

The body stores a reserve of granulocytes for about 11 days. The bone marrow releases granulocytes, and so there is a constant level in the circulation. However, when infection is present, their level may increase dramatically. This is regulated by granulocyte colony stimulating factor (G-CSF). Its receptor is found on immature neutrophils. In severe infection, G-CSF levels can increase by over 10,000 times. This increase of G-CSF is a result of G-CSF secretion by the bone marrow stroma (which produces G-CSF in health conditions) and secretion by other white cells (which accelerate G-CSF production in infection). G-CSF binds to its receptors (found on progenitors of the neutrophil line) and regulates their proliferation, maturation, and survival. It also moves neutrophils from the bone marrow into blood circulation. This shift makes rapid response to the growth factor possible. Granulocyte macrophage colony stimulating factor (GM-CSF) contributes to the development of granulocytes and macrophages.

One of the most important functions of the granulocytes and macrophages is the phagocytosis of foreign bodies. The function of phagocytes can be divided into phases: namely, chemotaxis (directed motility after recognition), diapedesis (phagocytes pass the endothelium to leave the circulation), endocytosis (of the damaging agent with formation of a phagosome), degranulation (content of granules digests ingested particles), and killing of the invader.

In addition, mature neutrophils carry receptors for growth factors (e.g., G-CSF). These receptors transduce signals from outside the cell and protect the cells from apoptosis. The granulocyte functions are also regulated by growth factors.

Growth factors for platelets

It has long been known that there must be an agent that specifically controls and accelerates platelet synthesis—a so-called thrombopoietin (megapoietin). This cytokine attaches to a platelet receptor called c-Mpl. It was not until the late 1980s that an agent was detected which acted as cytokine in megakaryosynthesis. This agent was named c-Mpl ligand. In 1994, the natural c-Mpl ligand was purified. This proved to be the thrombopoietin that had been looked for (also called megakaryocyte colony stimulating factor) [1]. It is one of the most potent stimulators of megakaryocyte production, size, and expression of platelet membrane glycoprotein. It acts almost specifically on the megakaryocyte line. However, it has a limited effect on red cell production by enhancing proliferation and survival of erythroid progenitors and on other primitive hematopoietic stem cells.

The native thrombopoietin precursor protein is synthesized primarily in the liver (and possibly also in stroma cells in the bone marrow). It consists of two domains: one for attaching to its receptor and the other one to maintain its stability. The liver seems to produce a constant amount of thrombopoietin. When autologous platelets are present, thrombopoietin attaches to the c-Mpl receptor of platelets and possibly to their precursors, and is incorporated into them. The thrombopoietin plasma level diminishes. The same is true when allogeneic platelets are transfused [1]. In contrast, when thrombocytopenia exists, thrombopoietin is not taken up by the platelets to the same degree and thrombopoietin plasma levels are increased. This leads to a stimulation of megakaryocyte synthesis.

As predicted, thrombopoietin is a potent megakaryocyte colony stimulating factor and increases the size and number of megakaryocytes. Thrombopoietin acts synergistically with other growth factors to increase myeloid and erythroid precursors, among them are many interleukins. Native thrombopoietin in physiological concentrations does not seem to cause a delay in megakaryocyte maturation and platelet shedding. Thrombopoietin (as well as some other growth factors) increases aggregation of platelets only in unphysiological doses.

Animal experiments suggest that there must be other stimulants for thrombopoiesis, since animals without thrombopoietin do not bleed to death, although thrombocytopenic and with reduced numbers of white and red cell precursors.

Recombinant or synthetic analogues of thrombopoietin and other c-Mpl agonists can be used to stimulate natural pathways that result in increased platelet production or enhanced platelet function.

Recombinant human thrombopoietin

Understanding the role of thrombopoietin in megakaryosynthesis helped in the engineering of recombinant agents that were able to attach to the c-Mpl receptor. Among them is recombinant human thrombopoietin (rhuTPO). It is the full-length recombinant form of native thrombopoietin. It is produced in mammalian cells. It mimics the action of native thrombopoietin when it increases the number of megakaryocytes progenitors and hastens the synthesis of platelets. Its effect on the red cell and white cell line is not consistent and is clinically often negligible.

rhuTPO has been used successfully to mobilize peripheral blood progenitor cells for autologous reinfusion. It has been used in doses of 0.6–5.0 mcg/kg intravenously. rhuTPO was also given to accelerate platelet recovery after chemotherapy. When rhuTPO was given together with GM-CSF, platelet and granulocyte recovery after chemotherapy was accelerated and red cell and platelet transfusions were reduced [2]. However, rhuTPO's delayed action has prevented most physicians from using it in acute thrombocytopenia.

Therapy with rhuTPO is usually well tolerated. If given intravenously, it does not seem to cause neutralizing antibody production.

Pegylated recombinant human megakaryocyte growth and development factor

Another recombinant c-Mpl agonist is pegylated recombinant human megakaryocyte growth and development factor (PEG-rhuMGDF). In contrast to rhuTPO, the recombinant PEG-rhuMGDF is shortened and holds only one domain of the native thrombopoietin, namely, its functional part that binds to its receptor [3]. This domain is bound to polyethylene glycol (PEG). PEG-rhuMGDF

is produced by *Escherichia coli* bacteria. As in its natural counterpart, thrombopoietin, PEG-rhuMGDF enhances the production of platelets, but also of other hematopoietic progenitors. Its effects are enhanced by coadministration of G-CSF.

PEG-rhuMGDF has been used extensively in humans. It brings about a dose-related increase in platelet counts in healthy volunteers and in patients prior to chemotherapy. It increases the life span of platelets in healthy volunteers, and in vitro experiments, it was shown that it increases platelet aggregability [4]. In animal experiments, the increase in aggregability did not lead to increased thrombosis formation. PEG-rhuMGDF has been used for the treatment of thrombocytopenia in aplastic anemia, myelosuppression of a variety of origins (chemotherapy), and in other disease-related or iatrogenic states of thrombocytopenia. The sooner PEG-rhuMGDF is administered after myelosuppression, the better the results seem to be as residual hematopoietic progenitors are still present [5]. PEG-rhuMGDF has also proven safe for patients on longterm treatment.

After initial promising results, the development of PEG-rhuMGDF came to a halt in the United States in 1998. Some patients developed neutralizing antibodies against it. Immunoglobulin G antibodies to PEG-rhuMGDF, which cross-reacted with endogenous thrombopoietin and neutralized its biological activity, were responsible [6]. Although the antibodies were rarely accompanied by the development of low platelet counts, research on PEG-rhuMGDF was stopped in some countries. However, in other countries, research continues and the results are still promising.

Interleukin 11 (oprelvekin)

Interleukin (IL) 11 is a multifunctional cytokine that has a profound effect on the synthesis of megakaryocytes. IL-11 enhances the growth and maturation of megakaryocyte progenitors, but proliferation remained almost unaffected. IL-11 works synergistically with other early promoters of hematopoiesis, such as IL-3 and stem cell factor. It also accelerates red cell and neutrophil production. However, as seems to be the case with thrombopoietin, IL-11 is not essential for hematopoiesis. Besides, it has immunological effects. IL-11 seems to stimulate growth of enterocytes, modifies autoimmune phenomena, and maintains female fertility [6].

Recombinant human interleukin 11 (rhuIL-11, oprelvekin) is now available for therapy. rhuIL-11 increases platelet counts in a dose-related fashion. The increase starts 5–9 days after the start of therapy and peaks 14–19 days thereafter. rhuIL-11 does not seem to influence platelet function, but it increases fibrinogen and von Willebrand factor levels.

Practice tip

rhuIL-11 is administered subcutaneously. Adults are administered a once-daily dose of 50 mcg/kg and children 75–100 mcg/kg, due to an accelerated clearance.

---

rhuIL-11 (oprelvekin) is certified for the prophylaxis of chemotherapy-induced thrombocytopenia in non-myeloid malignancies [7]. It is given as a prophylactic agent, starting 6–24 hours after chemotherapy, before thrombocytopenia develops. rhuIL-11 has also been used as treatment for thrombocytopenia in patients with myelodepression, undergoing chemotherapy or radiation therapy, stem cell infusion, and autologous bone marrow transplant. rhuIL-11 has successfully been used to treat thrombocytopenia in hypersplenic thrombocytopenia due to hepatic cirrhosis [8].

rhuIL-11 is generally well tolerated. However, it stimulates renal sodium absorption and therefore increases plasma volume by approximately 20%. This results in edema (which can be treated with diuretics), dyspnea, and cardiac arrythmia in susceptible individuals. Since native IL-11 is a pluripotent agent, acting on many organ systems, it is no surprise that it may cause side effects in many organ systems. These include hyperbilirubinemia, anemia, flu-like symptoms, and hypotension.

Other growth factors for platelets

Many more cytokines have been used therapeutically to enhance megakaryopoiesis. However, none of them is used routinely in clinical practice. Table 5.1 summarizes important features of these drugs [9–16].

Combinations

Mimicking nature, scientists have tried to use a combination of cytokines, either given together or sequentially, to speed up platelet recovery. Combinations of GM-CSF and IL-3, IL-3, and IL-6, as well as IL-3 and IL-11 were tried in animal experiments. Also, the combination of thrombopoietin and stem cell factor is intriguing. As a new development, their coexpression in one chimeric protein in *E. coli* is being tried [17].

Growth factors for leukocytes

Granulocyte colony stimulating factor

G-CSF is a naturally occurring glycoprotein that supports neutrophil maturation and function. It is synthesized in monocytes, macrophages, fibroblasts, bone marrow stroma, and the endothelium in response to other cytokines. Its levels are increased during infection. It enhances not only the proliferation but also the function of mature granulocytes. G-CSF stimulates progenitors of granulocytes, monocytes, megakaryocytes, and lymphocytes. It has, by far, the greatest effect on granulocytes. Its effects on cell lines other than the neutrophils are clinically negligible.

There are several recombinant forms of G-CSF available for clinical use. They differ from the natural form by their protein sequence or by their glycosylation. Glycosylation adds to the stability of the agent under differing temperatures and pHs and slows its degradation in the blood.

Practice tip

Therapeutic doses of rhuG-CSF usually range between 5 and 32 mcg/kg body weight/day.

The following recombinant G-CSF's are commonly used in clinical practice:
- *Filgrastim* (r-methuG-CSF) is a recombinant non-glycosylated protein expressed in *E. coli*. Its half-life is about 3.5 hours. It can be given intravenously or subcutaneously.
- *Pegfilgrastim* (= sustained delivery filgrastim SD/01, PEG-r-methuG-CSF) is produced by adding a PEG residue to the filgrastim molecule (pegylation). This pegylation prolongs the half-life to 15–80 hours and so less frequent doses, as compared to filgrastim, are required. In equivalent doses, it is equally effective as filgrastim.
- *Lenograstim* is the glycosylated recombinant form of human colony stimulating factor that is synthesized in Chinese hamster ovary cells [18]. Lenograstim seems to be as effective as filgrastim in stimulating leukocyte production during chemotherapy and peripheral blood stem cell transplantation [19].
- *Nartograstim* is a further recombinant form of G-CSF. In comparison to native G-CSF, its N-terminal amino

Table 5.1 Miscellaneous growth factors for megakaryopoiesis.

Name	Description	Biologic activity	Use	Side effects
Interleukin 3 (IL-3) and analogues (multi-CSF or multipoietin; daniplestim, synthokine (SC-55494), rhuIL-3)	Multilineal cell growth factor; it is secreted by lymphocytes, epithelial cells, and astrocytes	Stimulates clonal proliferation and differentiation of various hematological cell lines; enhances function of mature blood cells	Reactivates megakaryosynthesis after chemotherapeutic myelosuppression; used with mixed results in chemotherapy-induced thrombocytopenia, myelodysplastic syndrome, and aplastic anemia; promising in congenital megakaryocytic thrombocytopenia to reduce bleeding and transfusions	Low-dose regimen: mild flu-like effects (controlled with propranolol); high therapeutic doses: severe side effects limiting the use
Interleukin 1 (IL-1)	Soluble factor produced by monocytes and macrophages	Supports proliferation and differentiation of megakaryocyte progenitors; stimulates platelet production in two phases (peaking day 8 and 17 after application); reduces neutropenia; enhances the effect of other hematological growth factors; stimulates secretion of cytokines from other cells	Used in patients to reduce thrombocytopenia in chemotherapy patients	Severe side effects (high fever, severe flu-like syndromes, pain syndromes, and hypotension) limit use
Interleukin 6 (IL-6) (= interferon β2, B-cell stimulatory factor 2, plasmocytoma, hybridoma growth factor, hepatocyte-stimulating factor, cytotoxic T-cell differentiation factor)		Induces primitive progenitor cells; suppresses erythropoiesis; stimulates megakaryocyte progenitor growth and maturation (together with IL-3); does not affect the megakaryocyte progenitor number; causes smaller platelets to develop	Accelerates platelet production in chemotherapy patients; results mixed	Causes anemia and, due to its many physiological actions, a variety of severe side effects
Granulocyte macrophage colony stimulating factor (GM-CSF)		Stimulates megakaryocyte colonies	Used to increase platelet count and speed up platelet recovery after autologous transplantation in Hodgkin's disease, myelodysplastic syndrome, and aplastic anemia; results mixed; promising when used in combination with other hematopoietic growth factors	Mild
Xanthocillins and similar compounds	Small molecules made from fungal cultures	Agonists of thrombopoietin receptors	Promising to increase megakaryosynthesis in vitro and in vivo	Not Known

acid sequence is altered. It therefore has a threefold higher affinity to the G-CSF receptor.

The side effects of recombinant G-CSF are mild to moderate. Immediately after G-CSF is injected, the neutrophil count decreases, with a subsequent marked increase in granulocytes. Other side effects are similar to those of GM-CSF mentioned below. Overall, both G-CSF and GM-CSF are well tolerated. Up to 30% of patients experience flu-like symptoms with fever, musculoskeletal pain, diarrhea, and headaches. Occasionally, splenomegalia developed. Rashes may occur, but overt allergic reactions are rare [20].

Granulocyte macrophage colony stimulating factor

The endogenous GM-CSF is not as restricted to the neutrophil white cell line as is G-CSF. GM-CSF was shown to enhance growth and differentiation of neutrophils, eosinophils, monocytes, megakaryocytes, and erythrocytes. It also stimulates the phagocytosis and enzymatic function of mature granulocytes. GM-CSF is naturally synthesized in lymphocytes, monocytes, fibroblasts, bone marrow stroma, and endothelium.

GM-CSF has been produced in a recombinant form and is available for therapy. Commonly used recombinant forms of GM-CSF include the following:

Sargramostim: It differs from the natural GM-CSF in its amino acid sequence and its glycosylation. Sargramostim's half-life is about 2.7 hours, when given subcutaneously.

Molgramostim: It is the nonglycosylated variant of endogenous GM-CSF.

Regramostim: It is the fully glycosylated variant of endogenous GM-CSF.

Recombinant GM-CSF can be administered subcutaneously or intravenously. When given intravenously, its half-life is 1–3 hours. It is prolonged to about 10 hours after being given subcutaneously [21].

Apart from the above-mentioned side effects, higher doses of GM-CSF may lead to a capillary leakage syndrome with the development of edema as well as pleura and pericardial effusions. Thrombosis was also reported. However, these incidents are rare.

The clinical use of G-CSF and GM-CSF

For the majority of patients with neutropenia, G-CSF is the standard therapy. The following conditions associated with neutropenia can also be treated with G-CSF or GM-CSF.

G-CSF is effective in preventing chemotherapy-induced neutropenia. It can also be used to treat this syndrome [22]. Nevertheless the survival rate was not improved for cancer patients undergoing chemotherapy plus G-CSF or GM-CSF.

Also, patients undergoing stem cell transplantation benefited from G-CSF [23, 24]. G-CSF mobilizes stem cells into the blood and speeds up the hematological recovery of patients after transplantation.

Patients with myelodysplastic syndromes and neutropenia also benefited from G-CSF. However, concern has been raised that G-CSF may accelerate the development of the myelodysplastic syndrome into an overt leukemia. Currently, these concerns have not been substantiated. Nevertheless, it was recommended that only under certain circumstances, patients with myelodysplastic syndromes could receive G-CSF. These circumstances would include severe neutropenia associated with infection, a high risk of infection due to other than neutropenic risk factors (e.g., old age), and in conjunction with erythropoietin to enhance its efficacy to support red cell recovery. Under such circumstances, G-CSF is given only intermittently.

G-CSF is also indicated in selected cases of leukemia therapy to enhance neutrophil recovery. This does not improve the survival rate either.

Patients with acquired aplastic anemia may benefit from G-CSF (or GM-CSF) [25]. It was a theoretical concern that growth factors could accelerate the rate of transformation of aplastic anemia to myelodysplastic syndromes or to acute myeloic leukemia. A large database review did not confirm this worry. However, the continuous use of G-CSF is currently not recommended and it should be restricted to intermittent episodes of infection [26].

Patients with other forms of bone marrow failure or with diseases that include neutropenia may also benefit from G-CSF or GM-CSF. Among these are Fanconi anemia, dyskeratosis congenita [27], severe chronic neutropenia (as infantile agranulocytosis), cyclic neutropenia, idiopathic neutropenia, Shwachman–Diamond syndrome, Felty syndrome, Chediak–Higashi syndrome, autoimmune neutropenia, and glycogen storage disease 1b. In such conditions, the response rate of G-CSF or GM-CSF is very high, and it has been shown that the continuous use of the agents over years is possible and beneficial.

Neutropenia induced by intoxication (e.g., autumn crocus) [28] and that due to adverse reaction to drug therapy [29] can be successfully managed with G-CSF or GM-CSF.

Neutropenia, in HIV (human immunodeficiency virus) infection and HIV antiviral therapy, is also ameliorated by G-CSF or GM-CSF [30].

G-CSF and GM-CSF in combination with other hematological growth factors are used to treat accidental or therapeutic radiation injury. It speeds up bone marrow recovery. The sooner it is given after the irradiation, the better is the hematological response [21].

Monocyte colony stimulating factor

Monocyte colony stimulating factor (M-CSF) regulates the proliferation and differentiation of monocyte and macrophage progenitors. Natural M-CSF is produced in the fibroblasts, endothelium, osteoblasts, keratinocytes, and in the monocytes themselves.

There is a recombinant form of human M-CSF (rhuM-CSF) available. It is a glycoprotein produced in *E. coli* bacteria. rhuM-CSF is not widely used. It may, theoretically, be beneficial in increasing the monocyte count and with it the cells that produce other growth factors. The therapy of fungal infections may be enhanced by administration of rhuM-CSF. However, since rhuM-CSF may cause thrombocytopenia, its use is limited.

Pluripotent, multilineal growth factors

To a certain degree, all known hematopoietic growth factors seem to be multilineal agents and are pluripotent. However, the degree to which they influence organ systems other than a single line of hematopoiesis varies. This may be due to the fact that not much is known about the biological effects of the agents under consideration, or the agent's activity may indeed be restricted to a few hematopoietic actions. Table 5.2 discusses growth factors that are known to have a pluripotent effect on hematopoiesis [21, 31–34].

General concerns about growth factor use

Although growth factors enhance only a natural pathway, some concerns were raised about the use of growth factors [35]. This was the case for nearly all growth factors. The most pronounced concern is that growth factors might induce or enhance cancer growth. Growth factors, acting mainly on the white cell lines, raised a special concern about the induction of leukemia. It was indeed shown that patients with long-term use of white cell growth factors developed leukemia. But large databases (Severe Chronic Neutropenia International Registry) do not support the conclusion that this is due to the therapy [36]. Rather, at this point it seems that some of the underlying diseases

of chronic neutropenia naturally develop into leukemia in a certain percentage of cases, and the development of leukemia is now a recognized complication of congenital neutropenia and of aplastic anemia.

Another concern was raised regarding the antigenicity of growth factors. As was shown with erythropoietin, antibody formation is a realistic concern. Growth factors of the white cell lines and of the megakaryocyte line rarely induce antibody formation. And if so, they very rarely seem to cross-react with the respective endogenous growth factors.

A third concern is the lineage steal. Worries were voiced that the accelerated proliferation of one cell line with a growth factor does not leave enough progenitor cells for the other cell lines. While neutropenia, anemia, and thrombocytopenia have been observed during therapy with erythropoietin, IL-6, and G-CSF, large-scale studies did not confirm that a lineage steal is a common clinical problem.

Further concerns were raised regarding side effects of supranormal concentrations of growth factors. Many of the factors are proinflammatory. They increase the phagocytosis and chemotaxis of white cells. While this may be beneficial in some instances, it may theoretically lead to damage of the lung and the intestines. Other growth factors downregulate inflammatory responses. Skin reactions, vasculitis, and splenomegalia with rare atraumatic rupture have been observed after the use of some growth factors. Such reactions seem to be rare.

Growth factors in blood management

Management of thrombocytopenia

A variety of diseases cause thrombocytopenia and thrombocytopenia-related bleeding. While it is standard therapy for many of them to be treated with platelet transfusions, this has severe setbacks. Appropriate blood management therefore seeks to avoid thrombocytopenia and its associated bleeding and enhances endogenous platelet production and function. General measures to treat thrombocytopenic patients seem to be useful to improve the clinical outcome of the therapy (Table 5.3) [37]. To a certain degree, growth factors contribute to this as well. As shown above, several hematopoietic growth factors with thrombopoietic activity have been discovered over the last decades: GM-CSF, stem cell factor, IL-1, IL-3, IL-6, and IL-11, and thrombopoietin. The recombinant counterparts of some of them show promise as therapeutic

Table 5.2 Growth factors with known pluripotent effects on hematopoiesis.

Name	Description	Biological function	Use	Side effects
Stem cell factor (SCF, steel factor, c-kit ligand, ancestim)	Produced in stroma of bone marrow; ligand for c-kit, a growth factor receptor	Supports survival of hematopoietic cells; stimulates early proliferation and growth of hematopoietic progenitors	Used in experimental settings in patients to induce hematopoiesis; to mobilize peripheral stem cells for future autologous transplantation	Frequent; also due to mast cell activation, therefore antiallergy prophylaxis desirable
Leridistim	Myelopoietin, chimeric growth factor consisting of IL-3 and G-CSF receptor agonists, produced by *E. coli* bacteria		Enhances white cell and platelet recovery in radiated monkeys and reduces their use of red cell transfusions; not widely used in humans	Not known
SC-68420	Myelopoietin, consisting of IL-3 and G-CSF, but different to leridistim		Used in animal experiments to recover neutrophil counts	Not known
PIXY 321	Genetical product of an artificial fusion of the genes for GM-CSF and IL-3	Attaches to neither the GM-CSF nor the IL-3 receptor, but to a receptor that attracts both GM-CSF and IL-3	In chemotherapy patients and bone marrow failure induces a slight increase in platelets, white cells, and red cells	Rash, fever, and erythema at the injection site. The effects were reported to be tolerable
Promegapoietin (PMP)	Family of chimeric products, consisting of a thrombopoietin receptor ligand and an IL-3 receptor ligand		Used in animal studies to increase neutrophil and platelet counts	Highly immunogenic, its development has been halted
Flt3 ligand	Fetal liver tyrosine kinase 3 (Flt 3) (receptor found in hematopoietic progenitors, mature blood cells and the heart, the lungs, the spleen, and muscle tissue) ligand produced in bone marrow stroma	Proliferation, survival of primitive stem cells; supports development of lymphocytes and macrophages; synergistic with G-CSF and GM-CSF, erythropoietin and IL-3 and 11 and many other interleukins	Enhances white cell counts; much more potent when given together with G-CSF	Not known
Progenipoietin	Synthetic combination of Flt3 (fetal liver tyrosine kinase 3) and G-CSF receptor agonists	Induce proliferation of multiple hematological cell lines	Not available for human use	Not known

Table 5.3 General asanguine measures to treat thrombocytopenic patients.

All severely thrombocytopenic (<30,000 platelets) patients receive
Vitamin K
Antifibrinolytic agents, (e.g., aminocaproic acid 1 g every 4 h i.v., or p.o.)
No anticoagulation, acetyl salicylic acid
Proton pump inhibitors
Stool softeners
Early removal of vascular catheters
If thrombocytopenic patients start to bleed:
Increase antifibrinolytic agent (e.g., aminocaproic acid 4 g every 4 h i.v. or p.o.)
DDAVP
Nasal vasoconstrictors
Hormonal agents in females to prevent excessive blood loss via menses

---

agents, among them are rhuTPO, PEG-rhuMGDF, and rhuIL-11. It was shown that some of them were able to prevent and treat thrombocytopenia and bleeding. Some of the growth factors have been shown to reduce platelet and other allogeneic blood transfusions.

Patients suffering from thrombocytopenia, caused by different diseases, have benefited from therapy with platelet growth factors.

Patients with thrombocytopenia due to aplastic anemia have benefited from long-term therapy with PEG-rhuMGDF. Case reports have shown that the application increases platelet levels, reduces bleeding episodes, and platelet transfusions were stopped [38]. As a side effect of the platelet growth factor therapy, red cell levels increase and red cell transfusions decrease.

Patients with various forms of idiopathic thrombocytopenic purpura may also benefit from thrombopoietic agents, even if they are not considered standard therapy. Even long-term therapy (with PEG-rhuMGDF) is feasible. Platelet production increases and bleeding episodes decrease [39–42]. This was shown in animal experiments [43] as well as in human studies [39], even when the therapeutic agent was given for several years. Patients with idiopathic thrombocytopenic purpura have benefited from PEG-rhuMGDF [39, 44], rhuTPO [40], and rhuTPO in combination with rhuIL-11 [45].

Radiation- and chemotherapy-related thrombocytopenia are other areas where platelet growth factors have been employed. PEG-rhuMGDF, rhuTPO, and rhuIL-11 have proven successful in reducing thrombocytopenia and transfusions in patients undergoing myelosuppressive or

ablative therapeutic regimen [2, 46–48]. However, the results of clinical trials in patients undergoing chemotherapy or radiation therapy with platelet growth factor support are not consistent. The reason for this discrepancy is not fully understood. There are some common factors in patients who respond favorably and those who do not. In general, when the thrombopoietic agents are administered before chemotherapy, a dose-related increase in platelet count can usually be observed [49]. Also, red cell and platelet transfusions were reduced when thrombopoietic agents are given before stem cell transplantation in order to stimulate stem cells [2]. However, when the agents are administered after the start of chemotherapy, and especially after the onset of thrombocytopenia, an accelerated hematologic recovery is not consistently observed. Under such circumstances, some studies were able to demonstrate that rhuTPO, PEG-rhuMGDF, and rhuIL-11 reduce platelet transfusions and reduce the time to platelet recovery [50–53]. In contrast, other studies were disappointing regarding the reduction of platelet transfusions or improvement in the platelet count [52, 54]. Further reasons for the differences in study results seem to be found in the chosen chemotherapy regimen (myeloablative versus nonmyeloablative) and by differences in the underlying disease (solid tumors versus leukemia). Patients undergoing nonmyeloablative chemotherapy often seem to experience an increase in platelet levels. However, transfusions in these patients were not always reduced significantly. This is probably because nonmyeloablative chemotherapy regimens do not necessarily cause severe thrombocytopenia and only some studies in such patients showed a reduction of transfusions [55]. Patients undergoing myeloablative chemotherapy, stem cell transplantation [52, 56–58], and leukemia chemotherapy [59] often do not respond well. Despite all progress made in the hematopoietic support for chemotherapy and radiation therapy patients, the overall efficacy of the thrombopoietic agents in myelosuppressive and myeloablative therapy still needs major improvement.

Platelet growth factors also reduced the thrombocytopenia in selected patients with other diseases. Some (as yet not well defined) patients with myelodysplastic syndrome benefit from PEG-rhuMGDF [60] and other thrombopoietic agents. The patients respond to such therapy with increased platelet counts, and some of them demonstrate a multilineal response. Case studies about patients with myelodysplastic syndrome, who were administered thrombopoietic agents in a long-term fashion, did indeed demonstrate substantial and durable improvement in platelet and even in red cell count, thus eliminating the use of transfusions [61]. HIV infections and its treatment can cause thrombocytopenia, and PEG-rhuMGDF is able to reverse this effect. Also, the reduced production of native thrombopoietin in severe liver disease may be eligible for treatment with thrombopoietic agents, e.g., to prepare such patients for liver transplantation. Thrombopoietic agents have also been suggested as treatment for neonatal thrombocytopenia [62].

Some animal experiments suggest the use of thrombopoietic agents for yet other thrombocytopenic conditions. For instance, preoperative treatment with PEG-rhuMGDF has proven effective in animal models of surgical extracorporeal circulation to reduce bleeding and thrombocytopenia [63]. Also, platelet counts were increased in animals with Kasabach–Merrit syndrome, and PEG-rhuMGDF has been recommended for use in this setting [64].

The use of thrombopoietic growth factors in the future might also have a bearing on blood management. Current investigations try to use ex vivo maintenance and expansion of megakaryocyte progenitors (from harvested peripheral stems cells or umbilical cord blood stem cells) for infusion after chemotherapy and radiation therapy for speeding up platelet recovery [65, 66].

Some of the growth factors mentioned have been listed under the subheading "Platelet transfusion and alternatives to transfusion" [67]. Indeed, some of the growth factors are effective in increasing platelet counts and reducing transfusions. They do not seem to be the perfect agents we need, since they do not acutely increase platelet counts. Foresight, prevention, and earliest possible therapy with those agents are therefore mandatory in preventing platelet counts from falling too low. Whether it is beneficial for patients to receive thrombopoietic agents in an acute thrombocytopenic condition, by simply assuming that the function of the residual platelets is enhanced, cannot be said.

Management of neutropenia

A low neutrophil count is associated with infections. When falling below 1000/mcL the risk for infection is increased, and it is especially high if the count is below 100/mcL. The longer the time a patient is exposed to neutropenia, the higher is the risk of acquiring infections. In addition to antibiotics, granulocyte transfusions were favored. However, they come with severe side effects and their efficacy to improve patient outcome is far from proven. Actually,

granulocyte transfusions are not more than experimental. Nevertheless, severe neutropenia is life-threatening and calls for intervention. A variety of synthetic growth factors are available to do so. rhuG-CSF and rhuGM-CSF are the agents with a relatively long and reassuring efficacy and safety record.

Patients who might be given a leukocyte transfusion are apt candidates for therapy with rhuG-CSF or rhuGM-CSF. Patients who relapse after stem cell transplantation are typically given leukocyte transfusions. rhuG-CSF seems to be a better therapeutic option with less side effects [68]. Patients with aplastic anemia or congenital chronic neutropenia, who are considered candidates for white cell transfusion, can be successfully managed with white cell growth factors [20]. rhuG-CSF alone or in combination with rhuGM-CSF or EPO was shown to improve stem cell mobilization into the peripheral blood and accelerate hematological recovery after stem cell transplantation. This translates into fewer transfusions given [23, 69, 70].

rhuG-CSF and rhuGM-CSF reduce the duration of neutropenia, shorten hospitalization, and reduce antibiotic therapy in patients undergoing chemotherapy. Whether white cell transfusions can be reduced by the use of rhuG-CSF or rhuGM-CSF is not easy to say. It must be remembered that as yet the indications for white cell transfusions are controversial and their efficacy is not established. Since white cell transfusions are not widely used, not even in cases where rhuG-CSF and rhuGM-CSF are routinely given, it cannot be said whether leukopoietic agents actually reduce white cell transfusions.

Management of multilineal hematological failure

Many forms of hematological failures are multilineal failures. This is true for diseases such as myelodysplastic syndrome and aplastic anemia. Multilineal failure is also common as a result of chemotherapy and radiation therapy. Therefore, we must aim at preventing such multilineal failure or finding an effective treatment for it. Some approaches resort to treating every line failure separately, while other approaches try to address the multilineal failure collectively, using early acting factors or the interactions of hematopoietic growth factors.

The approaches that treat the lines with their respective agents typically use recombinant erythropoietin (rhuEPO) for red cell line failure, G-CSF or GM-CSF for white cell line failure, and possibly rhuIL-11 or rhuTPO to enhance megakaryosynthesis. However, since this approach, as straightforward as it may sound, may not invariably result in the desired effects, other approaches have been tried. Some early or multifunctional agents were proposed for the treatment of multilineal bone marrow failure. These include IL-3 and stem cell factor. This therapy was of some success. For instance, recombinant human IL-3 has shown a clear effect in improving chemotherapy-induced bone marrow failure, but with a variable response [71].

Another approach to multilineal failure is to use a combination of hematopoietic agents to achieve a synergistic action on hematopoiesis. In nature, there is clearly a synergistic action of a variety of factors. Certain factors act only in certain phases of hematopoiesis or on certain lines, while other factors seem to act on more or all hematopoietic lines and act almost throughout the whole hematopoietic process. Mimicking the interaction of so many factors is difficult. It is therefore understandable that progress in research has not (yet) yielded the desired universal agent(s) to successfully treat multilineal failures.

A combination of hematopoietic agents can be applied by either administering several single agents to the same patient, or to synthesize chimeric agents. Some combinations indeed achieve a better effect than single factors alone, e.g., rhuEPO and rhuGM-CSF combined for myelodysplastic syndrome to stimulate erythropoietic response. Other combinations have not proven successful, e.g., rhuEPO in combination with rhuIL-3 [72]. Yet, most proposed combinations did not keep what they promised. In trials using a variety of growth factors or early acting factors, it was seen that some patients reacted with a limited or even substantial improvement of their condition, even reducing or eliminating their transfusions. However, overall, there is no consistent success.

Key points

• Hematopoietic growth factors have tremendously improved selected patient's hematological status.
• A few growth factors seem to reduce neutropenia, but do not improve survival in most of the patients.
• Growth factors for platelets are available, but their use is mainly limited by their delayed action.
• Many more growth factors are under scrutiny for clinical use, but currently, none of them are developed enough so as to change blood management in the near future.

Questions for review

• Which growth factors act primarily on white cell production and which on platelet production? Which ones act on both lines?
• Which growth factors are already available for therapy and which ones are still in the experimental stage?
• What is the role of hematopoietic growth factors in blood management? Are thrombopoietic and leukopoietic agents able to reduce the patient's exposure to allogeneic blood?
• What conditions have benefited from therapy with thrombopoietic agents?

Suggestions for further research

Use Fig. 5.1 and insert the growth factors in the boxes of the cell types on which they act (as seen with the example of the pluripotent stem cell). If necessary, use further literature to perform this task.

Exercises and practice cases

Perform a literature search. What growth factors may be relevant for the therapy of patients with the following diseases: sepsis with *Aspergillus*, Diamond–Blackfan anemia, cyclic immune thrombocytopenia?

Homework

Find out what hematopoietic growth factors are available in your hospital and in your country. Are there any growth factors licensed or are they used in experimental settings only? Note who produces and markets them.

References

1 Kuter, D.J. and C.G. Begley. Recombinant human thrombopoietin: basic biology and evaluation of clinical studies. *Blood*, 2002. **100**(10): p. 3457–3469.
2 Somlo, G., *et al.* Recombinant human thrombopoietin in combination with granulocyte colony-stimulating factor enhances mobilization of peripheral blood progenitor cells, increases peripheral blood platelet concentration,

and accelerates hematopoietic recovery following high-dose chemotherapy. *Blood*, 1999. **93**(9): p. 2798–2806.

3 Neumann, T.A. and M. Foote. Megakaryocyte growth and development factor (MGDF): an Mpl ligand and cytokine that regulates thrombopoiesis. *Cytokines Cell Mol Ther*, 2000. **6**(1): p. 47–56.

4 Harker, L.A., *et al*. Effects of megakaryocyte growth and development factor on platelet production, platelet life span, and platelet function in healthy human volunteers. *Blood*, 2000. **95**(8): p. 2514–2522.

5 Miyazaki, H. and T. Kato. Thrombopoietin: biology and clinical potentials. *Int J Hematol*, 1999. **70**(4): p. 216–225.

6 Fetscher, S. and R. Mertelsmann. Supportive care in hematological malignancies: hematopoietic growth factors, infections, transfusion therapy. *Curr Opin Hematol*, 1999. **6**(4): p. 262–273.

7 Reynolds, C.H. Clinical efficacy of rhIL-11. *Oncology (Williston Park)*, 2000. **14**(9, Suppl 8): p. 32–40.

8 Ustun, C., P.M. Dainer, and G.B. Faguet. Interleukin-11 administration normalizes the platelet count in a hypersplenic cirrhotic patient. *Ann Hematol*, 2002. **81**(10): p. 609–610.

9 Guinan, E.C., *et al*. Effects of interleukin-3 and granulocyte-macrophage colony-stimulating factor on thrombopoiesis in congenital amegakaryocytic thrombocytopenia. *Blood*, 1993. **81**(7): p. 1691–1698.

10 Smith, J.W., II, *et al*. The effects of treatment with interleukin-1 alpha on platelet recovery after high-dose carboplatin. *N Engl J Med*, 1993. **328**(11): p. 756–761.

11 Vadhan-Raj, S., *et al*. Effects of interleukin-1 alpha on carboplatin-induced thrombocytopenia in patients with recurrent ovarian cancer. *J Clin Oncol*, 1994. **12**(4): p. 707–714.

12 Kaushansky, K. The thrombocytopenia of cancer. Prospects for effective cytokine therapy. *Hematol Oncol Clin North Am*, 1996. **10**(2): p. 431–455.

13 D'Hondt, V., *et al*. Thrombopoietic effects and toxicity of interleukin-6 in patients with ovarian cancer before and after chemotherapy: a multicentric placebo-controlled, randomized phase Ib study. *Blood*, 1995. **85**(9): p. 2347–2353.

14 Sakai, R., *et al*. Xanthocillins as thrombopoietin mimetic small molecules. *Bioorg Med Chem*, 2005. **13**(23): p. 6388–6393.

15 Safonov, I.G., *et al*. New benzimidazoles as thrombopoietin receptor agonists. *Bioorg Med Chem Lett*, December 20, 2005.

16 Cwirla, S.E., *et al*. Peptide agonist of the thrombopoietin receptor as potent as the natural cytokine. *Science*, 1997. **276**(5319): p. 1696–1699.

17 Zang, Y., *et al*. Expression, purification, and characterization of a novel recombinant fusion protein, rhTPO/SCF, in *Escherichia coli*. *Protein Expr Purif*, Nov 16, 2005.

18 Dunn, C.J. and K.L. Goa. Lenograstim: an update of its pharmacological properties and use in chemotherapy-induced neutropenia and related clinical settings. *Drugs*, 2000. **59**(3): p. 681–717.

19 Huttmann, A., *et al*. Comparison of lenograstim and filgrastim: effects on blood cell recovery after high-dose chemotherapy and autologous peripheral blood stem cell transplantation. *J Cancer Res Clin Oncol*, 2005. **131**(3): p. 152–156.

20 Balint, B. Renewed granulocyte support practice and its alternatives. *Vojnosanit Pregl*, 2004. **61**(5): p. 537–545.

21 Thierry, D., *et al*. Haematopoietic growth factors in the treatment of therapeutic and accidental irradiation-induced bone marrow aplasia. *Int J Radiat Biol*, 1995. **67**(2): p. 103–117.

22 Johnston, E.M. and J. Crawford. Hematopoietic growth factors in the reduction of chemotherapeutic toxicity. *Semin Oncol*, 1998. **25**(5): p. 552–561.

23 Olivieri, A., *et al*. Combined administration of alpha-erythropoietin and filgrastim can improve the outcome and cost balance of autologous stem cell transplantation in patients with lymphoproliferative disorders. *Bone Marrow Transplant*, 2004. **34**(8): p. 693–702.

24 Bishop, M.R., *et al*. A randomized, double-blind trial of filgrastim (granulocyte colony-stimulating factor) versus placebo following allogeneic blood stem cell transplantation. *Blood*, 2000. **96**(1): p. 80–85.

25 Jeng, M.R., *et al*. Granulocyte-macrophage colony stimulating factor and immunosuppression in the treatment of pediatric acquired severe aplastic anemia. *Pediatr Blood Cancer*, 2005. **45**(2): p. 170–175.

26 Heuser, M. and A. Ganser. Colony-stimulating factors in the management of neutropenia and its complications. *Ann Hematol*, 2005. **84**(11): p. 697–708.

27 Erduran, E., S. Hacisalihoglu, and Y. Ozoran. Treatment of dyskeratosis congenita with granulocyte-macrophage colony-stimulating factor and erythropoietin. *J Pediatr Hematol Oncol*, 2003. **25**(4): p. 333–335.

28 Gabrscek, L., *et al*. Accidental poisoning with autumn crocus. *J Toxicol Clin Toxicol*, 2004. **42**(1): p. 85–88.

29 Kotanagi, H., *et al*. Pancytopenia associated with 5-aminosalicylic acid use in a patient with Crohn's disease. *J Gastroenterol*, 1998. **33**(4): p. 571–574.

30 Scadden, D.T. Cytokine use in the management of HIV disease. *J Acquir Immune Defic Syndr Hum Retrovirol*, 1997. **16**(Suppl 1): p. S23–S29.

31 Blaise, D., *et al*. Rescue of haemopoiesis by a combination of growth factors including stem-cell factor. *Lancet*, 2000. **356**(9238): p. 1325–1326.

32 Farese, A.M., *et al*. Leridistim, a chimeric dual G-CSF and IL-3 receptor agonist, enhances multilineage hematopoietic recovery in a nonhuman primate model of radiation-induced myelosuppression: effect of schedule, dose, and route of administration. *Stem Cells*, 2001. **19**(6): p. 522–533.

33 Farese, A.M., *et al*. Promegapoietin-1a, an engineered chimeric IL-3 and Mpl-L receptor agonist, stimulates hematopoietic recovery in conventional and abbreviated schedules following radiation-induced myelosuppression in nonhuman primates. *Stem Cells*, 2001. **19**(4): p. 329–338.

34 Drexler, H.G. and H. Quentmeier. FLT3: receptor and ligand. *Growth Factors*, 2004. **22**(2): p. 71–73.

35 Carr, R. and N. Modi. Haemopoietic growth factors for neonates: assessing risks and benefits. *Acta Paediatr Suppl*, 2004. **93**(444): p. 15–19.

36 Hubel, K. and A. Engert. Clinical applications of granulocyte colony-stimulating factor: an update and summary. *Ann Hematol*, 2003. **82**(4): p. 207–213.

37 Ford, P. Stem cell transplantation without the use of blood products. In *First European Congress on Blood Conservation*, Vienna, Austria. 2005.

38 Yonemura, Y., *et al.* Long-term efficacy of pegylated recombinant human megakaryocyte growth and development factor in therapy of aplastic anemia. *Int J Hematol*, 2005. **82**(4): p. 307–309.

39 Nomura, S., *et al.* Effects of pegylated recombinant human megakaryocyte growth and development factor in patients with idiopathic thrombocytopenic purpura. *Blood*, 2002. **100**(2): p. 728–730.

40 Zhao, Y.Q., *et al.* A multi-center clinical trial of recombinant human thrombopoietin in chronic refractory idiopathic thrombocytopenic purpura. *Zhonghua Nei Ke Za Zhi*, 2004. **43**(8): p. 608–610.

41 George, J.N. Idiopathic thrombocytopenic purpura: current issues for pathogenesis, diagnosis, and management in children and adults. *Curr Hematol Rep*, 2003. **2**(5): p. 381–387.

42 von dem Borne, A., *et al.* The potential role of thrombopoietin in idiopathic thrombocytopenic purpura. *Blood Rev*, 2002. **16**(1): p. 57–59.

43 Shibuya, K., *et al.* Marked improvement of thrombocytopenia in a murine model of idiopathic thrombocytopenic purpura by pegylated recombinant human megakaryocyte growth and development factor. *Exp Hematol*, 2002. **30**(10): p. 1185–1192.

44 Rice, L., *et al.* Cyclic immune thrombocytopenia responsive to thrombopoietic growth factor therapy. *Am J Hematol*, 2001. **68**(3): p. 210–214.

45 Liao, X., *et al.* The effects of thrombopoietin and interleukin-11 on bone marrow megakaryocytic progenitors in patients with chronic idiopathic thrombocytopenic purpura in vitro. *Hua Xi Yi Ke Da Xue Xue Bao*, 2001. **32**(4): p. 572–575.

46 Basser, R.L., *et al.* Enhancement of platelet recovery after myelosuppressive chemotherapy by recombinant human megakaryocyte growth and development factor in patients with advanced cancer. *J Clin Oncol*, 2000. **18**(15): p. 2852–2861.

47 Tepler, I., *et al.* A randomized placebo-controlled trial of recombinant human interleukin-11 in cancer patients with severe thrombocytopenia due to chemotherapy. *Blood*, 1996. **87**(9): p. 3607–3614.

48 Turner, K.J., *et al.* The role of recombinant interleukin 11 in megakaryocytopoiesis. *Stem Cells*, 1996. **14**(Suppl 1): p. 53–61.

49 Gordon, M.S., *et al.* A phase I trial of recombinant human interleukin-11 (neumega rhIL-11 growth factor) in women with breast cancer receiving chemotherapy. *Blood*, 1996. **87**(9): p. 3615–3624.

50 Bai, C.M., *et al.* The clinical study of recombinant human thrombopoietin in the treatment of chemotherapy-induced severe thrombocytopenia. *Zhonghua Yi Xue Za Zhi*, 2004. **84**(5): p. 397–400.

51 Angiolillo, A.L., *et al.* A phase I clinical, pharmacologic, and biologic study of thrombopoietin and granulocyte colony-stimulating factor in children receiving ifosfamide, carboplatin, and etoposide chemotherapy for recurrent or refractory solid tumors: a Children's Oncology Group experience. *Clin Cancer Res*, 2005. **11**(7): p. 2644–2650.

52 Schuster, M.W., *et al.* The effects of pegylated recombinant human megakaryocyte growth and development factor (PEG-rHuMGDF) on platelet recovery in breast cancer patients undergoing autologous bone marrow transplantation. *Exp Hematol*, 2002. **30**(9): p. 1044–1050.

53 Wang, X.Y., *et al.* Phase II clinical trial on China manufactured recombinant human interleukin-11 derivative in the prevention and treatment of chemotherapy-induced thrombocytopenia. *Zhonghua Zhong Liu Za Zhi*, 2005. **27**(6): p. 373–376.

54 Geissler, K., *et al.* Prior and concurrent administration of recombinant human megakaryocyte growth and development factor in patients receiving consolidation chemotherapy for de novo acute myeloid leukemia—a randomized, placebo-controlled, double-blind safety and efficacy study. *Ann Hematol*, 2003. **82**(11): p. 677–683.

55 Vadhan-Raj, S., *et al.* Recombinant human thrombopoietin attenuates carboplatin-induced severe thrombocytopenia and the need for platelet transfusions in patients with gynecologic cancer. *Ann Intern Med*, 2000. **132**(5): p. 364–368.

56 Fields, K.K., *et al.* Use of PEG-rHuMGDF in platelet engraftment after autologous stem cell transplantation. *Bone Marrow Transplant*, 2000. **26**(10): p. 1083–1088.

57 Bolwell, B., *et al.* Phase 1 study of pegylated recombinant human megakaryocyte growth and development factor (PEG-rHuMGDF) in breast cancer patients after autologous peripheral blood progenitor cell (PBPC) transplantation. *Bone Marrow Transplant*, 2000. **26**(2): p. 141–145.

58 Vredenburgh, J.J., *et al.* A randomized trial of recombinant human interleukin-11 following autologous bone marrow transplantation with peripheral blood progenitor cell support in patients with breast cancer. *Biol Blood Marrow Transplant*, 1998. **4**(3): p. 134–141.

59 Archimbaud, E., *et al.* A randomized, double-blind, placebo-controlled study with pegylated recombinant human megakaryocyte growth and development factor (PEG-rHuMGDF) as an adjunct to chemotherapy for adults with de novo acute myeloid leukemia. *Blood*, 1999. **94**(11): p. 3694–3701.

60 Geissler, R.G., P. Schulte, and A. Ganser, Treatment with growth factors in myelodysplastic syndromes. *Pathol Biol (Paris)*, 1997. **45**(8): p. 656–667.

61 Kizaki, M., Y. Miyakawa, and Y. Ikeda. Long-term administration of pegylated recombinant human megakaryocyte growth and development factor dramatically improved cytopenias in a patient with myelodysplastic syndrome. *Br J Haematol*, 2003. **122**(5): p. 764–767.

62 Murray, N.A. Evaluation and treatment of thrombocytopenia in the neonatal intensive care unit. *Acta Paediatr Suppl*, 2002. **91**(438): p. 74–81.

63 Nakamura, M., *et al.* Recombinant human megakaryocyte growth and development factor attenuates postbypass thrombocytopenia. *Ann Thorac Surg*, 1998. **66**(4): p. 1216–1223.

64 Verheul, H.M., *et al.* Treatment of the Kasabach-Merritt syndrome with pegylated recombinant human megakaryocyte growth and development factor in mice: elevated platelet counts, prolonged survival, and tumor growth inhibition. *Pediatr Res*, 1999. **46**(5): p. 562–565.

65 Decaudin, D., *et al.* Ex vivo expansion of megakaryocyte precursor cells in autologous stem cell transplantation for relapsed malignant lymphoma. *Bone Marrow Transplant*, 2004. **34**(12): p. 1089–1093.

66 Mo, W.J., *et al.* Ex vivo expansion of megakaryocyte progenitor cells from human cord blood in serum-free culture. *Zhongguo Shi Yan Xue Ye Xue Za Zhi*, 2004. **12**(2): p. 133–137.

67 Vaickus, L., *et al.* Platelet transfusion and alternatives to transfusion in patients with malignancy. *Stem Cells*, 1995. **13**(6): p. 588–596.

68 Bishop, M.R., *et al.* Filgrastim as an alternative to donor leukocyte infusion for relapse after allogeneic stem-cell transplantation. *J Clin Oncol*, 2000. **18**(11): p. 2269–2272.

69 Nademanee, A., *et al.* High-dose therapy followed by autologous peripheral-blood stem-cell transplantation for patients with Hodgkin's disease and non-Hodgkin's lymphoma using unprimed and granulocyte colony-stimulating factor-mobilized peripheral-blood stem cells. *J Clin Oncol*, 1994. **12**(10): p. 2176–2186.

70 Schmitz, N., *et al.* Randomised trial of filgrastim-mobilised peripheral blood progenitor cell transplantation versus autologous bone-marrow transplantation in lymphoma patients. *Lancet*, 1996. **347**(8998): p. 353–357.

71 Rinehart, J., *et al.* Phase I trial of recombinant interleukin 3 before and after carboplatin/etoposide chemotherapy in patients with solid tumors: a southwest oncology group study. *Clin Cancer Res*, 1995. **1**(10): p. 1139–1144.

72 Miller, A.M., *et al.* Limited erythropoietic response to combined treatment with recombinant human interleukin 3 and erythropoietin in myelodysplastic syndrome. *Leuk Res*, 1999. **23**(1): p. 77–83.

6 Fluid therapy

Circulating intravascular volume is essential for survival. Therefore, fluid therapy is one of the first measures taken to resuscitate a patient. In the blood management context, fluids serve several purposes as they expand the plasma volume. Fluids keep the heart going by means of the Frank–Starling mechanism. Fluids carry red cells and transport oxygen. Furthermore, they carry nutrients, metabolic by-products, and drugs. Some intravenous solutions are able to mobilize interstitial fluids into the intravascular space and keep them there. All intravascular fluids have a profound impact on the water and electrolyte balance of the body. Additionally, fluids cause changes in the microvasculatory system, in the coagulation profile, and rheology. Since fluid therapy is potentially lifesaving in the framework of modern blood management, it is worth getting an in-depth understanding of this subject.

Objectives of this chapter

1 Know the reasons why fluids are used in blood management.
2 Learn about the role of blood products in volume therapy.
3 Explain different models that try to determine when and how much fluid is to be given.
4 Know how the choice of fluids influences blood transfusions.

Definitions

Plasma substitutes: Plasma substitutes are any liquids that are used to replace blood plasma. Sometimes, the term *plasma substitute* refers only to colloid solutions.
Crystalloids: Crystalloids are solutions that contain electrolytes or other small solutes. Their molecular weight does not exceed 30,000 Dalton. By definition, crystalloids have zero colloid osmotic pressure.

Colloids: Colloids are solutions that contain substances with a molecular weight exceeding 30,000 Dalton. The dispersed particles are between 10^{-7} and 10^{-4} cm in diameter and cannot be separated by filtration or gravity. Colloids exert a colloid-osmotic pressure.
Volume therapy: Volume therapy means the replacement or expansion of plasma volume to achieve an optimal intravascular fluid level, to restore osmotic pressure, and to influence rheology. The flow in the microvascular system is also influenced.

A brief look at history

The history of intravenously administered fluids started with Christopher Wren. He described the first vascular access by quill and bladder. He and his colleagues at the Royal Society, England, experimented with different fluids as "blood substitutes," including wine, beer, and milk. This was in the middle of the seventeenth century.

A more scientific approach to fluid management was chosen about 200 years later. O'Shaughnessy and Brooke observed pathophysiological changes in cholera patients. They wrote: "The blood drawn in the worst of cases of the cholera . . . has lost a large proportion of its water . . . . It has lost also a great proportion of its neutral saline ingredients . . . ." [1]. Based on this observation, Thomas Latta used a saline solution as therapeutic measure. One source wrote: "The great desideratum of restoring the natural current in the veins and arteries, of improving the color of the blood, and recovering the functions of the lungs, in Cholera Asphyxia, may be accomplished by injecting a weak saline solution into the veins of the patient. To Dr Thomas Latta . . . is due the merit of first having recourse to this practice . . . . To produce the effect referred to, a large quantity must be injected, from *five to ten pounds in an adult*" [2].

Some years later, in 1860, normal saline was used by Barnes and Little to treat hemorrhage. Bull and colleagues recommended the use of saline as a transfusion substitute for blood [3].

In 1880, Sydney Ringer, who experimented with frog hearts, used normal saline as well. Not being content with the results, he added other electrolytes to normal saline, forming a more physiological electrolyte solution. Consequently, he became the father of Ringer's solution. In the 1930s, Alexis Hartmann added a lactate buffer to an electrolyte solution to treat metabolic acidosis. The result was Hartmann's solution.

Today's sophisticated solutions are the result of innumerable refinements in the type and amount of ions added. Different, more or less similar, solutions have been developed up to our day. Finally, as the results of Penfield's work, the first successful use of hypertonic saline solutions for medical purposes was reported in 1919. But it was not until 1980 that DeFelippe and colleagues did systematic investigations on the clinical use of hypertonic sodium chloride solutions.

The history of the colloids began in 1861 when Thomas Graham experimented with different solutions. He made them pass through a membrane. Some fluids were not able to pass through the membrane. Graham called these fluids colloids, coming from the Latin word "collo," meaning glue.

The medical use of colloids began in the early part of the twentieth century. During the First World War, Arabian Gum Solutions were advocated for the treatment of severe hemorrhage. However, the toxicity of such solution made them fall into disrepute by the late 1930s. A more successful approach to volume substitution with a colloid was the use of gelatin. It has been in clinical use since 1915 [4]. In the beginning, gelatin was produced by boiling the connective tissues of animals, which developed a jelly-like fluid. These solutions had the advantage of having a significant oncotic effect. Unfortunately, they tended to gel when becoming colder—something that makes infusion difficult. To overcome this unwanted effect, modified gelatin solutions were introduced. These became known as new-generation gelatins.

During the Second World War, polyvinylpyrrolidone (PVP), a synthetic polymer of vinyl pyrrolidone, was used as a colloid. PVP was soon abandoned as it became known that PVP is stored permanently in the reticuloendothelial system. Attention was moved to other colloids. Dextran solutions appeared to be an alternative. Sponsored by the sugar industry, Swedish chemists performed research on sugar beets and found dextran. In order to detect even small amounts of this sugar, they tried to produce antibodies by injecting dextran into rabbits. However, no matter how hard they tried, the rabbits just did not develop antibodies. At the same time and in the same place, other researchers tried to dry blood plasma to ship it into regions where World War I was raging. During conversations of both groups of researchers, the idea was born to use dextran as a plasma expander, since it seemed non-antigenic. The urgent need for such a product was speeding up the research and, very soon, the first clinical investigations started [5]. Raw dextran solutions were first used in 1943 in animals. It had a very high molecular weight and was highly antigenic. Reducing the size of the dextran molecules by hydrolysis made it fit for human use. In 1947, "Macrodex," a dextran type with an average molecular weight of about 75,000 Da was introduced into clinical practice.

Finally, starch solutions were modified and proved to be a usable colloid. Hydroxyethyl starch (HES) was introduced as plasma replacement in 1957 by Wiedersheim. Its career in clinical use began in the late 1960s and continues to this day.

Why do we need fluid therapy?

Adequate fluid therapy correlates with a favorable outcome [6]. Restoration of blood volume, blood pressure, and cardiac output is what classically is aimed at and indicates macrovascular resuscitation. The ultimate goal of volume therapy, though, is to deliver oxygen and to prevent inadequate tissue perfusion, which results in tissue hypoxia. Additionally, "adequate capillary blood flow is necessary to remove metabolic waste products which, if allowed to accumulate exert toxic effects" [7].

In their advertising, the Red Cross claims: "Blood Saves Life." However, it would be more accurate to state: "Blood Volume Saves Life." The body tolerates considerable loss of blood cell mass whereas it does not tolerate major volume loss. Actually, low cardiac output is more dangerous than anemia itself. Restoring the blood flow by means of optimizing the cardiac output is therefore the primary goal in acute anemia. Restoring the red cell mass is secondary.

At first glance, treating like with like, namely treating blood loss and anemia with blood transfusions seems reasonable. But if increasing the cardiac output is the goal, transfusing red cells and whole blood is not the treatment of choice. Cellular fluids increase the viscosity of blood. Whole blood and erythrocyte transfusions sometimes even reduce blood flow and increase oxygen deficiency in tissue [8, 9].

Then, what should be used if not blood? The primary treatment of volume depletion and anemia is not transfusion but volume therapy. We just need to use an acellular fluid to restore plasma volume. There are many different agents for volume therapy. If applied properly, all of them can restore the macrocirculatory blood flow. Most recently, efforts were made to provide intravenous fluids that even restore microcirculatory blood flow. The following paragraphs will discuss different fluids suitable for plasma volume expansion.

Basics of volume household and intravenous fluids

A very simple model of the human fluid household helps to understand what happens when a particular fluid is infused. This model estimates that the total body water makes up 50–60% of the fat-free body mass. About 15% of this is found in connective tissue and bones. Water exchange within those fluids takes a long time and in an acute situation, these fluids can be neglected. Three spaces relevant for clinical considerations regarding fluid management are left:

- the intracellular fluids (ICF) that make up 55% of total body fluid,
- the interstitial fluids (ISF) that make up 20% of total body fluid, and
- the intravascular fluids (IVF) volume that is about 7.5% of total body fluid.

Based on these estimates, it is assumed that the following volume ratios are true:

ICF/ECF about 2:1

ISF/IVF about 3:1 (approx. 75% of the extracellular fluid is in the interstitium and 25% is in the vessels)

These assumptions are used later to explain the behavior of the various fluids after being infused.

Before starting the discussion of various fluids, please check Table A.6 in the Appendix A. It contains some definitions of terms that are used in the following paragraphs.

Crystalloid solutions

Since a wide variety of crystalloids exist for medical use, attempts have been made to classify them. One way is to group them according to their use. There are replacement fluids, maintenance fluids, and fluids for special purposes. Replacement fluids are used to replace fluids lost in the extracellular space. They do this without significantly increasing the fluid volume. Their sodium content is similar to that of the fluid they replace. Maintenance fluids make water available, expanding the extracellular and intracellular spaces. Special fluids are used to correct selected pathologies, e.g., bicarbonate solutions for the treatment of acidosis.

Another way to classify crystalloids is to differentiate between balanced and unbalanced solutions. Balanced solutions are those with electrolyte concentrations similar to normal human plasma. Logically, balanced fluids are recommended for plasma (volume) replacement. Balanced solutions may have fewer side effects than unbalanced solutions.

Sodium chloride 0.9% (normal saline)

Normal saline is the prototype of crystalloid solutions. It contains 154 mmol sodium and 154 mmol chloride. Although normal saline is referred to as "physiological" sodium chloride solution, it is not at all physiological. The sodium level is a little higher than in normal plasma and the chloride level is much higher. Thus, normal saline is not a physiologically balanced solution.

What happens to 1 L of normal saline after rapid intravenous infusion? As already mentioned, the sodium content of normal saline is similar to that of extracellular fluid. This limits its distribution to the extracellular space. The infused solution distributes according to the distribution of the extracellular fluid—namely, 25% intravascular volume and 75% interstitial fluid. Only 25% of the infused liter remain in the vascular system and expand it by about 250 mL. This is the reason for recommending substituting 1 L of blood loss with 3–4 L of normal saline.

Ringer's, Hartmann's & Co.

Besides sodium and chloride, other ions may be added to a crystalloid solution—constituting a distinct solution or brand, e.g., Ringer's solution, Hartmann's solution, E153, and Plasmalyte. Among those added ions are potassium, calcium, and magnesium. Sometimes bicarbonate is added to these solutions. Lactate, gluconate, or acetate may be added as well. They are bicarbonate precursors that are metabolized to bicarbonate in the liver.

The distribution of all replacement solutions is similar to that of normal saline as discussed above.

Glucose solutions

Glucose is a small organic molecule. If dissolved in water, it also constitutes a crystalloid solution. Isotonic glucose solutions (about 5% glucose in water) are used to treat dehydration by providing free water. Hypertonic glucose solutions (>10%) are used to provide metabolic substrate or to treat hyperkalemia (together with insulin).

Glucose solutions are not suitable for volume substitution. Why? Consider what happens to 1 L of 5% glucose solution. Glucose—given intravenously—is rapidly metabolized, leaving free water behind. This free water distributes throughout the whole body water space. Each space gets its share in proportion to its contribution to total body water. We know that only 7.5% of the total body water is in the blood vessels. Consequently, only 7.5% of the liter of glucose solution remains in the blood stream, i.e., only 75 mL. You see, this is less than ideal when it comes to plasma volume expansion. That is why glucose solutions are not a good choice for volume substitution.

There are still other arguments against the use of glucose as mere volume replacement. Severely sick patients may not be able to metabolize glucose properly. That is why glucose may act as a "toxin" after transformation to lactate. Accumulation of glucose itself exerts osmotic pressure and leads to cell dehydration. Additionally, CO_2 production during metabolism may be problematic to patients on ventilation.

Hypertonic fluids

Hypertonic fluids contain an unphysiologically high percentage of electrolytes and come at varying osmolarities (500–2400 mOsm/kg). There are many different hypertonic fluids available. Among them are NaCl 1.8% and 7.5%. Rapid volume expansion occurs after infusion of small amounts of such hypertonic fluids (e.g., 250 mL). This effect, however, is only transient. The addition of colloids is thought to prolong the duration of action of the hypertonic solutions since colloids may be able to hold fluid in the intravascular system. Dextran and hetastarch are used for this purpose.

Hypertonic solutions come at relatively low costs. It is even possible to prepare hypertonic solutions on the spot.

Practice tip

Preparing a hypertonic solution
  You can prepare a 1.8% NaCl solution by adding 150 mEq NaCl to 1 L of normal saline (NaCl 0.9%).

The way hypertonic fluids work is very simple. The sodium content of the solution limits its distribution to the extracellular space, since sodium cannot cross cell membranes easily. Water, in contrast, crosses cell membranes with ease and follows the osmotic gradients. The intravenous injection of hypertonic sodium chloride results in an increase of plasma sodium concentration and creates an osmotic gradient. As a sponge put in a pot of water, hypertonic sodium chloride draws water into the vessels. Endogenous intracellular fluids are mobilized and the intravascular volume increases. This is a kind of autotransfusion, tapping on the total body water which is a huge reservoir amounting to more than 30 L in the adult.

Volume expansion is not the only effect hypertonic solutions have. Due to the resulting volume expansion, cardiac output increases. Possible vasodilatatory effects in combination with venoconstriction lead to a drop in the afterload and overall changes in vascular tone. Taken together, oxygen delivery improves. Besides this effect, myocardial performance improves since an increased serum osmolarity acts as an inotrope. Other beneficial effects discussed are an enhanced renal perfusion, induction of diuresis, mobilization of third-space fluid, improvement of blood fluidity, reestablishment of spontaneous arteriolar vasomotion, and activation of the sympathetic nervous system. Beneficial effects of hypertonic saline or even more so of hypertonic saline with dextran were also reported regarding microcirculation. Since hypertonic saline draws water out of cells into vessels, swelling of the endothelial cell lining in the vasculature is reduced. Small vessels that were blocked by this swelling open again. This improves tissue perfusion. Adhesion and activation of neutrophils is reduced by hypertonic solutions as well. Substances that damage the endothelium are released less by neutrophils. However, this positive effect was observed only if hypertonic solutions were given early after a physiological insult, such as a trauma, before the activation of neutrophils.

Unfortunately, hypertonic fluids also cause some unwanted effects. Infusion leads to electrolyte imbalance, resulting in hypernatremia, hyperchloremia, hyperosmolarity, and hypokalemia. Rapid infusion is to be avoided due to the danger of causing cardiac arrhythmias and cardiac failure. Severe hypernatremia and other electrolyte imbalances may lead to neurological sequelae. This risk is only theoretical, though, since using only 250 mL of a 7.5% solution has not caused neurological damage when administered to patients.

Hypertonic fluids irritate the vessel wall occasionally, resulting in pain at the injection site and thrombophlebitis. Coagulation disorders, due to added dextran, are possible but not likely because the solution is given only in increments of 250 mL. There is also the potential danger of excessive blood loss when the hypertonic solution is given before active hemorrhage is stopped. Increased intravascular volume increases vascular wall tension and interferes with clotting. When hemorrhage is controlled, hypertonic solutions might be more effective than isotonic solutions.

Hypertonic solutions are used for so-called small-volume resuscitation. When compared with isotonic crystalloids, less infusion volume is needed to provide equal volume expansion. Less edema formation was observed. The volume-sparing effect of hypertonic solutions is especially desirable in cardiac patients and in patients undergoing extensive procedures, which normally require large amounts of fluids.

Despite more than 20 years of research yielding encouraging results, small-volume resuscitation does not have the place in clinical practice it probably deserves. Trials were conducted in prehospital trauma patients, after cardiac bypass surgery, burns, endotoxic shock, brain edema, and others. Despite a mass of literature, fluid therapy with hypertonic solutions is only recommended for a selected group of patients. In the prehospital trauma setting, improved survival rate was shown when compared with conventional treatment. Currently, though, small-volume resuscitation is limited to single dose administrations. It was recommended to give initially one dose of 7.5% NaCl/dextrose and then to continue with conventional fluids if the trauma patient is hypotensive.

Colloid solutions

In normal human plasma, proteins are the major colloids present. Colloids are important since they exert osmotic forces across the wall of the blood vessel. Due to their size, usually only small amounts of colloids leave the intact vessel. (However, when the vessel wall is damaged, capillary leakage results, and relatively large molecules may leave the blood vessel and travel to the interstitial space.) Synthetic colloids are called "plasma substitutes" since they replace plasma volume and act as a substitute for the osmotic effects of endogenous albumin and other blood proteins.

The origin of therapeutically used colloids varies. There are naturally occurring colloids, such as albumin, and synthetically produced colloids, such as gelatin, dextran, and starch. Albumin is a molecule that has a relatively constant molecular weight. As the molecules in the solution are all of about the same size, such solutions are called monodisperse. In contrast, the molecular weight of synthetic colloid molecules varies. The molecular weight follows the Gaussian distribution. That is why these solutions are called polydisperse. The given molecular weight of such solutions denotes the average weight of all molecules in a bottle.

The intravascular molecular weight is clinically more important than the average molecular weight in the bottle. Small molecules of a polydisperse colloid are rapidly excreted. Other molecules may easily be broken down by blood enzymes. Such molecules do not contribute to the volume effect. What counts are the molecules that actually remain in the circulation for a given time.

Not the size, but the number of molecules present are responsible for the osmotic, water-binding effect. The abbreviation Mn denotes the average weight of the solution—and is related to the oncotic pressure. Mw indicates molecular weight, determining the size of the molecule and, therefore, the viscosity of a solution.

Hydroxyethyl starch

Hydroxyethyl starch is a synthetic colloid which is made from corn or potato starch. This starch is the basis for the production of amylopectin, a glucose chain. (Corn starch is preferred because it consists of more than 95% amylopectin. Potato starch has only 80% amylopectin.) Hydroxyethyl groups are added to amylopectin to get the final product. Hydroxylation acts a protection from degradation of the HES molecules in the blood through amylases.

The pharmacology of HES varies greatly from one solution to another, depending on its properties. To distinguish them, certain characteristics are described, namely, the molecular weight, degree, and pattern of substitution and concentration (Table 6.1). Labels of bottles with HES solutions state the characteristics of the fluids in formulas such as HES 6% (130/0.4). The number behind the term HES gives the concentration of the starch solution, in this example, 6%. The first number in parentheses denotes the molecular weight. The molecular weight in HES solutions follows Gaussian distribution, where the number given as molecular weight is the average of all molecules present in the bottle. In vivo, the weight changes by enzymatic breakdown of the starch molecule and due to the excretion of small molecules. The second number in the parentheses is the substitution degree of the starch solution. The "substitution degree" of an HES tells how many glucose units on average are substituted, that is, hydroxylated. A substitution degree of 0.4 means that there are an average of 4 hydroxyethyl groups per 10 glucose molecules. A fourth characteristic of HES solutions is the pattern of substitution. The pattern of substitution is determined by the

Table 6.1 Classification of HES.

Characteristic	Classification	Definition
Molecular weight	High	450–480 kDa
	Medium	130–200 kDa
	Low	40–70 (<100) kDa
Concentration	High	10%
	Low	3–6%
Degree of substitution	High	0.6–0.7
	Low	0.4–0.5
Pattern of substitution	High	>8
(C2/C6 ratio)	Low	<8

kDa, kilo Dalton.

position of the glucose groups on the entire HES molecule. It is sometimes expressed as the C2/C6 ratio. A high ratio means that there are many glucose molecules on the second carbon atom in the HES molecules. The more glucose substitution on a C2-molecule in a HES molecule, the longer is the duration of the starch in the circulation. The reason is that the glucose in the C2-position hinders the breaking down of the HES molecule by amylases. The less hydroxylation, the shorter is the stay in the circulation.

The molecular size and degree of substitution determine how long the starch solution remains in the blood vessels. The breakdown of the starch molecules depends on how easily amylase binds to the molecule (determined by degree of substitution and pattern of substitution). After HES infusions, serum amylases increase. This is not a sign of pancreatitis but rather the reaction to the HES infusion.

HES is a polydisperse solution. That means that there is a mix of molecules, with different molecular weight, in the bottle. Small molecules are rapidly excreted by the kidneys, if they are below the renal threshold of 50–60 kDa. Large molecules are hydrolyzed into smaller molecules. If this is hindered by the size and substitution pattern of the molecule, accumulation of HES occurs. Accumulation is responsible for many of the side effects of HES: renal and immunological impairment, pruritus (especially in long-term administration), changes in the coagulation system, and an increase in blood viscosity. Pruritus is especially troubling for patients. It commences several weeks after HES administration and the effects can last as long as 2 years, with no therapy being effective [10].

HES solutions have an effect on the microvasculature. Some experimental evidence exists for the beneficial effect of HES. Some HES reduce the extravascular leakage of albumin. The underlying mechanism is not clear. Initially, it was believed HES has a sealing effect on the capillaries. More probably, though, the effect is related to the inhibition of endothelial activation during sepsis or the reduction of xanthine oxidase after reperfusion [11]. HES may also modify severe inflammatory responses and reduce endothelial dysfunction. It may therefore be organ protective in sepsis and surgeries that elicit severe systemic inflammatory responses [12–14].

Acetylstarch

Acetylstarch is a new synthetic colloid. It is—like HES—a derivative of starch, namely, an acetylamylopectin. Acetyl groups, instead of glucose, are bound to a glucose frame. Acetic acid is bound by a weak ester linkage in vivo. Esterases easily liberate the acetyl groups from the glucose chains, and glucosidases hydrolyze the remaining glucose chain to glucose. This relatively rapid degradation of acetylstarch is responsible for the shorter half-life (compared with HES) and the decrease of side effects related to long-term storage of starch solutions in the reticuloendothelial system and other tissues.

Dextran

Dextran is a glucose polymer. It is synthesized by enzymes of the *Leuconostoc mesenteroides* bacteria. The bacteria produce dextran of very high molecular weight. Hydrolytic breakdown and fractionation finally lead to different dextran preparations. Dextran solutions are available as dextran 40 (average molecular weight of 40,000 Da) and dextran 70 (average molecular weight of 70,000 Da). They come in concentration of 3–10%.

Initially, dextran has an excellent volume-increasing effect but the effect is only short-lived. Because of the small molecule size, dextran is excreted rapidly. Dextran 40 increases plasma volume more and acts shorter than dextran 70.

Although initial experiments with dextran failed to demonstrate the antigenicity of dextran, antibodies are developed occasionally. To prevent anaphylactic reactions, a monovalent hapten, dextran 1, is usually given prior to the infusion of dextran 40 or 70 to block possible antibodies.

Gelatin solutions

Gelatins available today are so-called new-generation gelatins. They are modified polypeptides from bovine collagen. Three different modifications are used: cross-linked gelatin (e.g., Gelifundol), urea-linked gelatin (e.g., Polygelin), and succinylated gelatin (e.g., Gelofusine). Gelatin solutions differ with regard to their electrolyte concentrations. This is of clinical importance. Urea-linked gelatin has a high calcium and potassium concentration while the succinylated preparations are low in calcium and potassium. Gelatin is available in concentrations of 4, 6, and 10% solutions and is dissolved in sodium chloride solution.

The average molecular weight of gelatin is 30–35 kDa. This is way below the renal threshold of approximately 60 kDa. Gelatin is therefore rapidly excreted. The plasma half-life is only short, namely about 2 hours. Repeated doses are needed to maintain an appropriate intravascular volume.

High-viscosity fluids: alginate solutions

Alginate solutions are not new. Already in the 1950s, studies with these agents were launched [15]. They were not widely used in patients. The interest in alginate was rekindled recently when searching for an agent to increase the viscosity of blood. In animal experiments, high-viscosity alginates are currently under investigation for use as a plasma expander [16].

Last but not least: the albumin story

Albumin is a naturally occurring colloid. It is a blood protein that is responsible for approximately 75% of the colloid-osmotic pressure. Albumin solutions for clinical use are prepared from pooled human plasma. Commercially available solutions are either isooncotic (4/5%) or hyperoncotic (20/25%).

Some think of albumin as the gold standard of colloid therapy. Others are absolutely against it [17]. Why? The rationale for the use of albumin is to correct hypoalbuminemia. It is true to say that the serum albumin level of critically ill patients correlates with their outcome. A low albumin level predicts a bad outcome. Nevertheless, the artificial correction of the albumin level by albumin infusion does not improve the outcome. On the contrary, albumin substitution, in critically ill patients, is associated with worse outcome [18]. Hypoalbuminemia is best corrected with sufficient nutrition and treatment of the underlying condition.

Another reason for albumin use is the attempt to treat edema since albumin is a colloid that binds water. However, this is not the case. The reason for this is easy to understand when we consider that albumin is also present in the interstitial space. Also, when intravenously administered, albumin disperses freely in the interstitium, an effect that is even more pronounced in critically ill patients with capillary leakage. That is why albumin may even cause edema.

Albumin has no proven advantages over HES in volume substitution. Studies show that HES is equal or even superior to albumin in fluid management. HES therefore can replace albumin as a volume substitute. Although there is no proven indication for human albumin, it is sometimes recommended. Why? Professor von Bormann, an expert in volume therapy, claims that albumin is used on an emotional basis only [19]. There is also a strong interest of the albumin industry to find uses for their product [20]. By now, the use of albumin as a volume substitute is not justified in the general patient population.

Side effects of volume therapy

Despite decades of research on fluid therapy, the choice of a resuscitation fluid is often nothing more then a creed. Taking into consideration what side effects the fluids have may make it easier to decide on the therapy of an individual patient.

Coagulation

In one way or the other, every fluid has the potential to impair hemostasis. Besides specific effects on factors in the coagulation system, all fluids dilute clotting factors. However, crystalloids also enhance hemostasis. They were shown to cause a mild hypercoagulopathy, lasting several hours. In contrast, colloids seem not to enhance coagulation.

Albumin was thought of as the gold standard as regards fluid therapy, since it was postulated that it does not cause coagulopathy. Nevertheless, it was also shown that albumin impairs coagulation [21]. The same is true of gelatines. They were also thought not to influence coagulation, even in higher doses. However, specialized clotting tests (e.g., ristocetin time) were able to show some influence of gelatin on coagulation [22]. Even so, the influence of albumins and gelatins on the body's ability to clot is not as pronounced as in dextran or some HES [23].

Dextran is known for its inhibition of thrombocyte aggregation by coating platelets (inhibition of factor VIII) and its ability to increase fibrinolysis. Further, it reduces blood viscosity. Such properties may not be favorable when it comes to bleeding patients but they can be used to prevent thrombosis and to treat rheological complications.

HES are able to cause an acquired von-Willebrand syndrome. These may also alter the platelet's ability to participate effectively in the clotting process. Some HES decrease the expression of platelet receptors, while others increase it. The extent to which this is true depends on the type of HES studied [22]. DDAVP (1-deamino-8-D-arginine vasopressin) can offset some of the ill effects of HES on coagulation [24, 25]. There is a historical restriction of the amount of HES given. To prevent coagulopathy, HES infusions were restricted to 20 mL/kg body weight/ day. This recommendation was given in the early days of HES therapy, when only HES with a high molecular weight and a high substitution ratio were available. Medium-molecular-weight HES with low substitution ratio and HES with low molecular weight can be used in higher quantities, without causing relevant coagulation disturbances. Yet, higher doses are needed because they do not stay intravascularly as long as the high-molecular-weight agents. A long overlooked factor in the work of HES is the solution in which HES is dissolved. There are starch solutions with balanced and with unbalanced solutions. Changes in the coagulation profile may be partially due to the solvent and not only to the starch itself. A lack of calcium was proposed to be the mechanism behind this observation. Starch in balanced solutions (containing calcium) may influence coagulation less than that in unbalanced solutions [26].

Kidney function

Albumin and gelatins seem not to impair kidney function. HES, though, if not given with enough crystalloid fluids, may cause problems in patients with kidney disease, especially when the creatinine level is already increased. In patients with renal insufficiency, HES should only be given in low concentration and with sufficient fluids as to prevent kidney damage.

Allergic reactions

According to a study by Laxenaire [27], the following incidence of anaphylactoid reactions after colloid infusion occurred: 0.345% for gelatin, 0.273% for dextran, 0.099% for albumin, and 0.058% for HES. In 20% of the cases, these reactions were serious. Especially patients with a history of drug allergies were at risk of developing an anaphylactoid reaction. Gelatins and dextrans therefore should be avoided in patients with a known history of drug allergies.

Hyperchloremic metabolic acidosis

Hyperchloremic metabolic acidosis is a nonrespiratory acidosis with an increase of chloride in plasma. The most common avoidable cause of this acidosis is an intravenous fluid with a high chloride content as it is found in unbalanced fluids and especially in normal saline. Balanced fluids do not cause this derangement. Hyperchloremic metabolic acidosis was reported to have many effects on red cells, coagulation, the gastrointestinal tract, and renal function. Although the clinical relevance of those effects is controversial, it was stated that balanced solutions could be superior to unbalanced solutions.

Fluids at work: when do we take what fluid and how much?

When?

Does the timing of fluid resuscitation play a role? In general, the earlier the patient has an adequate fluid status, the better it is. In the surgical patient, early fluid optimization is more efficacious than delayed resuscitation in maintaining or restoring normal tissue function. Especially the first 6 hours after a physical insult resulting in volume depletion are a "window of opportunity" for resuscitation [6]. However, a recent trend, questioning early liberal fluid management can be observed in the current literature [28]. It was claimed that restrictive intraoperative fluid management (with fluid therapy in major visceral surgery being as low as 4 mL/kg /h) could improve the outcome. It was shown that patients on the restrictive fluid regimen had improved bowel function and higher hematocrit levels and left the hospital earlier. Whether this trend actually improves outcome of the patients is currently subject to debate.

An alternate resuscitation strategy claims that it is beneficial for the surgical patient to first undergo a restrictive fluid regime. Fluid therapy is held back until surgical hemorrhage is over. Toward the end of surgery, the lost fluid is fully replaced. This strategy has been proposed to reduce intraoperative blood loss. A similar strategy was proposed under the name "delayed resuscitation," to be used in actively hemorrhaging trauma victims and those suffering from gastrointestinal bleeding. Aggressive volume therapy favors bleeding when administered before definitive surgical hemostasis is achieved. The resulting increase in blood pressure disturbs the body's mechanisms to clot. Therefore, the delayed resuscitation model proposes the following: In the actively bleeding patient it may be wise

Table 6.2 Volume effects of fluids.

Solution	Intravascular volume effect (% of infused volume)
Ringer's solution	25
NaCl 0.9%	25
Glucose 5%	<10
NaCl 7.5%	300–400
6% dextran 60	120
6% HES 450/0.7	100
6% HES 200/0.62	100
10% dextran 40	200
6% HES 200/0.5	100
10% HES 200/0.5	130
6% HES 70/0.5	70
3% gelatin	70
5% albumin	70–90
6% HES 130/0.4	100

to give only a limited amount of fluid just to raise the blood pressure to a tolerable level. Then, bleeding should be stopped as soon as possible, after which the fluid level should be optimized.

What?

Neither blood nor albumin are suitable liquids for fluid resuscitation, leaving only synthetic fluids as an option. The discussion whether crystalloids or colloids are to be preferred seems to be a never-ending story. Both kinds of solutions increase the cardiac output appropriately if administered correctly, that is, with the right substitution ratio (crystalloids, 1:3–4; colloids, 1:1–1.5). To date, no conclusions can be drawn whether crystalloids or colloids are preferred when only overall mortality is considered [29]. The final decision of the kind of fluid administered is determined by volume effects required (Table 6.2), the side effects, costs, etc. With the knowledge we have to date, the most important thing is not whether crystalloid or colloid is used but the fact that the patient is actually volume-resuscitated.

How much?

Hypovolemia is detrimental since it precipitates tissue hypoxia. Giving too much fluids may be just as detrimental. Hypervolemia may lead to pulmonary edema and paralytic ileus. Tissue edema can lead to tissue hypoxia as well. That is why it would be beneficial to know the optimum fluid level of any individual.

Monitoring the volume status of individual patients is an art. There is no number or symptom which tells whether a patient will benefit from further volume or not. Good clinical judgment is needed to find the best possible volume level for an individual patient. As a rule of thumb, it is assumed that hypovolemia is present when there is orthostatic hypotension (which may indicate an estimated volume loss of at least 20%) or when there is supine hypotension (which may indicate an estimated volume loss of at least 30%). In a particular patient, though, basic vital signs do not say much about whether the patient has reached the optimum volume level or not.

There are quite a few monitoring tools available to target volume therapy. Traditionally, intravascular pressures such as the arterial blood pressure, the central venous pressure, and the pulmonary capillary wedge pressure are measured. Low pressure may indicate hypovolemia. Normal pressure, however, does not rule out hypovolemia and tissue hypoxia. Intravascular pressures may be useful if their trends are considered, but a single given pressure reading does not tell how to proceed with the volume therapy. Measuring variables of the global blood flow, e.g., cardiac output, stroke volume, oxygen delivery, and oxygen consumption, may be better. Optimizing the cardiac output is associated with a better outcome. Such monitoring is preferred over static pressure measurements. However, neither intravascular pressures nor variables of the global blood flow answer the important question: Do I optimize tissue perfusion and oxygenation with my current therapy regime? Since tissue oxygenation and perfusion is the ultimate goal of volume therapy, monitoring of this can be more helpful. Currently, only gastric tonometry—an indirect estimate of mucosa perfusion—is available in clinical practice to provide an estimate of tissue oxygenation.

Influence of fluid therapy on blood management

The last question in this chapter is: Does the choice of fluids affect the use of allogeneic blood products, bleeding, and the final outcome? Well, it does in so far that blood is not a volume replacement. It is not necessary to transfuse a drop of blood for the sole reason of volume replacement. Acellular fluids are actually superior to blood as far as their ability to facilitate tissue oxygenation is concerned.

Physiologically balanced fluids seem to cause less blood loss than unbalanced fluids and to decrease the use of transfusions. Lactated Ringer's solution is superior to normal saline in blood management [30] and so is HES in a balanced solution when compared to HES in normal saline. Actually, high-molecular-weight HES, in normal saline, increases blood loss and transfusions in surgical patients when compared to HES in a balanced solution. In contrast, when a low-molecular-weight HES is used, blood loss may not be more pronounced than that when using gelatin [31].

Choosing a resuscitation fluid with regard to its influence on hemostasis may also reduce blood loss and allogeneic transfusions. It was suggested that blood loss can be reduced by choosing a HES solution with a relatively low in vivo molecular weight and a low degree of hydroxyethylation [32]. However, studies are inconclusive with respect to whether HES causes increased bleeding and blood transfusions if used correctly. It must be kept in mind that greater volumes of lower molecular weight HES solutions are needed to expand the plasma volume for prolonged periods of time since the intravascular half-life of lower molecular weight solutions is not as long as the one of higher molecular weight solutions. The increased amount of the lower molecular weight HES infused may also increase the side effects, e.g., bleeding. In contrast to HES, gelatin does not seem to cause unnecessary blood loss by impairment of hemostasis [33].

Another important factor for blood management is the plasma expander's ability to preserve microcirculation during bleeding and in anemic states. Animal experiments did show that HES, in a balanced solution, is able to preserve microcirculation better than crystalloids [34]. This effect was shown also when the delayed resuscitation model was employed [35].

Fluids in severely anemic patients: blood is thicker than water

Expanding the blood volume with a low-viscosity fluid, such as a crystalloid, reduces the blood viscosity. This is beneficial in patients with sufficient cardiac compensation, since the reduced viscosity increases the blood flow. When the heart is not able to compensate for the reduction in hemoglobin, traditionally, transfusions are considered. However, a better approach is to increase the viscosity of blood. Effects of decreased oxygen delivery can be compensated by increased plasma viscosity. Viscosity increases the shear stress on the microvasculature system and more nitric oxide (NO) is produced. Vessels dilate and the functional capillary density increases [36]. Under experimental conditions in anemic animals, it was shown that microvascular blood flow and tissue oxygenation improve when the

viscosity was increased to achieve values similar to that of whole blood. This was accomplished with a high-viscosity solution such as dextran 500, HES, or alginate solutions [16, 36]. In addition, the combination of an artificial oxygen carrier (hemoglobin) with viscosity similar to that of blood is a very promising approach to resuscitation after hemorrhage. "The results show that a low-dose oxygen carrier, with a high viscosity and high colloid osmotic pressure might be superior to . . . blood in returning the organism to normal conditions after hemorrhagic shock and that a small amount of this type of hemoglobin in plasma is required to obtain similar or better results than those obtained with blood transfusion" [7].

Key points

- Restoring blood volume in hypovolemic patients is more important than correcting anemia. Crystalloids and colloids are equally effective in optimizing the cardiac output, if the correct dose is given.
- Whole blood and erythrocytes have no use as sole volume therapeutics.
- Albumin rarely is indicated for volume therapy, if at all.
- The choice of fluid therapy may influence the total blood loss. Physiologically balanced fluids are superior to unbalanced fluids. HES and other high-viscosity fluids may improve the microcirculation. Improving the blood viscosity in states of severe hemodilution maintains tissue perfusion and oxygenation.

Questions for review

- What is the difference between crystalloids and colloids?
- What crystalloids are there and how do they differ from each other?
- What colloids are there?
- What do the following terms mean: polydisperse, substitution degree, hypertonic, replacement fluid?
- What four terms are typically used to describe HES?

Exercises and practice cases

A boxer weighing 100 kg experiences severe epistaxis. He loses 1.5 L of blood. How much of the following solutions are needed to restore his blood volume?—normal saline, lactated Ringer's, HES 6% (450/0.7); 10% dextran 40, gelatin 3%, NaCl 7.5%.

Suggestions for further research

What solutions are suitable plasma substitutes for therapeutic plasma exchange, e.g., in myasthenic crisis?
What specific considerations are needed for fluid therapy in babies?
What fluids are acceptable to strict vegetarians?

Homework

List all available fluids in your hospital, classify them as being a crystalloid or a colloid, and make a table containing all fluids and their content of electrolytes, molecular weights, substitution degree, etc.

Find out where you can get the best available colloids and the best available crystalloids. Record the contact information of the sources (e.g., a pharmacy or a pharmaceutical company) in the address book in the Appendix E.

References

1 O'Shaughnessy, D. and W. Brooke. Experiments on the blood in cholera [letter]. *Lancet*, 1831. (1): p. 490.

2 Lewins, R. and T. Latta. Injection of saline solutions in extraordinary quantities into the veins in cases of malignant cholera. *Lancet*, 1831. **32**(2): p. 243–244.

3 Bull, W.T. On the intra-venous injection of saline solutions as a substitute for transfusion of blood. *Med Rec*, 1884. p. 6–8.

4 Gruber, U.F. Blutersatz. *Fortschr Med*, 1969. **87**: p. 631–634.

5 Gronwall, A. and B. Ingelman. The introduction of dextran as a plasma substitute. *Vox Sang*, 1984. **47**(1): p. 96–99.

6 Levett, D.Z.H., M.P.W. Grocott, and M.G. Mythen. The effects of fluid optimization on outcome following major surgery. *TATM*, 2002. **4**: p. 74–79.

7 Wettstein, R., *et al.* Resuscitation with polyethylene glycol-modified human hemoglobin improves microcirculatory blood flow and tissue oxygenation after hemorrhagic shock in awake hamsters. *Crit Care Med*, 2003. **31**(6): p. 1824–1830.

8 Silverman, H.J. and P. Tuma. Gastric tonometry in patients with sepsis. Effects of dobutamine infusions and packed red blood cell transfusions. *Chest*, 1992. **102**(1): p. 184–188.

9 Marik, P.E. and W.J. Sibbald. Effect of stored-blood transfusion on oxygen delivery in patients with sepsis. *JAMA*, 1993. **269**(23): p. 3024–3029.

10 Bork, K. Pruritus precipitated by hydroxyethyl starch: a review. *Br J Dermatol*, 2005. **152**(1): p. 3–12.

11 Oz, M.C., *et al.* Attenuation of microvascular permeability dysfunction in postischemic striated muscle by hydroxyethyl starch. *Microvasc Res*, 1995. **50**(1): p. 71–79.

12 Tian, J., *et al.* Influence of hydroxyethyl starch on lipopolysaccharide-induced tissue nuclear factor kappa B activation and systemic TNF-alpha expression. *Acta Anaesthesiol Scand*, 2005. **49**(9): p. 1311–1317.

13 Rittoo, D., *et al.* The effects of hydroxyethyl starch compared with gelofusine on activated endothelium and the systemic inflammatory response following aortic aneurysm repair. *Eur J Vasc Endovasc Surg*, 2005. **30**(5): p. 520–524.

14 Rittoo, D., *et al.* Randomized study comparing the effects of hydroxyethyl starch solution with Gelofusine on pulmonary function in patients undergoing abdominal aortic aneurysm surgery. *Br J Anaesth*, 2004. **92**(1): p. 61–66.

15 Tomoda, M. and K. Inokuchi. Sodium alginate of lowered polymerization (alginon). A new plasma expander. *J Int Coll Surg*, 1959. **32**: p. 621–635.

16 Cabrales, P., A.G. Tsai, and M. Intaglietta. Alginate plasma expander maintains perfusion and plasma viscosity during extreme hemodilution. *Am J Physiol Heart Circ Physiol*, 2005. **288**(4): p. H1708–H1716.

17 Pape, H.C., R. Meier, and J.A. Sturm. Physiological changes following infusion of colloids or crystalloids. *Int J Intensive Care*, 1999: p. 47–53.

18 Foley, E.F., *et al.* Albumin supplementation in the critically ill. A prospective, randomized trial. *Arch Surg*, 1990. **125**(6): p. 739–742.

19 von Bormann, B. and J. Weiler. Hypalbuminämie: Therapieren oder tolerieren? *J Anaesth Intensivbehandlung*, 2001. (**1**, Quart 1): p. 271–272.

20 Yamey, G. Albumin industry launches global promotion. *BMJ*, 2000. **320**: p. 533.

21 Boldt, J. Volume replacement in critically ill intensive-care patients. No classic review. *Anaesthesist*, 1998. **47**(9): p. 778–785.

22 Thaler, U., E. Deusch, and S.A. Kozek-Langenecker. In vitro effects of gelatin solutions on platelet function: a comparison with hydroxyethyl starch solutions. *Anaesthesia*, 2005. **60**(6): p. 554–559.

23 Niemi, T.T. and A.H. Kuitunen. Artificial colloids impair haemostasis. An in vitro study using thromboelastometry coagulation analysis. *Acta Anaesthesiol Scand*, 2005. **49**(3): p. 373–378.

24 Conroy, J.M., *et al.* The effects of desmopressin and 6% hydroxyethyl starch on factor VIII:C. *Anesth Analg*, 1996. **83**(4): p. 804–807.

25 Lazarchick, J. and J.M. Conroy. The effect of 6% hydroxyethyl starch and desmopressin infusion on von Willebrand factor: ristocetin cofactor activity. *Ann Clin Lab Sci*, 1995. **25**(4): p. 306–309.

26 Gan, T.J., *et al.* Hextend, a physiologically balanced plasma expander for large volume use in major surgery: a randomized phase III clinical trial. Hextend Study Group. *Anesth Analg*, 1999. **88**(5): p. 992–998.

27 Laxenaire, M.C., C. Charpentier, and L. Feldman. Anaphylactoid reactions to colloid plasma substitutes: incidence, risk factors, mechanisms. A French multicenter prospective study. *Ann Fr Anesth Reanim*, 1994. **13**(3): p. 301–310.

28 Nisanevich, V., *et al.* Effect of intraoperative fluid management on outcome after intraabdominal surgery. *Anesthesiology*, 2005. **103**(1): p. 25–32.

29 Choi, P.T., *et al.* Crystalloids vs. colloids in fluid resuscitation: a systematic review. *Crit Care Med*, 1999. **27**(1): p. 200–210.

30 Waters, J.H., *et al.* Normal saline versus lactated Ringer's solution for intraoperative fluid management in patients undergoing abdominal aortic aneurysm repair: an outcome study. *Anesth Analg*, 2001. **93**(4): p. 817–822.

31 Van der Linden, P.J., *et al.* Hydroxyethyl starch 130/0.4 versus modified fluid gelatin for volume expansion in cardiac surgery patients: the effects on perioperative bleeding and transfusion needs. *Anesth Analg*, 2005. **101**(3): p. 629–634, table of contents.

32 Treib, J., A. Haaß, G. Pindur, E. Wenzel, and K. Schimrigk. Blutungskomplikationen durch Hydroxyethylstärke sind vermeidbar. *Dtsch Arztebl*, 1997. **1997**(94): p. C1748–C1752.

33 Boldt, J., S. Suttner, B. Kumle, and I. Hüttner. Cost analysis of different volume replacement strategies in anesthesia. *Infus Ther Transfus Med*, 2000. **27**: p. 38–43.

34 Komori, M., *et al.* Effects of colloid resuscitation on peripheral microcirculation, hemodynamics, and colloidal osmotic pressure during acute severe hemorrhage in rabbits. *Shock*, 2005. **23**(4): p. 377–382.

35 Handrigan, M.T., *et al.* Choice of fluid influences outcome in prolonged hypotensive resuscitation after hemorrhage in awake rats. *Shock*, 2005. **23**(4): p. 337–343.

36 Tsai, A.G., *et al.* Elevated plasma viscosity in extreme hemodilution increases perivascular nitric oxide concentration and microvascular perfusion. *Am J Physiol Heart Circ Physiol*, 2005. **288**(4): p. H1730–H1739.

7 The chemistry of hemostasis

All bleeding eventually stops, but it is a matter of timing whether the patient experiences this phenomenon dead or alive. The faster, the more complete, and the more proficient the hemostasis is, the better are the patient's chances for recovery. Mere chemistry may help to achieve such timely surgical hemostasis.

Systemically administrable drugs are available to enhance endogenous coagulation factor production and release. Some drugs are able to modify fibrinolysis and intensify platelet contribution to hemostasis. There are also drugs that enhance local hemostasis. Systemically as well as locally acting hemostatic drugs have been shown to reduce bleeding and patient exposure to donor blood.

Objectives of this chapter

1 Describe ways how blood loss can be reduced by systemically administering drugs.
2 Explain the mode of action and use of agents that promote local hemostasis.
3 Define the use of hemostatically acting drugs in blood management and their impact on the use of blood products.

Definitions

Antifibrinolytics: Antifibrinolytics are agents that prevent fibrinolysis or lysis of a thrombus by prohibiting the conversion of plasminogen to plasmin and the action of plasmin itself. The drugs are used to prevent and control hemorrhage and to enhance hemostasis.
Vitamin K-group (antihemorrhagic factors): The vitamin K-group comprises a group of compounds with a naphthoquinone ring and different side chains. Vitamins of the K group are important for the posttranslational γ-carboxylation of blood clotting factors.
Conjugated estrogens: Conjugated estrogens are mixtures of compounds containing water-soluble female

hormones derived from urine of pregnant mares or synthetically from estrone and equilin with other concomitant conjugates including 17-α-dihydroequilin, 17-α-estradiol, and 17-β-dihydroequilin.
Tissue adhesive or sealant: Tissue adhesive or sealant (formerly called tissue glue) is any substance that polymerizes to an extent to glue tissues together and prevent leakage of body fluids including blood [1].
Hemostatics: Hemostatics are agents that arrest bleeding either by forming an artificial clot or by providing the matrix for physiological clot formation.

A brief look at history

The oldest methods used to stop a hemorrhage were probably implemented directly onto the bleeding spot. A wide variety of agents were used to achieve hemostasis. Among them were agents that initiated clotting using a variety of mechanisms such as providing a matrix for endogenous platelets to aggregate (flour, cotton ashes), agents that reduced the blood flow to the site of bleeding (ice, water, cocaine), some that added exogenous clotting factors (freshly slaughtered chicken meat, snake venoms), others that changed the coagulation medium in the wound (lemon juice) or acted as caustic agents (hot oil, animal and plant products). Some of these agents proved very effective in locally reducing hemorrhage.

Adding to the local treatment of wounds, systemically administered drugs for hemostasis were later added to the armamentarium of the physician attempting to stop a hemorrhage. In 1772, William Hewson noted that blood collected under stress clotted rapidly. This finding triggered a series of animal experiments that clarified the role of the stress hormone responsible for this phenomenon: adrenaline. Almost 200 years later it was found that a release of coagulation factor VIII (FVIII) followed the injection of adrenaline—with no change in other known clotting factors. The concept of treating a coagulation disorder simply by releasing the patient's own FVIII was taunting, but the means to do it were lacking. Furthermore, adrenaline injections were followed by too many side effects. Subsequent research also found that vasopressin and insulin were able to induce FVIII release. However, these substances also had too many side effects in order to be used therapeutically in the setting of coagulation disorders. In 1974, desmopressin, the synthetic analogue of vasopressin, was shown to release FVIII and von Willebrand's factor (vWF). Since the side effects of desmopressin are mild, the substance proved to be the long-looked-for drug to be used in certain clotting factor deficiencies, with the first human use soon to follow [2]. Desmopressin was first shown to be useful in von Willebrand's disease (vWD) and hemophilia in 1977 in Italy [2, 3]. After some more studies in other countries were published, the WHO took up desmopressin in its list of essential drugs. Since 1986, desmopressin has also been evaluated for its use as a drug that reduces patient exposure to donor blood [2].

Vitamin K was discovered by Henrik Dam in 1935. He was experimenting with cholesterol synthesis and observed that chicken fed with a cholesterol-deficient diet developed a coagulation disorder. The discovery of a vitamin that was obviously related to coagulation followed. The vitamin was called vitamin K since it has such a close relation to the process of koagulation, the Danish term for coagulation.

In the 1930s, Kraut *et al.* and Kunitz *et al.* worked on aprotinin, which was shown to be an inhibitor of trypsin and kallikrein. This drug was shown to reduce fibrinolysis as well. Other antifibrinolytic drugs were discovered soon thereafter, among them are carbazochrome (1954), hemocoagulase (1966), amniocaproic acid (1962), and tranexamic acid (1965). The development of hemostatic drugs came to a halt in the late 1960s and a trend toward the development of antithrombotic and fibrinolytic drugs developed, probably spurred on by the increase in thromboembolic cardiovascular events. The blood-sparing effect of the invented hemostatic drugs received renewed attention in the 1980s when drugs were needed to reduce the use of transfusions.

The history of the unconjugated estrogen mixture Premarin, an example of another hemostatically acting drug, teaches us that drugs, although potent, are often not completely understood. Premarin is derived from the urine of pregnant mares and contains several different estrogens. At the time of the drug's approval by the US Food and Drug Administration in 1942, Premarin was known to contain two estrogens, estrone, and equilin. It was known that additional estrogens were present in smaller amounts.

In 1970, the United States Pharmacopeia published the first standards for conjugated estrogens, describing conjugated estrogens as containing sodium estrone sulfate and sodium equilin sulfate. In 1975, another compound in Premarin was identified, namely δ-(8,9)-dehydroestrone sulfate. Recent findings regarding this estrogen compound showed that, although representing only a small percentage (4.4%) of the estrogenic compounds present in the product, it becomes a major compound when considering those compounds actually absorbed into the bloodstream. The amount, the mechanism of action, and the role of yet other estrogens in the mixture are not fully disclosed as well. Despite this lack of knowledge, the drug works and reduces bleeding in a variety of settings.

Systemic hemostatic drugs

Antifibrinolytics

Physiology of fibrinolysis

Ideally, the coagulation process and fibrinolysis are balanced, and so neither a bleeding diathesis nor an exaggerated intravascular thrombosis occur. Since blood clots are not meant to be durable structures, they need to be dissolved as soon as the damaged tissues are sufficiently repaired. Fibrin in the clot is the prime target of plasmin, a serine protease that is able to cleave the fibrin molecules. Plasminogen, the plasmin precursor, diffuses through water channels into the fibrin clot. There it is responsible for the fibrinolysis. Tissue plasminogen activator (t-PA), which is released from the vascular endothelium, converts plasminogen to plasmin. Plasminogen binds to the lysine residues of fibrin, where it is converted to plasmin by t-PA, which simultaneously binds to fibrin.

Plasmin, mainly, is active when bound to fibrin. When it is free in plasma, it is rapidly inactivated by α2-antiplasmin. Plasmin seems to be the central antagonist of coagulation. Apart from cleaving fibrin, it also impairs other processes in hemostasis (degradation of cofactor Va and VIIIa, proteolysis of platelet receptors, consumption of α2-antiplasmin, and degradation of fibrinogen).

The role of fibrinolysis in blood management

A variety of procedures and conditions are associated with an increased fibrinolysis or the presence of plasminogen activators. The use of a tourniquet for surgery leads to the local activation of fibrinolysis, which may increase postoperative blood loss. During liver transplantation, there is a time period during which the body does not have a functioning liver synthesis and clearance of metabolites (anhepatic phase). Fibrinolysis is increased due to the anhepatic phase. Many body compartments contain naturally occurring plasminogen activators. Among them are the urine and the mucosa in the urinary tract, the cervical tissue, the iris and the choroid, as well as the gastrointestinal tract including the mouth and saliva. Placental abruption activates the fibrinolytic system as well as the lack of C1-esterase inhibitor, as is the case in hereditary angioneurotic edema. Surgery in all these areas may benefit from the use of antifibrinolytics to reduce bleeding.

Patients undergoing a cardiac procedure with cardiopulmonary bypass show signs of increased coagulation and fibrinolysis, which are stimulated not only by the surgery itself, but also by the use of the bypass machine. This activation leads to the consumption of clotting factors, which may lead to excessive postoperative bleeding. In cardiac surgery, the use of an antifibrinolytic agent seems to improve this condition by at least preventing accelerated clot lysis.

Aprotinin

Aprotinin is a natural serine protease inhibitor. It occurs in bovine lungs. Such lungs are the source for drug production.

The mechanisms of action of aprotinin are not completely identified. It is known, however, that it reversibly forms enzyme–drug complexes with enzymes carrying a serine site. Many enzymes that play roles in the process of coagulation, fibrinolysis, and inflammation carry such serine sites, e.g., trypsin, plasmin, and kallikrein. Therefore, aprotinin prevents the plasmin-mediated fibrinolysis. It inhibits the contact activation of blood components (especially important in areas where blood is in contact with foreign material for a prolonged time). Aprotinin preserves the adhesive glycoproteins in the platelet membrane (glycoprotein GPIb). This makes the platelets resistant to damage from increased plasmin levels and mechanical injury. Additionally, aprotinin attenuates the heparin-induced platelet dysfunction. The net effect is that fibrinolysis and the turnover of coagulation factors are decreased. Aprotinin also has anti-inflammatory and antioxidant properties as well as a weak anticoagulant effect.

Aprotinin given orally is quickly degraded. Therefore, the parenteral route has to be used, typically the intravenous one. After injection, aprotinin distributes rapidly into the extracellular space. After distribution, it has a plasma half-life of 150 minutes. Aprotinin is cleared by the kidneys and reabsorbed in the proximal tubuli. Lysosomal enzymes slowly degrade aprotinin. Aprotinin has a low toxicity and even large doses are well tolerated. Until recently, the concern about increased thrombosis after administration of aprotinin was not confirmed in studies. Neither myocardial infarction rate, incidence of deep vein thrombosis, graft occlusion, nor mortality after cardiac surgery were shown to increase after aprotinin administration [4]. However, a recent study strongly suggests that aprotinin use is associated with renal failure, myocardial infarction, heart failure, stroke, and encephalopathy in patients who underwent cardiac surgery [5]. Incidences of hypersensitivity occur in 0.1–0.6% of patients treated with aprotinin and seem to happen more often in patients with repeated exposure to the drug (especially when the drug is repeated within a 6-month period) [6].

Units of aprotinin
1 mg = 0.15 µmol
1 mg = 7.143 KIU
KIU = kallikrein inactivator/inhibitor unit

Several dose regimen of aprotinin have been reported. The most commonly used regimen for heart surgery is the high-dose regimen, occasionally called Hammersmith high-dose regimen. It consists of a loading dose of 280 mg (= 2 million KIU), 280 mg added to the cardiopulmonary bypass prime, and an infusion of 70 mg/h for the duration of the operation. Lower dosages were also tried, commonly half of the respective doses of the Hammersmith regimen. Conventional high doses of aprotinin are slightly more effective in reducing transfusions in cardiac patients compared with low-dose regimen [7]. High-dose regimens are used to inhibit kallikrein and plasmin and thereby attenuate the inflammatory effects. Low-dose regimens are used to lower costs but are not able to achieve the full anti-inflammatory effects.

Aprotinin was extensively studied in cardiac surgery. It was shown to significantly reduce blood loss (33–66%), transfusions (31–85%), and thorax drainage volume [4]. It has also been successfully used in patients who have to undergo surgery despite being on antiplatelet therapy such as clopidogrel and aspirin. Instead of stopping the medications, they can be continued when aprotinin is given. Under such circumstances, aprotinin reduces bleeding and transfusions as well [8]. Compared to lysine analogues (see below), aprotinin was slightly more effective to reduce transfusions in cardiac surgery [7].

After cardiac indications [9], noncardiac surgeries were also evaluated regarding the use of aprotinin in order to reduce blood loss and exposure to donor blood. Patients undergoing hip, spine, and other major orthopedic surgery benefited from aprotinin [10]. The transfusion frequency was reduced [11–13]. Also, in patients undergoing liver transplantation, aprotinin was used. Large doses of the drug (according to the Hammersmith high-dose regimen) were not more effective in reducing transfusions than was a low-dose regimen, consisting of 500000 KIU, followed by an infusion of 150000 KIU/h [14]. Another indication for aprotinin (and other antifibrinolytics) is heavy bleeding after thrombolytic therapy.

There is still debate about the use of aprotinin in patients with a moderate risk to receive allogeneic blood. Compared to other drugs such as lysine analogues, aprotinin is expensive. Aprotinin is typically used in patients at high risk for transfusions, and alternative approaches are used when the risk to bleed extensively is moderate [11].

Tranexamic acid

Tranexamic acid is a synthetic derivative of the amino acid lysine. It is similar to EACA (see below), but binds 6–10 times more potently to plasminogen. Tranexamic acid reversibly blocks lysine-binding sites on plasminogen. The saturation of this site with tranexamic acid prevents the binding of plasminogen to the surface of fibrin. This delays fibrinolysis.

After intake, tranexamic acid diffuses in the mother's milk and into joints. It can also cross the blood–brain barrier and the placental barrier. Tranexamic acid is generally well tolerated. Seldom, patients complain of nausea and vomiting or orthostatic reactions. The theoretical concern about increased thrombotic events was not confirmed in studies. A rare reaction to the drug is disturbance of color vision. In this event, the drug must be discontinued. To prevent drug-induced hypotension, intravenous application should be slow, not exceeding 100 mg/min.

Tranexamic acid is available as injectable solution, as tablets, and as syrup. An example of possible dosages in various indications is provided in Table 7.1 [15–17]. Since tranexamic acid is excreted primarily by the kidneys, its dosage needs to be reduced in patients with impaired kidney function.

Tranexamic acid is used to reduce perioperative bleeding in patients undergoing a variety of surgeries. Tranexamic acid was shown to reduce postoperative blood loss, e.g., via mediastinal drains, and the red cell

Table 7.1 Dose recommendations for tranexamic acid.

Indication	Dosage
Local fibrinolysis	500 mg–1 g i.v.: 3×/day or 1.0–1.5 g p.o.: 2–3×/day
General fibrinolysis	Single dose of 1 g or 10 mg/kg i.v.
Patients undergoing cardiopulmonary bypass	10 mg/kg before bypass and infusion of 1 mg/(kg h) afterward or 10 g i.v. over 20 min as a single shot before sternotomy 30 mg/kg after induction of anesthesia and same dose added to the prime solution of cardiopulmonary bypass 15 mg/kg after systemic heparinization followed by an infusion of 1 mg/(kg h) until the end of the surgery
Upper gastrointestinal bleeding	1.5 g 3×/day to 1 g 6×/day for 5–7 days; first i.v., then p.o.
Patients with hemophilia for oral surgery	1–1.5 g 3×/day
Patients under oral anticoagulants for oral surgery	4.8–5.0% mouthwash used for 2 min 4×/day for 7 days
Transurethral prostatectomy	6–12 g p.o. daily for 4 days
Liver transplantation	40 mg/(kg h) as i.v. infusion
Menorrhagia	1–1.5 g p.o. 3–4×/day for 3–4 days
Hereditary angioneurotic edema	1.5 g p.o. 3×/day
Acute promyeloic leukemia	4–8 g p.o. in 3–4 doses/day

p.o., per os; i.v., intravenous.

transfusions [15, 18] in cardiac surgery. Patients undergoing other surgeries such as total knee [19] and hip [20] arthroplasty, spinal surgery [21, 22], oral surgery [23, 24], transurethral prostatectomy, and liver transplantation [25] also benefited from tranexamic acid. Also in gynecological patients for cervix conizatio or those suffering from blood loss due to menorrhagia or placental abruption, tranexamic acid proved beneficial by reducing blood loss. Tranexamic acid can also reduce the rebleeding rate in a variety of conditions, such as intracranial bleeding [26], ocular trauma, and upper gastrointestinal hemorrhage [27]. Tranexamic acid is also effective in reducing the number and severity of attacks in patients with hereditary angioedema. Both, adult and pediatric patients can be treated with tranexamic acid.

Practice tip

Two tablets of tranexamic acid (= 1 g) can be easily given orally before surgery with anticipated major blood loss [28]. This is a simple means to reduce blood loss in a variety of settings. Suggesting this measure of blood conservation may help a newcomer to see that blood management is indeed simple.

Tranexamic acid can also be combined with desmopressin, e.g., in patients with vWD or in other conditions that warrant maximal enhancement of hemostasis. Tranexamic acid is contraindicated in hemorrhages of the upper urinary tract because of the risk of clotting in the urinary system.

ε-Aminocaproic acid

ε-Aminocaproic acid (EACA) is another lysine analogue used as an antifibrinolytic agent. It mainly inhibits plasminogen activators and has a slight antiplasmin activity. The mechanism by which EACA treats bleeding in thrombocytopenic patients is not known.

When there is a fibrinolytic component to the bleeding of a patient, EACA can be used successfully. Such has been observed in cardiac surgery with or without cardiopulmonary bypass, abruptio placentae, liver cirrhosis, surgery in the urinary tract (prostatectomy, nephrectomy), and hematuria due to severe trauma, shock, or anoxia. EACA was also successfully used in bleeding patients with thrombocytopenia due to immune and nonimmune processes. It has been used in bleeding thrombocytopenic patients with hemophilia, aplastic anemia, or acute leukemia, as well as in patients with Kasabach–Merritt syndrome [29].

EACA can be given orally or intravenously. It is taken up rapidly from the gastrointestinal tract. It distributes in the extravascular and intravascular compartments and diffuses into red cells and tissues. The drug is excreted with the urine. The intravenous standard dose is 0.1 g/kg administered over 30–60 minutes (or a loading dose of 5 g), followed by 8–24 g/day or 1 g every 4 hours. When the bleeding ceases, 1 g is usually given every 6 hours. The same dose regimen is used when the patient is able to take the drug per os.

Side effects of EACA are rare. Nasal stuffiness, abdominal complaints with nausea and diarrhea, headaches, allergic reactions, dizziness, and arrhythmias are among them.

If given rapidly intravenously, hypotension and bradycardia can occur. A syndrome characterized by myopathy and necrosis of muscle fibers has been described in some patients. If it occurs, the drug has to be stopped for the symptoms to disappear. However, on reexposure, the same usually happens again.

p-Aminomethylbenzoic acid

A third lysine derivative is *p*-aminomethylbenzoic acid (PAMBA) [30–33]. Saturation of the lysine-binding sites of plasminogen with this inhibitor displaces plasminogen from the fibrin surface. Thereby, PAMBA inhibits fibrinolysis [34]. On a molar basis, tranexamic acid is twice as potent as PAMBA.

There is not much literature that deals with the role of PAMBA in the transfusion arena. The scarce information that can be gathered is that PAMBA may be effective in reducing rebleeding after subarachnoidal hemorrhage when given intrathecally [35–37]. It has also been used for perioperative and peripartum bleeding [38, 39]. No valid claim can be made about PAMBA's ability to reduce a patient's exposure to blood products.

Desmopressin

Desmopressin (also called 1-deamino-8-D-arginine vasopressin or DDAVP) is a synthetic analogue of the natural antidiuretic hormone L-arginine vasopressin which has been altered so that the plasma half-life is prolonged. DDAVP binds to vasopressin receptors of the V2 type, located in the renal tubule and the endothelium. It releases the content of endogenous storage sites for the clotting factors (e.g., the Weibel–Palade bodies, which are the secretory granules of the endothelium, and the sinusoid liver endothelia cells). Consequently, the blood levels of vWF, FVIII, and t-PA increase. This effect is observed in factor-deficient patients as well as in healthy individuals. For some coagulation factor deficiencies—vWD and hemophilia A—DDAVP could be likened to an autologous replacement therapy. The expected release of vWF and FVIII depends on the baseline level of the patient and his/her individual response to the drug. The factor levels usually increase three to five times baseline (range: 1.5–20.0 times) [2]. Platelet reactivity and adhesiveness, presumably due to the release of vWF, glycoprotein Ib/IX, and other, yet unknown mechanisms, increase as well [40]. DDAVP also has a fibrinolytic effect (by the release of t-PA) and is therefore sometimes administered in association with an antifibrinolytic drug, such as ε-aminocaproic acid [41] or tranexamic acid. Whether this is necessary or not is controversial, since the released t-PA is rapidly complexed and supposedly does not produce fibrinolysis in blood [2]. Occasionally, DDAVP is also given for thromboprophylaxis [42].

DDAVP is a safe and affordable therapy for patients with vWD [43–45]. This disease is characterized by the lack or malfunctioning of von Willebrand factor. Three main types of vWD were discovered. Type 1 is the most common with 80% of all cases. Most patients with type 1 vWD respond favorably to DDAVP. In contrast, type 2 patients have a functional abnormality of vWF which is not correctable by desmopressin. However, there are reports of patients with type 2 A vWD who responded with a shortened bleeding time to DDAVP. In a subtype of type 2 vWD, vWD type 2B, DDAVP is considered to be contraindicated, because release of the abnormal vWF can cause platelet aggregation and thrombocytopenia. This, however, is not unanimously agreed upon, since some patients with vWD type 2B respond favorably to the drug [2]. Patients with vWD type 3 do not have any vWF and, therefore, do not respond to DDAVP with a release of vWF.

DDAVP also releases FVIII into the bloodstream. Therefore, hemophiliacs with hemophilia A also benefit from the use of DDAVP. Mild to moderate cases can be successfully treated with this drug rather than with blood-derived or recombinant clotting factors.

The response to DDAVP administration in hemophilia A and vWD differs from patient to patient, but is consistent over time. This finding can be used when a test dose is given to patients who potentially benefit from DDAVP. The magnitude of the increase of the factor under investigation (vWF, FVIII) can also be observed in subsequent administrations, especially when time has elapsed between the test dose and the therapeutic dose [46].

Patients with a variety of platelet disorders respond favorably to the use of DDAVP, namely, by an increase of platelet adhesiveness. Congenital defects of the platelets (e.g., in Bernard–Soulier's syndrome, but not Glanzmann's thrombasthenia) can be treated with DDAVP. Patients with acquired platelet defects can be treated with DDAVP instead of platelet transfusions [47]. DDAVP has been used in bleeding due to drug-induced platelet dysfunctions such as those caused by aspirin, dextran [42], ticlopidin, or heparin [46]. Patients with platelet dysfunction due to uremia or liver cirrhosis (with usually normal to high levels of FVIII or vWF) [48] are also good candidates for DDAVP treatment.

Thrombocytopenic bleeding also responds to desmopressin [49]. The mechanism of action of DDAVP in this setting is not clear. Probably an increase in platelet adhesiveness in the remaining platelets contributes to the effect. DDAVP also shortens bleeding time in patients with isolated and unexplained prolongations of their bleeding time [2].

It has been claimed that desmopressin also reduces blood loss and the use of transfusions in patients without congenital platelet abnormalities. However, most of the available studies were unable to demonstrate a significant reduction of blood loss or transfusions in patients with uncomplicated cardiac surgery and in patients without congenital or acquired platelet defects [7, 46]. Cardiac surgery patients benefited from DDAVP only if they had such platelet defects, either due to drugs or prolonged cardiopulmonary bypass [50].

Desmopressin is available as an injectable pharmaceutical form for intravenous or subcutaneous administration, as well as a spray or liquid formulation for intranasal use. For home treatment, e.g., women with menorrhagia due to vWD, the intranasal route is the most convenient. Two intranasal "standard puffs" of a total of 300 μg DDAVP is all that is needed to reduce blood loss due to menorrhagia. If needed, the spray can be used repeatedly, typically after an 8–12 hour interval. Even a low dose of 10–20 μg DDAVP spray seems to be effective, as shown in uremic children [51]. In the perioperative phase, intravenous administration is recommended. The intravenous route provides slightly better results than the intranasal route. An intravenous or subcutaneous dose of 0.3 μg/kg achieves optimal results in the majority of patients. Perioperatively, DDAVP should be given at least twice, the second dose administered 6–8 hours after the first one.

A reported effect of DDAVP is tachyphylaxis, i.e., a reduced response to treatment when repeated in short succession. However, Lethagen [46] claims: "In the clinical use of desmopressin, tachyphylaxis is, . . . rarely a problem, even if prolonged treatment is given." When DDAVP is given three to four times per 24 hours, the response of FVIII is reduced by about 30% [2].

Desmopressin is a safe drug. Serious side effects are rare. Facial flushing and mild lightheadedness are commonly observed [41]. DDAVP does not exert the vasopressive action of its mother substance vasopressin, but has an antidiuretic effect that continues for about 24 hours after the last administered dose. Patients should be advised to reduce their water intake, especially when repeated doses are needed. Although there are reports of arterial thrombosis in patients treated with DDAVP, studies and a metaanalysis did not show an increased risk of arterial thrombosis after administration of the drug [52].

Table 7.2 Vitamin K complex.

Vitamin K	Description
K_1: Phylloquinone (phytonadione, phytonactone)	Natural form, found in green plants, part of healthy diet
K_2: Menaquinone (group of menaquinones)	Natural form, synthesized by intestinal bacteria
K_3: Menadione (menodoine/ menaphthone)	Synthetically derived, used as dietary supplements, esp. for babies, lipid-soluble
K_4: Menadiol (Acetomenaphthone and others)	Synthetically derived, water-soluble dietary supplements for farm animals, food preservatives
K_{5-9}, K-S, MK etc.	Synthetically derived, dietary supplements for farm animals, food preservatives

Vitamins of the K-group

Vitamin K is the collective term for different compounds with a common naphthoquinone ring structure and different side chains (Table 7.2).

Vitamins K_1, K_2, and K_3 are the only ones used for human therapy. Upon administration, vitamin K_1 is converted to vitamin K_2. Vitamin K_1 has the quickest onset of action, the most prolonged duration, and is the most potent of all the Vitamin K forms.

The natural forms of vitamin K are lipid-soluble and are stored in the liver. Healthy adults need at least 65–80 µg of vitamin K per day. Children need about one-third of the adult requirements. Approximately half of the vitamin K requirements needed by humans is produced by intestinal bacteria. The other half is taken up in a healthy diet. The excretion of absorbed vitamin K occurs mainly in the feces, but some is also excreted in the urine.

Proteins involved in the coagulation process undergo posttranslational changes. Certain glutamate molecules are γ-carboxylated and so the factors finally carry γ-carboxyglutamate residues. The posttranslational γ-carboxylation of the coagulation factors II (prothrombin), VII (proconvertin), IX (Christmas factor), X (Stuart–Prower factor), and the anticoagulant proteins C, S, and Z depends on the presence of vitamin K. If the γ-carboxyglutamate is missing, coagulation factors are synthesized, but lack the carboxy-groups which are essential for the interaction between coagulation factors and calcium. Such deficient factors are called des-γ-carboxy

molecules or PIVKA (proteins induced by vitamin K absence). By a yet unknown mechanism, vitamin K also influences platelet aggregation. In vitamin K deficiency, the prothrombin time and the activated partial thromboplastin time are prolonged.

Vitamin K is the prophylaxis of choice to prevent hemorrhagic disease of the newborns. Coagulation factors do not cross the placenta barrier and have to be synthesized by the baby itself. During normal gestation, the level of vitamin K-dependent coagulation factors is about half that of the adult level, while the other factors reach adult level at birth. After birth, vitamin K provided by mother's milk is marginally sufficient. In case of increased need, in case of prematurity or if the mother took drugs that interfere with vitamin K metabolism (antibiotics, anticonvulsants, tuberculostatics, vitamin K antagonists), the level of vitamin K-dependent factors may be insufficient for the baby. This may result in gross hemorrhage, a condition easily preventable by peripartal vitamin K therapy. Vitamin K can be given either to the child or to the expectant mother [53]. The baby is usually administered 1.0 mg of the lipid-soluble form orally or intramuscularly. This dose may even be excessive, since 1–5 µg have been shown to be sufficient [54].

Several other conditions may cause a lack of vitamin K and its dependent factors. Among the common ones are treatment with vitamin K antagonists, such as warfarin, and the absolute lack of vitamin K due to gastrointestinal disturbances, inadequate diet, impaired lipid absorption, malabsorption, and excess intake of fat-soluble vitamins and salicylates. In their effort to rid the body of foreign bacteria, antibiotics may also destroy the normal intestinal flora needed for vitamin K synthesis, causing a deficiency of the vitamin.

Therapeutic doses of vitamin K rapidly normalize the hemostatic disorder, given the liver can provide the factors. The response is so rapid that even emergency surgery can be performed when patients present with a coagulation disturbance due to a lack vitamin K. Traditionally, fresh frozen plasma was used to provide the needed factors. However, in many cases vitamin K serves the same purpose. Even if fresh frozen plasma is deemed necessary, vitamin K has to be given to correct the underlying problem.

Given a normal or residual liver function, vitamin K-dependent coagulation factors can be synthesized, once the vitamin is given. For adults, the vitamin K dose in case of bleeding due to a lack of vitamin K-dependent factors is 2.5–10 mg. If a more rapid response is needed, 10–20 mg (up to 50 mg) may be administered. The response to the vitamin K is fairly rapid and clinical bleeding may subside quickly. However, a measurable improvement in the prothrombin time takes at least 2 hours.

Vitamin K can be given intravenously, intramuscularly, subcutaneously, or orally. In case of an emergency, the intravenous route is preferred [55]. In other cases, oral administration may be sufficient and may even be superior to the subcutaneous route [56].

Side effects of vitamin K depend on the preparation given. Natural vitamins K_1 and K_2 seem to cause much less side effects than the synthetic vitamin K_3. A severe hemolytic anemia is occasionally observed in newborns, but not in adults. This reaction may be due to overdosing which occurred in babies who were given up to 80 mg/kg, whereas the effective prophylactic dose is less than 1.0 mg/kg. The water-soluble vitamin K_3 seems to have a greater ability to induce hemolysis than the natural, lipid-soluble vitamin K_1. In addition, liver damage, deafness, and severe neurological problems, including retardation in infants have been reported after vitamin K_3 therapy. Care must be taken with intravenous injections of vitamin K, since they can cause facial flushing, excessive perspiration, chest tightness, cyanosis, and shock.

Conjugated estrogens and other hormones

It is well known that estrogens increase the risk of thrombotic events. It was also observed that some women with vWD showed a marked improvement in their bleeding diathesis when pregnant or when taking contraceptives. Bleeding resumed once the baby was born or contraception discontinued. Obviously, estrogens have an impact on the coagulation system.

Conjugated estrogens increase the level of prothrombin and factors VII, VIII, IX, X, and decrease fibrinolysis and the level of antithrombin III. Additionally, they increase the norepinephrine-induced platelet aggregability. Estrogens also have a weak anabolic effect.

Conjugated estrogens can be given intravenously, intramuscularly, or orally. They are rapidly absorbed from the gastrointestinal tract. Estrogens are widely distributed in the body and moderately bound to plasma proteins. They are metabolized and inactivated primarily in the liver and eliminated in the urine. Some estrogens are excreted into the bile; however, they are reabsorbed by the intestine and returned to the liver.

Side effects of a short-term course of conjugated estrogens are uncommon. When the drug is given only for about 5–7 days, hormonal activity is negligible. When given for a prolonged time, gallbladder disease, thromboembolic events, hepatic adenoma, elevated blood pressure, glucose intolerance, hypercalcemia, and other symptoms typically occurring in hormonal therapy (increased water retention, changed skin pigmentation, changes in sexual function, depression, etc.) develop.

Abnormal uterine bleeding due to hormonal imbalance in the absence of organic pathology is the typical indication for conjugated estrogens in blood management. One 25-mg injection, intravenously or intramuscularly, may be sufficient. The intravenous route is preferred when a rapid response is needed. Repeated doses every 6–12 hours can be administered, if necessary.

Case reports have shown that patients with vWD benefit from oral contraception or another form of estrogen therapy [57], i.e., control of postmenopausal symptoms. Such patients also benefit from a short course of estrogens given perioperatively, reducing the use of allogeneic blood products. Another potential area for estrogen therapy is in patients with end-stage liver disease with coagulation abnormalities.

Conjugated estrogens shorten prolonged bleeding time and reduce bleeding in patients with uremia. The mechanism of action is unknown. In uremic patients, single daily infusions of 0.6 mg/kg for 4–5 days shorten the bleeding time for at least 2 weeks. Given orally, 50 mg of conjugated estrogens shorten the bleeding time after about 7 days [58]. The effect of the conjugated estrogens lasts 10–15 days [2] and therefore makes the drug ideal when long-term hemostasis needs to be achieved [59]. In uremia, conjugated estrogens are a long-acting alternative to DDAVP.

Other hormones have been used in blood management. As multiple case reports demonstrate, patients with bleeding due to gastrointestinal vascular abnormalities, Osler–Rendu–Weber disease, and angiodysplasia benefited from a certain combination of estrogens and progesterone. Actually, ethynylestradiol (30 mg) and norethisterone (1.0–1.5 mg/day) decreased or eliminated blood transfusions in a subset population of patients [60–62].

Other hemostatic drugs

The above-mentioned drugs are commonly used (Table 7.3) [2, 7, 11–13, 15, 17, 18, 21, 23–25, 29, 42, 46, 48, 49, 54, 63–77]. In addition to them, a great variety of other hemostatic drugs have been advocated over the years [78]. Quite a few of them are still in clinical use. Extensive efficacy and safety studies are lacking for most of them. The following points outline some of the distinct features of such drugs.

Table 7.3 What is proven and what is recommended.

Drug	Fields in which reduction of transfusions was shown	Other settings in which the drug is recommended
Aprotinin	Cardiac surgery in patients with preoperative aspirin; cardiac surgery in general; hip and major orthopedic surgery; pediatric spinal surgery	Liver transplantation
Tranexamic acid	Cardiac surgery in general; knee arthroplasty; liver transplantation; hip arthroplasty; spinal surgery	Hyperfibrinolytic disseminated intravascular coagulation; oral surgery, also in patients on oral anticoagulants or with hemophilia; transurethral prostatectomy; upper gastrointestinal bleeding; menorrhagia, bleeding after placental abruptio and cervix conization, bleeding after cesarean section; ocular hemorrhage after traumatic hyphema; hereditary angioedema; rebleeding after subarachnoidal hemorrhage; acute promyeloic leukemia; bleeding patients with factor XI deficiency (in conjunction with rhFVIIa)
EACA	Cardiac surgery in general	Hemophilia, aplastic anemia, or acute leukemia with thrombocytopenia, Kasabach–Merritt syndrome, spinal fusion, hip arthroplasty, hyperfibrinolysis in liver cirrhosis.
DDAVP	Cardiac surgery in patients with preoperative aspirin or other nonsteroidal antirheumatic drugs; patients for cardiac surgery with expected major blood loss and confirmed platelet abnormality	Patients with congenital platelet disorders, e.g., platelet TxA2 receptor abnormality and vWD; drug-induced platelet disorders causing bleeding (aspirin, ticlopidin, heparin, dextran, clopidogrel); thrombocytopenic bleeding due to immune and nonimmune causes; bleeding due to cirrhosis.
Vitamins of the K-group	Patients with a lack of vitamin K	Hemorrhagic disease of the newborn; patients with liver disease lacking vitamin K-dependent factors.
Conjugated estrogens	Liver transplantation	Uremic coagulopathy; dysfunctional uterine bleeding.

EACA, ε-aminocaproic acid; DDAVP, 1-deamino-8-D-arginine vasopressin; rhFVIIa, recombinant human factor VIIa; vWD, von Willebrand's disease.

1 *Tissue extracts* have a thromboplastin-like action. After intravenous administration, they may accelerate coagulation. Extracts from animal brain, for instance, have been used for this purpose.

2 *Oxalic and malonic acid* were once proposed as hemostatic agents, but they were never extensively clinically tested.

3 *Tetragalacturonic acid ester* was obtained from apple pectin. It was recommended for topical and oral use as a hemostatic agent. This substance may inhibit fibrinolysis, but clinical trials have not been performed.

4 *Naphthionine* is related to Congo red. It was claimed to be useful in normal and thrombocytopenic patients. The mechanism of action is supposed to be the shifting of the isoelectric point of fibrinogen, thereby favoring the gel state.

5 *Ethamsylate* is also a derivative of Congo red. Although its mode of action is still vaguely defined, it seems to increase platelet adhesiveness and capillary resistance. It may also have an antihyaluronidase activity and may inhibit prostacyclin. Clinical trials propose its use in menorrhagia as well as in bleeding after dental extraction, adenotonsillectomy, and transurethral prostatectomy.

6 *Naftazone* was shown to reduce the use of transfusions in patients undergoing prostatectomy. However, there are only a limited number of clinical trials to support its use.

7 *Adrenochrome, carbazochrome*: Adrenochrome is a derivative of adrenaline. When complexed with a salicylate, it increases its stability (carbazochrome). It was claimed to reduce blood loss, but the evidence is sparse.

Local hemostatic agents

Local hemostasis depends on a variety of factors and processes which, under physiological conditions, provide a stepwise approach to tissue repair. Vasoconstriction is an early mechanism to stop bleeding. Activated platelets contribute to this vasoconstriction by releasing vasoactive compounds at the site of injury. Thereupon, vessels constrict and blood flow is reduced. Platelets activated at the site of tissue injury contribute many more hemostyptic effects. They adhere to injured vessels where they begin to form a physical barrier to blood flow. They also change their outer membrane in a way to facilitate the formation of a blood clot. They also release compounds that activate plasmatic clotting, including calcium ions. Finally, thrombin is generated which cleaves fibrinogen to fibrin fibers, the latter of which are stabilized by factor XIII. The interaction of platelets, tissue components, red cells, and plasmatic components of the clotting process finally forms a stable clot and promotes tissue healing. Tissue healing is accompanied by changes in vessel structures. Bigger ones are often recanalized by proteolyzing the blood clot. Smaller ones obliterate and growth factors promote the vascularization with new vessels in the repaired tissue.

Chemical local hemostatic agents are valuable adjuncts to the physical means of hemostasis. The use of physical means sometimes depends on visualization of distinct bleeding vessels to ligate them. Other physical means for hemostasis use heat to cauterize vessels. This heat may spread sideward and be detrimental to delicate tissues such as neural structures. While chemical agents to stop bleeding are rarely effective in brisk bleeding from big vessels, they are very effective in stopping bleeding from small venous and capillary vessels and from the surface of parenchymatous structures where suturing is difficult. Chemical hemostatic agents may also be effective when a coagulopathic patient is unable to provide for hemostasis. Chemical hemostatic agents can be used in addition to physical means, hence being useful even when brisk bleeding occurs. As for all medical treatments, the success of hemostasis and the avoidance of side effects of hemostatic agents depends on the expertise of the clinicians and their in-depth knowledge of the abilities and potential complications of the agents used.

All of the below-mentioned agents have been used with the intent to reduce bleeding. Empirically, they indeed do so. However, randomized controlled trials are absent for the majority of the discussed agents. While many of the agents were shown to have a hemostatic effect, only a minority of them have been shown to reduce patient exposure to blood transfusions [79–90] (Table 7.4).

Tissue adhesives and other agents accelerating clot formation locally

Tissue adhesives, also referred to as tissue glues, are a heterogenous group of compounds that all have the ability to stick to tissues and to seal them, either by their own action or by promoting physiological processes. In doing so, they

Table 7.4 The effects of tissue adhesives on blood loss and use of transfusions.

Field of use	Tissue adhesives	Effect on blood loss and use of transfusions
Cardiothoracic surgery	Fibrin sealant	Reduces postoperative blood loss
Aortic dissection	Fibrin sealant	Blood loss reduced
Cardiac surgery	Fibrin spray	Reduces bleeding
Femoral artery cardiac catheterizations	Fibrin sealant given per sheath at the end of procedure (animal study)	Reduces bleeding
Cardiac surgery in pediatrics	Fibrin sealant	Reduces bleeding and transfusions
Hepatic surgery	Microcrystalline collagen powder, fibrin glue	Reduces bleeding
Bleeding gastroduodenal ulcers	Fibrin sealant vs. polidocanol	Reduces bleeding
Bone bleeding	Gelatin foam paste, gelatin sponge with thrombin, microfibrillar collagen	Reduces bleeding
Knee replacement	Fibrin spray applied	Reduces blood loss and transfusions
Spinal instrumentation	Fibrin glue	Reduces blood loss, no patients who received fibrin glue was transfused
Burns	Fibrin sealant	Eliminated transfusions

can also promote wound healing, seal tissues to prevent leakage of tissue fluids or air, support sutures, and deliver drugs (e.g., chemotherapeutics, antibiotics) to the target tissues. Above all, they can promote hemostasis.

Fibrin sealants

Probably the most commonly used tissue adhesives are fibrin sealants. They mimic the natural process of clotting by providing the needed physiological material for clot formation. This makes fibrin sealants biodegradable; that is, it is broken down by fibrinolysis. The two main components of fibrin glues are thrombin and fibrinogen. Thrombin may be derived from human plasma or bovine blood. Fibrinogen is typically taken from human blood. In addition to these two main components, factor XIII (for added clot strength), calcium (for the clotting process itself), and antifibrinolytics (for prevention of early clot lysis) may be added. The more fibrinogen is found in glue, the higher the tensile strength. The more thrombin is found, the more rapid is the clot formation.

Fibrin-based tissue adhesives have a very low complication rate. They are biocompatible and do not cause local irritation, inflammation, or foreign body reactions. Occasionally, allergic reactions to one of its ingredients have been described. Bovine thrombin rarely causes immunologic complications. While most of these complications are of allergic origin, they may also result in a coagulopathy. In this case, neutralizing antibodies to human factor V, which have been formed after exposure to bovine thrombin, are the cause of coagulopathy. Another kind of side effect of fibrin glues is the transmission of infectious agents. Since commercial fibrin sealants are made from allogeneic blood, they have been shown to transmit diseases. To date, however, the only published complications were a series of parvovirus B19 infections. Since the source plasma for fibrin adhesive production is treated by several virus inactivation steps, the risk of infection with HIV and hepatitis viruses is almost nonexistent.

Fibrin and thrombin when used together, effectively and rapidly promote hemostasis. However, this also brings a challenge since as soon as both agents mix, they clot. Delivery systems are needed that mix those agents where the adhesive is expected to form the clot. Double-barrel syringes are typically used when commercial preparations are applied. It is also possible to attach a spray mechanism to this syringe. When large surfaces are to be sprayed, fibrinogen may be sprayed first, followed by thrombin. When no double-barrel syringe is available, the two components

of the fibrin sealant can also be attached to one of the ports of a double-lumen central line, and the tip of the line is placed into the wound.

Commercially available fibrin sealants made from donor blood are rather consistent in their action. They have predictable levels of ingredients, and the levels are often supranormal. In contrast, when the glue is self-made, e.g., from cryoprecipitate or from autologous blood prior to surgery, the clotting factor levels are variable and not as highly concentrated. Nevertheless, autologous glue may be an attractive alternative to avoid disease transmission and immunologic reactions. Besides, it may be the only sealant available in countries where they are not permitted or otherwise not available. In the future, recombinant fibrinogen and thrombin may eliminate the use of allogeneic blood products altogether.

Indications for the use of fibrin sealants are diverse, including bleeding in cardiac surgery, parenchymatous organs (liver and spleen surgery), bleeding gastroduodenal ulcers, burns, and many other situations. Fibrin glue is also useful in coagulopathic patients with hemophilia A, B, von Willebrand syndrome, anticoagulant therapy, etc., since it provides for the missing clotting factors [91]. While there are not many high-quality studies of fibrin sealants and their effectiveness to reduce blood transfusions, a Cochrane metaanalysis strongly suggests that fibrin glue reduces patient exposure to allogeneic blood [92]. It was also suggested that hemophiliac patients are not exposed to as many clotting factor concentrates when fibrin glue is used.

Albumin-based compounds

Another group of tissue adhesives is made of albumin and a glue-like substance. There are a handful of variants to them: gelatin-resorcinol-formaldehyde glue, gelatin-resorcinol-formaldehyde-glutaraldehyde glue, and glutaraldehyde glue. Albumin-based tissue sealants are biodegradable. Compared with fibrin sealants, their hemostatic activity is weaker. However, these enhance fibroblastic proliferation and thus produce greater tensile strength than fibrin sealants. Therefore, these are mainly used where tissues need strength, as in aortic dissection surgery.

Bone wax

Bone wax is a mix of beeswax and Vaseline. It melts slightly when it comes into contact with the warm hand of the surgeon. Bone wax can be applied to bleeding bones, and there it stops blood flow by being a mechanical barrier. Bone wax is an inert substance and is not absorbed. It therefore hinders the healing of bones and should not be used when two bone parts are expected to fuse. Bone wax can also cause foreign body reactions. It should be used only for the time needed to achieve hemostasis and excess wax must be removed. It must not be used for infected wounds.

Cyanoacrylates

Cyanoacrylates are a group of compounds that have strong tissue adhesive properties. However, they are not biodegradable and their use is akin to the implantation of a foreign body. They can provoke immunologic and inflammatory responses, including tissue necrosis. They may even be cancerogenic. These adhesives are almost exclusively used to approximate skin. Since they are bacteriostatic, they can also be used in dental procedures. However, they should not be used internally.

Hydrogels

Hydrogels mainly are based on polyethylene glycol polymers. These agents are water soluble and biodegradable. Some of their brands need to be activated by light and so they are not useful for urgent hemostasis.

Gelatin

Gelatin is an animal product that is made from animal skin. The product is boiled and supplied as a paste or sponge. It can be whipped foamy and can be dried into a spongy substance. It is also available as powder. When applied alone, it works as a matrix for coagulation. When combined with agents such as thrombin, it actively promotes clot formation.

Gelatin sticks readily to tissues. It can easily be applied with wet pads. However, it is also easily dislodged when soaked in blood. When hemostasis is achieved, residual material should be removed. Since gelatin is resorbable, it is a good alternative to bone wax in sites where fusion is needed.

Gelatin foam has some reported side effects when applied to neuronal tissues, such as inflammatory reactions, paresthesias, pain, and neurological deficiencies. It was reported to induce toxic shock syndrome when used in the nose. Gelatin must not remain in a closed space since it can swell and cause pressure injury to adjacent tissues. Gelatin

also accelerates bacteria growth and therefore must not be used in infected areas.

Collagen

Hemostatic collagen is obtained from the collagen of bovine corium. It is available in various forms, e.g., microfibrillar collagen (MFC) and microcrystalline collagen powder. Collagen serves as the matrix that promotes platelet aggregation. It seems to be effective in heparinized patients, but less so in thrombocytopenia. It readily adheres to the tissues and provides rapid hemostasis. MFC is very sticky, and it is stickier on rubber gloves than on the tissue. Therefore, it must be applied with instruments, and not with gloved hands. It does not swell extensively. Since collagen can increase infection and interferes with the healing process, it should be removed from the surgical site before closure.

Hemostatic collagen can be combined with a variety of other hemostatics to enhance its performance. A mix of collagen and thrombin is available. A composite of MFC and polyethylene glycol has been marketed to treat bone bleeding. It is biodegradable and does not interfere with bone healing.

Oxidized cellulose and oxidized regenerated cellulose

Cellulose is made from wood pulp. During preparation it is formed into a fibrillar material that can be knit into meshes. Cellulose promotes clot formation and hemostasis by mechanical means. It can swell or form a gel. Oxidized cellulose also promotes activation of corpuscular and humoral components of the clotting system. It has a low pH and acts as a caustic. The low pH may be the reason why it works as an antiseptic. This makes oxidized cellulose appropriate for use in infected areas.

Oxidized regenerated cellulose (ORC) should be used dry for maximum hemostasis. It should not be combined with thrombin in order not to interfere with ORC's action. Since it swells, it must not be packed in closed spaces. Bipolar vessel sealing can be used even through ORC layers. After hemostasis is achieved, it can be removed from the wound.

Microporous polysaccharide hemosphere

Microporous polysaccharide hemosphere comes as a powder, which is applied in wounds. It soaks water out of the bleeding wound and concentrates endogenous clotting factors. The powder seems to work only in deep wounds where blood is pooling. When it is applied to heavily bleeding superficial wounds, the blood flow washes the powder away.

Mineral zeolite

As is the case with microporous polysaccharide hemosphere, mineral zeolite powder absorbs liquids in the wound and concentrates clotting factors in the wound, and seems to be effective only in wounds where blood is pooling. Mineral zeolite acts in an exothermic reaction, which increases the temperature in the wound rapidly to 40–42°C. Burns have been reported after its use.

Physics meets chemistry

A smart way to achieve hemostasis is to combine physical and chemical measures. Applying pressure with hemostatic-coated packs adds the physical component of tamponade to the chemical component of clot formation. The packs may either be removed after application and clot formation or remain in situ, given they are absorbable. Such combinations make for a robust hemostatic. They can be applied to major bleeding vessels without impairing blood flow beyond the hemostatic. They can also be applied to bleeding parenchymatous organs. Such hemostatic packs are especially valuable in the preclinical setting [93–96].

A hemostatic pack that has been available for decades is a bandage coated with extremely high concentrations of dry fibrinogen and thrombin. When applied to the wound, it accelerates clot formation. In animal studies, it has proven successful in reducing blood loss and has shown promise clinically. However, it is very expensive. Besides, it has to be handled with care since it breaks easily. That is why it cannot be applied to deep wounds in the prehospital setting.

Another, less expensive hemostatic pack employs chitin or its deacetylated form, chitosan. These agents are derivatives from algae products, which seem to have a vasoconstrictive effect and mobilize clotting factors in the wound. Some evidence supports that a pack with chitin or the more efficacious chitosan may reduce blood loss from trauma [97].

A further dressing uniting chemical and physical means to achieve hemostasis is a dressing with a microporous polyacrylamide core. This core absorbs fluids and has the potential to absorb 1400 times its weight in fluids. Doing so, it expands and turns heavy. When applied to a wound, it creates local pressure to stop the bleeding, and by its absorption of fluids it may accelerate coagulation.

Practical recommendations for the use of tissue adhesives

Choice of the tissue adhesive

Apart from the intrinsic properties of available agents, two major considerations should be taken into account before a suitable tissue adhesive is chosen. The first point to consider is whether the adhesive is needed urgently or not. If it is urgent, preparations that are supplied in frozen form are not suitable since it takes time to thaw them. Autologous glues, which require the patient to be phlebotomized, are also not suitable when there is an emergency. In case of emergency, ready-to-use preparations are indicated. The second point to consider should be the patient's intrinsic ability to form a clot. In coagulopathic patients, tissue adhesives that merely concentrate and accelerate physiological clotting effects are not suitable. In this case, adhesives that exhibit their own clotting ability should be used.

Method of application

Hemostatic agents come in many different forms, i.e., spray, powder, gel, mesh, or wool. Sprays and powders are more suitable for larger areas to be treated. Gels can be precisely targeted and seem not to dislodge easily in wet areas. Meshes and wools are positioned strategically, and the swelling effect can be used to apply pressure to a bleeding spot. Some hemostatic agents need a dry field for application. Since this is sometimes difficult to achieve, prophylactic use is recommended to prevent anticipated bleeding. Prophylactic use of some tissue sealants may allow for completed polymerization of the agent and maximum clot strength before it is challenged by blood flow. For instance, the sealant can be applied to vascular anastomoses before the clamps are released. When the sealant is finally polymerized, the clamps are opened and blood flow can start.

Vasoconstrictors

Mimicking the first physiological step in hemostasis, namely vasoconstriction, is a simple and effective means to reduce blood loss and transfusions. As the gold standard, epinephrine is the agent of choice for hemostatic vasoconstriction. Depending on the mode of application, it is typically used in dilutions of 1:10,000–1:2,000,000.

Other than epinephrin, vasoconstrictors may also achieve hemostatic vasoconstriction, including vasopressin, terlipressin, norepinephrine, and phenylephrine. The agents are either injected locally or are applied directly to the wound, mucosa, or the peritoneum. Sprays, sponges, tamponade material, or glues have served as vectors for the application of the vasoconstrictors. Epinephrine can also be nebulized to treat hemorrhage in the oropharynx [98].

Vasoconstrictors have been very successful in reducing bleeding in burn surgery [99, 100] and in breast surgery [101–103]. In addition, many other minor and major surgeries have used the hemorrhage reduction induced by vasoconstrictors. They have been proven useful in such diverse interventions as pilonidal sinus surgery [104], bone graft harvest [105], bleeding peptic ulcers [106], head and neck surgery [107, 108], gynecological procedures [109], and postpartum hemorrhage [110].

Usually, local vasoconstrictors are simple and safe to use. However, systemic absorption of the drugs may cause cardiovascular, neurological, and immunological side effects (changes in heart rate and blood pressure, cardiac arrhythmias, myocardial infarction, seizures, allergic reactions, etc.).

Miscellaneous topical agents used to stop bleeding

A heterogenous group of agents have been used to stop bleeding locally. Among them are the above-mentioned fibrinolytics. Aprotinin, aminocaproic acid, and tranexamic acid have successfully been used to irrigate bleeding areas, resulting in reduction in bleeding. Such therapy has been shown to be successful in heart surgery [111, 112], spinal surgery, bleeding colitis as an enema, epistaxis, before tonsillectomy and as irrigation for bladder hemorrhage, and after transurethral resection of the prostate. Antifibrinolytics have also been instilled into the pleural cavity to treat hemoptysis. Tranexamic acid as a 5% solution can be used as mouthwash [113] to reduce bleeding after surgery of patients on oral anticoagulants. Hot water has also been proposed to stop bleeding, e.g., in epistaxis [114].

Apart from antifibrinolytics, a variety of other substances have been shown to reduce bleeding. Among them are barium preparations given as enema for diverticular bleeding [115] and aluminum salts for bladder hemorrhage [116]. Also, calcium alginate, silver nitrate, trichloroacetic acid [117], and Monsel's solution (20% ferric subsulfate) [118] have been used to locally stop bleeding. Some of them are caustic; they leave a layer of damaged tissue that stops bleeding.

An increasingly recommended hemostatic agent is formalin. Instillation of the 4% solution is an effective treatment for patients bleeding from hemorrhagic cystitis or proctitis. It has a caustic effect, and therefore, all tissues not bleeding should be protected from the solution. The perineum can be protected by jelly and formalin-soaked sponge sticks can be used to apply the solution directly to the bleeding bowel, preventing spread of the solution more proximally [119, 120]. The procedure is not without complications but may be helpful in selected cases.

Key points of this chapter

• Antifibrinolytics are indicated in patients bleeding from exaggerated fibrinolysis. Some of the antifibrinolytics are also effective in thrombocytopenic bleeding.
• Desmopressin is helpful in bleeding due to many congenital and acquired platelet disorders as well as in thrombocytopenia.
• Vitamin K, not fresh frozen plasma, is the therapeutic of choice in patients with vitamin K deficiency, given that there is sufficient time for the vitamin to be effective and a liver that is able to synthesize the factors.
• There are a wide variety of local hemostatic agents. They act as topical sealants, matrix for endogenous clotting, vasoconstrictors, caustics, or by other mechanisms. All of them can reduce bleeding and some have been shown to reduce the use of transfusions. Maximum benefit results when the health-care practitioner is acquainted with their use.

Questions for review

• What is the role of fibrinolysis in blood management?
• What are the essential and the adjunct ingredients of fibrin sealants?
• What different kinds of tissue sealants are available and what are the indications for their use?
• What agents are available for local hemostasis?

Suggestions for further research

Collect different recipes on how to prepare autologous fibrin sealants. Apart from a patient's blood, what other ingredients are required for the preparation? Which methods are used to prepare fibrin concentrates? How long does it take to prepare autologous sealants?

Exercises and practice cases

Give recommendations for the pharmacological treatment of the following patients. Prescribe one or more drugs you deem beneficial to reduce bleeding. Relate the exact dosing, timing, and route of administration.

1 A 54-year-old patient has been on chronic hemodialysis for the past 3.5 years. He is scheduled for emergency laparotomy for peritonitis due to a suspected ruptured appendix.

2 A 98-year-old healthy patient fell when he was on a hiking tour and broke his arm. He is scheduled for open reduction and internal fixation of his humerus.

3 A 14-year-old girl is admitted to the hospital for open correction of her scoliosis.

4 You see a 33-year-old female with menorrhagia. She does not have any apparent anatomical lesions in her genitalia.

5 A 55-year-old patient presents in the emergency room because he has severe chest pain. During cardiac catheterization he shows severe stenosis of his coronary arteries. The patient agrees to have coronary artery bypass surgery. He did not take any drugs until now.

6 A known 61-year-old lady comes for coronary artery bypass graft and aortic valve replacement. She was on aspirin until 3 days ago.

7 A 76-year-old lady fell in her bathroom and broke her hip. She is scheduled for hip replacement tomorrow. She currently takes Coumadin® for a preexisting atrial fibrillation. Her current INR is 2.9.

8 A 40-year-old fat female with vWD presents for cholecystectomy.

9 A 24-year-old patient with hemophilia A needs to have his wisdom teeth removed. His factor A level is 2.5%.

10 A patient with recurrent epistaxis is known to have liver cirrhosis.

Homework

Visit different surgical departments of your hospital and inquire about the use of tissue sealants, vasoconstrictors, and other locally acting hemostatic agents. Note the current indications for the agents used.

Go to the pharmacy and note all available means to improve hemostasis. Jot down the package size and the price and ask for a package insert of the available products. When you have a complete list of the available products, compare them with the products mentioned in this chapter. Note all missing products and try to find out whether there is a way to get them in the country where you live. Record all your findings in the address book in the Appendix E.

If there is somebody in your hospital who prepares autologous fibrin sealants, ask to join him/her when he/she is preparing it next time.

Check different delivery devices for tissue adhesives and try to master their assembly procedure and their use.

References

1 Reece, T.B., T.S. Maxey, and I.L. Kron. A prospectus on tissue adhesives. *Am J Surg*, 2001. **182**(2 Suppl): p. 40S–44S.

2 Mannucci, P.M. Desmopressin (DDAVP) in the treatment of bleeding disorders: the first 20 years. *Blood*, 1997. **90**(7): p. 2515–2521.

3 Cattaneo, M. Review of clinical experience of desmopressin in patients with congenital and acquired bleeding disorders. *Eur J Anaesthesiol Suppl*, 1997. **14**: p. 10–14; discussion 14–18.

4 Rich, J.B. The efficacy and safety of aprotinin use in cardiac surgery. *Ann Thorac Surg*, 1998. **66**(5 Suppl): p. S6–S11; discussion S25–S28.

5 Mangano, D.T., I.C. Tudor, and C. Dietzel. The risk associated with aprotinin in cardiac surgery. *N Engl J Med*, 2006. **354**(4): p. 353–365.

6 Peters, D.C. and S. Noble. Aprotinin: an update of its pharmacology and therapeutic use in open heart surgery and coronary artery bypass surgery. *Drugs*, 1999. **57**(2): p. 233–260.

7 Levi, M., *et al.* Pharmacological strategies to decrease excessive blood loss in cardiac surgery: a meta-analysis of clinically relevant endpoints. *Lancet*, 1999. **354**(9194): p. 1940–1947.

8 Akowuah, E., *et al.* Comparison of two strategies for the management of antiplatelet therapy during urgent surgery. *Ann Thorac Surg*, 2005. **80**(1): p. 149–152.

9 Smith, P.K. and A.S. Shah. The role of aprotinin in a blood-conservation program. *J Cardiothorac Vasc Anesth*, 2004. **18**(4 Suppl): p. 24S–28S.

10 Kokoszka, A., *et al.* Evidence-based review of the role of aprotinin in blood conservation during orthopaedic surgery. *J Bone Joint Surg Am*, 2005. **87**(5): p. 1129–1136.

11 Samama, C.M. Aprotinin and major orthopedic surgery. *Eur Spine J*, 2004. **13**(Suppl 1): p. S56–S61.

12 Haas, S. Aprotinin—an allogeneic transfusion sparing drug. *Anasthesiol Intensivmed Notfallmed Schmerzther*, 2003. **38**(1): p. 38–40.

13 Murkin, J.M., *et al.* Aprotinin decreases exposure to allogeneic blood during primary unilateral total hip

replacement. *J Bone Joint Surg Am*, 2000. **82**(5): p. 675–684.

14 Soilleux, H., *et al.* Comparative effects of small and large aprotinin doses on bleeding during orthotopic liver transplantation. *Anesth Analg*, 1995. **80**(2): p. 349–352.

15 Dunn, C.J. and K.L. Goa. Tranexamic acid: a review of its use in surgery and other indications. *Drugs*, 1999. **57**(6): p. 1005–1032.

16 Armellin, G., *et al.* Tranexamic acid in primary CABG surgery: high vs low dose. *Minerva Anestesiol*, 2004. **70**(3): p. 97–107.

17 Seto, A.H. and D.S. Dunlap. Tranexamic acid in oncology. *Ann Pharmacother*, 1996. **30**(7–8): p. 868–870.

18 Karski, J.M., *et al.* Prevention of bleeding after cardiopulmonary bypass with high-dose tranexamic acid. Double-blind, randomized clinical trial. *J Thorac Cardiovasc Surg*, 1995. **110**(3): p. 835–842.

19 Cid, J. and M. Lozano. Tranexamic acid reduces allogeneic red cell transfusions in patients undergoing total knee arthroplasty: results of a meta-analysis of randomized controlled trials. *Transfusion*, 2005. **45**(8): p. 1302–1307.

20 Yamasaki, S., K. Masuhara, and T. Fuji. Tranexamic acid reduces postoperative blood loss in cementless total hip arthroplasty. *J Bone Joint Surg Am*, 2005. **87**(4): p. 766–770.

21 Neilipovitz, D.T. Tranexamic acid for major spinal surgery. *Eur Spine J*, 2004. **13**(Suppl 1): p. S62–S65.

22 Sethna, N.F., *et al.* Tranexamic acid reduces intraoperative blood loss in pediatric patients undergoing scoliosis surgery. *Anesthesiology*, 2005. **102**(4): p. 727–732.

23 Zellin, G., *et al.* Evaluation of hemorrhage depressors on blood loss during orthognathic surgery: a retrospective study. *J Oral Maxillofac Surg*, 2004. **62**(6): p. 662–666.

24 Morimoto, Y., *et al.* Haemostatic management of intraoral bleeding in patients with von Willebrand disease. *Oral Dis*, 2005. **11**(4): p. 243–248.

25 Boylan, J.F., *et al.* Tranexamic acid reduces blood loss, transfusion requirements, and coagulation factor use in primary orthotopic liver transplantation. *Anesthesiology*, 1996. **85**(5): p. 1043–1048; discussion 30A–31A.

26 Sorimachi, T., et al. Rapid administration of antifibrinolytics and strict blood pressure control for intracerebral hemorrhage. *Neurosurgery*, 2005. **57**(5): p. 837–844.

27 Henry, D.A. and D.L. O'Connell. Effects of fibrinolytic inhibitors on mortality from upper gastrointestinal haemorrhage. *BMJ*, 1989. **298**(6681): p. 1142–1146.

28 Zohar, E., *et al.* The postoperative blood-sparing efficacy of oral versus intravenous tranexamic acid after total knee replacement. *Anesth Analg*, 2004. **99**(6): p. 1679–1683, table of contents.

29 Bartholomew, J.R., R. Salgia, and W.R. Bell. Control of bleeding in patients with immune and nonimmune thrombocytopenia with aminocaproic acid. *Arch Intern Med*, 1989. **149**(9): p. 1959–1961.

30 Hellinger, J. The significance of local fibrinolysis increase in symptomatic hematuria and its inhibition by *p*-aminomethylbenzoic acid. *Z Urol Nephrol*, 1966. **59**(9): p. 633–639.

31 Hellinger, J. The treatment of severe fibrinolytic bleeding after prostatectomy with *p*-aminomethylbenzoic acid. *Urol Int*, 1966. **21**(1): p. 61–67.

32 Hellinger, J. Fibrinolytic hemorrhage in surgery and its treatment with *p*-aminomethylbenzoic acid. *Folia Haematol Int Mag Klin Morphol Blutforsch*, 1967. **87**(1): p. 32–40.

33 Hellinger, J. and G. Vogel. On the clinical features and therapy of fibrinolytic hemorrhages in surgery with special consideration of the new antifibrinolytic agent *p*-aminomethylbenzoic acid (PAMBA). *Bruns Beitr Klin Chir*, 1966. **213**(4): p. 478–487.

34 Westlund, L.E., R. Lunden, and P. Wallen. Effect of EACA, PAMBA, AMCA and AMBOCA on fibrinolysis induced by streptokinase, urokinase and tissue activator. *Haemostasis*, 1982. **11**(4): p. 235–241.

35 Kassell, N.F., E.C. Haley, and J.C. Torner. Antifibrinolytic therapy in the treatment of aneurysmal subarachnoid hemorrhage. *Clin Neurosurg*, 1986. **33**: p. 137–145.

36 Hindersin, P., *et al.* Current status of intrathecal antifibrinolytic therapy with *p*-aminomethylbenzoic acid (PAMBA) in subarachnoid hemorrhages. *Psychiatr Neurol Med Psychol (Leipz)*, 1985. **37**(12): p. 686–689.

37 Heidrich, R., *et al.* Antifibrinolytic therapy of subarachnoid hemorrhage by intrathecal administration of *p*-aminomethylbenzoic acid. *J Neurol*, 1978. **219**(1): p. 83–85.

38 Shukla, K.K., *et al.* Use of antifibrinolytic therapy in prostate surgery. *Int Surg*, 1979. **64**(2): p. 79–81.

39 Yang, H., S. Zheng, and C. Shi. Clinical study on the efficacy of tranexamic acid in reducing postpartum blood lose: a randomized, comparative, multicenter trial. *Zhonghua Fu Chan Ke Za Zhi*, 2001. **36**(10): p. 590–592.

40 Gordz, S., *et al.* Effect of desmopressin (DDAVP) on platelet membrane glycoprotein expression in patients with von Willebrand's disease. *Clin Hemorheol Microcirc*, 2005. **32**(2): p. 83–87.

41 Kobrinsky, N.L., *et al.* Shortening of bleeding time by 1-deamino-8-D-arginine vasopressin in various bleeding disorders. *Lancet*, 1984. **1**(8387): p. 1145–1148.

42 Lethagen, S., *et al.* Effects of desmopressin acetate (DDAVP) and dextran on hemostatic and thromboprophylactic mechanisms. *Acta Chir Scand*, 1990. **156**(9): p. 597–602.

43 Srivastava, A. von Willebrand disease in the developing world. *Semin Hematol*, 2005. **42**(1): p. 36–41.

44 Rodeghiero, F. and G. Castaman. Treatment of von Willebrand disease. *Semin Hematol*, 2005. **42**(1): p. 29–35.

45 Mannucci, P.M. Management of von Willebrand disease in developing countries. *Semin Thromb Hemost*, 2005. **31**(5): p. 602–609.

46 Lethagen, S. Desmopressin in the treatment of women's bleeding disorders. *Haemophilia*, 1999. **5**(4): p. 233–237.

47 Powner, D.J., E.A. Hartwell, and W.K. Hoots. Counteracting the effects of anticoagulants and antiplatelet agents during neurosurgical emergencies. *Neurosurgery*, 2005. **57**(5): p. 823–831; discussion 823–831.

48 Cattaneo, M., *et al.* Subcutaneous desmopressin (DDAVP) shortens the prolonged bleeding time in patients with liver cirrhosis. *Thromb Haemost*, 1990. **64**(3): p. 358–360.

49 Kobrinsky, N.L. and H. Tulloch. Treatment of refractory thrombocytopenic bleeding with 1-desamino-8-D-arginine vasopressin (desmopressin). *J Pediatr*, 1988. **112**(6): p. 993–996.

50 Despotis, G.J., *et al.* Use of point-of-care test in identification of patients who can benefit from desmopressin during cardiac surgery: a randomised controlled trial. *Lancet*, 1999. **354**(9173): p. 106–110.

51 Ozen S.S.U., A. Bakkaloglu, S. Ozdemir, O. Ozdemir, and N. Besbas. Low-dose intranasal desmopressin (DDAVP) for uremic bleeding. *Nephron*, 1997. **75**: p. 119–120.

52 Douglas, J.T. and J. Shaw. High-dose desmopressin in bleeding disorders. *Eur J Anaesthesiol Suppl*, 1997. **14**: p. v–vi.

53 Suzuki, S., G. Iwata, and A.H. Sutor. Vitamin K deficiency during the perinatal and infantile period. *Semin Thromb Hemost*, 2001. **27**(2): p. 93–98.

54 Zipursky, A. Prevention of vitamin K deficiency in newborns. *Br J Haematol*, 1999. **106**(1): p. 256.

55 Alparin, J.B. Transfusion medicine issues in the practice of anesthesiology. *Transfus Med Rev*, 1995. **9**(4): p. 339.

56 Crowther, M.A., *et al.* Oral vitamin K lowers the international normalized ratio more rapidly than subcutaneous vitamin K in the treatment of warfarin-associated coagulopathy. A randomized, controlled trial. *Ann Intern Med*, 2002. **137**(4): p. 251–254.

57 Alperin, J.B. Estrogens and surgery in women with von Willebrand's disease. *Am J Med*, 1982. **73**(3): p. 367–371.

58 Mannucci, P.M. Hemostatic drugs. *N Engl J Med*, 1998. **339**(4): p. 245–253.

59 Heunisch, C., *et al.* Conjugated estrogens for the management of gastrointestinal bleeding secondary to uremia of acute renal failure. *Pharmacotherapys*, 1998. 18(1): p. 210–217.

60 Tran, A., *et al.* Treatment of chronic bleeding from gastric antral vascular ectasia (GAVE) with estrogen-progesterone in cirrhotic patients: an open pilot study. *Am J Gastroenterol*, 1999. **94**(10): p. 2909–2911.

61 Coppola, A., *et al.* Long-lasting intestinal bleeding in an old patient with multiple mucosal vascular abnormalities and Glanzmann's thrombasthenia: 3-year pharmacological management. *J Intern Med*, 2002. **252**(3): p. 271–275.

62 Knudsen, H.E. and P. Ott. Treatment of chronic transfusion-requiring watermelon stomach with oral contraceptives. *Ugeskr Laeger*, 2002. **164**(25): p. 3364–3366.

63 Flordal, P.A. Pharmacological prophylaxis of bleeding in surgical patients treated with aspirin. *Eur J Anaesthesiol Suppl*, 1997. **14**: p. 38–41.

64 Sedrakyan, A., T. Treasure, and J.A. Elefteriades. Effect of aprotinin on clinical outcomes in coronary artery bypass graft surgery: a systematic review and meta-analysis of randomized clinical trials. *J Thorac Cardiovasc Surg*, 2004. **128**(3): p. 442–448.

65 Cole, J.W., *et al.* Aprotinin reduces blood loss during spinal surgery in children. *Spine*, 2003. **28**(21): p. 2482–2485.

66 Baldry, C., *et al.* Liver transplantation in a Jehovah's Witness with ankylosing spondylitis. *Can J Anaesth*, 2000. **47**(7): p. 642–646.

67 Johansson, T., L.G. Pettersson, and B. Lisander. Tranexamic acid in total hip arthroplasty saves blood and money: a randomized, double-blind study in 100 patients. *Acta Orthop*, 2005. **76**(3): p. 314–319.

68 Husted, H., *et al.* Tranexamic acid reduces blood loss and blood transfusions in primary total hip arthroplasty: a prospective randomized double-blind study in 40 patients. *Acta Orthop Scand*, 2003. **74**(6): p. 665–669.

69 Riewald, M. and H. Riess. Treatment options for clinically recognized disseminated intravascular coagulation. *Semin Thromb Hemost*, 1998. **24**(1): p. 53–59.

70 Gai, M.Y., *et al.* Clinical observation of blood loss reduced by tranexamic acid during and after caesarian section: a multicenter, randomized trial. *Eur J Obstet Gynecol Reprod Biol*, 2004. **112**(2): p. 154–157.

71 O'Connell, N.M. Factor XI deficiency. *Semin Hematol*, 2004. **41**(1, Suppl 1): p. 76–81.

72 Daily, P.O., *et al.* Effect of prophylactic epsilon-aminocaproic acid on blood loss and transfusion requirements in patients undergoing first-time coronary artery bypass grafting. A randomized, prospective, double-blind study. *J Thorac Cardiovasc Surg*, 1994. **108**(1): p. 99–106; discussion 106–108.

73 Florentino-Pineda, I., *et al.* The effect of amicar on perioperative blood loss in idiopathic scoliosis: the results of a prospective, randomized double-blind study. *Spine*, 2004. **29**(3): p. 233–238.

74 Gunawan, B. and B. Runyon. The efficacy and safety of epsilon-aminocaproic acid treatment in patients with cirrhosis and hyperfibrinolysis. *Aliment Pharmacol Ther*, 2006. **23**(1): p. 115–120.

75 Fuse, I., *et al.* DDAVP normalized the bleeding time in patients with congenital platelet TxA2 receptor abnormality. *Transfusion*, 2003. **43**(5): p. 563–567.

76 Nacul, F.E., *et al.* Massive nasal bleeding and hemodynamic instability associated with clopidogrel. *Pharm World Sci*, 2004. **26**(1): p. 6–7.

77 Frenette, L., *et al.* Conjugated estrogen reduces transfusion and coagulation factor requirements in orthotopic liver transplantation. *Anesth Analg*, 1998. **86**(6): p. 1183–1186.

78 Verstraete, M. Haemostatic drugs. In Forbes, C.D., A.L. Bloom, D.P. Thomas, E.G.D. Tuddenham (eds.) *Haemostasis and Thrombosis*. Churchill Livingstone, Edinburgh, Scotland, 1994. p. 607–617.

79 Kahalley, L., A.R. Dimick, and R.W. Gillespie. Methods to diminish intraoperative blood loss. *J Burn Care Rehabil*, 1991. **12**(2): p. 160–161.

80 Rousou, J., *et al.* Randomized clinical trial of fibrin sealant in patients undergoing resternotomy or reoperation after cardiac operations. A multicenter study. *J Thorac Cardiovasc Surg*, 1989. **97**(2): p. 194–203.

81 Ismail, S., *et al.* Reduction of femoral arterial bleeding post catheterization using percutaneous application of fibrin sealant. *Cathet Cardiovasc Diagn*, 1995. **34**(1): p. 88–95.

82 Mankad, P.S. and M. Codispoti. The role of fibrin sealants in hemostasis. *Am J Surg*, 2001. **182**(2 Suppl): p. 21S–28S.

83 Kohno, H., *et al.* Comparison of topical hemostatic agents in elective hepatic resection: a clinical prospective randomized trial. *World J Surg*, 1992. **16**(5): p. 966–969; discussion 970.

84 Rutgeerts, P., *et al.* Randomised trial of single and repeated fibrin glue compared with injection of polidocanol in treatment of bleeding peptic ulcer. *Lancet*, 1997. **350**(9079): p. 692–696.

85 Harris, W.H., *et al.* Topical hemostatic agents for bone bleeding in humans. A quantitative comparison of gelatin paste, gelatin sponge plus bovine thrombin, and microfibrillar collagen. *J Bone Joint Surg Am*, 1978. **60**(4): p. 454–456.

86 Seguin, J.R., *et al.* Fibrin sealant improves surgical results of type A acute aortic dissections. *Ann Thorac Surg*, 1991. **52**(4): p. 745–748; discussion 748–749.

87 Levy, O., *et al.* The use of fibrin tissue adhesive to reduce blood loss and the need for blood transfusion after total knee arthroplasty. A prospective, randomized, multicenter study. *J Bone Joint Surg Am*, 1999. **81**(11): p. 1580–1588.

88 Tredwell, S.J. and B. Sawatzky. The use of fibrin sealant to reduce blood loss during Cotrel-Dubousset instrumentation for idiopathic scoliosis. *Spine*, 1990. **15**(9): p. 913–915.

89 McGill, V., *et al.* Use of fibrin sealant in thermal injury. *J Burn Care Rehabil*, 1997. **18**(5): p. 429–434.

90 Spotnitz, W.D., *et al.* Reduction of perioperative hemorrhage by anterior mediastinal spray application of fibrin glue during cardiac operations. *Ann Thorac Surg*, 1987. **44**(5): p. 529–531.

91 Martinowitz, U. and S. Schulman. Fibrin sealant in surgery of patients with a hemorrhagic diathesis. *Thromb Haemost*, 1995. **74**(1): p. 486–492.

92 Carless, P.A., D.A. Henry, and D.M. Anthony. Fibrin sealant use for minimising peri-operative allogeneic blood transfusion. *Cochrane Database Syst Rev*, 2003. (2): p. CD004171.

93 Holcomb, J.B., *et al.* Effect of dry fibrin sealant dressings versus gauze packing on blood loss in grade V liver injuries in resuscitated swine. *J Trauma*, 1999. **46**(1): p. 49–57.

94 Holcomb, J., *et al.* Efficacy of a dry fibrin sealant dressing for hemorrhage control after ballistic injury. *Arch Surg*, 1998. **133**(1): p. 32–35.

95 Kheirabadi, B.S., *et al.* Hemostatic efficacy of two advanced dressings in an aortic hemorrhage model in Swine. *J Trauma*, 2005. **59**(1): p. 25–34; discussion 34–35.

96 Poretti, F., *et al.* Chitosan pads vs. manual compression to control bleeding sites after transbrachial arterial catheterization in a randomized trial. *Rofo*, 2005. **177**(9): p. 1260–1266.

97 Vournakis, J.N., *et al.* The RDH bandage: hemostasis and survival in a lethal aortotomy hemorrhage model. *J Surg Res*, 2003. **113**(1): p. 1–5.

98 Rowlands, R.G., L. Hicklin, and A.E. Hinton. Novel use of nebulised adrenaline in the treatment of secondary oropharyngeal haemorrhage. *J Laryngol Otol*, 2002. **116**(2): p. 123–124.

99 Sheridan, R.L. and S.K. Szyfelbein. Staged high-dose epinephrine clysis is safe and effective in extensive tangential burn excisions in children. *Burns*, 1999. **25**(8): p. 745–748.

100 Beausang, E., *et al.* Subcutaneous adrenaline infiltration in paediatric burn surgery. *Br J Plast Surg*, 1999. **52**(6): p. 480–481.

101 Bell, M.S. The use of epinephrine in breast reduction. *Plast Reconstr Surg*, 2003. **112**(2): p. 693–694.

102 Armour, A.D., B.W. Rotenberg, and M.H. Brown. A comparison of two methods of infiltration in breast reduction surgery. *Plast Reconstr Surg*, 2001. **108**(2): p. 343–347.

103 O'Donoghue, J.M., *et al.* An infiltration technique for reduction mammaplasty: results in 192 consecutive breasts. *Acta Chir Plast*, 1999. **41**(4): p. 103–106.

104 Aysan, E., *et al.* Efficacy of local adrenalin injection during sacrococcygeal pilonidal sinus excision. *Eur Surg Res*, 2004. **36**(4): p. 256–258.

105 Cheeseman, G.A. and A. Chojnowski. Use of adrenaline and bupivacaine to reduce bleeding and pain following harvesting of bone graft. *Ann R Coll Surg Engl*, 2003. **85**(4): p. 284.

106 Garrido Serrano, A., *et al.* Local therapeutic injection in bleeding peptic ulcer: a comparison of adrenaline to adrenaline plus a sclerosing agent. *Rev Esp Enferm Dig*, 2002. **94**(7): p. 395–405.

107 Sorensen, W.T., *et al.* Beneficial effect of low-dose peritonsillar injection of lidocaine-adrenaline before tonsillectomy. A placebo-controlled clinical trial. *Auris Nasus Larynx*, 2003. **30**(2): p. 159–162.

108 Dunlevy, T.M., T.P. O'Malley, and G.N. Postma. Optimal concentration of epinephrine for vasoconstriction in neck surgery. *Laryngoscope*, 1996. **106**(11): p. 1412–1414.

109 Bartos, P., *et al.* Adrenalin versus terlipressin: blood loss and cardiovascular side-effects in the vaginal part of laparoscopically-assisted vaginal hysterectomy or vaginal hysterectomy. *Clin Exp Obstet Gynecol*, 2000. **27**(3–4): p. 182–184.

110 Lurie, S., Z. Appelman, and Z. Katz. Intractable postpartum bleeding due to placenta accreta: local vasopressin may save the uterus. *Br J Obstet Gynaecol*, 1996. **103**(11): p. 1164.

111 Yasim, A., R. Asik, and E. Atahan. Effects of topical applications of aprotinin and tranexamic acid on blood loss

after open heart surgery. *Anadolu Kardiyol Derg*, 2005. **5**(1): p. 36–40.

112 Mand'ak, J., V. Lonsky, and J. Dominik. Topical use of aprotinin in coronary artery bypass surgery. *Acta Medica (Hradec Kralove)*, 1999. **42**(4): p. 139–144.

113 Carter, G. and A. Goss. Tranexamic acid mouthwash—a prospective randomized study of a 2-day regimen vs 5-day regimen to prevent postoperative bleeding in anticoagulated patients requiring dental extractions. *Int J Oral Maxillofac Surg*, 2003. **32**(5): p. 504–507.

114 Seidman, M.D. Hot-water irrigation in the treatment of posterior epistaxis. *Arch Otolaryngol Head Neck Surg*, 1999. **125**(11): p. 1285.

115 Koperna, T., *et al.* Diagnosis and treatment of bleeding colonic diverticula. *Hepatogastroenterology*, 2001. **48**(39): p. 702–705.

116 Hongo, F. and M. Saitoh. Intravesical instillation of Maalox for the treatment of bladder hemorrhage due to prostate cancer invasion: report of two cases. *Hinyokika Kiyo*, 1999. **45**(5): p. 367–369.

117 Kucuk, M. and T.K. Okman. Intrauterine instillation of trichloroacetic acid is effective for the treatment of dysfunctional uterine bleeding. *Fertil Steril*, 2005. **83**(1): p. 189–194.

118 Jetmore, A.B., J.W. Heryer, and W.E. Conner. Monsel's solution: a kinder, gentler hemostatic. *Dis Colon Rectum*, 1993. **36**(9): p. 866–867.

119 Tsujinaka, S., *et al.* Formalin instillation for hemorrhagic radiation proctitis. *Surg Innov*, 2005. **12**(2): p. 123–128.

120 Fu, L.W., *et al.* Formalin treatment of refractory hemorrhagic cystitis in systemic lupus erythematosus. *Pediatr Nephrol*, 1998. **12**(9): p. 788–789.

8 Recombinant blood products

Biotechnology is a promising science, also for blood management. It furnishes a variety of methods that are useful to mimic nature in order to provide patients with proteins not derived from allogeneic blood. Among them are recombinant clotting factors, albumin, and recombinant hemoglobin (rHb). This chapter will address the chances and challenges biotechnology offers. Above all, it will discuss what biotechnologically manufactured blood proteins will contribute to optimal blood management.

Objectives of this chapter

1 Learn how biotechnology contributes to blood management.
2 Know how recombinant blood products are synthesized.
3 List current and future recombinant products and how they relate to blood management.

Definitions

Biotechnology: Biotechnology is the integration of natural sciences and engineering sciences in order to achieve the application of organisms, cells, parts thereof, and molecular analogues for products and science (European Federation of Biotechnology, 1989). Or, put simply, biotechnology is about adapting and using resources found in plants and animals.

Recombinant drugs: Recombinant drugs are medicines that are produced by employing recombinant DNA technology. In this process, DNA is altered, joining genetic materials from two different sources.

A brief look at history

Honolulu, Hawaii, is the birthplace of the recombinant sector of biotechnology. This was in 1972. During a conference on biochemistry, two professors reported the results of their research. Stanley Cohen told the audience that it is possible to introduce foreign DNA into *Escherichia coli* bacteria. Herbert Boyer described an enzyme that is able to split DNA in such a way that the strands have identical ends. Near Waikiki Beach, those men met and discussed the potential to combine their discoveries. Some months later, they were able to present their work. They had been able to introduce foreign DNA into the genome of *E. coli*. Recombinant DNA was invented and the recombinant sector of biotechnology took off [1].

Hemophilia patients were the first group of patients that benefited from recombinant blood proteins. Born with a defect in their plasmatic coagulation, they suffer from recurrent bleeding into muscles and joints, which leads to a subsequent destruction of their tissues, leaving them disabled. The advent of blood-derived coagulation products in the 1970s aroused the hope that such crippling consequences of hemophilia can be prevented. However, blood products were obtained by pooling thousands of plasma sources, and hepatitis B and C were invariably detectable in antihemophiliac preparations. Almost all hemophiliac patients were infected with hepatitis, which was considered acceptable in comparison with the benefits the clotting factors provided. In the 1980s, 60–70% of hemophiliac patients were also infected with HIV. For this reason, plasma-derived products were scrutinized and virus-inactivation steps were included in their production, which made the factor concentrates safer. Another quantum leap in making factor concentrates safer was provided by biotechnology. In 1984, the gene for factor VIII was cloned and the recombinant protein extracted. Four years later, recombinant factor concentrates were tested in clinical trials. These factor concentrates were thought to be safer than plasma-derived products. But they still had parts of plasma-derived proteins in their formulation, namely, albumin. Efforts were made to eliminate albumin from this formulation. The second-generation factors do not contain albumin any more and a third generation of recombinant clotting factors do not contain human or animal products at all.

As recombinant antihemophilia preparations entered the market, other recombinant blood proteins were developed. Some of them are now being marketed, while others are still in different stages of investigation. There is still an immense potential for further recombinant drugs to be developed, some of which will be used for blood management.

Basics of recombinant drugs

Producing a recombinant drug starts with the detection of the gene locus that encodes the protein of interest. By means of restriction enzymes, the DNA of interest is cut out. The isolated gene sequence is introduced into a vector, such as a virus or the plasmid of bacteria. Via this vector, the DNA sequence is introduced into the genome of another organism. The organism will soon produce the protein that the DNA encodes for, given that available vital factors, such as a promoter, are present. For some proteins, this is all that is required. But for most drugs used in blood management this is not enough. Blood proteins that are used for therapeutic reasons often have a very complex structure. Vitamin K-dependent clotting factors, for instance, undergo a series of changes after their translation from the DNA, such as γ-carboxylation, phosphorylation, and glycosylation. Posttranslational changes are required to endow the proteins with their typical properties. Such changes are performed by enzyme systems in the medium that is used to extract the recombinant protein. Bacteria often lack vital enzyme systems for the posttranslational changes, while mammalian cells may have what is needed. Baby hamster kidney cells and the Chinese hamster ovary (CHO) cells, for instance, are able to synthesize proteins with their posttranslational changes.

Today's recombinant drugs are often produced in the laboratory. Cultures of yeast, bacteria, or mammalian cells serve as factories for the proteins. The maintenance of mammalian cell cultures is very costly and only a small amount of drugs can be produced. It was shown that transgenic animals are a good source of recombinant drugs as well. The human genes of the needed drug can be introduced into the genome of animals. Depending on where the genes are inserted, the recombinant drug can be secreted in the milk of animals, can be expressed in the blood, or can be found in their eggs. The synthesized protein can be purified and marketed. Sheep, cows, goats, and pigs are often used as protein factories. Proteins of human blood can be produced in this fashion. These include antithrombin III, fibrinogen, protein C, hemoglobin, and human serum albumin.

Animal farming for pharmacological purposes—also called pharming—is a lucrative business. The value of transgenic animals is immense. Additionally, the animals can multiply, the volume of the stock can be adapted to the current needs, and the maintenance of the herds is not as cumbersome as that of maintaining mammalian cell cultures. According to an interesting calculation, it takes only one transgenic cow to produce 2 kg of blood clotting factor IX per year [2].

A further step toward the production of the unlimited production of blood proteins is the use of transgenic plants. Under the subheading "Blood from a Plant," it was reported that thrombin, factor XIII, and coagulation factor VIII can be expressed in tobacco plants [2]. There are different ways to introduce foreign genes into the genome of the plant. One way to do it is by using *Agrobacterium tumefaciens* bacteria. This bacterium contains a plasmid, called the Ti plasmid. It is integrated into the plant's genome, once the plant is infected by the bacterium. Biotechnologically altered Ti plasmids, which are transferred back to the bacterium, are inserted into the plant, once it is infected. Other ways to introduce foreign DNA into plants include the Biolistic Particle Delivery System ("gene gun"). Small DNA-coated metal particles are shot into the plant cell. Some cells incorporate the foreign DNA into their genome. Such cells are selected and used to grow transgenic plants. Electroporation, by making holes in cells, using specific electrical impulses, is used as well. DNA can penetrate the cells with holes and after discontinuation of the electrical impulses; the DNA is trapped in the cell. Microinjection of liposome-coated DNA is a further way to introduce foreign DNA into cells. Cells that incorporate the DNA, which was artificially introduced into their genome, are used to produce the transgenic plants.

Although the mass production of blood proteins in transgenic plants still lies in the future, considerable progress has been made. It is already possible to produce immunoglobulins ("plantibodies") in soybeans. Tomato and tobacco plants can be used to produce human serum albumin [3, 4]. Hemoglobin can also be expressed in tobacco plants. The output of such transgenic floral systems needs to be increased further. Nevertheless, plants are an interesting alternative to allogeneic blood as a source of therapeutics.

Problems with the production of recombinant drugs

While some posttranslational changes, which normally occur in humans, are of minor importance to the work of the proteins in the body, many of them are not. This makes it especially difficult to produce proteins in the laboratory. Chances are that the cells used as factory for the proteins are not able to reproduce the posttranslational changes that the protein would normally undergo in the human body. Furthermore, recombinant proteins may either lose their activity in the process of production, purification, transport, and storage or they may be activated by it—both of which reduce their value. Additionally, it may even cause adverse effects if such proteins are used for therapeutic reasons. Proteins may become immunogenic or they do not perform the required activity. Actually, the tiniest differences between human and recombinant proteins may have a big impact on the clinical use of the proteins.

Safety of recombinant blood proteins

Recombinant blood proteins are widely considered as being safer than plasma-derived products. Nevertheless, there is still room for concern. The use of human or animal plasma components in first-generation recombinant clotting factors still holds the potential for disease transmission. Animal and human products have been used in the culture medium and during the purification process. For instance, mouse monoclonal antibodies are used in the purification process of recombinant proteins. These leave some remnants in the final product. Furthermore, cell lines can become infected by viruses. The orbivirus, bluetongue virus, and the minute virus all have infected cell lines derived from the CHO (a commonly used source of recombinant blood products).

Another factor that threatens the safety of recombinant drugs is albumin. It is widely used to stabilize the final recombinant product and was also shown to be the source of viral contamination. TT virus particles, for instance, were detected in recombinant clotting factors stabilized with albumin. The particles were less in factors without albumin.

Second-generation products avoid foreign proteins, such as albumin in their final formulation. This adds to their safety. However, human or animal proteins are still used during the production process of the second-generation products. The complete elimination of foreign proteins in the production process led to third-generation recombinant proteins. In this method of production, no human or animal protein is used in the production process, nor in the final product. To be on the safe side, whenever possible, a product should be chosen that contains the least amount of animal or human protein [5].

Use of recombinant blood proteins in blood management

While there are many recombinant proteins available for clinical use, we want to restrict our discussion to those that have the potential to reduce the patient's exposure to allogeneic blood products.

Classical antihemophilia factors

Octocog: recombinant factor VIII

As mentioned in the beginning of this chapter, patients with hemophilia A, i.e., patients lacking factor VIII, were the first group to benefit from recombinant clotting factor concentrates.

Initial recombinant clotting factor concentrates of factor VIII resembled closely the natural pattern. The natural factor VIII consists of s series of domains ([N-terminal]-A1-a1-A2-a2-B-a3-A3-C1-C2-[C-terminal]) [6]. In the 1990s it became possible to express the whole protein of factor VIII, and several brands of factor VIII concentrates entered the market [7]. However, the production process of full-length factor VIII limits its availability since the expression of this drug in cell lines is insufficient to meet the needs of all patients. A variant of full-length factor VIII is secreted more readily in cell cultures and is less sensitive to degradation. This variant lacks the B-domain of the protein (B-domain deleted, BDD-FVIII), which is not mandatory for its hemostatic ability [8, 9]. BDD-FVIII is now available for the treatment of hemophilia A [10, 11].

Another variation of recombinant factor VIII may be available in the future. It is known that the domains A2 and C2 of factor VIII tend to be more immunogenic than the domains A1 and B. This fact is used to work on recombinant factors that are less immunogenic and that reduce the incidence of inhibitor development. Attempts are made to delete the more immunogenic domains on the protein if they do not participate in the coagulation activity.

The choice of an antihemophiliac concentrate depends on different factors. While many blood-derived clotting factor concentrates may enhance clotting in hemophilia A patients, they may no longer be first choice of therapy.

If substitution is required nowadays, recombinant factor VIII is the treatment of choice in patients with hemophilia A [5].

Recombinant factor IX

Patients with hemophilia B are lacking factor IX. Treatment with factor IX concentrates is the treatment of choice. The advent of recombinant clotting factor concentrates of factor IX has made therapy for hemophilia B patients safer.

Recombinant factor IX (rFIX) concentrates, which are available, do not use animal or human proteins in their production process and formulation. This makes factor IX concentrate a safe alternative to serum-derived formulations. The high purity of the recombinant product eliminates unnecessary thrombotic complications that occur with crude plasma-derived therapeutics for hemophilia B therapy (such as prothrombin complex concentrates (PCC) and factor IX concentrates). According to current recommendations, in a variety of countries [5], rFIX concentrates are the treatment of choice in patients with hemophilia B.

Eptacog: recombinant factor VIIa

A very special drug is made from recombinant factor VIIa (rFVIIa), also called eptacog. Due to its unique properties, it once was termed the "universal hemostatic agent." There are two main hypotheses to explain why eptacog may be such a help to hemophilic patients. The first theory is that the action of rFVIIa depends on the presence of tissue factor to initiate clotting. Tissue factor is not normally present in blood. However, when vessels are injured, tissue factor comes into contact with blood and coagulation can be initiated at the site of injury. This hypothesis supports the notion that rFVIIa works mainly at the site of injury and does not cause widespread thrombosis. An alternative hypothesis of rFVIIa's action claims that the recombinant factor binds to platelet surfaces and activates FX there—quite independent of the presence of tissue factor. By this action, rFVIIa enhances thrombin formation on the surface of platelets. Probably, rFVIIa works by a variety of modes of action. This is supported by the variety of clinical clotting disturbances in which it successfully reduces or stops bleeding.

Recombinant human factor VIIa was originally used in the therapy of hemophilia A or B patients who had developed inhibitors. These inhibitors inactivate infused factor concentrate and leave the patient refractory to treatment. Formerly, PCC, activated PCC, porcine clotting factors, or high-dose human factor concentrates in combination with plasmapheresis or other techniques to lower inhibitor load were used. It was shown that rFVIIa is effective for prophylaxis as well as for treatment of bleeding episodes in hemophiliac patients with inhibitors. Therefore, when available, rFVIIa is the treatment of choice in patients unresponsive to factor concentrates [12].

In contrast to recombinant variants of clotting factors VIII and IX, the use of rFVIIa is not restricted to the therapy of patients with a single clotting factor deficiency. It is also beneficial in patients who have a combined lack of clotting factors. The most commonly encountered is the lack of vitamin K-dependent clotting factors (II, VII, IX, X, protein S, protein C). (as in the therapy with Vitamin K antagonists). Among them, FVII is affected to the greatest extent by vitamin K antagonists [12]. Under the influence of oral anticoagulation, patients may bleed spontaneously or need reversal of the drug for a surgical procedure. The traditional approach to this problem is the use of human plasma products such as fresh frozen plasma (FFP) and activated or inactivated PCC. There are a couple of problems associated with such treatment. FFP, though it may be effective if given in large quantities, has a variable content of vitamin K-dependent coagulation factors, causes volume overload, and requires time to be effective. PCC may cause disseminated intravascular coagulation, thrombosis, and/or myocardial infarction. Both products carry the inherent risks of allogeneic human blood products. To circumvent the patient's exposure to those allogeneic blood products, rFVIIa has proven successful. Replacing the defective FVII by rFVIIa provides almost immediate hemostasis of bleeding caused by vitamin K antagonists [13]. For this indication, doses lower than 90 μg/kg (as low as 20 μg/kg) may provide adequate hemostasis [14, 15]. rFVIIa is also effective when reversal of anticoagulation prior to surgery is required. If patients on vitamin K antagonists are scheduled for an elective surgical procedure, they are typically required to come into the hospital for heparinization and concomitant discontinuation of their anticogulant therapy. rFVIIa can eliminate the need for prior hospitalization. The drug, infused directly prior to surgery, acts within minutes. Given in sufficient doses, the effect of rFVIIa lasts about 10–12 hours. During this time, surgery can be performed. After that, rFVIIa application can be repeated as needed, or the patient can return to the anticoagulated state.

Patients with liver disease such as cirrhosis may also suffer from coagulopathy, which is due to a combined lack of vitamin K-dependent clotting factors. It is also partially due to defective platelets or thrombocytopenia. It was shown that coagulopathic patients with liver disease benefit from rFVIIa. Traditionally, coagulopathic patients with liver diseases are treated with FFP to restore their hemostatic capacity. With this approach, it is possible to increase the level of clotting factors in the patient's serum. However, the defects in the platelets are not treated by transfusion of FFP. Unlike FFP, rFVIIa can control bleeding due to a lack of plasmatic coagulation factors as well as thrombocytopenia and thrombasthenia. So, it is no wonder that patients with coagulopathy caused by liver disease benefit from rFVIIa. Patients with acute upper gastrointestinal bleeding, cirrhotic patients undergoing partial hepatectomy, and cirrhotic patients undergoing endoscopic polypectomy were successfully treated with rFVIIa, either prophylactically or therapeutically [16].

Since rFVIIa obviously also enhances the action of platelets, it has been used in a variety of settings where thrombocytes were either lacking or dysfunctional. The increased efficiency of thrombin generation by pharmacological doses of rFVIIa seems to compensate for the lack of functional platelets. rFVIIa is effective in thrombocytopenic and thrombocytopathic patients and can stop bleeding in such patients.

A variety of other settings saw the use of rFVIIa. In fact, there is an enormous potential for the use of rFVIIa in the arena of blood management. However, many of the proposed indications are not supported by randomized clinical trials. Case reports and case studies are often the only support for the use of rFVIIa in bleeding patients. rFVIIa was used successfully for achieving hemostasis in trauma and surgical patients, in patients with congenital or acquired factor deficiencies or other coagulopathies, with intracerebral hemorrhage, and in patients bleeding under the influence of anticoagulants. Table 8.1 gives an overview of the extensive off-label use of rFVIIa [5, 17–56].

Although this drug sounds wonderful, it is very expensive. Therefore, recommendations have been published regarding the use of rFVIIa. In the "Model Consensus Recommendations for the Use of Recombinant, Activated Human Factor VII in Adult Patients" [57], formulated by the Society for the Advancement of Blood Management and the University Health System Consortium expert panel, three groups of situations were defined where rFVIIa is recommended or may be appropriate. However, the expert panel did not formulate recommendations for

pediatric patients and for patients who cannot receive allogeneic blood products.

1 First-line treatment (without prior allogeneic clotting product use) of patients who present with new onset (<4 h) of a nontraumatic intracranial bleeding. The drug may also be appropriate as first-line treatment or prophylaxis for bleeding induced by major liver surgery or in expanding traumatic intracranial bleeding.

2 Patients on Coumadin or on low-molecular-weight heparin who have traumatic intracranial bleeding should receive rFVIIa. It may also be appropriate when they present with nontraumatic intracranial bleeding (not subarachnoidal bleeding) after the above-mentioned 4 hours have elapsed.

3 rFVIIa is appropriate as rescue therapy when the patient is bleeding and clotting factor replacement has failed to arrest hemorrhage: rFVIIa was recommended under such circumstances, when the following were present: cardiac or (thoracic) aortic surgery, major liver surgery, spinal surgery, postpartum or posthysterectomy bleeding, polytraumatized patients, gastrointestinal bleeding in hepatic failure, or pending invasive procedures. A rescue therapy may or may not be appropriate in retroperitoneal bleeding or in patients with thrombocytopenia.

Apart from the recommendations about the medical conditions that may warrant the use of rFVIIa, some general background information may help in the decision about the appropriate use of rFVIIa.

• Hypothermia decreases the activity of rFVIIa. This is consistent with the common temperature dependence of enzymatic activity. This effect, though, does not abolish rFVIIa's ability to reduce bleeding altogether. While it is beneficial to maintain or restore normothermia, hypothermic patients may still benefit from rFVIIa.

• Acidosis drastically reduces the activity of rFVIIa. A drop of the pH from 7.4 to 7.0 virtually abolishes the activity of rFVIIa. Severely acidotic patients are therefore not likely to benefit from rFVIIa. It remains to be seen whether correction of acidosis prior to the infusion of rFVIIa reestablishes its ability to provide hemostasis [58].

• Scoring systems for massively hemorrhaging patients, used to screen for patients most likely to benefit from rFVIIa [59, 60], are under investigation. Although it was shown that bleeding is reduced or even stopped in the majority of patients, mortality is still high in patients receiving rFVIIa, especially since most patients are in extremis when they receive their first dose of the drug. Patient characteristics associated with an unfavorable response to the drug include revised trauma score <4, prothrombin

Table 8.1 Off-label use of recombinant factor VIIa concentrates.

Setting	Remarks
Bleeding due to necrotizing pancreatitis	
Bleeding from the gastrointestinal tract	Used in patients with different etiologies of upper gastrointestinal bleeding as rescue therapy after transfusions failed
Bleeding from the lung	Used after standard treatment failed, used in adults and pediatric patients
Bleeding intracranial	Due to trauma or anticoagulant use
Bleeding postpartum	Due to DIC, HELLP syndrome, etc., given after allogeneic transfusion
Coagulopathy after head injury	Used as first-line treatment and after FFP failed
Coagulopathy due to cirrhosis and other liver diseases	Given when bleeding occurs or prior to intervention, in adults and in children
Coagulopathy due to DIC	e.g., during sepsis
Coagulopathy due to dilution during surgery	Used in spinal surgery of children
Deficiency of single coagulation factors or in the presence of inhibitors	Used in patients with inhibitors to, or a lack of FIX or with inhibitors or von Willebrand factor
Dengue fever	Demonstrated in a placebo-controlled trial in bleeding children
Platelet dysfunction	Glanzmann's thrombasthenia: used in pediatric and adult patients, for prophylaxis as well as for treatment of bleeding; Bernard–Soulier syndrome
Reversal of anticoagulants in bleeding patients	Rescue therapy for bleeding by the use of clopidogrel, fondaparinux, warfarin, and bivalirudin
Surgery of congenital vascular lesions	Case report of pediatric patient with bleeding vascular malformation; drug stopped bleeding, made surgery easier
Surgery, cardiac with cardiopulmonary bypass in adults and pediatric patients; e.g., valve replacement, coronary artery bypass grafting, aortic surgery	In excessive postoperative bleeding that met the criteria for reexploration; used after allogeneic transfusions failed or just at the onset of bleeding without prior transfusion; used as last resort in bleeding after cardiopulmonary bypass, reduced blood products use, and bleeding
Surgery, liver transplantation	Used in patients who cannot receive any allogeneic transfusions
Surgery, prostatectomy	When given prophylactically, in sufficient dosing, it eliminates transfusion
Thrombocytopenia	Even effective in platelet count $\geq 2 \times 10^9$ platelets/L; different thrombocytopenic settings: refractory thrombocytopenia after multiple platelet transfusions, autoimmune thrombocytopenia without prior transfusion, heparin-induced thrombocytopenia
Trauma, as last resort	Case reports, case series, and randomized controlled trials: used after massive transfusion; standard or lower than standard dose reduced allogeneic blood exposure or effected cessation of bleeding; blunt trauma seems to benefit more than penetrating trauma, it provides rapid and often lasting hemostasis, reducing patient's exposure to donor blood, and may or may not improve outcome.

DIC, disseminated intravascular coagulation; FFP, fresh frozen plasma.

time >18 seconds, elevated lactate levels, and profound acidosis.

• Pediatric patients tend to have a clearance of rFVIIa that is almost twice as high as that of adults. Children, therefore, require higher doses or more frequent administration to achieve a satisfying hemostasis. The clearance of rFVIIa diminishes over prolonged administration and the doses can be reduced over time.

• The route of administration of rFVIIa is typically intravenous. To prevent phlebitis at the site of injection, it is recommended to have saline running parallel to rFVIIa. Heparin should not be added into the bag of rFVIIa since it diminishes the activity of the drug. Antifibrinolytics as concomitant therapy is sometimes recommended.

• Different dosing strategies for the use of rFVIIa were recommended: high-dose bolus injection, continuous infusion, or high-dose continuous infusion. The most commonly used regimen is bolus injection. Higher doses may be used to increase the application interval and possibly also the total requirement of rFVIIa. Since rFVIIa has a short half-life of about 2–3 hours, frequent injections are required. This raised the interest in the feasibility of continuous infusions of rFVIIa. A more constant plasma level may help to achieve a reliable hemostasis. Continuous infusion is easier to apply than bolus injection and may decrease the total requirement of the drug. Continuous infusion of rFVIIa is initiated with a bolus injection of a standard dose and then continued with a calculated amount. To achieve the required hemostasis, additional bolus injections may be added. High-dose regimens promise a more rapid, improved response to rFVIIa infusion.

• The timing of administration of rFVIIa also plays an important role. rFVIIa has often been used as rescue treatment, after transfusing immense amounts of allogeneic blood products. However, multiple examples of Jehovah's Witnesses who received rFVIIa demonstrate that the drug can be used, also without prior use of allogeneic blood products. Several approaches have been proposed as to how long to wait until the factor is given, e.g., after 6 or 10 units of red cells. Current investigations explore the use of rFVIIa as the first means of treatment. This is even true for the use of rFVIIa in prehospital settings, where blood products are not available [50, 61, 62]. Actually, the earlier the treatment with rFVIIa starts, the better it seems to act. "Current treatment strategies emphasize the benefits of early use of . . . (rFVIIa). There is now good evidence that the earlier . . . (rFVIIa) treatment is initiated after the onset of a bleeding episode, the better the response rate, and the fewer the doses required, with subsequent cost savings" [12].

• High costs of rFVIIa may preclude its use in patients who may not likely benefit from the drug, such as moribund patients.

Recombinant human factor VIIa appears to have remarkably few side effects. Low-grade fever, anaphylactic and skin reactions, as well as hypertension were reported. High doses, of up to 300 μg/kg, have been given with no reported side effects. rFVIIa therefore seems to have a wide safety margin. There is a theoretical concern about disseminated intravascular coagulation, thrombosis, and a possible increase of inhibitor titers. In clinical practice, neither thrombosis nor pulmonary embolism or myocardial infarction are common, although some reports about such events are presented in the literature.

Although rFVIIa is a promising agent to be used in a variety of clinical bleeding disorders, its full potential has not yet been explored. More work is needed to define the correct place that the current preparation has in clinical practice. Apart from the already available concentrate, variants of rFVIIa are being developed. The aim is to increase its intrinsic activity [63]. The addition of other agents, e.g., platelet membrane fragments, to further enhance rFVIIa ability to arrest bleeding is under investigation [64].

Practice tip

Dose regimen for recombinant clotting factor concentrates:

rFVIIa:

For inhibitor treatment: 90 (150–200) μg/kg body weight i.v. in adults, 90–120 μg/kg in children

For the initial 48 h, repeat dose every 2–3 h or as needed, afterward increase dosing intervals

Infusion rate (IU/(kg/h)) = clearance (mL/(kg/h)) × steady state concentration (IU/mL)

Target: rFVII:C is 10–30 U/mL or higher

rFVIII:

Required units of rFVIII = (desired level − initial level) × plasma volume*

Maintenance: 50% of initial dose every 12 h (half-life of rFVIII is 12 h)

rFIX:

Required units of rFIX = ((desired level − initial level) × plasma volume*) × 2

Maintenance: 50% of initial dose every 24 h (half-life of rFIX is 18–24 h)

Since rFIX has a greater distribution volume than rFVIII, more concentrate needs to be given to reach a certain plasma level.

*plasma volume = (kg weight × 66 mL/kg for males (60 mL/kg for females)) × (1 − Hct)

Other recombinant clotting factors

Recombinant factor XIII, fibrinogen, and thrombin

Not only factors VII, VIII, and IX are available as recombinant products but many other blood proteins related to the clotting process have been synthesized in a recombinant fashion. Of special interest are recombinant human fibrinogen, recombinant human thrombin, and recombinant factor XIII (rFXIII). Human recombinant fibrinogen can be expressed in the milk of transgenic animals [65]. Recombinant thrombin and its precursor prethrombin can be synthesized using CHO cells or *E. coli* cells [66] and rFXIII is produced in yeast [67] or plants [68].

All three recombinant clotting factors are in development phase. Should they become available for common use, they may have significant impact on blood management. The combination of the three recombinant factors fibrinogen, thrombin, and factor XIII forms a stable clot. It has the potential to be used as fibrin glue, which does not use any allogeneic blood products at all. Patients with congenital deficiencies of the respective clotting factors may benefit as well from these recombinant proteins. Also, acquired factor deficiencies could be treated with the recombinant products.

Of special interest is rFXIII. Naturally, it stabilizes blood clots by cross-linking fibrinogen and protects it from destruction by plasmin. It also enhances wound healing [69]. When it is lacking, blood clots turn to be fragile and patients tend to bleed. There is a congenital disorder in which patients have insufficient factor XIII levels. Under certain conditions, patients may also acquire a lack of factor XIII. Patients undergoing cardiopulmonary bypass (CPB) typically have a reduced level of factor XIII after the end of the CPB and the blood clot strength is reduced. The lower the levels of factor XIII, the more the postoperative bleeding. Adding rFXIII in vitro increases the clot strength of blood exposed to CPB [70]. rFXIII is licensed in some countries as a drug for patients with congenital factor XIII deficiency. Trials are under way to explore its role in acquired factor XIII deficiencies such as after CPB.

Recombinant human antithrombin

Antithrombin (AT) is a natural inhibitor of coagulation. It inhibits serine proteases, mainly thrombin and FXa. It probably also has some antiviral and immunomodulatory properties.

Antithrombin can be produced in a recombinant fashion (recombinant human antithrombin, rhAT) as well.

Certain animals are transfected with the gene of human antithrombin and excrete it in their milk. Several steps of purification finally lead to the product. Since rhAT is excreted in milk and not derived from blood, there is a theoretical advantage as regards safety. Animals as well as milk are screened for viruses [71]. rhAT can also be produced in yeasts or in CHO cells.

Apart from spontaneously resolving skin hyperpigmentation at the injection site, no side effects are reported. Neither increased bleeding nor antibody formation have been observed [72].

rhAT also plays a role in blood management. Hereditary deficiency of antithrombin increases the risk of thrombosis. Patients with this disorder are treated with oral anticoagulation, once they have had at least one thrombotic event. During pregnancy and in preparation for surgery, oral anticoagulation is stopped. This may increase the risk of thrombosis. Although there is no clear evidence for the use of antithrombin in patients with deficiency of this protein, traditionally antithrombin concentrates prepared from human plasma are given to prevent thrombosis, once anticoagulation needs to be stopped or is insufficient. Recombinant human AT therefore may eliminate the use of human-blood-derived AT concentrates.

rhAT concentrates also seem to be useful in surgical patients who depend on heparin for treatment, e.g., for the use of the CPB. When such patients develop a heparin unresponsiveness, FFP is sometimes used. Recombinant human AT can restore heparin responsiveness in patients undergoing CPB without exposing them to allogeneic blood products [73].

Recombinant human serum albumin

About 60% of protein in human serum is albumin. This is a globular protein that consists of three domains. The albumin content of serum is one of the important determinants of the osmotic pressure in the circulation. Furthermore, albumin is able to bind and transport a variety of ligands, among them many drugs.

Recombinant human serum albumin (rHSA) can be produced in yeast cultures. Some yeast species are able to express only parts of the albumin molecule. *S. cerevisiae* (even beer has its scientific side), for instance, is able to express domains I and III of albumin, but not domain II. Another yeast, *Pichia pastoris*, has been shown to be an excellent medium for the expression of complete albumin molecules. Sixty-five to three hundred mg of albumin can be yielded per liter yeast solution [74]. After expression in the yeast, the albumin is purified. Several purification methods are combined. Ultrafiltration, phenyl-sepharose hydrophobic chromatography, and immunoadsorbent chromatography are used to bring rHSA to electrophoretic purity [75]. The resulting product is structurally equivalent to blood-derived albumin.

Albumin is often used for volume expansion. However, there is no evidence that this benefits the patient. On the contrary, there is some evidence that albumin used for volume replacement may even increase morbidity and mortality. Additionally, serum-derived albumin is used as an adjunct in drug therapy. Many first- and second-generation recombinant drugs contain serum-derived albumin. As outlined above, this does not contribute to the safety of the drug. Attempts have been made to produce third-generation recombinant drugs that do not contain serum-derived albumin. Recombinant albumin can be added to vaccines (e.g., measles, mumps, and rubella vaccine) and other drugs as a stabilizer. It can also be used as a coating for medical devices. Several biotechnological procedures can use rHSA. Cell cultures can be fed or stabilized with rHSA [76]. rHSA can also be used in vivo. Animal research supports that recombinant human albumin may be useful to treat ascites [77, 78]. And preliminary tests, in humans, have shown rHSA's safety and tolerability [79]. The next step is to use recombinant instead of blood-derived albumin in humans.

Recombinant hemoglobin

The idea of hemoglobin as a source of infusible oxygen carriers is not new. But attempts to use lysed red cells and their hemoglobin were hampered by severe side effects, such as allergic reactions, renal failure, severe gastrointestinal side effects, and hypertension. Furthermore, using red cells as a hemoglobin source makes this kind of oxygen carrier dependent on a limited blood supply. A fully recombinant hemoglobin would have potential advantages over blood-derived hemoglobin: It would be independent of blood donations, it could be produced without the threat of remnants of erythrocyte stroma (which was accused of being one of the responsible factors for the side effects), it excluded blood-borne diseases, and the hemoglobin molecule could be tailored to have certain characteristics that improve oxygen delivery.

It is possible to synthesize recombinant human hemoglobin (rHb). It can be expressed in different substrates, such as yeast [80], bacteria [81], milk, animal blood, tobacco plants etc. However, most of the rHbs are not currently ready for clinical use.

For a better understanding, let us have a closer look at one product, rHb 1.1 [82], which was used in animals and humans [83]. The solution is a hemoglobin-based oxygen carrier. The hemoglobin was produced in *E. coli*. It is a challenging task to coexpress two different protein chains in one single cell, to assemble two nonidentical protein chains (alpha and beta), and to have them finally incorporate the heme molecule. *E. coli* is able to perform this miracle. After expression of human hemoglobin in *E. coli*, the bacteria are lysed, and the rHb is purified by a series of chromatographical steps [84]. The resultant hemoglobin molecule has similar functional characteristics as human hemoglobin Ao. Nevertheless, there are some differences between normal human hemoglobin and the recombinant variant. One is that the two alpha-chains are attached to each other, to prevent rapid dissociation (which is not needed in normal hemoglobin that is naturally protected from dissociation by the red cell membrane). Another genetic modification is the exchange of the amino acid Asn to Lys, as it is found in a natural mutant of hemoglobin (Presbyterian hemoglobin variant). This modification decreases the oxygen affinity of hemoglobin to facilitate oxygen delivery. The P50 of this modified hemoglobin is 33 mm Hg. The reduction of the hemoglobin's oxygen affinity is essential. Hemoglobin in red cells is influenced by the presence of 2,3-diphosphoglycerate, which lowers the oxygen affinity of hemoglobin and enables it to release oxygen into the tissue. Hemoglobin outside the red cell does not have the needed 2,3-diphosphoglycerate and has, therefore, a very high oxygen affinity. This means that the hemoglobin can carry oxygen but cannot unload it in the tissue. Therefore, rHbs need some changes to make them a useful oxygen carrier. Recombinant technology makes it possible to a certain extent to tailor hemoglobin molecules to the needs of the patients.

Although rHb 1.1 has favorable characteristics, as it regards oxygen unloading and dissociation, side effects were reported during the use in humans, such as gastrointestinal upset. Furthermore, most of the first-generation hemoglobin solutions caused hypertension, which is thought to be due to nitric oxide scavenging and other mechanisms. The second-generation rHb solutions address this problem as well by changing the hemoglobin's affinity for nitric oxide.

Currently, many other rHb variants are synthesized (Table 8.2). They are in early experimental stages where attempts to produce hemoglobin variants with desired properties are going on. The size of the hemoglobin molecule, its conformation, oxygen- and CO-binding and release abilities, the strength of joining globin chains, its susceptibility to oxidative damage, and its NO-binding capacity are all varied and studied [85–87]. Unfortunately,

Table 8.2 Examples of recombinant variants of hemoglobin produced.

normal HbAo	(Adult hemoglobin—the basis for the below mentioned changes in protein structure to achieve the recombinant variants)
rHb 0.0	• Val to Met changes at the N-termini of the alpha- and beta-chain • No other changes
rHb 0.1	• Val to Met changes at the N-termini of the alpha- and beta-chain • Extra amino acid added to the C-terminal arginine of the alpha-chain (fuses alpha-chains, prevents dissociation, and prolongs half-life of hemoglobin)
rHb 1.0	• Val to Met changes at the N-termini of the alpha- and beta-chain • Asn to Lys mutation (as in hemoglobin Presbyterian, decreases oxygen affinity)
rHb 1.1	• Val to Met changes at the N-termini of the alpha- and beta-chain • Extra amino acid added to the C-terminal arginine of the alpha-chain (fuses alpha-chains, prevents dissociation, and prolongs half-life of hemoglobin) • Asn to Lys mutation (as in hemoglobin Presbyterian, decreases oxygen affinity)
rHb 2.0	• Polyethylene glycol polymerized (to prevent dissociation and prolong half-life) • Changed amino acid sequence in the distal heme pocket (to reduce nitric oxide affinity of hemoglobin)

rHb, recombinant hemoglobin.

none of the tested recombinant human hemoglobins are currently available for use in blood management.

Vaccines, sera, and immunoglobulins

Several vaccines, sera, and immunoglobulins are derived from human or animal plasma. For the production of antivenom to treat bites of poisonous animals, horses and sheep are traditionally used. They receive injections of animal venoms (e.g., from poisonous snakes or scorpions). This arouses an immunological response and they, finally, synthesize immunoglobulins in their blood. The animals are phlebotomized and their serum is used as antivenom. Since the purification of the antivenoms is cumbersome and has a low yield, antivenoms are often not purified. Therefore, antivenoms are a crude mixture of polyvalent antibodies with many different other horse or sheep proteins. Understandably, anaphylactic reactions, pyrogen reactions, and serum sickness are not uncommon.

An interesting alternative to animal-serum-derived immunoglobulins is avian antibodies. The eggs of normal hens are a convenient means to harvest antibodies [88]. In analogy to the production process of horse-blood-derived sera, hens are given shots with animal venom and they produce antibodies against it. These, however, need not be harvested from their blood. Eggs contain plenty of proteins, among them immunoglobulins. As early as 12 days after injection, antibodies are detectable in the eggs and remain so for up to 100 days thereafter. Some simple steps of purification from the egg yolk (such as freezing and

thawing) are needed to receive a purified immunoglobulin that is ready for use. This method is an efficient and gentle means for preparing antivenoms. Also, it is an efficient and cost-effective alternative. It has been reported that one egg may contain as much antibodies as 300 mL of rabbit blood [89]. About 75–100 mg of antivenom can be yielded per egg.

Antibodies are also synthesized in humans and are used as therapeutics, once they are fractionated from donor blood. To circumvent the use of human blood to obtain immunoglobulins, recombinant technology probably will be able to provide antibodies. While still in the experimental phase, it has been shown that transgenic tobacco plants, for instance, are a potential source of antibodies against a herpes virus. Other antibodies are produced using other recombinant resources. When this mode of antibody production is finally used for marketed products, this may further reduce the use of allogeneic blood products.

Key points

• Most blood-derived proteins can be synthesized by biotechnological methods (Table 8.3).
• The safety of recombinant blood proteins is perceived to be greater than that of blood-derived products. However, blood-derived stabilizers such as albumin added to the recombinant product adds risk to the product. Second- and third-generation products try to minimize or avoid

Table 8.3 Comparison of recombinant and plasma-derived blood proteins.

	Recombinant products	Blood-derived products
Safety	Third-generation products are made without blood proteins; therefore, no transmission of blood-borne diseases possible; first- and second-generation products are made with animal (and human) products in the production process, transmission of animal (and human) diseases possible	Virus inactivation employed in some products, blood-borne diseases still transmittable, until now undetected pathogens in products likely
Efficacy	Depends on the quality of product; less than blood-derived product when posttranslational changes inadequate; potentially higher than blood-derived products since protein is more homogenous than blood-derived product (no products of alternative splicing or mutant variations)	If not standardized, its efficacy may vary with the factor content of the donor blood; product more heterogenous than recombinant product
Production of antibodies against protein	Possible	Possible
Costs	Comparable to blood-derived products, occasionally higher trend: costs will probably decrease due to mass production	Comparable to recombinant products, occasionally less trend: costs will increase because of decreasing donor supply and increasing demand on safety
Use as standard treatment	Preferred over blood-derived products in most countries, recommended in the United Kingdom and Italy	Should be used only when recombinant products not available or indicated

this risk by reducing or eliminating human and animal protein from the manufacturing process.
• Whenever possible, hemophiliacs should be treated with recombinant factor concentrates.
• rFVIIa is considered a universal hemostatic agent.

Questions for review

• What is the use of recombinant factors VIII and IX?
• What was the original indication for which rFVII was developed?
• Which scenarios have been described where rFVII has been used off-label?
• What factors influence the efficacy of rFVII. Which of them are treatable?
• What other blood proteins are developed using biotechnology? What is their current use?

Suggestions for further research

What indications for albumin therapy are evidence-based?

Exercises and practice cases

Calculate the dose of recombinant clotting factor concentrate for a male patient with hemophilia A (compare Table A.7). He has a body weight of 70 kg, a hematocrit of 0.40, and a factor level of 1%. He is undergoing liver surgery.

How much clotting factor concentrate do you give initially? Would you repeat the therapy with clotting factors after the initial dose? If so, when and with what dose?

Imagine, the same patient did not have hemophilia A, but hemophilia B. How would you now answer the above questions?

Compare the evidence-based recommendations for the use of rFVIIa with the scenarios of off-label use listed in Table 8.1. In what areas is further research warranted?

Homework

List all available recombinant blood proteins in your country. Record what animal or human proteins are used for their production. Record the product and the suppliers contact information in the address book in the Appendix E of this book.

References

1 Special Report. *Nature*, 2003. **421**(January 23): p. 456–457.

2 "Blood from a plant" available at: http://biology.about.com/library/weekly/aa080599.htm. Accessed: May 8, 1999.

3 Sijmons, P.C., *et al.* Production of correctly processed human serum albumin in transgenic plants. *Biotechnology (N Y)*, 1990. **8**(3): p. 217–221.

4 Fernandez-San Milan, A., *et al.* A chloroplast transgenic approach to hyper-express and purify human serum albumin, a protein highly susceptible to proteolytic degradation. *Plant Biotechnol J*, 2003. **1**(2): p. 71.

5 United Kingdom Haemophilia Centre Doctors' Organisation (UKHCDO). Guidelines on the selection and use of therapeutic products to treat haemophilia and other hereditary bleeding disorders. *Haemophilia*, 2003. **9**: p. 1–23.

6 Mannucci, P.M. and E.G. Tuddenham. The hemophilias—from royal genes to gene therapy. *N Engl J Med*, 2001. **344**(23): p. 1773–1779.

7 McCormack, P.L. and G.L. Plosker. Octocog alfa, plasma/albumin-free method. *Drugs*, 2005. **65**(18): p. 2613–2620.

8 Lusher, J.M. and D.A. Roth. The safety and efficacy of B-domain deleted recombinant factor VIII concentrates in patients with severe haemophilia A: an update. *Haemophilia*, 2005. **11**(3): p. 292–293.

9 Lusher, J.M., *et al.* The safety and efficacy of B-domain deleted recombinant factor VIII concentrate in patients with severe haemophilia A. *Haemophilia*, 2003. **9**(1): p. 38–49.

10 Josephson, C.D. and T. Abshire. The new albumin-free recombinant factor VIII concentrates for treatment of hemophilia: do they represent an actual incremental improvement? *Clin Adv Hematol Oncol*, 2004. **2**(7): p. 441–446.

11 Kessler, C.M., *et al.* B-domain deleted recombinant factor VIII preparations are bioequivalent to a monoclonal antibody purified plasma-derived factor VIII concentrate: a randomized, three-way crossover study. *Haemophilia*, 2005. **11**(2): p. 84–91.

12 Shapiro, A. Inhibitor treatment: state of the art. *Dis Mon*, 2003. **49**(1): p. 22–38.

13 Kessler, C. Haemorrhagic complications of thrombocytopenia and oral anticoagulation: is there a role for recombinant activated factor VII? *Intensive Care Med*, 2002. **28**(Suppl 2): p. S228–S234.

14 Erhardtsen, E., *et al.* The effect of recombinant factor VIIa (NovoSeven) in healthy volunteers receiving acenocoumarol to an International Normalized Ratio above 2.0. *Blood Coagul Fibrinolysis*, 1998. **9**(8): p. 741–748.

15 Deveras, R.A.E. and C.M. Kessler. Recombinant factor VIIa (rFVIIa) successfully and rapidly corrects the excessively high international normalized ratio (INR) and prothrombin times induced by warfarin. *Blood*, 2000. **96**: p. A2745.

16 Anantharaju, A., *et al.* Use of activated recombinant human factor VII (rhFVIIa) for colonic polypectomies in patients with cirrhosis and coagulopathy. *Dig Dis Sci*, 2003. **48**(7): p. 1414–1424.

17 Svartholm, E., V. Annerhagen, and T. Lanne. Treatment of bleeding in severe necrotizing pancreatitis with recombinant factor VIIa. *Anesthesiology*, 2002. **96**(6): p. 1528.

18 Vilstrup, H., *et al.* Recombinant activated factor VII in an unselected series of cases with upper gastrointestinal bleeding. *Thromb Res*, December 1, 2005.

19 Hoffman, R., *et al.* Successful use of recombinant activated factor VII in controlling upper gastrointestinal bleeding in a patient with relapsed acute myeloid leukemia. *J Thromb Haemost*, 2003. **1**(3): p. 606–608.

20 Pastores, S.M., *et al.* Diffuse alveolar hemorrhage after allogeneic hematopoietic stem-cell transplantation: treatment with recombinant factor VIIa. *Chest*, 2003. **124**(6): p. 2400–2403.

21 Leibovitch, L., *et al.* Recombinant activated factor VII for life-threatening pulmonary hemorrhage after pediatric cardiac surgery. *Pediatr Crit Care Med*, 2003. **4**(4): p. 444–446.

22 Steiner, T., J. Rosand, and M. Diringer. Intracerebral hemorrhage associated with oral anticoagulant therapy: current practices and unresolved questions. *Stroke*, 2006. **37**(1): p. 256–262.

23 Segal, S., *et al.* The use of recombinant factor VIIa in severe postpartum hemorrhage. *Acta Obstet Gynecol Scand*, 2004. **83**(8): p. 771–772.

24 Zupancic Salek, S., *et al.* Successful use of recombinant factor VIIa for massive bleeding after caesarean section due to HELLP syndrome. *Acta Haematol*, 2002. **108**(162–163).

25 Bouwmeester, F.W., *et al.* Successful treatment of life-threatening postpartum hemorrhage with recombinant activated factor VII. *Obstet Gynecol*, 2003. **101**(6): p. 1174–1176.

26 Moscardo, F., *et al.* Successful treatment of severe intra-abdominal bleeding associated with disseminated intravascular coagulation using recombinant activated factor VII. *Br J Haematol*, 2001. **114**(1): p. 174–176.

27 Morenski, J.D., J.D. Tobias, and D.F. Jimenez. Recombinant activated factor VII for cerebral injury-induced coagulopathy in pediatric patients. Report of three cases and review of the literature. *J Neurosurg*, 2003. **98**(3): p. 611–616.

28 Pettersson, M., *et al.* Recombinant FVIIa in children with liver disease. *Thromb Res*, 2005. **116**(3): p. 185–197.

29 Bernstein, D.E., *et al.* Recombinant factor VIIa corrects prothrombin time in cirrhotic patients: a preliminary study. *Gastroenterology*, 1997. **113**(6): p. 1930–1937.

30 Tobias, J.D. Synthetic factor VIIa to treat dilutional coagulopathy during posterior spinal fusion in two children. *Anesthesiology*, 2002. **96**(6): p. 1522–1525.

31 Bern, M.M., *et al.* Treatment of factor XI inhibitor using recombinant activated factor VIIa. *Haemophilia*, 2005. **11**(1): p. 20–25.

32 O'Connell, N.M. Factor XI deficiency—from molecular genetics to clinical management. *Blood Coagul Fibrinolysis*, 2003. **14**(Suppl 1): p. S59–S64.

33 Chuansumrit, A., *et al.* Control of bleeding in children with Dengue hemorrhagic fever using recombinant activated factor VII: a randomized, double-blind, placebo-controlled study. *Blood Coagul Fibrinolysis*, 2005. **16**(8): p. 549–555.

34 Hennewig, U., *et al.* Bleeding and surgery in children with Glanzmann thrombasthenia with and without the use of recombinant factor VII a. *Klin Padiatr*, 2005. **217**(6): p. 365–370.

35 Peters, M. and H. Heijboer. Treatment of a patient with Bernard-Soulier syndrome and recurrent nosebleeds with recombinant factor VIIa. *Thromb Haemost*, 1998. **80**(2): p. 352.

36 von Heymann, C., *et al.* Clopidogrel-related refractory bleeding after coronary artery bypass graft surgery: a rationale for the use of coagulation factor concentrates? *Heart Surg Forum*, 2005. **8**(1): p. E39–E41.

37 Lisman, T., *et al.* Recombinant factor VIIa reverses the in vitro and ex vivo anticoagulant and profibrinolytic effects of fondaparinux. *J Thromb Haemost*, 2003. **1**(11): p. 2368–2373.

38 Deveras, R.A. and C.M. Kessler. Reversal of warfarin-induced excessive anticoagulation with recombinant human factor VIIa concentrate. *Ann Intern Med*, 2002. **137**(11): p. 884–888.

39 Stratmann, G., *et al.* Reversal of direct thrombin inhibition after cardiopulmonary bypass in a patient with heparin-induced thrombocytopenia. *Anesth Analg*, 2004. **98**(6): p. 1635–1639, table of contents.

40 Waner, M. Novel hemostatic alternatives in reconstructive surgery. *Semin Hematol*, 2004. **41**(1, Suppl 1): p. 163–167.

41 Pychynska-Pokorska, M., *et al.* The use of recombinant coagulation factor VIIa in uncontrolled postoperative bleeding in children undergoing cardiac surgery with cardiopulmonary bypass. *Pediatr Crit Care Med*, 2004. **5**(3): p. 246–250.

42 Tobias, J.D., *et al.* Recombinant factor VIIa to control excessive bleeding following surgery for congenital heart disease in pediatric patients. *J Intensive Care Med*, 2004. **19**(5): p. 270–273.

43 von Heymann, C., *et al.* Recombinant activated factor VII for refractory bleeding after cardiac surgery—a retrospective analysis of safety and efficacy. *Crit Care Med*, 2005. **33**(10): p. 2241–2246.

44 Stratmann, G., I.A. Russell, and S.H. Merrick. Use of recombinant factor VIIa as a rescue treatment for intractable bleeding following repeat aortic arch repair. *Ann Thorac Surg*, 2003. **76**(6): p. 2094–2097.

45 Jabbour, N., *et al.* Recombinant human coagulation factor VIIa in Jehovah's Witness patients undergoing liver transplantation. *Am Surg*, 2005. **71**(2): p. 175–179.

46 Friederich, P.W., *et al.* Effect of recombinant activated factor VII on perioperative blood loss in patients undergoing retropubic prostatectomy: a double-blind placebo-controlled randomised trial. *Lancet*, 2003. **361**(9353): p. 201–205.

47 Goodnough, L.T. Experiences with recombinant human factor VIIa in patients with thrombocytopenia. *Semin Hematol*, 2004. **41**(1, Suppl 1): p. 25–29.

48 Vidarsson, B. and P.T. Onundarson. Recombinant factor VIIa for bleeding in refractory thrombocytopenia. *Thromb Haemost*, 2000. **83**(4): p. 634–635.

49 Kristensen, J., *et al.* Clinical experience with recombinant factor VIIa in patients with thrombocytopenia. *Haemostasis*, 1996. **26**(Suppl 1): p. 159–164.

50 Holcomb, J.B. Use of recombinant activated factor VII to treat the acquired coagulopathy of trauma. *J Trauma*, 2005. **58**(6): p. 1298–1303.

51 Rizoli, S.B. and T. Chughtai. The emerging role of recombinant activated factor VII (rFVIIa) in the treatment of blunt traumatic haemorrhage. *Expert Opin Biol Ther*, 2006. **6**(1): p. 73–81.

52 Khan, A.Z., *et al.* Recombinant factor VIIa for the treatment of severe postoperative and traumatic hemorrhage. *Am J Surg*, 2005. **189**(3): p. 331–334.

53 Udy, A., *et al.* The use of recombinant activated factor VII in the control of haemorrhage following blunt pelvic trauma. *Anaesthesia*, 2005. **60**(6): p. 613–616.

54 Boffard, K.D., *et al.* Recombinant factor VIIa as adjunctive therapy for bleeding control in severely injured trauma patients: two parallel randomized, placebo-controlled, double-blind clinical trials. *J Trauma*, 2005. **59**(1): p. 8–15; discussion 15–18.

55 Mayer, S.A., *et al.* Recombinant activated factor VII for acute intracerebral hemorrhage. *N Engl J Med*, 2005. **352**(8): p. 777–785.

56 Ciavarella, N., *et al.* Use of recombinant factor VIIa (Novo-Seven) in the treatment of two patients with type III von Willebrand's disease and an inhibitor against von Willebrand factor. *Haemostasis*, 1996. **26**(Suppl 1): p. 150–154.

57 Society for the Advancement of Blood Management (SABM) and the University Health System Consortium (UHC) Expert Panel. *Model Consensus Recommendations for the Use of Recombinant, Activated Human Factor VII in Adult Patients*, Washington, DC, July 16–18, 2004. P&T 2005. 30 (11) (www.PTcommunity.com)

58 Meng, Z.H., *et al.* The effect of temperature and pH on the activity of factor VIIa: implications for the efficacy of high-dose factor VIIa in hypothermic and acidotic patients. *J Trauma*, 2003. **55**(5): p. 886–891.

59 Stein, D.M., *et al.* Determinants of futility of administration of recombinant factor VIIa in trauma. *J Trauma*, 2005. **59**(3): p. 609–615.

60 Biss, T.T. and J.P. Hanley. Recombinant activated factor VII (rFVIIa/NovoSeven(R)) in intractable haemorrhage: use of a clinical scoring system to predict outcome. *Vox Sang*, 2006. **90**(1): p. 45–52.

61 Lynn, M., *et al.* Early use of recombinant factor VIIa improves mean arterial pressure and may potentially decrease mortality

in experimental hemorrhagic shock: a pilot study. *J Trauma*, 2002. **52**(4): p. 703–707.

62 Jeroukhimov, I., *et al*. Early injection of high-dose recombinant factor VIIa decreases blood loss and prolongs time from injury to death in experimental liver injury. *J Trauma*, 2002. **53**(6): p. 1053–1057.

63 Persson, E., Variants of recombinant factor VIIa with increased intrinsic activity. *Semin Hematol*, 2004. **41**(1, Suppl 1): p. 89–92.

64 Tonda, R., *et al*. Platelet membrane fragments enhance the procoagulant effect of recombinant factor VIIa in studies with circulating human blood under conditions of experimental thrombocytopenia. *Semin Hematol*, 2004. **41**(1, Suppl 1): p. 157–162.

65 Butler, S.P., *et al*. Secretion of recombinant human fibrinogen by the murine mammary gland. *Transgenic Res*, 2004. **13**(5): p. 437–450.

66 Soejima, K., *et al*. An efficient refolding method for the preparation of recombinant human prethrombin-2 and characterization of the recombinant-derived alpha-thrombin. *J Biochem (Tokyo)*, 2001. **130**(2): p. 269–277.

67 Bishop, P.D., *et al*. Expression, purification, and characterization of human factor XIII in *Saccharomyces cerevisiae*. *Biochemistry*, 1990. **29**(7): p. 1861–1869.

68 Gao, J., B.S. Hooker, and D.B. Anderson. Expression of functional human coagulation factor XIII A—domain in plant cell suspensions and whole plants. *Protein Expr Purif*, 2004. **37**(1): p. 89–96.

69 Schroth, M., *et al*. Recombinant factor XIII reduces severe pleural effusion in children after open-heart surgery. *Pediatr Cardiol*, August 3, 2005.

70 Chandler, W.L., *et al*. Factor XIIIA and clot strength after cardiopulmonary bypass. *Blood Coagul Fibrinolysis*, 2001. **12**(2): p. 101–108.

71 Edmunds, T., *et al*. Transgenically produced human antithrombin: structural and functional comparison to human plasma-derived antithrombin. *Blood*, 1998. **91**(12): p. 4561–4571.

72 Konkle, B.A., *et al*. Use of recombinant human antithrombin in patients with congenital antithrombin deficiency undergoing surgical procedures. *Transfusion*, 2003. **43**(3): p. 390–394.

73 Avidan, M.S., *et al*. Recombinant human antithrombin III restores heparin responsiveness and decreases activation of coagulation in heparin-resistant patients during cardiopulmonary bypass. *J Thorac Cardiovasc Surg*, 2005. **130**(1): p. 107–113.

74 Dockal, M., D.C. Carter, and F. Ruker. The three recombinant domains of human serum albumin. Structural characterization and ligand binding properties. *J Biol Chem*, 1999. **274**(41): p. 29303–29310.

75 Qiu, R.D., *et al*. High expression and purification of recombinant human serum albumin from *Pichia pastoris*. *Sheng Wu Hua Xue Yu Sheng Wu Wu Li Xue Bao (Shanghai)*, 2000. **32**(1): p. 59–62.

76 Chuang, V.T., U. Kragh-Hansen, and M. Otagiri. Pharmaceutical strategies utilizing recombinant human serum albumin. *Pharm Res*, 2002. **19**(5): p. 569–577.

77 Tsukada, M., *et al*. Effects of recombinant human serum albumin on ascites in rats with puromycin aminonucleoside-induced nephropathy. *Gen Pharmacol*, 1998. **31**(2): p. 209–214.

78 Horie, S., *et al*. Effectiveness of recombinant human serum albumin in the treatment of ascites in liver cirrhosis: evidence from animal model. *Gen Pharmacol*, 1998. **31**(5): p. 811–815.

79 Bosse, D., *et al*. Phase I comparability of recombinant human albumin and human serum albumin. *J Clin Pharmacol*, 2005. **45**(1): p. 57–67.

80 Adachi, K., *et al*. Oxygen binding and other physical properties of human hemoglobin made in yeast. *Protein Eng*, 1992. **5**(8): p. 807–810.

81 Vasseur-Godbillon, C., *et al*. High-yield expression in *Escherichia coli* of soluble human {alpha}-hemoglobin complexed with its molecular chaperone. *Protein Eng Des Sel*, January 3, 2006.

82 Looker, D., *et al*. A human recombinant haemoglobin designed for use as a blood substitute. *Nature*, 1992. **356**(6366): p. 258–260.

83 Viele, M.K., R.B. Weiskopf, and D. Fisher. Recombinant human hemoglobin does not affect renal function in humans: analysis of safety and pharmacokinetics. *Anesthesiology*, 1997. **86**(4): p. 848–858.

84 Hoffman, S.J., *et al*. Expression of fully functional tetrameric human hemoglobin in *Escherichia coli*. *Proc Natl Acad Sci U S A*, 1990. **87**(21): p. 8521–8525.

85 Vasseur-Godbillon, C., *et al*. Recombinant hemoglobin betaG83 C-F41Y. *Febs J*, 2006. **273**(1): p. 230–241.

86 Wiltrout, M.E., *et al*. A biophysical investigation of recombinant hemoglobins with aromatic B10 mutations in the distal heme pockets. *Biochemistry*, 2005. **44**(19): p. 7207–7217.

87 Choi, J.W., *et al*. Characteristic of aromatic amino acid substitution at alpha 96 of hemoglobin. *J Biochem Mol Biol*, 2005. **38**(1): p. 115–119.

88 Zhu, L., *et al*. Production of human monoclonal antibody in eggs of chimeric chickens. *Nat Biotechnol*, 2005. **23**(9): p. 1159–1169.

89 Devi, C.M., *et al*. Development of viper-venom antibodies in chicken egg yolk and assay of their antigen binding capacity. *Toxicon*, 2002. **40**: p. 857–861.

9 Artificial blood components

Re-creating blood, the fluid of life, is a human dream that dates back thousands of years. However, myth and reality met when the first unsuccessful attempts were made to actually resuscitate patients. From the humble beginnings up to this day it has not been possible to even come close to re-creating a blood component, let alone whole blood. However, as the result of decades of research, several drugs have been developed that are able to mimic some of the properties of blood components. This chapter will give an overview of science's quest for re-creating the fluid of life.

Objectives of this chapter

1 Describe the main qualities of hemoglobin-based oxygen carriers (HBOCs).
2 Describe the main qualities of perfluorocarbons (PFCs).
3 Explain how different artificial blood components may substitute for lacking platelets.

Definitions

Artificial oxygen carriers: Artificial oxygen carriers (AOCs) are drugs that can carry significant amounts of oxygen, e.g., with the bloodstream.
Perfluorocarbons: These are inert chemical compounds consisting of carbon and fluorine that are able to dissolve gases. PFCs are the basis for artificial-oxygen-carrying drugs.
Hemoglobin-based oxygen carriers: These are AOCs based on hemoglobin as the carrier entity.

A brief look at history

The first attempts to infuse solutions carrying oxygen were made at the beginning of the twentieth century. In 1916, the British Dr Tunnicliffe used saline to infuse oxygen. He reported: "For some time it has been the practice . . . , when using saline venous injections, either simple nutrient (glucose and lecithin) or medicated, to use . . . oxygenated saline solution" [1]. Although this therapy somehow seemed to work, Dr Tunnicliffe acknowledged the limitations of his approach: "We are quite aware that the quantity of oxygen introduced by this method is very small as compared with the oxygen requirement of the subject, nevertheless cyanosis is rapidly alleviated by the use of such solutions . . . " [1]. These early attempts to use saline as an oxygen carrier proved that something different was needed to infuse oxygen, something that could carry much more oxygen than saline. Logical choices were hemoglobin solutions, solutions with the molecule especially designed to transport oxygen.

In the 1930s, experiments were undertaken to resuscitate a total exsanguinated sheep with a hemoglobin solution made from cow blood [2]. Human experiments with hemoglobin solutions started in the 1940s [3]. Amberson and colleagues [3] infused cell-free hemoglobin into humans. The solutions both researcher groups used were simply hemoglobin from lysed red cells, coming with considerable amounts of red cell membrane and stroma residues. The side effects of such solutions were tremendous, with renal failure and high blood pressure being the most prominent. In addition, coagulopathies have been attributed to stromal contaminants. The earlier researchers figured that the reasons for the side effects of hemoglobin solutions were the remaining parts of red cell membrane and stroma. Therefore, purification was the logical consequence to reduce the risks of hemoglobin solutions.

After adding a purification step to the preparation of the early crude hemoglobin solutions, new experiments were performed on humans. In 1970, Rabiner treated hemorrhagic shock with stroma-free hemoglobin [4]. A test performed in 1978, by Savitsky [5], found only limited side effects after infusion of hemoglobin solutions into healthy volunteers. Also purified solutions had major disadvantages, still including renal toxicity and a short intravascular half-life.

To reduce the side effects further, hemoglobin was chemically altered. Modifications made in the 1980s aimed at making the solutions more stable and thus reduced the side effects resulting from hemoglobin chains that had disassembled.

Another group of compounds entered the race for a usable AOC when in the 1960s, Dr Leland Clark started experiments with PFCs. Gollan and Clark demonstrated in 1966 that mice submerged completely into perfluorochemicals could survive for a prolonged time [6]. This was due to the oxygen-carrying capacity of the PFCs. After about two decades of research, the first chemically manufactured oxygen carrier entered the market. The first-generation perfluorochemical, Fluosol-DA™—a product of the Green Cross in Japan—was approved in the United States for medical use in 1989. It was primarily used as an adjunct to percutaneous transluminal coronary angioplasty. The production of Fluosol-DA stopped when catheter techniques improved. Fluosol-DA has also been used as an AOC. However, due to the low content of the perfluorochemical in the product and due to other properties, trials with the new drug in the therapy of severe anemia were disappointing.

As with many products used in blood management, the military had a keen interest in AOCs. Much was invested to have an AOC for the battlefield. Especially during the Vietnam War, efforts for such a product were intensified. However, no suitable product could be developed at that time. Also today, the military is interested in AOCs. Once available, an HBOC is likely to be included in the therapy algorithm developed by the military initiative STORMACT' (strategies to reduce military and civilian transfusion) [7].

Artificial oxygen carriers

AOCs were initially thought to serve as a "blood substitute" or as a substitute for red cells. They were designed to be an alternative for donor blood. It was hoped they would be simple, safe, and fast to apply. Besides, it was felt that such "artificial blood" should have no infectious risks and other side effects, should have a sufficient intravasal half-life and a long shelf life, and that they should be universally applicable, independent of blood groups. Such AOCs were thought to provide an unlimited supply of blood substitutes to overcome blood shortages. However, decades of intensive research did not yield a product that is even close to the expectations of the early enthusiastic advocates of artificial blood. The early enthusiasm gave way to the notion that re-creating blood is beyond the scope of human ability. At best, humans are able to mimic some of the features of blood, with more or less severe side effects.

Currently, two major groups of AOCs have been developed: HBOCs and PFCs.

Hemoglobin-based oxygen carriers

Sources of hemoglobin

Hemoglobin for infusion can be obtained in a variety of ways. Outdated human red cell concentrates can be used as a source. However, their supply is limited and blood shortages cannot be overcome by the use of human blood as basis for AOCs. It is also possible to use animal blood, e.g., from pigs or cows. This source of hemoglobin is potentially unlimited. Besides, bovine hemoglobin does not need 2,3-diphosphoglycerate (2,3-DPG) to unload oxygen and naturally has a P50 value of about 30 mm Hg, which is very similar to that of human hemoglobin in red cells. However, concerns include antigenicity and the transmission of animal diseases, such as bovine spongiform encephalitis.

Probably the best, yet most complicated, way to get hemoglobin is the recombinant route. Hemoglobin molecules can be expressed in yeast, *Escherichia coli* bacteria, plants or in transgenic animals [8, 9]. The risk of disease transmission is very low, supply is potentially unlimited, and it is possible to modify the hemoglobin molecule to get a product that has the required qualities. However, up to now, there seems to be no technology that provides enough hemoglobin to satisfy the market once a product has been developed which gets approval.

Modified hemoglobin solutions

Native, cell-free hemoglobin is able to transport oxygen; at the same time not being as antigenic as red cells are (antigenic determinants are mainly embedded in the red cell membrane). However, the loss of the surrounding cell leaves the hemoglobin molecule "unprotected, helpless and too small for the job." The natural environment of the hemoglobin molecule provides it with everything it needs to do its assigned job. The cell protects the molecule from oxidative damage and provides systems to undo oxidation (superoxide dismutase, catalase, met-hemoglobin reductase, glutathione). The cell also provides 2,3-DPG which hemoglobin needs to unload oxygen. Last but not least, the cell keeps hemoglobin molecules intact, as tetramers, and keeps the single hemoglobin tetramers together in a package that is big enough not to escape an intact circulation and to exert all its needed effects to regulate blood flow and oxygen delivery, e.g., by exerting shear stress and by a graded interaction with nitric oxide (NO). All these interactions of the red cell and the hemoglobin molecule are lost when hemoglobin is freed from the red cell. Clinically useful HBOCs have to consider this and have to try to overcome the obstacles associated with the loss of the red cell environment. Free, native hemoglobin, therefore, comes with several problems:

1 The hemoglobin tetramer rapidly disintegrates into its four protein chains. This leads to (a) nephrotoxicity, (b) escape into the extravascular space, and (c) a short intravascular half-life.

2 Since there is no 2,3-DPG with the free hemoglobin, it cannot unload its oxygen normally and the hemoglobin's oxygen affinity is too high to be a clinically useful HBOC (P50 about 10–15 mm Hg).

3 Protective enzymes are lacking. The hemoglobin molecule is therefore easily autooxidized and methemoglobin is formed.

4 Hemoglobin reacts much easier than when in a red cell. Therefore, it (a) easily scavenges NO (free hemoglobin reacts 1000 times faster with NO than hemoglobin in a red cell) and (b) it may interchange oxygen in tissue more rapidly.

Different methods had to be devised to produce HBOCs, which cause less of the above-mentioned problems associated with free hemoglobin.

SURFACE-MODIFIED HEMOGLOBIN (CONJUGATED HEMOGLOBIN)

Surface-modified hemoglobins are combinations of hemoglobin molecules with large molecules like dextran, polyoxyethylene, or polyethylene glycol. This co-work increases the size of the particle, increases the amount of water bound to the molecule, and increases the intravascular half-life. Besides, modified hemoglobin has a reduced antigenicity, a high oncotic pressure, and a high viscosity. Infusion of such HBOCs also results in plasma volume expansion.

INTRAMOLECULAR CROSS-LINKED HEMOGLOBIN

Cross-linking of the hemoglobin chains within a hemoglobin tetramer (e.g., by pyridoxylation or diacetylation) prevents the early diffusion of the hemoglobin tetramer into dimers. The size of the tetrameric hemoglobin molecule does not change considerably.

POLYMERIZED HEMOGLOBIN

Single hemoglobin reacts with chemical cross-linkers and so hemoglobin polymers develop (polyHb). Sebacyl chloride and glutaraldehyde were first used in the 1960s to cross-link hemoglobin for polymerization [10]. o-Raffinose, a new cross-linker, also serves this purpose. The size of the polyHb differs, depending on how many single hemoglobin molecules are coupled to each other. The polymerized hemoglobins have a longer plasma half-life, but come with a higher antigenicity than natural hemoglobin molecules.

ENCAPSULATED HEMOGLOBIN

Natural hemoglobin can be encapsulated in synthetic liposomes made from natural lecithin or synthetic phospholipids [11] (liposome-encapsulated hemoglobin, LEH). It is also possible to include enzymes or other substances into the liposomes, so that some of the side effects of free hemoglobin can be overcome. The LEH mimic natural red cells and are therefore called "neohemocytes." However, their production is complicated. LEH are taken up by macrophages and hepatocytes. Components of LEH (especially the capsule), and their breakdown products, lead to lasting damage of the cells. Further work is needed to improve the capsule of the particles to make it biodegradable. Polyactide, a material already used to make resorbable surgical suture material, can be degraded to water and carbon dioxide by the body. Also, polyglycolide is biodegradable. These compounds are currently under investigation to serve as capsules for hemoglobin [10, 12].

HEMOGLOBIN SOLUTIONS WITH ANTIOXIDANT PROPERTIES

Free hemoglobin is lacking the antioxidant systems that typically protect it in its natural environment, the red cells. To overcome this, certain antioxidant principles have been added to the hemoglobin molecules in the HBOCs. Enzymes such as superoxide dismutase (SOD), carbonic anhydrase, and catalase (CAT) can be added either by cross-linking the polyHb molecule (PolyHb-SOD-CAT) or by encapsulation together with the hemoglobin molecule. In addition, the polynitroxylation of hemoglobin molecules improves the antioxidant status.

Effects of hemoglobin solutions

As outlined above, freeing hemoglobin from red cells changes its properties. Besides, during attempts to overcome these changes and to adapt the final drug to the needs of the consumer, the HBOCs develop certain properties.

Some of them are common to all or a group of HBOCs, while others are specific for one product.

As nowadays, all tested hemoglobin solutions use highly purified hemoglobin; theoretically, stroma, viruses, and endotoxins are not a concern.

OXYGEN AFFINITY

Most natural free hemoglobin molecules have a high oxygen affinity. To change their affinity to more normal values, hemoglobin has been modified. Pyridoxylation (adding pyridoxal-5-phosphate) [13] or cross-linking (e.g., by 3,5-dibromosalicylate) [14] increases the oxygen affinity of hemoglobin. The cross-linker, o-raffinose, modifies the 2,3-DPG pocket of the hemoglobin, resulting in a higher P50. However, it is not clear whether it is really beneficial to have free hemoglobin with an oxygen affinity near to normal. It is thinkable that the more rapid reaction of oxygen with free hemoglobin as opposed to hemoglobin in the red cell may offset the effects of an increased oxygen affinity. A higher oxygen affinity may ensure that the microcirculation is not unduly affected by high oxygen levels.

ONCOTIC EFFECTS

Red cell transfusions, per se, do not exert relevant oncotic pressure. In contrast, free hemoglobin does. This is a two-edged sword. To draw fluids from tissues into the circulation (plasma expansion) may be beneficial in hemorrhaging patients or in patients with ischemia due to tissue swelling. However, in cases where additional intravascular fluids are detrimental, the oncotic effects of HBOCs may be harmful.

The extent of the oncotic effects encountered depends on the number, not on the size of the particles. Therefore, many small particles (as in intramolecularly cross-linked hemoglobins) exert a much greater oncotic pressure than fewer, yet bigger particles with the same amount of hemoglobin (as in LEH).

RHEOLOGICAL PROPERTIES, VISCOSITY

A circulating viscous fluid in the vessels exerts a shear stress on the vessel wall. This results in the release of NO, a vasodilator. By this mechanism, whole human blood with a viscosity of about 4 cPoise (cP) is able to regulate the perfusion of the microvasculature. Artificial infusion solutions, including HBOCs, also exert certain effects on the microvascular system. However, since some HBOCs have a lower viscosity than blood, they may impair the microvascular blood flow. This effect is especially pronounced when a patient is so anemic that an increase in

cardiac output cannot compensate for the decreased red cell level and viscosity. Since exactly that situation is the classical indication for HBOC therapy, the low viscosity of HBOCs may be detrimental. The rheological properties have to be taken into account when designing a solution [15]. Newer HBOCs do just that [16].

VASOPRESSOR EFFECTS

Right from the early experiments with hemoglobin solutions, it was obvious that there is a strong vasopressor effect of free hemoglobin. There are two theories to explain this phenomenon [10]. The first relates the vasoactivity to the interaction of hemoglobin with NO (and endothelin, a strong vasoconstrictor). Hemoglobin in red cells can scavenge NO, but the extent is limited due to the red cell membrane acting as a barrier. Free hemoglobin can scavenge NO as well. This capability being stronger, when the red cell membrane—which formerly worked as barrier to NO diffusion—is missing [17]. Besides, small hemoglobin molecules can leave the vessels and interact directly with NO in the perivascular space. Modifications in the production of HBOCs can reduce the vasoconstrictive effect of hemoglobin. These modifications address the binding capacity of hemoglobin and NO, as well as the size of the hemoglobin molecules. Encapsulated hemoglobin may have a limited vasoactivity, since the neohemocytes mimic some effects of the red cells. This way, the hemoglobin cannot easily diffuse into the perivascular space anymore and cannot react that easily with NO [18]. The interaction of hemoglobin and NO has also been altered by chemical modification of the hemoglobin sites where NO is typically bound. Besides, recombinant hemoglobin can be designed in a way that reduces its NO-scavenging properties. The NO-binding site of the recombinant hemoglobin molecule can be modified, making it difficult for NO to bind to hemoglobin [19]. In addition, tetrameric hemoglobin molecules, which are small and therefore diffuse outside the vasculature to scavenge NO, can be eliminated from the final HBOC. Vasoactive side effects of hemoglobin solution have been reduced in some products when tetrameric hemoglobin was removed [12]. The less tetrameric hemoglobin, the less vasoconstrictive side effects and the more HBOC can be infused.

The second theory used to explain the vasoconstrictive effects of HBOCs is the inference of regulative mechanisms of the microvasculature. Precapillary arterioles sense the oxygen level in the blood coming toward the capillaries and, depending on the oxygen content, constrict or dilate. Since free hemoglobin can react much faster than hemoglobin bound in red cells, oxygen may be released from the hemoglobin to the arterioles easily and prematurely, giving the arterioles the illusion there is plenty of oxygen available. As a result, arterioles may not dilate as they would if red cells would arrive. This may impair the microcirculation. In this context, hemoglobin with a higher oxygen affinity than that of red cells may be beneficial [20].

RENAL EFFECTS

Normal human hemoglobin is a tetramer. In the red cell it is stable, but it easily disassembles into dimers, once it leaves the cell. The dimers pass through the glomeruli in the kidney and cause renal damage.

INTRAVASCULAR HALF-LIFE

Compared with red cells, the intravascular half-life of HBOCs is very short. Therefore, repeated infusions are needed to provide sufficient oxygen-carrying capacity. In order to prolong the stability and intravascular half-life of acellular hemoglobin, intramolecular cross-linking, polymerization, encapsulation, or conjugation with macromolecules has been employed in the current generation of HBOCs. Besides, recombinant hemoglobin does not disintegrate easily, prolonging its half-life [13]. By these means, plasma half-life of HBOCs is about 5–40 hours. Further work on HBOCs attempts to increase the intravascular half-life even more.

INFECTIOUS RISKS AND EFFECTS ON THE IMMUNE SYSTEM

It is believed that the production process of HBOCs excludes every possibility of viral contamination coming from the original hemoglobin source. Moreover, since the cross-linking process of hemoglobin stabilizes the protein, heat-sterilization is possible as well [14]. HBOCs are therefore thought to be free from infectious agents.

Of greater concern is the effect of HBOCs on the immune system of the recipient. HBOCs may overload the reticuloendothelial system, impair bactericidal activities, and may promote bacterial growth by the iron content of HBOCs. Besides, these may potentiate the detrimental effects of endotoxin in the patients.

Antigenicity from red cell membranes does not occur with purified hemoglobins. Therefore, HBOCs can be administered independent of the blood group of the recipient. Another form of antigenicity may evolve with the use of HBOCs. Reactions to polymerized hemoglobin molecules or to molecules from other species are of (theoretical) concern. During trials with the only bovine

product, IgE production was not observed and only moderate levels of IgG were seen [21].

OXIDATIVE DAMAGE

Superfluous delivery of oxygen may come with side effects. Oxygen may cause oxidative damage. Reperfusion injury may occur after therapy of conditions with prolonged ischemia, e.g., stroke, myocardial infarction, and severe prolonged hemorrhage. Also, blood cells are not immune to the damaging effects of oxygen. The iron of free hemoglobin is prone to oxidation and so met-hemoglobin builds up easily. Besides, peroxides and other oxidative products may accumulate and result in the damage of hemoglobin and in endothelial damage. Red cells have enzymes that protect them from the influence of oxygen. SOD and CAT found in red cells may ameliorate the damaging effects of oxygen. The early HBOCs did not contain these enzymes. To control the oxygen-related damage to hemoglobin, the mentioned enzymes were added to the molecules, resulting in polyHb-SOD-CAT. These compounds were shown to remove free oxygen radicals and stabilize the hemoglobin molecule. Other approaches to add an antioxidant principle to hemoglobin are possible (adding Tempol to form polynitroxylated α-α-Hb) as well. Such protecting enzymes can also be included in the liposomes of LEH [22]. Simultaneous application of antioxidant agents (ascorbic acid, riboflavin) can protect from oxidative damage to the HBOCs [21].

HEMOSTASEOLOGICAL ALTERATIONS

Both thrombocytopenia and thrombocytopathy have been observed after infusion of certain HBOCs. These effects have been thought to be due to the NO-scavenging effects of hemoglobin. When scavenged, not enough NO is available to exert its antiplatelet effects. Besides, activation of the complementary system may lead to the thrombocytopenia—sometimes observed after HBOC infusion (especially LEH).

EFFECTS ON ERYTHROPOIESIS

It has been suggested that HBOCs stimulate erythropoiesis [23, 24].

SHELF LIFE

While red cells can be stored for a maximum of 49 days under standard conditions (about 4°C), HBOCs are stored much longer. Some HBOCs can be refrigerated; others are stabile even under room temperature. Also, storage after lyophilization of the HBOC is possible [12]. This prolongs their shelf life to 1–2 years or longer.

OTHER SIDE EFFECTS

In healthy volunteers, infusion of HBOCs resulted in gastrointestinal upset (with increased motility and sphincter spasms) and flu-like symptoms (fever, chills, headaches, and backaches) [25]. As a physiological response to infusion of hemoglobin, jaundice occurs. After administration of some HBOCs, liver enzyme levels increase.

Current products

Several types of HBOCs have been developed and are in different phases of clinical trials [12, 20, 21, 26, 27]. Table 9.1 summarizes the HBOCs developed and their properties. A comparison of the products demonstrates that they differ tremendously in one feature or the other. Obviously, HBOCs are a heterogenic group of drugs rather than the sole and perfect blood substitute.

Potential indications

Apart from use in blood management, HBOCs have been proposed and experimentally tested in a variety of settings. With that, HBOCs have the potential to become a drug rather than a blood substitute.

In animal experiments, HBOCs were used to improve the outcome of animals subjected to brain ischemia [21]. HBOCs may be clinically useful in focal or global ischemia of the brain, cardiopulmonary-bypass-induced brain lesions, and in brain trauma. These notions, however, are only supported by animal studies [28]. In studies involving humans, the potential increase in strokes in patients treated with HBOCs has stopped one trial using HBOCs.

The vasoconstrictive and NO-scavenging "side effects" of certain HBOCs can be used in septic patients who are hypotensive. It is hoped that the microvascular alterations developing during sepsis may be influenced beneficially by HBOCs. In studies on septic animals, HBOCs did not alter the regional perfusion profoundly, as would be the case with other antihypotensive agents, such as catecholamines [29]. Studies are expected to demonstrate the benefits of HBOCs in humans with severe sepsis or septic shock.

HBOCs have also been used to provide oxygen to ischemic tissues. Tissue beyond a peripheral or coronary stenosis may benefit from oxygenation provided by HBOCs. Since the HBOC particles are much smaller than red cells, a residual blood flow may suffice to provide the poststenotic tissue with oxygen [30]. HBOCs have also

been proposed in acute pancreatitis to improve microcirculation and to avoid tissue damage [31].

An improved oxygenation of organs by HBOCs is also beneficial to preserve organs reserved for transplantation. Oxygenation of tumors by HBOC infusion may improve the efficacy of anticancer treatment, which depends on the presence of oxygen in the tumor.

Further developments

After overcoming the first problems with stroma and dissociation of hemoglobin tetramers, a few first-generation HBOCs have been developed and refined and are more or less ready for use. However, while tested in thousands of patients, apart from a single exception, none of the products is approved for clinical use.

HBOCs are now developed, but mostly not in the area for which they were initially intended to be used, namely, to replace blood transfusions. Most of the first-generation HBOCs have been tested for indications that came up during development ("We have the solution, where is the problem?"). Likely, HBOCs can be used for the preservation of microcircular perfusion in ischemic areas (stroke, heart attack, sickle cell crises), as antihypotensive therapy (sepsis), for organ preservation (transplantation), and as an ultrasound contrast medium [32].

Some of the problems of HBOCs have obviously turned into a useful property. Nevertheless, we seem not to have found what we were looking for in the first-generation products, namely, a red cell substitute for acute (let alone chronic) anemia. Second-generation HBOCs are about to address the problems that prevent HBOCs' use in those settings. The hypertensive effects, short intravasal half-life, and antioxidative challenges of HBOCs must be addressed before we can use them the way we originally intended. However, during the years of research, much has been learned about hemoglobin as well as about anemia tolerance. Maybe we really do not need to have any more of what we originally wanted. Perhaps we just need an agent with a higher viscosity than the traditionally used plasma expanders. A lower hemoglobin level may suffice, given other conditions as viscosity and blood volume are taken into account. New products are in the pipeline, and time will show how much they will change the blood management.

ALBUMIN–HEME CONJUGATES AS ARTIFICIAL
OXYGEN CARRIERS

Recombinant human albumin can be engineered so that it includes up to eight heme molecules. These conjugates

Table 9.1 HBOCs and their properties.

	Class	Intravascular $t_{1/2}$	Oncotic pressure	Viscosity	Vasoactive	Source of Hgb
MP4, Hemospan (Sangart)	Malemide-PEG-conjugated = MalPEG-Hb	ca. 43 h	High (55 ± 20)	High (2.5 ± 1 cP)	Low	Human
VTR-PHP (Apex Bioscience)	Surface-modified polyoxyethylene-conjugated, pyridoxylated	ca. 40 h	Moderate to high	Moderate to high	Mild	Human
PEG Hgb (Enzon)	Surface-modified	44 h	Moderate to high	Moderate to high	Mild	Bovine
Liposome-encapsulated (Terumo)		16 h (rodent)	0.7			Bovine
Polyheme (Northfield)	GA-polymerized, pyridoxylated	24 h	Low (20–25)	Low	Moderate to low	Human
Hemolink (Hemosol)	o-Raffinose polymerized	14–24 h	Low (COP 26 mm Hg)	Low (1.15 cP)	Moderate	Human
Hemopure (Biopure) similar to HBOC-201, HBOC-301, HbGlutoamer250bovine (Oxypure for veterinarian use approved)	GA-polymerized	9–24 h	Low (17)	Low (1.3)	Moderate	Bovine
Optro (Baxter) (rHb 1.1)	α-α-cross-linked recombinant hemoglobin from E. coli		Low	Low	Marked	Recombinant human, Presbyterian mutant of Hgb
HemAssist (Baxter)	Intramolecular cross-linked with diaspirin (DCLHb)	2–14 h (dose-dependent)	(COP 42 mm Hg)	Low (1.0)	Marked	Human

PEG, polyethylene glycol; GA, glutaralydehyde; Hgb, Hemoglobin; GI, gastrointestinal; COP, colloid osmotic pressure; AST, aspartate transaminase.

have been shown to transport and release oxygen [33, 34] and have an intravascular half-life of about 36 hours. Rats were able to survive a substantial exchange of their blood volume with albumin–heme conjugates, while the control group did not [35]. These early trials with albumin–heme conjugates show promise for a future generation of AOCs.

HEMOGLOBIN AQUASOMES

Hemoglobin aquasomes consisting of hemoglobin molecules attached to a hydroxylapatite core have recently been synthesized [36]. These have been successfully tested

in animals to transport oxygen and may be another attempt to prepare a useful oxygen carrier.

Perfluorocarbons

The second group of AOCs is PFCs. They are greenhouse gases that develop during the production of aluminum. Chemically, they are related to Teflon®. PFCs consist of carbohydrate chains with 8–10 carbon atoms. Most of the atoms are substituted with fluorine. Some of the carbon atoms may also be substituted with bromine.

P50	Met-Hgb%	% Hgb tetramer	Hgb g/dL	Use	Stable	Side effects	Status
6 ± 2	<0.5		4.2 g/dl		Stable at −20°C	GI and vasoactive effects very low to absent	Phase I clinical trials
20	3		10	NO-induced shock (sepsis)			
15	<5		6	Cancer (radiosensitizer)			Trials suspended
18	12		10				
28–30	<3	<1	10	Trauma, perioperative	At room temperature >1 yr	No GI, no vasoconstrictive	
39 ± 12	<10–25	30–36	10	Cardiac, general surgery, anemia		Marked GI, purification improved this, rise in blood pressure	
38–43	<10	<5	13	Perioperative, hemodilution, anemia	At room temperature stable	Chest pain (problem resolved), jaundice, mild increase in blood pressure, AST and lipase increased	Approved in South Africa in 2001
30–33	<5		5	Surgery, trauma, hemodilution		Fever, headaches, rising blood pressure, purification has improved the situation, amylase, lipase increased	Pulled off market in 1998
30–32	4–18		10	Surgery, organ failure, trauma, stroke			Pulled off market in 1998

PFCs can dissolve and thus carry gases. About 40–50 mL of oxygen can be dissolved in 100 mL of a PFC. The oxygen-carrying characteristics of PFCs are like the ones of saline or other liquids. They follow the physical principles as mentioned in Chapter 2 on oxygen physiology. The higher the partial pressure of a gas above the PFC, the more gas is dissolved in it. This characteristic is unlike hemoglobin which dissolves oxygen in a pH-dependent manner and cooperatively, as is depicted in hemoglobin's S-shaped oxygen-binding curve (see Fig. 2.1). In contrast, the oxygen-binding curve of PFCs is a linear function. In clinical practice, this means that oxygen can be trans-ported in relevant amounts in PFC only when the inspirations oxygen fraction is high enough. That is why patients on PFCs always need supplemental oxygen.

PFCs are insoluble in water. Therefore, they come emulsified. The first-generation PFCs were dissolved in pluronic F-68. Since complement activation was associated with this compound, second-generation PFCs are now dissolved in a lecithin (and cholesterol) solution.

The intravasal half-life of PFCs is very short, some hours only. However, the biological half-life is much longer. PFC particles are chemically and physically inert. They are taken up by phagocytosis by components of the reticuloendothelial system (spleen, liver, and lung). There, the lecithin emulator is metabolized and the PFCs remain inert and are slowly given back into the bloodstream to be excreted by the lung. There is concern regarding the PFC blocking the reticuloendothelial system, which may immunocompromise the patient transiently. Furthermore, the emulgator of the PFC may be toxic to elements of the immune system. Therefore, there is a maximum dose of PFCs that should not be overstepped. Especially in patients with sepsis or an active infection, care must be taken. However, some beneficial effects of PFCs on the immune system have been postulated, since these may diminish the reperfusion damage in myocardial infarction or apoplexia. Overall, the clinical relevance of the immunomodulative effects is not yet clear.

Apart from immunosuppression, PFC administration may lead to fever 4–6 hours after infusion, shaking, nausea, and transient leukopenia. A transient thrombocytopenia is observed 2–3 days after infusion. It is usually not severe (<20% from baseline) and seems to be self-limiting after about 7 days. The thrombocytopenia occurs

without proof of platelet function problems or prolongation of prothrombin time and partial thromboplastin time in healthy volunteers [37]. The second-generation PFCs do not show relevant immunogenic reactions or complement activation (Table 9.2) [21, 26, 38, 39].

Oxygen delivery by perfluorocarbons

Normal blood with a hematocrit of about 45% and at a PO_2 of 100 mm Hg carries about 20 mL of oxygen/100 mL blood. About 25%, that is, 5 mL is released during the blood's trip through a normal, resting organism. The venous blood that returns to the heart has about 75% of oxygen left in it. When PFC is given, the body first takes oxygen from the PFC, since this is easier than taking oxygen from the "neatly packed" oxygen in the red cells. Before red cells can unload the oxygen and transfer it through their membrane, PFC already filled the needs of the tissue. Therefore, if enough PFCs are in the blood, the blood may not need to unload any oxygen and may return with nearly 100% of the oxygen it had when it left the lungs.

Table 9.2 Characteristics of perfluorocarbons.

	Fluosol-DA (Green Cross Corp., Osaka, Japan)	Oxygent (Alliance)
Generation	First	Second
Active constituents	14% perfluorodecalin and 6% perfluorotripropyl amine	58% perflubron (perfluorooctyl bromide, PFOB; C8F17 Br) and 2% perfluorodecyl bromide (PFDB, C10 F21 Br)
Emulgator	Pluronic F-68, egg yolk phospholipid	Lecithin (in phosphate-buffered aqueous electrolyte solution)
Size of particles		0.16–0.18 mcm
Intravasal half-life	12–18 h	4–15 h
Biological half-life	7 days	4 days
Dose	30 mL/kg	2.7 g PFC/kg (1.4 mL PFC/kg)
Oxygen dissolved in the presence of pure oxygen and STPD	6 mL/dL	17 mL/dL
Viscosity		ca. 4 cP
Hemoglobin equivalency		4.0 ±/ 2.7 g/dL in a dose of 2.7 g/kg (recommended clinical dose)
Storage	Frozen, mix before use	About 2 yr with standard refrigeration or room temperature

More PFCs have been developed, among them are products based on perfluorodecalin (Synthetic Blood International and Sanguine Corp.; available for use in Russia since 1996 as Perftoran™) and emulsified perfluorodichloro octane (Oxyfluor™, HemaGEN).
STPD, standard temperature and pressure, dry.

In contrast, the PFCs deliver most of their oxygen. In fact, about 91% (under $PaO_2 = 500$ mm Hg) of the oxygen bound to PFCs is unloaded during one circulation [38].

The different characteristics of oxygen unloading make it difficult to compare hemoglobin and PFCs. The clinicians typically want to know how much oxygen is theoretically available to the patient. Since most clinicians are comfortable with knowing that the patient has a hemoglobin level sufficient to meet the oxygen needs, they have a problem when there is not enough hemoglobin, yet there is an agent that may mimic the hemoglobin's function. To make matters easier, the concept of "hemoglobin equivalency" has been developed. It tells how much of a PFC is equivalent to a certain amount of hemoglobin as regards to oxygen transportation ability. It relates the percentage of whole body oxygen consumption (VO_2) from PFC to that from hemoglobin. For example: A patient with a hemoglobin level of 8 g/dL uses 50% of oxygen from hemoglobin and 25% from the PFC. This means that the PFC contributes half the amount of oxygen of that of hemoglobin to the tissue (25% is half of 50%.). Therefore, the PFC is equivalent to 4 g/dL of hemoglobin (since half of 8 g/dL is 4 g/dL) [38]. Another term used in this connection is the "effective hemoglobin," which is the sum of the hemoglobin of the patient plus the hemoglobin equivalent of the PFC.

PFCs also have effects on oxygen delivery that are beyond that of increased intravascular oxygen transport. PFCs increase the availability of oxygen in the tissue, a phenomenon called "diffusion facilitation". It is not clear how this occurs. It is thought that PFCs can travel into very small vessels in the tissue which the red cells cannot reach. Besides, PFCs may help red cells to deliver their oxygen. Since the PFCs flow near the vessel wall, and the red cells are near the center of the vessel, PFCs may serve as a bridge between red cells and the tissue ("near wall phenomenon") [40].

Tested and potential indications

PFCs are promising in blood management (see below). Additionally, PFCs can be of potential benefit in other areas. PFC particles are many times smaller than red cells. This enables them to travel to tissues that are ischemic and where red cells can no longer travel, e.g., in myocardial infarction and ischemic limbs due to a tourniquet. PFCs are also used to avoid tissue ischemia during the repair of cerebral aneurysms and to improve the outcome of cardiopulmonary bypass (microbubbles, thought to cause problems, can be readily absorbed by

PFC). PFCs augment tumor oxygenation and can preserve transplant organs [39]. PFCs were also proposed to be used in liquid ventilation in acute respiratory distress syndrome or acute lung injury, or as an ultrasound-imaging medium [21].

Artificial oxygen carriers in blood management

The original impetus to develop AOCs has been to provide a solution, which substitutes for red cell transfusions. To a certain, limited extent, AOCs are able to do so. The following paragraphs outline how AOCs can be used in blood management—instead of red cell transfusions or in other areas related to blood management.

Perfluorocarbons

SEVERE ANEMIA
Fluosol-DA, the first-generation PFC, has been used in severely anemic patients as an AOC. It was able to reverse the clinical signs of oxygen deficiency [40, 41]. However, the intravascular half-life was too short and, as a result, it was not able to improve the survival of the anemic patients. Therefore, it has not been developed further into an agent suitable for blood management [21, 30].

A second-generation PFC was shown in animal studies to be useful in resuscitation from hemorrhagic shock. Oxygen delivery can be maintained or reestablished with PFCs, so that tissues submitted to severe anemia can continue with aerobic metabolism and the organ function is preserved [42, 43]. After a PFC became available in Russia, extensive use of this PFC has been made in humans with severe anemia and it seems that the PFC can improve tissue oxygenation under such circumstances [44].

AUGMENTED ACUTE NORMOVOLEMIC HEMODILUTION[TM]
Oxygent[TM], a second-generation PFC, is not an approved drug. However, several trials have been performed, many of which directly relate to blood management. As learnt from the early trials with the first-generation PFCs, in severe anemia, current PFC products are not able to remain in the circulation long enough to work until the patient's own erythropoiesis has provided the missing red cell mass. Many publications, therefore, discuss PFCs mainly in settings where short times of decreased oxygen delivery are to be bridged. The most prominent indication in this connection is augmented acute normovolemic hemodilution (A-ANH[TM]) [45]. Intraoperatively, PFCs have been shown to reverse signs of anemia ("the transfusion trigger") more effectively than the infusion of autologous blood or

colloids. Besides, when used in conjunction with A-ANH™, the transfusion rate of noncardiac surgical patients, with a high intraoperative blood loss (defined as > 20 mL/kg), can be reduced [46, 47].

Despite the beneficial effects in reducing the transfusion of red cells, clinical trials with Oxygent™ were stopped in 2001. The reason was that in a trial with Oxygent™, the treatment group had a higher incidence of stroke, compared to the control group.

SICKLE CELL ANEMIA

Patients with sickle cell anemia may benefit from PFCs when severe sickle cell-induced vasoocclusion occurs. Since vasoocclusion is often only partial and allows for a residual flow, small PFC molecules can still travel to the ischemic areas and ameliorate the effects of sickle cell crises. It was suggested that oxygenated PFC could even unsickle and dislodge red cells and thereby reduce the vasoocclusion [48].

Hemoglobin-based oxygen carriers

TRAUMA AND HEMORRHAGIC SHOCK

In theory, HBOCs are the ideal solutions for resuscitation of patients with trauma and in hemorrhagic shock [49]. In fact, in the emergency setting and in prehospital care, HBOCs can be used to treat catastrophic blood loss [14] without resorting to allogeneic blood transfusions.

Early trauma trials with an HBOC consisting of diaspirin-cross-linked hemoglobin demonstrated an increased mortality in severely hemorrhaging trauma patients treated with this agent. This was, likely, the result of the strong vasoactive properties of the product. In contrast, Polyheme™ (see Table 9.1), which is much less vasoactive, has been used successfully to resuscitate trauma patients who do not receive red cells. Up to 20 units of the HBOC was given, and the 30-day mortality was clearly reduced to 25%, compared with 64% in a control group [50]. Despite these and other encouraging results of animal trials, HBOCs are not licensed in most countries. More experience needs to be gained regarding the use of HBOCs in trauma patients [51]. Until then, patients in only a few countries can benefit from HBOCs.

WHEN RED CELLS ARE NOT AN OPTION

HBOCs have also been used to treat patients with severe anemia who cannot take donor blood transfusions [52–54]. The use of the HBOCs is often done in a "compassionate use protocol." The inherent problem with this use

of HBOCs in severe anemia is the short half-life of the HBOCs. Due to this, serial infusions over several days were necessary, until autologous erythropoiesis provided enough red cells. Initially, HBOCs were used for short periods only. Several case reports suggest that long-term survival is also possible by exclusively using HBOCs instead of red cells, as shown in reports of patients with sickle cell crisis [55], autoimmune hemolytic anemia [56], and leukemia [57].

ACUTE NORMOVOLEMIC HEMODILUTION

In analogy to A-ANH™ using PFCs, HBOCs have been used to perform A-ANH™. HBOCs can extend the tolerance of anemia during acute normovolemic hemodilution.

SURGICAL BLOOD LOSS

As a bridge until blood is available, different HBOCs have been used to substitute surgical blood loss in the setting of general, cardiac, and vascular surgery [58–62]. As a result, red blood cell transfusions have been reduced [62, 63]. Hemopure™ (see Table 9.1), which has been approved in South Africa for the therapy of patients with major surgical blood loss, avoided red cell transfusions in 34, 27, 43, and 60% of patients undergoing cardiopulmonary bypass, abdominal aortic reconstruction, general surgery, and orthopedic surgery, respectively [64].

SICKLE CELL ANEMIA

In the event of ischemic complications of sickle cell disease, such as acute chest syndrome, exchange transfusions are recommended. As an alternative approach, HBOCs have been used in selected cases to treat anemia and sickle cell complications [55, 65].

Artificial platelet substitutes

It has not only been tried to re-create red cells, but also attempts to re-create artificial platelets have been done. Platelets are a very complex entity. Although already much is known about the importance of platelets, their modes of action are only marginally understood. It is obvious how difficult it is to produce platelet substitutes artificially.

In analogy to human HBOCs, outdated platelets have been used as source material for platelet substitutes. Nonviable platelets, platelet microvesicles (membrane fragments), and even membrane phospholipids have been tested as to their ability to support clotting [66]. Even such tiny microvesicles, as those used, have been shown to carry platelet receptors and to be able to enhance endogenous clotting or clotting processes induced by recombinant clotting factors [67].

Attempts have been made to use known elements of platelets to create a product that at least mimics some of the platelet's function. A plateletsome consisting of a liposome with a lipid bilayer has been employed as a carrier. Integrated in the lipid layer, platelet-derived receptors (e.g., for von Willebrand factor, fibrinogen, and thrombospondin) have been added. Infusion and topical application of the plateletsome solutions have been shown to decrease clinical bleeding in animals [68]. Such basic experiments aim at defining which components of platelets are needed to trigger a favorable response in bleeding. With the prospect of being able to produce the needed receptors in a recombinant fashion, the research is promising.

Another "artificial platelet substitute" called Synthocytes (Andaris Group Ltd., Quadrant Healthcare plc, Nottingham, UK) consists of albumin microcapsules with fibrinogen [69]. Since fibrinogen on the surface of Synthocytes can interact with receptors on platelets and activates platelets, Synthocytes, together with residual platelets in thrombocytopenia, may contribute to hemostasis [69]. It was hoped they would selectively target sites of hemorrhage. And indeed, in animal experiments, Synthocytes were shown to reduce bleeding.

Many other platelet substitutes, e.g., rehydrated, lyophilized platelets or thromboerythrocytes [70], are in the developing phase and are currently undergoing trials as to their usefulness as a clinically effective platelet substitute [71, 72]. It was considered that in the "far future, procoagulant cell surface transformation may be influenced by topical application of inhaled thrombomodulin-loaded liposomes or by sense or antisense oligonucleotides inducing thrombomodulin expression or suppressing tissue factor expression, respectively" [73].

However, since research on platelet substitutes is in a very early stage, basic parameters have to be established to evaluate the final products as to their ability to reduce bleeding. To this end, the Food and Drug Administration of the United States has compiled recommendations for the testing of such products in humans [74].

Key points

- It is impossible for human beings to re-create blood.
- First-generation AOCs have a very short half-life and come with unwanted side effects that make them unsuitable for general use as a blood substitute. AOCs are promising drugs with well-described indications and contraindications.

Questions for review

- What are AOCs and what are their indications in blood management?
- What are the sources of hemoglobin used for the production of HBOCs?
- What are the differences between (a) hemoglobin in the viable red cell, (b) hemoglobin free after lysis of red cells, and (c) hemoglobin attached to polyethylene glycol?
- What are common side effects of HBOCs and how have they been engineered to reduce them?
- What is the source of PFCs?
- How do PFCs transport oxygen?
- What different platelet substitutes have been described?

Suggestions for further research

What is the current status of HBOCs and PFCs? Check the Internet and medical literature for more information.

Exercises and practice cases

Read the case report of Cothren and colleagues [75]. Discuss the management of the described patient. What indicators have there been to support the claim that (a) the patient benefited from HBOC and (b) the patient did not benefit from HBOC. What lessons do you learn from this report about the oxygen transport of HBOCs?

Homework

1 Find out whether there is somebody in your vicinity who uses AOCs. Record his/her contact information in the address book in the Appendix E.
2 Is it possible in your country to get AOCs? If so, record the contact information of the provider(s) in the address book in the Appendix E.

References

1 Tunnicliffe, F.W. and G.F. Stebbing. The intravenous injection of oxygen gas as a therapeutic measure. *Lancet*, 1916. (August 19): p. 321–323.

2 Amberson, W., *et al.* On the use of Ringer–Locke solutions containing hemoglobin as a substitute for normal blood in mammals. *J Cell Comp Physiol*, 1937. **5**: p. 359–382.

3 Amberson, W.R., *et al.* Clinical experience with hemoglobin-saline solution. *J Appl Physiol*, 1949. **1**: p. 469–489.

4 Rabiner, S.F., *et al.* Further studies with stroma-free hemoglobin solution. *Ann Surg*, 1970. **171**(4): p. 615–622.

5 Savitsky, J.P., *et al.* A clinical safety trial of stroma-free hemoglobin. *Clin Pharmacol Ther*, 1978. **23**(1): p. 73–80.

6 Clark, L.C., Jr. and F. Gollan. Survival of mammals breathing organic liquids equilibrated with oxygen at atmospheric pressure. *Science*, 1966. **152**(730): p. 1755–1756.

7 Strategies to reduce military and civilian blood transfusions. *Anesthesiology News*, September 2002, p. 1–7.

8 Hoffman, S.J., *et al.* Expression of fully functional tetrameric human hemoglobin in Escherichia coli. *Proc Natl Acad Sci USA*, 1990. **87**(21): p. 8521–8525.

9 Looker, D., *et al.* A human recombinant haemoglobin designed for use as a blood substitute. *Nature*, 1992. **356**(6366): p. 258–260.

10 Chang, T.M. Hemoglobin-based red blood cell substitutes. *Artif Organs*, 2004. **28**(9): p. 789–794.

11 Sakai, H. and E. Tsuchida. Performances of PEG-modified hemoglobin-vesicles as artificial oxygen carriers in microcirculation. *Clin Hemorheol Microcirc*, 2006. **34**(1–2): p. 335–340.

12 Chang, T.M. Oxygen carriers. *Curr Opin Investig Drugs*, 2002. **3**(8): p. 1187–1190.

13 Rabinovici, R. The status of hemoglobin-based red cell substitutes. *Isr Med Assoc J*, 2001. **3**(9): p. 691–697.

14 Baron, J.F. Haemoglobin therapy in clinical practice: use and characteristics of DCLHb. *Br J Anaesth*, 1998. **81**(Suppl 1): p. 34–37.

15 Intaglietta, M. Microcirculatory basis for the design of artificial blood. *Microcirculation*, 1999. **6**(4): p. 247–258.

16 Wettstein, R., *et al.* Resuscitation with polyethylene glycol-modified human hemoglobin improves microcirculatory blood flow and tissue oxygenation after hemorrhagic shock in awake hamsters. *Crit Care Med*, 2003. **31**(6): p. 1824–1830.

17 Reiter, C.D., *et al.* Cell-free hemoglobin limits nitric oxide bioavailability in sickle-cell disease. *Nat Med*, 2002. **8**(12): p. 1383–1389.

18 Bucci, E., *et al.* Cell-free hemoglobin, oxygen off-load and vasoconstriction. *Anasthesiol Intensivmed Notfallmed Schmerzther*, 2001. **36**(Suppl 2): p. S123–S124.

19 Malhotra, A.K., *et al.* Resuscitation with a novel hemoglobin-based oxygen carrier in a Swine model of uncontrolled perioperative hemorrhage. *J Trauma*, 2003. **54**(5): p. 915–924.

20 Creteur, J. and J.L. Vincent. Hemoglobin solutions. *Crit Care Med*, 2003. **31**(12 Suppl): p. S698–S707.

21 Dinkelmann, S. and H. Northoff. Artificial oxygen carriers—a critical analysis of current developments. *Anasthesiol Intensivmed Notfallmed Schmerzther*, 2003. **38**(1): p. 47–54.

22 Chang, T.M. Future generations of red blood cell substitutes. *J Intern Med*, 2003. **253**(5): p. 527–535.

23 Lindahl, S.G. Thinner than blood. *Anesth Analg*, 1995. **80**(2): p. 217–218.

24 Hughes, G.S., Jr., *et al.* Hematologic effects of a novel hemoglobin-based oxygen carrier in normal male and female subjects. *J Lab Clin Med*, 1995. **126**(5): p. 444–451.

25 Viele, M.K., R.B. Weiskopf, and D. Fisher. Recombinant human hemoglobin does not affect renal function in humans: analysis of safety and pharmacokinetics. *Anesthesiology*, 1997. **86**(4): p. 848–858.

26 Mazer, C.D. Review of clinical trials of oxygen therapeutics. *TATM*, 2000. **S1**: p. 27–31.

27 Bjorkholm, M., *et al.* A phase I single blind clinical trial of a new oxygen transport agent (MP4), human hemoglobin modified with maleimide-activated polyethylene glycol. *Haematologica*, 2005. **90**(4): p. 505–515.

28 Lenz, C. and F. Waschke. Artificial oxygen carriers and the cerebral circulation. *Anasthesiol Intensivmed Notfallmed Schmerzther*, 2001. **36**(Suppl 2): p. S110–S113.

29 Bone, H.G. Hemoglobin-based oxygen carriers in sepsis. *Anasthesiol Intensivmed Notfallmed Schmerzther*, 2001. **36**(Suppl 2): p. S114–S116.

30 Kale, P.B., *et al.* Fluosol: therapeutic failure in severe anemia. *Ann Pharmacother*, 1993. **27**(12): p. 1452–1454.

31 Strate, T., *et al.* The potential of HBOC in acute pancreatitis. *Anasthesiol Intensivmed Notfallmed Schmerzther*, 2001. **36**(Suppl 2): p. S119–S120.

32 Creteur, J., W. Sibbald, and J.L. Vincent. Hemoglobin solutions—not just red blood cell substitutes. *Crit Care Med*, 2000. **28**(8): p. 3025–3034.

33 Wang, R.M., *et al.* Human serum albumin bearing covalently attached iron(II) porphyrins as O_2-coordination sites. *Bioconjug Chem*, 2005. **16**(1): p. 23–26.

34 Komatsu, T., *et al.* O_2 and CO binding properties of artificial hemoproteins formed by complexing iron protoporphyrin IX with human serum albumin mutants. *J Am Chem Soc*, 2005. **127**(45): p. 15933–15942.

35 Komatsu, T., *et al.* Exchange transfusion with synthetic oxygen-carrying plasma protein "albumin-heme" into an acute anemia rat model after seventy-percent hemodilution. *J Biomed Mater Res A*, 2004. **71**(4): p. 644–651.

36 Khopade, A.J., S. Khopade, and N.K. Jain. Development of hemoglobin aquasomes from spherical hydroxyapatite cores precipitated in the presence of half-generation poly(amidoamine) dendrimer. *Int J Pharm*, 2002. **241**(1): p. 145–154.

37 Leese, P.T., *et al.* Randomized safety studies of intravenous perflubron emulsion. I. Effects on coagulation function in healthy volunteers. *Anesth Analg*, 2000. **91**(4): p. 804–811.

38 Faithfull, N.S. Fluorocarbon formulations and principles of oxygen delivery. *TATM*, 2001. **3**: p. 5–9.

39 Keipert, P.E. Perflubron emulsion (Oxygent(tm)): a temporary intravenous oxygen carrier. *Anasthesiol Intensivmed Notfallmed Schmerzther*, 2001. **36**(Suppl 2): p. S104–S106.

40 Welte, M. Current status of perfluorocarbons. *Anasthesiol Intensivmed Notfallmed Schmerzther*, 2001. **36**(Suppl 2): p. S165–S168.

41 Spence, R.K., *et al.* Perfluorocarbons as blood substitutes: the experience with Fluosol DA 20% in the 1980s. *Artif Cells Blood Substit Immobil Biotechnol*, 1994. **22**: p. 955–963.

42 Paxian, M., *et al.* Perflubron emulsion improves hepatic microvascular integrity and mitochondrial redox state after hemorrhagic shock. *Shock*, 2003. **20**(5): p. 449–457.

43 Kemming, G.I., *et al.* Oxygent as a top load to colloid and hyperoxia is more effective in resuscitation from hemorrhagic shock than colloid and hyperoxia alone. *Shock*, 2005. **24**(3): p. 245–254.

44 Maevsky, E., *et al.* Clinical results of Perftoran application: present and future. *Artif Cells Blood Substit Immobil Biotechnol*, 2005. **33**(1): p. 37–46.

45 Spahn, D.R., P.F. Willimann, and N.S. Faithfull. The effectiveness of augmented acute normovolemic hemodilution (A-ANH). *Anaesthesist*, 2001. **50**(Suppl 1): p. S49–S54.

46 Kemming, G., O. Habler, and B. Zwissler. Augmented acute normovolemic hemodilution (A-ANH(tm)) in cardiac and non-cardiac patients. *Anasthesiol Intensivmed Notfallmed Schmerzther*, 2001. **36**(Suppl 2): p. S107–S109.

47 Spahn, D.R., *et al.* Use of perflubron emulsion to decrease allogeneic blood transfusion in high-blood-loss non-cardiac surgery: results of a European phase 3 study. *Anesthesiology*, 2002. **97**(6): p. 1338–1349.

48 Kaul, D.K., X. Liu, and R.L. Nagel. Ameliorating effects of fluorocarbon emulsion on sickle red blood cell-induced obstruction in an ex vivo vasculature. *Blood*, 2001. **98**(10): p. 3128–3131.

49 Moore, E.E. Blood substitutes: the future is now. *J Am Coll Surg*, 2003. **196**(1): p. 1–17.

50 Gould, S.A., *et al.* The life-sustaining capacity of human polymerized hemoglobin when red cells might be unavailable. *J Am Coll Surg*, 2002. **195**(4): p. 445–452; discussion 452–455.

51 Sloan, E.P., *et al.* Diaspirin cross-linked hemoglobin (DCLHb) in the treatment of severe traumatic hemorrhagic shock: a randomized controlled efficacy trial. *JAMA*, 1999. **282**(19): p. 1857–1864.

52 Cothren, C., *et al.* Blood substitute and erythropoietin therapy in a severely injured Jehovah's Witness. *N Engl J Med*, 2002. **346**(14): p. 1097–1098.

53 Anton, N., J.K. Hitzler, and B.P. Kavanagh. Treatment of life-threatening post-haemorrhagic anaemia with cell-free haemoglobin solution in an adolescent Jehovah's Witness. *Br J Haematol*, 2002. **118**(4): p. 1183–1186.

54 Shander, A., *et al.* Use of a hemoglobin-based oxygen carrier in the treatment of severe anemia. *Obstet Gynecol*, 2004. **103**(5, Pt 2): p. 1096–1099.

55 Lanzkron, S., *et al.* Polymerized human Hb use in acute chest syndrome: a case report. *Transfusion*, 2002. **42**(11): p. 1422–1427.

56 Mullon, J., *et al.* Transfusions of polymerized bovine hemoglobin in a patient with severe autoimmune hemolytic anemia. *N Engl J Med*, 2000. **342**(22): p. 1638–1643.

57 Agrawal, Y.P., M. Freedman, and Z.M. Szczepiorkowski. Long-term transfusion of polymerized bovine hemoglobin in a Jehovah's Witness following chemotherapy for myeloid leukemia: a case report. *Transfusion*, 2005. **45**(11): p. 1735–1738.

58 Lamy, M.L., *et al.* Randomized trial of diaspirin cross-linked hemoglobin solution as an alternative to blood transfusion after cardiac surgery. The DCLHb Cardiac Surgery Trial Collaborative Group. *Anesthesiology*, 2000. **92**(3): p. 646–656.

59 Hill, S.E., L.I. Gottschalk, and K. Grichnik. Safety and preliminary efficacy of hemoglobin raffimer for patients undergoing coronary artery bypass surgery. *J Cardiothorac Vasc Anesth*, 2002. **16**(6): p. 695–702.

60 Levy, J.H., *et al.* Polymerized bovine hemoglobin solution as a replacement for allogeneic red blood cell transfusion after cardiac surgery: results of a randomized, double-blind trial. *J Thorac Cardiovasc Surg*, 2002. **124**(1): p. 35–42.

61 LaMuraglia, G.M., *et al.* The reduction of the allogeneic transfusion requirement in aortic surgery with a hemoglobin-based solution. *J Vasc Surg*, 2000. **31**(2): p. 299–308.

62 Schubert, A., *et al.* Diaspirin-crosslinked hemoglobin reduces blood transfusion in noncardiac surgery: a multicenter, randomized, controlled, double-blinded trial. *Anesth Analg*, 2003. **97**(2): p. 323–332, table of contents.

63 Anbari, K.K., J.P. Garino, and C.F. Mackenzie. Hemoglobin substitutes. *Eur Spine J*, 2004. **13**(Suppl 1): p. S76–S82.

64 Jacobs, E. Clinical update: Hemopure(r)—a room temperature stable hemoglobin oxygen carrier. *Anasthesiol Intensivmed Notfallmed Schmerzther*, 2001. **36**(Suppl 2): p. S121–S122.

65 Gonzalez, P., *et al.* A phase I/II study of polymerized bovine hemoglobin in adult patients with sickle cell disease not in crisis at the time of study. *J Investig Med*, 1997. **45**(5): p. 258–264.

66 Alving, B. Potential for synthetic phospholipids as partial platelet substitutes. *Transfusion*, 1998. **38**(11–12): p. 997–998.

67 Tonda, R., *et al.* Platelet membrane fragments enhance the procoagulant effect of recombinant factor VIIa in studies with circulating human blood under conditions of experimental thrombocytopenia. *Semin Hematol*, 2004. **41**(1, Suppl 1): p. 157–162.

68 Rybak, M.E. and L.A. Renzulli. A liposome based platelet substitute, the plateletsome, with hemostatic efficacy. *Biomater Artif Cells Immobilization Biotechnol*, 1993. **21**(2): p. 101–118.

69 Davies, A.R., *et al.* Interactions of platelets with Synthocytes, a novel platelet substitute. *Platelets*, 2002. **13**(4): p. 197–205.

70 Coller, B.S., *et al*. Thromboerythrocytes. In vitro studies of a potential autologous, semi-artificial alternative to platelet transfusions. *J Clin Invest*, 1992. **89**(2): p. 546–555.

71 Fischer, T.H., *et al*. Splenic clearance mechanisms of rehydrated, lyophilized platelets. *Artif Cells Blood Substit Immobil Biotechnol*, 2001. **29**(6): p. 439–451.

72 Levi, M., *et al*. Fibrinogen-coated albumin microcapsules reduce bleeding in severely thrombocytopenic rabbits. *Nat Med*, 1999. **5**(1): p. 107–111.

73 Scherer, R.U. Haemostaseological aspects of perioperative blood management. *Zentralbl Chir*, 2003. **128**(6): p. 473–480.

74 US Department of Health and Human Services, Food and Drug Administration, Center for Biologics Evaluation and Research (CBER), *Guidance for Industry for Platelet Testing Evaluation of Platelet Substitute Products*, 1999.

75 Cothren, C.C., *et al*. Large volume polymerized haemoglobin solution in a Jehovah's Witness following abruptio placentae. *Transfus Med*, 2004. **14**(3): p. 241–246.

10 Oxygen therapy

Oxygen can have tremendous effects on the human organism. Obviously, human life without oxygen is impossible. On the other hand, life is endangered when there is too much oxygen. Oxygen therapy, as a valuable adjunct to the therapy of hypoxia secondary to anemia, comes with great benefits, but also with side effects. It takes knowledgeable health-care providers to make oxygen another lifesaving piece in the armamentarium for blood management.

Objectives of this chapter

1 Describe why patients in a blood management program may be the candidates for inhalational or hyperbaric oxygen therapy.
2 Review the physiology, pathophysiology, and physics of oxygen.
3 Give basic advice on how to prescribe oxygen therapy, how to prepare the patient, and how to treat possible side effects of the therapy.

Definitions

Inhalational oxygen therapy: Inhalation of oxygen aimed at restoring any normal pathophysiological alterations of gas exchange in the cardiopulmonary system and at the tissue level.
Hyperbaric oxygen therapy: The patient breathes 100% oxygen intermittently, while the pressure of the treatment chamber is increased to greater than 1 atm. According to the Undersea and Hyperbaric Medical Society (UHMS), breathing 100% oxygen at 1 atm or the topical application of hyperbaric oxygen is not hyperbaric oxygen therapy.

A brief look at history

The use of gases for medical therapy dates back thousands of years. Actually, as with many other therapies, oxygen therapy has been prescribed before even the basic mechanism of action was known. Amazingly, oxygen therapy was used even before oxygen was discovered.

Medical use of oxygen initially built on the work divers had done. Since the lack of oxygen under water is the limiting factor for prolonged diving, the main problem of diving was to make additional oxygen available. Already in 320 BC, Alexander the Great used a glass vessel to dive into the Bosporus Straits during the siege of Tyre. Much later, in 1620, Cornelius Drebbel developed a normobaric diving bell. It became the forerunner of today's medical hyperbaric chambers.

The first medical use of a hyperbaric environment was reported in 1662. Henshaw, a British clergyman, used compressed air for the treatment of pulmonary disease. Using a system of organ bellows, he could adjust pressure within a sealed chamber called a "domicilium." Valves were placed so that air could be either compressed into the chamber or extracted from it. In the domicilium, increased pressure was used for the treatment of acute diseases, and reduced pressure for the treatment of chronic diseases. Although this concept may not be accepted today, the treatment of anemia probably would have benefited from it. Patients with symptoms of acute anemia would have gained from the additional oxygen, while chronically anemic patients may have been benefited by the increased erythropoietin production, due to the lack of oxygen under hypobaric conditions.

Scientific proof of the effectiveness of hyperbaric therapy was lacking at that time. The situation slowly changed. In 1670, Boyle gave the first description of decompression phenomena. Finally, oxygen, as a gas, was discovered independently by the Swedish apothecary Karl W. Scheele in 1772 and by the English chemist Joseph Priestley in 1774. Although Scheele was the first to discover oxygen, Priestley is credited with the discovery, since he published his findings in 1775, while Scheele published his work 2 years later. Priestley influenced a researcher named Lavoisier who eventually named the gas *oxygene*, meaning acid-former.

Priestley experimented with the new gases and reported about them in his work *Experiments and Observations on Different Kinds of Air*. Priestley seemed to be the first person ever to inhale air with a greater concentration of oxygen than normal. He describes that he, while breathing his "new air," "... fancied that (his) breast felt peculiarly light and easy for some time afterwards." He continued: "Hitherto only two mice and myself have had the privilege of breathing it" [1]. Priestley had already thought about the medical use of this gas. However, he also warned about its use. "From the greater strength and vivacity of the flame of a candle, in this pure air, it may be conjectured, that it might be peculiarly salutary to the lungs in certain morbid cases, ... But, perhaps, we may also infer from these experiments, that though (oxygen) might be very useful as a medicine, it might not be so proper for us in the usual healthy state of the body; for, as a candle burns out much faster in (oxygen) than in common air, so we might, as may be said, live out too fast."

During the first 100 years after Priestley's discovery, oxygen was employed for the treatment of many diseases. Quacks, as well as scientists, used this gas (or other gases supposed to be oxygen) for the cure of almost every disease, among them symptoms and diseases of the respiratory tract (tuberculosis, asthma, pneumonia, bronchitis, dyspnea), infectious conditions (cellulitis, pyemia, ulcers) and conditions possibly associated with shock (cholera, anemia, asphyxia, poisoning, eclampsia, septicemia). Curiously, oxygen has also been used in conditions like indigestion, albuminuria, diabetes, spermatorrhea, rheumatism, gout, hysteria, and menstrual irregularities.

In the 1800s, hyperbaric medicine was fashionable and institutions offering hyperbaric medicine flourished throughout Europe. Famous medical journals like the *Lancet* [2] and the *British Medical Journal* caught up on the topic of oxygen therapy. The interest in oxygen therapy was so great that societies were founded to further the use of oxygen. In 1798, the Pneumatic Institution for Inhalation Gas Therapy was founded by Thomas Beddoes. The engineer James Watt helped manufacture the gases. Actually, lower concentrations of oxygen were also thought to be beneficial. Patients with consumption, asthma, palsy, dropsy, and obstinate venereal complaints and others came to the institute for treatment. Patients were treated for free. The institute closed in 1802.

In 1879, a French surgeon named Fontaine built a fully equipped mobile hyperbaric operating room. He used the fact that the solubility of a gas in a liquid is proportional to the pressure of the gas over the solution. Under hyperbaric conditions, in the operating room, Fontaine increased the amount of oxygen in the patient's blood. It was claimed that patients did better when surgery was performed under hyperbaric conditions. They recovered from the anesthetic more rapidly, and cyanosis and asphyxia were reported to be less or absent. The chamber was also recommended for patients with anemia. Fontaine's work ended with a fatal accident at his work place.

Anemia was one of the indications for oxygen therapy. William Osler briefly recommended oxygen for anemia in his book *The Principles and Practice of Medicine* in 1892 [3]. J. Henry Davenport describes: "Oxygen here acts as a tonic, increasing the weight and strength, and visibly restoring the natural ruddy hue of the face in health. It has in this way been found valuable in ... anaemia .... three or four gallons are inhaled daily [4]. C.E. Ehinger confirmed his findings in oxygen therapy for anemia. However, the administered dose of oxygen was very low and oxygen was used only intermittently [5]. Therefore, the extent of the effects of oxygen therapy seems questionable from today's perspective.

By the end of the nineteenth century, oxygen therapy was becoming accepted by an ever-growing number of practitioners, although many still doubted its usefulness [6]. This is understandable when we see how oxygen was used. Oxygen was not only inhaled, but was also advocated as compound oxygen, that is, bound in chemical compounds [7], as enema [8], for intraabdominal and intrapleural insufflation [9], as well as injection into joints, veins [10], and into the subcutis [11]. Oxygen has also been used in shock, probably due to hemorrhage [9]. As Dr Howitt claims, subcutaneous administration does appear to help in urgent situations. The described modes of oxygen application may indeed have looked strange to the prejudiced observer.

Despite all the ridicule, oxygen therapy was never completely devoid of advocates. In 1918, Dr Orval Cunningham studied the differences between people living through or dying due to the flu epidemic in the Rocky Mountains. He noted people in the valley did better than people in the mountains. He reasoned that denser air in the valley helped people fight the infection. Cunningham used a small hyperbaric chamber, built next to his clinic, to test this hypothesis. He successfully treated a young colleague with influenza, who was near death, due to restricted lung function and secondary hypoxia. Positive results in patients suffering from pneumonia encouraged him to build other oxygen chambers. After experiencing an amazing cure of his kidney disease after hyperbaric therapy, a grateful patient built a huge chamber for Cunningham. This chamber was built in Kansas City in 1921.

It looked like a hollow steel ball of approximately 20 m in diameter. It was equipped with a smoking lounge, carpets, dining room, and private quarters. Seven years later, Cunningham built in Cleveland the world's largest functional hyperbaric chamber, a five-floor "hyperbaric hospital." However, Cunningham's hyperbaric hospital was closed during the Great Depression in the 1930s and was demolished for scrap metal for the impending war.

A turning point in the medical use of oxygen occurred after World War I. Haldane described the use of oxygen on victims of gas poisoning. His article was a landmark in oxygen therapy [12]. A further impetus for hyperbaric medicine came from the Dutch Boerema in 1956. He demonstrated that pigs could survive in a hyperbaric environment without any red cells. His article "Life without blood" was another landmark in the scientific work-up of the age-old subject of hyperbaric medicine [13,14]. In order to prolong operative time with a patient in cardiac arrest, Boerema and associates performed cardiac surgery in a hyperbaric chamber. Based on these experiences, in 1969, the (most probably) first case of hemorrhagic shock was reported to be treated successfully with hyperbaric oxygen therapy [15] instead of blood transfusions.

A widespread enthusiasm for hyperbaric medicine resulted in its use in cancer, stroke, and myocardial infarction. However, the scientific results were disappointing. In 1967, the Undersea and Hyperbaric Medical Society (UHMS) was founded in the United States. During the 1970s, the practice of hyperbaric oxygen therapy decreased, probably due to the lack of improvement in many of the treatments for which hyperbaric oxygen was used. In 1976, the UHMS established a Committee on Hyperbaric Oxygen Therapy. It helped to lay the scientific basis for hyperbaric medicine. A set of approved indications were put together. Hyperbaric medicine gained renewed interest. In March 2000, the American Board of Medical Specialties approved undersea and hyperbaric medicine as a subspecialty of both emergency medicine and preventive medicine.

Physics and physiology of oxygen

Under the climatic conditions where human life is possible, oxygen is a gas. It obeys gas laws and other related physical principles. Do you remember the following laws?

Dalton's Law: The total gas pressure is the sum of all partial pressures of the gases in a gas mixture ($P_T = P1 + P2 + P3 + \cdots + Pn$).

Table 10.1 Units for barometric pressure.

1 atm (atmosphere)
760 mm Hg (millimeters mercury) = Torr
1.470×10^1 psi (pounds per square inch = lbs/in.^{2})
1.033 kg/cm^2 (kilograms per square centimeters)
1.013 bar
3.305×10^1 fsw (feet or meters of seawater)
1.033×10^1 msw (meters of seawater)

Henry's Law: The degree to which a gas is dissolved in a solution is directly proportional to the pressure of the gas.

Boyle's Law: When temperature remains constant, the volume of a gas is inversely proportional to its pressure.

Charle's law: When volume remains constant, pressure is directly proportional to temperature. For example, when the pressure increases from 1 to 3 atm, the temperature also increases threefold.

Apart from knowing the above, it is also vital to know that the amount of gas dissolved in a liquid is determined by its solubility coefficient. This coefficient is specific for each fluid and is dependent on temperature. The lower the temperature, the more gas is dissolved. The solubility of oxygen in plasma at 37°C is 0.0214 mL of oxygen/mL plasma per atmosphere partial pressure of oxygen (PO_2).

In our environment in ambient air, the gas we breathe consists of approximately 21% oxygen and 78% nitrogen, with trace amounts of other gases. Expressed in medical terms, we would breathe with an inspiratory oxygen fraction (FiO_2) of 21%. At sea level, the gases exert a pressure of 1 atm, that is, 760 mm Hg (Table 10.1). The share of each one of the gases is exerted in relation to their percentage in the gas mixture. Since about 21% of the gas in our atmosphere is oxygen, oxygen exerts a partial pressure (PO_2) of 21% of 760 mm Hg, that is, approximately 160 mm Hg.

In the lung, the relationship of the gases changes. Carbon dioxide is added to the inhaled air mixture. Carbon dioxide exerts a partial pressure of 40 mm Hg. Water vapor is added as well. At normal body temperature (37°C), the air in the lungs is saturated with water. The water exerts a pressure of 47 mm Hg (= PH_2O, saturated water vapor pressure). Based on the alveolar gas equation (see below), on breathing room air, the oxygen partial pressure in the lung thus reduces from 160 mm Hg in open air to about 100–110 mm Hg in the alveoli.

How much oxygen finally reaches the blood stream is determined by the diffusion across the barrier between the alveoli and the vasculature. The alveolar to arterial gradient (A–a gradient) provides an assessment of this alveolar–capillary gas exchange and is the difference between the oxygen partial pressure in the alveoli (PAO_2) and the oxygen partial pressure in the arteries (PaO_2). The normal A–a gradient is calculated by adding 10 to the age of the patient and dividing this by 4. The A–a increases from 5 to 7 mm Hg for every 10% increase in FiO_2. Values between 20 and 65 mm Hg are normal. Severe respiratory distress may have an A–a gradient of >more than 400. Another way to estimate how much oxygen is transferred across the barrier between alveoli and arterioles is to assume that for every six parts of oxygen in the lung, five parts are found in the vessels.

Alveolar gas equation: $PAO_2 = (Pb - PH_2O \times FiO_2 - PACO_2 \times (FiO_2 + [(1 - FiO_2)/R])$ where
Pb is barometric pressure
PH_2O is saturated water vapor pressure
$PACO_2$ is alveolar PCO_2, assumed to be equal to arterial PCO_2
R is respiratory quotient, normally 0.8

Oxygen—friend and enemy

Oxygen is the single most important substance for life. It is essential in the pathway leading from food intake to energy production. The cells, as electrical systems, depend on oxygen to perform the electron transfer that is needed to produce energy. Besides, oxygen combines with protons to form water, another essential substance. Since oxygen is such an important substance for life, it is not surprising that a severe lack of oxygen is fatal. Therefore, the provision of oxygen to the tissue is the main goal of many therapies, and it proves lifesaving. However, oxygen also comes with effects that endanger life. Oxygen therapy therefore needs to be based on a thorough knowledge of the effects on the human body.

Effects of oxygen on the human body

Circulatory effects: Inhalation of greater than normal oxygen concentrations has a profound effect on the blood flow. The total peripheral resistance increases, and with it the systemic blood pressure. A redistribution of blood flow from the skeletal muscles to areas of the splanchnic vasculature occurs [16]. The blood flow to the kidneys increases as well [17]. Hyperoxic ventilation, in healthy persons with a normal hemoglobin level, increases the systemic vascular resistance and decreases the cardiac output (by decreasing both stroke volume and heart rate) and

oxygen consumption [18, 19]. Interestingly, the effects of normovolemic anemia modulate the vascular effects of oxygen. Anemia increases the blood flow, and with it the shear stress on the vessel walls. NO is released and vessels dilate. Oxygen reverses this vasodilatation.

Immunological effects: Oxygen can act as an antibiotic [20]. It facilitates the clearance of bacteria from the tissue since it supports the work of neutrophils. Normally, neutrophils phagocyte bacteria, resulting in a respiratory (oxidative) burst—the creation of oxygen radicals, which play their role in bactericidal activity. This respiratory burst increases the oxygen consumption of the tissue 15–20 times. The partial pressure of oxygen in the tissue containing the neutrophils is approximately 0–10 mm Hg. The side products of the neutrophils' respiratory burst damage the tissue. Adding oxygen to this scenario (that is, when the patient breathes more oxygen) facilitates the neutrophils' action, and the bacteria are cleared more effectively. Besides, tissue is provided with the needed oxygen. Therefore, necrosis of the tissue is minimized and scars tend to be smaller when formed under oxygen therapy [20]. Oxygen thus promotes wound healing and angiogenesis.

Metabolic effects: Free oxygen radicals are needed for the function of phagocytes to kill bacteria. The radicals can also lead to cell damage in the body. Free oxygen is toxic. It oxidizes sulfhydryl group bearing enzymes and increases the production of peroxides [21]. The inhibited enzymatic work disturbs the metabolic activity. Oxygen can damage tissue, when enzyme levels are not allowed to recover.

Ocular effects: Preterm children are often given oxygen to keep their arterial oxygen saturation at, at least, 90%. But, this causes side effects. Especially during the first weeks of life, supplemental oxygen causes eye damage. Since oxygen furthers angiogenesis, vessels may develop in the vitreous body, followed by fibrosis and retinopathy. This leads to blindness (retrolental fibroplasia). The risk of such a serious retinopathy [22] increases when the arterial oxygen saturation exceeds 80%.

Cerebral effects: Breathing oxygen either at a high FiO_2 or at a high ambient air pressure can cause cerebral damage. Generalized convulsions are a vivid expression of this damage. A direct toxic effect of oxygen, the accumulation of carbon dioxide and altered cerebral circulation, when combined, may lead to this cerebral damage [23].

Oxygen therapy may also reduce the drive to breathe. The reduced breathing leads to hypercapnia and may result in carbon dioxide narcosis.

Pulmonary effects: Inhalation of higher than normal concentrations of oxygen results, primarily, in pulmonary damage. First, an acute exudative phase, with interstitial and alveolar edema, hemorrhage, fibrinous exudate, formation of hyaline membranes, and the destruction of the capillary endothelial and type I alveolar epithelial cells, results. This phase is followed by a second, subacute, proliferative phase. Interstitial fibrosis and proliferation of fibroblasts and type II alveolar epithelium cells follow, together with the partial resolution of the effects of the exudative phase.

Clinically, the first sign of oxygen toxicity is tracheobronchitis. The patients develop a cough and chest pain. The tracheal symptoms gradually spread through the pulmonary branches. Auscultation shows rales, ronchi, and bronchial breath sounds and the patients develop fever. Animal experiments, with toxic levels of oxygen, show that further development of pulmonary damage results in dyspnea and respiratory insufficiency with hypoxia and death [24].

Atelectasis is also typical of pulmonary exposure to oxygen. Since the inspired gas consists mainly of oxygen, nitrogen is washed out of the lung. Nitrogen is an inert gas, which is not absorbed by the lung. Its presence means that there is always gas in the alveoli. This serves as a "pneumatic splint" for the alveoli, preventing them from collapsing. When this inert gas is no longer there, problems arise. Oxygen is taken up from the alveoli into the body and the inert gas is lacking. The alveoli collapse and atelectasis develops. Atelectasis is also facilitated by a lack of surfactant, which results from the damage exerted by toxic oxygen [24].

There are some factors that modify the effects of oxygen in the lungs. Probably, the most important factor is that intermittent exposure to high oxygen levels elicits an adaptive response. Intermittent exposure to a normal PO_2 is the most practical approach to minimize side effects of oxygen. Air breaks during hyperbaric oxygen therapy allow antioxidants to deal with free oxygen radicals and reduce oxygen toxicity.

A long list of drugs has been examined regarding their influence on the toxicity of oxygen. As a rule of thumb, factors that increase sympathetic influence enhance the toxic effects of oxygen, while increased vagal effects prove protective. Increased thyroid activity, cortisol, insulin, atropine, estrogen, hyperthermia, and catecholamines increase the detrimental effects of oxygen, while adrenergic blockers, antihistamines, antioxidants, cobalt, hypothermia, hypothyroidism, and starvation reduce the toxic effects of oxygen. Also, many general anesthetics protect against the toxic effects of oxygen, on the lung as well as on the brain [24].

Effects of pressurized oxygen on the human body

Hyperbaric oxygen therapy exerts its beneficial effects through two distinct features: an increase in oxygen tension and an increase in pressure.

The effects of an increase in oxygen tension have already been discussed above. The effects of oxygen exposure in normobaric and hyperbaric environments are essentially the same. But, since the magnitude of the oxygen-related effects depends on the oxygen partial pressure in the body and not on the inspiratory oxygen fraction, hyperbaric conditions magnify the oxygen effects at a given FiO_2. Under hyperbaric conditions, a decrease in heart rate (5–7%), stroke volume, and sympathetic tone have been observed [25]. This leads to a cardiac output decreased by 10–20% [25]. Hyperbaric oxygen therapy also leads to vasoconstriction, but the hyperbaric oxygenation of the tissues offsets any decrease in oxygen delivery by vasoconstriction [26].

Increased pressure drives more oxygen into the body fluids than the same FiO_2 at only 1 atm pressure. Resting tissues need 5–6 mL of oxygen/100 mL blood to sustain life. Human life is generally not possible when oxygen is solely delivered by physical solution in plasma. Hemoglobin is needed to provide the major portion of oxygen needed by the tissue. At 1 atm pressure, only 0.3 mL of oxygen is dissolved in 100 mL of plasma. When the FiO_2 is increased five times (by switching from inhalation of room air to inhalation of pure oxygen), the amount of oxygen dissolved in plasma is also five times greater, namely 1.5 mL/100 mL of plasma. Administering 100% oxygen at a pressure of 3 atm provides about 6 mL oxygen/100 mL of blood. (At a PO_2 of 3.5 atm, the PaO_2 is 2100 mm Hg.) This is enough to provide the tissue with the oxygen it needs, without using any hemoglobin [27].

Under hyperbaric and hyperoxic conditions, the carotid chemoreceptor activity is reduced. This reduces cerebral blood flow, and the concentration of CO_2 in the brain tissue is increased [28]. Carbon dioxide is retained and a slight acidosis develops. Since hyperbaric oxygen fully saturates hemoglobin with oxygen, no reduced hemoglobin is left for the transport of carbon dioxide. In case of hyperbaric oxygen therapy, other mechanisms are activated to transport CO_2. Under most conditions, these changes are not clinically significant. Just when other mechanisms add to CO_2 retention (in large right–left shunts and in inadequate ventilation), HBO_2 may be adding to the already precarious situation.

Effects exerted mainly by pressure follow Boyle's Law. According to this law, changes of pressure lead to changes of the volume of gas-filled cavities. When gas bubbles are at the root of a medical problem, such as in gas embolism, decompression sickness, and gas gangrene, hyperbaric therapy can be used to reduce the size of the gas collection and may speed up recovery. On the other hand, abnormal gas collections, or normal gas collections that do not participate in pressure equalization (pneumothorax, emphysema, blocked middle ears, and paranasal sinuses), may cause trouble and can cause barotrauma.

Normobaric oxygen inhalation therapy

Indications

Oxygen, as with all drugs, has its indications and contraindications. The indications for oxygen therapy have been summarized by the American College of Chest Physicians and National Heart, Lung, and Blood Institute, which include the following:

• Cardiac and respiratory arrest
• Hypoxemia with an oxygen saturation below 90% or a PaO_2 of less than 59 mm Hg
• Systolic blood pressure less than 100 mm Hg
• A low cardiac output and a metabolic acidosis
• Respiratory distress with a respiratory rate of more than 24/min
• Anesthesia

At the heart of all the indications is the prevention and treatment of hypoxemia (oxygen deficiency in arterial blood, $PaO_2 < 80$ mm Hg; arterial oxygen saturation, $SaO_2 < 90\%$) and hypoxia (the oxygen deficiency in the tissues). Hypoxia can be caused by hypoxemia (*hypoxic hypoxia*), low hemoglobin level (*anemic hypoxia*), and/or a diminished flow of blood with a normal amount of oxygen (*stagnant, ischemic hypoxia*). It can also be caused by a disruption of the use of oxygen in the cells (*toxic hypoxia*).

In blood management, oxygen therapy is warranted for the prevention and treatment of anemic hypoxia. In addition, other kinds of hypoxia may be present in anemic patients, contributing to the overall hypoxic state. Therefore, we must be aware of other factors that could worsen hypoxia. This is another example of the fact that blood management has to take the whole patient into consideration, not only the blood.

Diagnostic measures

Since hypoxia is the main indication of oxygen therapy, it is important that this is recognized as early as possible and events that may lead to hypoxia are foreseen and prevented.

Clinical features of hypoxia include altered mental status and respiration, arrhythmia, blood pressure alterations, peripheral vasoconstriction with sweaty extremities, and gastrointestinal upset. Such unspecific findings often do not reliably indicate hypoxia. Cyanosis may also be unreliable to indicate hypoxia. Cyanosis appears when more than 1.5 g of hemoglobin/100 mL blood is deoxygenated. In severely anemic patients, no cyanosis can develop.

Since clinical features are unreliable to detect hypoxia, adding one or more monitoring features to the diagnostic measures may help. Measuring the SaO_2 helps to monitor the need for oxygen. Noninvasive pulse oximetry is an elegant method to do this and is available in many countries. Invasive monitoring of blood gases may show the partial pressure of oxygen in the arterial blood (PaO_2). Hypoxia may still exist when arterial oxygen saturation and oxygen partial pressure are normal. This may be the case in patients with low cardiac output or in patients with anemia. In this case, the monitoring of the mixed venous oxygen partial pressure may be indicated in addition to SaO_2 and PaO_2 [29].

Although the mentioned monitoring tools may add to the diagnosis of hypoxia, the clinical response to the oxygen therapy is still a valuable guide to use oxygen in anemia. If the patient feels better with oxygen, his/her mind clears, and other clinical signs of hypoxia resolve, oxygen therapy is being applied correctly.

Technical background information

Oxygen supply

Oxygen, for therapy, is readily available. It comes in tanks, either as a gas or as a liquid. Compressed gas systems use cylinder tanks containing compressed oxygen. The oxygen is stored in tanks as a gas at room temperature. For a hospital that needs much oxygen, the tank system is cumbersome, since the tanks need to be refilled frequently and maintenance is costly. On the other hand, small, portable oxygen tanks are handy and allow easy transportation of patients undergoing continuous oxygen therapy.

When oxygen is cooled to less than $-118°C$, it turns from the gaseous state to the liquid state, thereby reducing the volume it occupies. The reduced volume under such conditions is helpful in transporting oxygen. Also, oxygen as a liquid can be stored at the facility needing the oxygen. Special, usually stationary, containers, so-called vacuum insulated evaporators, are needed to keep the oxygen cooled. The stationary tank can be refilled with commercially available liquid oxygen. The liquid system can either be used to refill oxygen tanks, which contain compressed gaseous oxygen, or can be attached to the hospital wall system that distributes oxygen throughout the facility [30].

To guarantee a constant supply of oxygen for the patients, a reliable source is mandatory. Where oxygen is not readily and reliably available, oxygen concentrators are a viable alternative for a hospital to provide the patients with oxygen. Oxygen concentrators take oxygen from the room air. Room air is drawn into the concentrator and pressurized to 4 atm. Then, the air is passed through a cylinder with zeolite (aluminum silicate). Nitrogen is bound to zeolite, and 95% of oxygen is available for inhalation. The zeolite cylinder is recovered by venting it to room air so that nitrogen is released. While the zeolite cylinder is recovering, the gas flow is switched to a second zeolite cylinder. A set of zeolite columns last approximately 20,000 hours [31]. Oxygen concentrators depend on electricity. Their use under conditions with frequent power outages requires a backup system for electricity supply. Apart from this requirement and the need for simple maintenance procedures, oxygen concentrators are a simple-to-use alternative to industrial oxygen.

Oxygen mixing

To receive the mix of gases needed to administer oxygen, two basic methods of air–oxygen mixing are defined.

One method is jet mixing. It is widely used, but the FiO_2 is variable and changes with the atmospheric pressure. Jet mixing is performed with an injector (Venturi mechanism) or with a jet-mixing device. The Venturi mechanism uses the Bernoulli effect to draw in (= entrain) a second gas through a side arm. The first gas passes though a tube, which has a narrowing. This narrowing in the tube makes the gas increase in speed as it passes through. Due to the increased speed, the pressure drops. A second gas is drawn into the low-pressure area [30].

The alternative to jet mixing is the use of a high-pressure blender, which blends air and oxygen. With this method, the FiO_2 is stable. It is a mechanical blending of compressed air and oxygen. Several valves ensure that air and oxygen mix at certain pressures, so that a chosen FiO_2 is reached.

Oxygen delivery systems

There is a great variety of systems delivering normobaric supplemental oxygen to the patient [29]. The FiO_2 delivered by some systems depends on the patient's breathing pattern (uncontrolled oxygen, noncapacitance systems), while, in others, it does not (controlled oxygen, large-capacitance systems). In an uncontrolled system, the amount of gas delivered to the patient depends on the flow rate of oxygen and on the patient's breathing. A patient breathing with a low minute volume has a high oxygen concentration at a given flow, and vice versa. Noncapacitance systems do not influence the gas mixture just by exhalation, since the exhaled gas cannot be stored.

The simplest of all oxygen delivery systems are nasal tubes or catheters. Nasal tubes are just held under the nostrils. Nasal catheters are inserted into the nose, down to the pharynx, and need to be taped to prevent migration into the esophagus. In emergencies, other soft fine catheters can be used as nasal catheters (e.g., nasogastric tubes, urinary catheters). Such simple oxygen delivery devices do not increase the amount of dead space. The FiO_2 increases by 3–4% per liter increased oxygen flow.

A more sophisticated method of oxygen delivery is by the use of facemasks.

A *simple facemask* acts like an increased anatomic reservoir out of which the patient is breathing. The mask does not have any valves or a reservoir. In order to reduce the rebreathing of exhaled gas, the oxygen flow must exceed the ventilation volume per minute of the patient. The FiO_2 depends on the respiratory activity of the patient.

A *partial rebreathing mask* contains an oxygen reservoir, out of which the patient breathes. It provides a relatively high FiO_2, while conserving oxygen. Oxygen flow is adapted so that about one-third (approximately the anatomic dead space of the patient) of the exhaled air distends the reservoir. After the first third of the exhaled volume has filled the reservoir, the remaining exhaled air escapes through holes in the sides of the mask. The mask reduces oxygen flow requirement by about 30%.

A *non-rebreathing mask* contains valves that direct oxygen flow. The valves ensure that exhaled gas is given out into the room, while no room air is inhaled. Other valves prevent expired gas from entering the reservoir. The oxygen flow is adjusted so that the reservoir bag is constantly filled.

Table 10.2 Oxygen delivery systems.

Method	Maximum achievable FiO$_2$
Nasal prong, catheter	0.45–0.50
Simple mask	0.35–0.50
Partial rebreathing mask	0.70–0.85
Non-rebreathing mask	0.8–0.95
Air entrainment mask	0.25–0.70
Oxygen tent	Near 1.0
Ventilator-assisted systems (endotracheal tube, larynx mask, etc)	Near 1.0

A *high-flow oxygen-enrichment mask* (*air entrainment mask*) works with a high flow of oxygen. A high-flow velocity oxygen stream entrains room air and dilutes the oxygen stream. The gas stream exceeds the minute volume of the patient. Therefore, no valves and reservoirs are needed. FiO$_2$ depends on flow and the amount of air entrained.

Many more oxygen delivery systems are in use (Table 10.2). Among them are face tents and whole body tents, tracheal cannulas, endotracheal tubes, larynx masks, and masks that are designed to deliver a very accurate amount of oxygen or pressure.

Practical recommendations for normobaric oxygen therapy

A safe prescription for oxygen includes the delivery system, the flow rate of oxygen, and the monitoring of the treatment.

There is a great variety of oxygen delivery systems available. The choice of the delivery system depends on the intended duration of oxygen therapy, the acceptance and condition of the patient, and, most importantly, the maximal FiO$_2$ required. Short-term, low FiO$_2$ use of supplemental oxygen can be achieved by nasal tubes, cannulas, or simple masks. Different mask models can administer not only oxygen, but can also provide positive pressure. When oxygen therapy is used continuously, over an extended period or at a high flow rate in a conscious patient, a transtracheal oxygen catheter may be recommended.

The flow rate of oxygen or the FiO$_2$ have to be prescribed as well. In fact, most patients do not need controlled oxygen therapy, that is, oxygen therapy with a limited, preset inspiratory oxygen fraction. Such a strict control is only indicated in patients with chronic obstructive pulmonary disease, who have a hypoxic drive, and in premature infants. All other patients in need of oxygen may be sufficiently treated when they receive an uncontrolled oxygen therapy.

The duration of oxygen therapy depends mainly on the clinical condition. It is known that side effects of oxygen therapy occur with prolonged and high-concentration oxygen, and lifesaving oxygen therapy cannot be denied solely on grounds of the potential hazards of oxygen. However, knowledge about the patient's resistance to oxygen and possible modifications of his/her oxygen tolerance is clinically important to minimize oxygen-related side effects. It is generally believed that the prolonged exposure to an FiO$_2$ of 0.55–0.60 does not cause severe side effects. However, the oxygen resistance and tolerance of the individual patient is difficult to assess. Attempts have been made to modify oxygen tolerance pharmacologically. Most of the drugs which were tested need to be given in unacceptably high doses to achieve the desired clinical effects on oxygen tolerance [24]. Antioxidant vitamins are an exception, since they can be administered in the needed dose without eliciting unacceptable side effects. Although their efficacy remains to be proven, antioxidant vitamins are used clinically to treat oxygen toxicity [25].

Hyperbaric oxygen

Indications

Hyperbaric oxygen therapy has a set of approved indications, issued by the Hyperbaric Oxygen Therapy Committee of the UHMS:
- Air or gas embolism
- Carbon monoxide poisoning (also in connection with cyanide poisoning)
- Gas gangrene (clostridial infection)
- Traumatic ischemias, such as crush injury, compartment syndrome
- Decompression sickness
- Wound healing for problem wounds
- Severe blood loss anemia
- Intracranial abscess
- Necrotizing soft tissue infections
- Refractory osteomyelitis
- Delayed radiation injury
- Skin grafts and flaps compromised in healing
- Thermal burns

As the above list demonstrates, hyperbaric oxygen therapy plays a role in blood management (albeit a small one). Increased pressure augments the effect of oxygen on the body. This effect is used as an adjunct for the therapy of severe anemia.

Contraindications

Untreated pneumothorax and bleomycin/doxorubicin or cisplatinum chemotherapy constitute contraindications for hyperbaric therapy.

Some other conditions are considered relative contraindications [28]. A history of a spontaneous pneumothorax or thoracic surgery may increase the likelihood of barotrauma to the lung. Infection of the upper respiratory tract as well as ear surgery may hinder pressure equalization in the middle ear and increases the risk for barotrauma. Severe emphysema, with hypercarbia, may cause respiratory arrest in the chamber. A history of epilepsy may increase the seizure risk under hyperbaric conditions. Also, a high fever may predispose to convulsions. Patients with hereditary spherocytosis may experience exaggerated hemolysis under hyperbaric conditions, and a history of optical neuritis may be a risk factor for a pressure-associated recurrence of the visual disturbance.

Pregnancy does not constitute a contraindication for hyperbaric oxygen therapy.

Technical background information

Hyperbaric oxygen is administered in so-called hyperbaric chambers. The early chambers were "multiplace" chambers. These large tanks can hold more than one person. Usually, a transfer chamber allows for the entering and leaving of persons without losing the pressure in the main chamber. The chambers are big enough that personnel can join patients and can care for them under hyperbaric conditions. Specially modified medical equipment can be used in such chambers so that intensive care of the critically ill is possible. The chambers can build up a pressure of 6 atm or more. Oxygen is delivered directly to the patient, using masks or ventilators. The chamber itself is filled with compressed air, to reduce fire hazards.

In contrast, "monoplace" chambers look like a bed surrounded by a tube made of metal and plastic. Only one person can be in the chamber at a time. The chambers are less costly than the big multiplace chambers and are often portable. Patients do not need to wear an oxygen mask. The whole chamber is filled with the gas that the patient is supposed to breathe. Since this is often 100%

oxygen, there is a high risk of explosion. Electronic equipment (ventilators and monitors) cannot be taken along into the chamber, unless they are especially designed for hyperbaric conditions. When intensive care is required for the patient in the monoplace chamber, noncollapsible intravenous tubes with unidirectional valves can be used as well as the mentioned ventilators and monitors. Pressure-sealed ports allow the treatment of the critically ill patient from outside the chamber [28].

Apart from the traditional monoplace and multiplace chambers, there is a wide variety of mobile monoplace chambers, designed for different uses [32]. An interesting example is the Gamow bag. A Gamow bag, which looks like a big sleeping bag, was designed as a portable hyperbaric chamber for the use by mountain climbers who suffer from high-altitude sickness. The original bags were made of lightweight fabric, which did not stand standard pressures for hyperbaric oxygen therapy. Modifications in the material used for the Gamow bag now make it possible to increase the pressure to 2 atm [33]. Oxygen and pressure are provided to the bag, using oxygen cylinders, scuba tanks, or hospital wall ports. Gamow bags provide an affordable, portable alternative to conventional chambers. Patients with carbon monoxide poisoning, who report to a hospital which does not have a hyperbaric chamber, have successfully been treated with the Gamow bag [34]. To our knowledge, to date nobody has tried a Gamow bag in blood management therapy.

Patterns of therapy sessions

Very different treatment patterns of hyperbaric oxygen are used, depending on the indications. When treatment of decompression sickness is required, initially, patients may be treated with pressures up to 6 atm. Such high pressures are not needed for the therapy of severe anemia. The UHMS gives recommendations for treatment protocols for the indications approved by the society. For exceptional blood loss anemia, the following recommendation was given: "Treatments are continued repetitively, as needed, at pressures dictated by clinical response. May be used in conjunction with erythropoietin, which has a lag time of 3–4 days. Average number of treatments: Until Hct >22.9% or based on clinical judgement" [28]. Whether this recommendation is of use to specialists in the field of blood management is debatable. But it gives a concept of hyperbaric oxygen therapy in blood management.

Severe anemia is usually treated with pressures up to a maximum of 2–3 atm. The time of pressurization lasts about 60–90 minutes. Depending on the clinical condition of the patient, the treatment is initially administered three times daily and the frequency is reduced as the patient becomes more stable. Other treatment modes are used at the discretion of the physician, depending on the clinical condition of the patient and the response to the treatment.

Practical recommendations for hyperbaric therapy

Before the therapy

• As with all treatments, hyperbaric therapy requires the consent of the patient. Before therapy is commenced, an explanation, tailored to the needs of the patient, should be given and the patient needs to consent to the treatment.

• If a patient is considered a candidate for hyperbaric therapy, he/she needs to be prepared, to avoid undue damage to his/her health [35]. A chest radiograph should rule out pneumothorax, severe obstructive lung disease, or other pathological gas-filled cavities. When a pneumothorax is present, a chest tube needs to be inserted and put on a water seal.

• Patients must be checked regarding their ability to equalize pressure in their middle ears to prevent rupture of the eardrums. Vasoconstrictive drops may help. Pressure equalization tubes must be inserted into the patients who cannot equalize pressure in their middle ears by themselves. In emergencies, with a nonresponsive patient, paracentesis is required.

• The pressure cuff of tubes, such as endotracheal tubes, changes in relation to the changes in the hyperbaric chamber. When the pressure increases, the volume of the cuff diminishes, no longer sealing the airway. This may lead to hypoventilation. When the pressure in the chamber is decreased, the cuff increases in size and may cause tracheal rupture. Therefore, saline should be used, rather than air, to fill the cuff tube. The same is true also for the balloons of bladder catheters.

• Since the density of a gas increases as the pressure increases, patients in the hyperbaric environment have to exert themselves more, in order to breathe. When patients breathe through a tube or a tracheal stoma, the widest possible tubes should be employed to offset the density-induced increased workload. Patients with dyspnea, or those who cannot maintain adequate ventilation, need to be intubated and put on ventilatory support. The largest possible size of tube should be used.

• In patients not hemodynamically stable, invasive monitoring with central lines, arterial lines, etc., should be established. On the other hand, all vascular accesses not needed should be discontinued to reduce the chance of air embolism.

• When the patient is in critical condition, monitoring or ventilation may be required. Equipment needs to be chosen that is fit for use under hyperbaric conditions.

• Patients need adequate pain control and sometimes sedation for anxiety control. Opioids and diazepam or other suitable benzodiazepines are optimal.

• The patient's current, or recent, medication needs to be revised. Steroids, thyroid hormones, and other drugs can increase the likelihood of oxygen toxicity and convulsions [36]. Patients receiving such drugs must be monitored closely for signs of convulsions. The medication of choice to treat and prevent convulsions is diazepam (or other suitable benzodiazepines). Patients on doxorubicin or cisplatinum are not to receive hyperbaric treatment, since it may be deadly. This is probably due to hyperbaric oxygen, which increases the cardiotoxic effects of the chemotherapeutics [37].

• Diabetics need to have a good control of their blood sugar. Availability of an adaptable insulin schedule and glucose helps to treat any disturbance of the blood sugar.

During the therapy

When the patient is in the chamber, some measures may have to be taken to prevent and treat side effects of the therapy [35, 38].

• When large amounts of pulmonary secretions are present, the patient needs to be suctioned, to prevent air being trapped in the lungs, leading to pulmonary barotrauma during ascent.

• A seizure during therapy, usually, is due to oxygen toxicity in the chamber. It occurs in 1.3 of 10,000 cases and it usually does not have adverse consequences, since there is no hypoxia present [21]. Seizures, during hyperbaric therapy, can be resolved by reducing the oxygen concentration in the chamber, but not the pressure. Pharmacological therapy is not required in the majority of cases.

• Physiological and pathological gas-filled cavities, in which pressure equalization cannot occur, are prone to develop barotrauma. The eardrums can rupture when it is not possible to equalize the pressure. To equilibrate the pressure, groaning, chewing, and swallowing or the valsalva maneuver can be encouraged.

• Barotrauma can also occur in the paranasal sinuses, teeth, gastrointestinal tract, and in pathological cavities like emphysema bullae or pneumothorax. The patient therefore needs to be monitored closely to detect any problems early enough to intervene.

• Diabetics must be monitored closely during hyperbaric treatment, since blood glucose levels may fall rapidly under hyperbaric conditions and hypoglycemia and insulin therapy dispose to increased oxygen toxicity and seizures.

After the therapy

• Patients may complain about numb fingers and myopia after their treatment. Neither of these symptoms are permanent, usually resolving within weeks or months.

Oxygen in blood management

Supportive treatment in anemia and hemorrhagic shock

Oxygen has long been used for the supportive treatment of severe hemorrhagia and hemorrhagic shock. It augments oxygen delivery and may improve the outcome. This has been accredited to increased arterial oxygen content and improved arterial blood pressure as well as to the redistribution of blood flow from the skeletal muscles to the splanchnic area [17].

Interestingly, hyperoxic ventilation, but not red cell transfusions, improves tissue oxygenation [39]. Therefore, hyperoxic ventilation adds further safety to a therapeutic regimen for anemia. It was shown in animal experiments that switching from breathing room air to hyperoxic ventilation not only reversed signs of hypoxic myocardial dysfunction, but also allowed considerable further blood loss without recurrence of signs of myocardial dysfunction in the ECG (electrocardiogram) [40]. Besides, hyperoxic ventilation improves survival in hemorrhagic shock patients with controlled hemorrhaging [41, 42]. In human trials, it was shown that brain function and heart rate return to normal when severely anemic volunteers breathe oxygen [43].

Beneficial effects of oxygen therapy in hemorrhage are not always observed. Patients with controlled hemorrhage, that is, stopped hemorrhage, clearly benefit from the effects of oxygen. Animal experiments suggest that the same is true for the individuals with uncontrolled hemorrhaging from small vessels [17]. However, victims of uncontrolled hemorrhaging from large vessels do not seem to benefit. Initially, the blood pressure rises, supposedly as an effect of the oxygen. However, the elevated blood pressure augments the hemorrhaging and the blood pressure drops soon afterward, due to accelerated hemorrhage.

This is in line with the findings of other studies which demonstrated that therapies administered to resuscitate patients (e.g., aggressive fluid resuscitation)—while beneficial when the hemorrhaging is controlled—may have adverse effects (increase the total blood loss) when hemorrhaging has not been controlled.

The oxygen-induced redistribution of blood to the splanchnic vasculature brings some theoretical benefit. In hemorrhagic shock, splanchnic perfusion is often impaired and ischemia may occur. This triggers a response that results in endothelial damage and a dysfunction of the epithelium and macrophages of the intestines. Bacterial translocation, endotoxinemia, and the resulting systemic response negatively affect the whole body. Oxygen may indeed be beneficial to reduce ischemia which would develop during hemorrhage periods.

Intraoperative hyperoxic ventilation

Oxygen is not only a measure to treat patients suffering from anemia or hemorrhage. Oxygen therapy can indeed reduce the patient's exposure to allogeneic blood. Hyperoxic ventilation in extreme hemodilution has been advocated [18]. Ventilating a patient with 100% oxygen rapidly increases the arterial oxygen content. The amount of oxygen dissolved in plasma is increased. This effect is enhanced in patients with anemia, since their plasma volume is expanded. Plasma, thus, becomes a significant source of oxygen. Using the concept of hyperoxic ventilation during acute normovolemic hemodilution helps to reduce allogeneic transfusions. Patients undergoing acute normovolemic hemodilution are hemodiluted down to the hemoglobin level that is acceptable. When further blood loss occurs, mainly due to surgical losses, signs of impaired oxygen delivery may appear (e.g., a reduced mixed venous oxygen partial pressure, ST-segment changes in the EKG). When this occurs, collected blood is given back, and allogeneic blood is administered when the autologous sources are depleted. Starting to transfuse before surgical hemostasis is achieved increases the use of allogeneic blood. To minimize allogeneic transfusions, the proposed approach in the event of signs of impaired oxygen delivery is to switch from low oxygen concentration in the ventilated gas to 100% oxygen. Now, enough oxygen is available to reverse the signs of impaired oxygen delivery and the surgery can continue. An average of 30 minutes can be bought by this approach [18]. This may bridge the time until surgical hemorrhaging is stopped. Afterward, the autologous blood is returned.

Hyperbaric oxygen in severe anemia

High oxygen content in the plasma can supplement or supplant the oxygen delivery by hemoglobin. Since the amount of a gas dissolved in a liquid is proportional to the pressure of the gas above the liquid, an increase in the ambient air pressure can greatly increase the amount of oxygen dissolved in plasma. When the hemoglobin-bound oxygen is not able to meet the needs of the body, hyperbaric oxygen therapy can dissolve enough oxygen into the plasma. In this way, hyperbaric oxygen therapy can maximize oxygen dissolved in the plasma while the patient synthesizes hemoglobin.

Hyperbaric oxygen therapy is a therapeutic option for patients with severe symptomatic anemia. Multiple case reports and case studies [15, 25, 44–46], but no controlled trials, testify this. Besides, a recent review of the available literature about the use of hyperbaric oxygen therapy in severe anemia summarized that "all publications report a positive result when HBO$_2$ is delivered as treatment for severe anemia" [47]. In particular, it has been shown that ischemic changes in the EKG (ST-segment changes), and corresponding clinical signs, such as angina pectoris, heart failure with pulmonary edema, metabolic acidosis, impaired mental status, and diminished kidney and bowel function, rapidly resolve after exposure to hyperbaric oxygen. Often, the beneficial effects of the temporarily increased oxygen delivery last for minutes to several hours after the therapy.

Hyperbaric oxygen in sickle cell crisis

Hyperbaric oxygen therapy has also been used in sickle cell crisis [48]. Patients with sickle cell disease experience vasoocclusive crisis when hemoglobin S is polymerized and sickling occurs. Such is seen under conditions that expose red cells to low oxygen tensions. Some of the red cells are irreversibly sickled, while others are disaturated but not irreversibly sickled. Sickled, stiff cells block the microcirculation and cause tissue ischemia and infarction. In patients with a developing crisis, hyperbaric oxygen can reduce the amount of sickle cells in peripheral blood. Hyperbaric treatments, when started within the first 24 hours after the onset of symptoms, may shorten total hospital stay of patients compared with those receiving conventional treatment [48].

Newer experiments did not demonstrate a direct effect of hyperbaric oxygen on the amount of sickle cells in blood samples. It was thought that other effects might, in vivo, contribute to the beneficial effect of hyperbaric oxygen

in sickle cell crisis [49]. Due to the lack of evidence, the UHMS does not list sickle cell crises as a recommended indication for hyperbaric oxygen therapy.

Key points

• Oxygen therapy can be lifesaving in the case of anemia.
• Severe cases of anemia can be treated with hyperbaric oxygen, especially when transfusions are not an option.
• The choice of the right oxygen delivery device influences how much oxygen the patient finally breathes.

Questions for review

• What laws govern the physical behavior of oxygen?
• How does the body react to oxygen in anemic and nonanemic states?
• What information is needed to safely prescribe inhalational oxygen therapy?
• What preparations are needed for a patient who is going to have hyperbaric oxygen treatment?
• What are the side effects of oxygen therapy?

Suggestions for further research

What role does oxygen play in reperfusion injury?
How does the position of the patient while breathing oxygen influence his/her arterial oxygen content (sitting, supine, prone, head-down, on his/her side)?

Exercises and practice cases

Calculate the oxygen partial pressure in the lung of a normal healthy young man who breathes room air at sea level. Do the same when he is breathing 100% oxygen.

You are asked to teach interns about oxygen therapy. How would you go about it? What information do you think will benefit them? How would you present the information? What demonstration material would you take along with you? Is there an article you would like to recommend to the students for further reading?

Homework

1 Get the address and phone number of the nearest hyperbaric chamber and think about how to transfer a patient there, if necessary (jot down the results of your research in the address book in Appendix E).

2 Find out how oxygen is provided to the patients in your facility:

(a) What color do the oxygen tanks have?

(b) Where does the hospital get the oxygen?

(c) What safety precautions are there

• to prevent explosion and

• to prevent errors in administration (to make sure that oxygen is administered and not another gas)?

References

1 Priestley, J. *Experiments and Observations on Different Kinds of Air and Other Branches of Natural Philosophy Connected with the Subject*, in three volumes. Printed by Th. Pearson, sold by J. Johnson, St. Paul's Church-Yard: Birmingham, London, 1790.

2 Birch, S.B. On the therapeutic use of oxygen. *Lancet*, 1857. (August 1): p. 112.

3 Osler, W. *The Principles and Practice of Medicine*. D. Appleton & Co., New York, 1892.

4 Davenport, J.H. Oxygen as a remedial agent. *Boston Med Surg J*, 1872. **10**(4): p. 61–64.

5 Ehinger, C.E. *Oxygen in Therapeutics: A Treatise Explaining the Apparatus, the Material and the Processes Used in the Preparation of Oxygen and Other Gases with Which It May Be Combined, Also, Its Administration and Effects, Illustrated by Clinical Experience of the Author and Others*. W.A. Chatterton & Co., Chicago, 1887.

6 Conklin, W.L. The therapeutic value of oxygen. *N Y State Med J*, 1899. (September 2): p. 338–341.

7 Starkey, P. *Compound Oxygen—Its Origin and Development*. 1529 Arch Street, Philadelphia, PA, 1888.

8 Kellogg, J.H. Oxygen enemata as a remedy in certain diseases of the liver and the intestinal tract. *JAMA*, 1888. **11**: p. 258–262.

9 Bainbridge, W.S. Oxygen in medicine and surgery—a contribution, with report of cases. *N Y State J Med*, 1908. **8**(6): p. 281–295.

10 Tunnicliffe, F.W. and G.F. Stebbing. The intravenous injection of oxygen gas as a therapeutic measure. *Lancet*, 1916. (August 19): p. 321–323.

11 Howitt, H.O. The subcutaneous injection of oxygen gas. *CMAJ*, 1914. **4**: p. 983–985.

12 Haldane, J.S. The therapeutic administration of oxygen. *BMJ*, 1917. (February 10): p. 181–183.

13 Boerema, I., *et al.* Life without blood. *Ned Tijdschr Geneeskd*, 1960. **104**: p. 949–954.

14 Boerema, I., N.G. Meyne, W.K. Brummelkamp, S. Bouma, M.H. Mensch, F. Kamermans, M. Stern Hanf, and W. Van Aalderen. Life without blood. A study on the influence of high atmospheric pressure and hypothermia on dilution of blood. *J Cardiovasc Surg*, 1960. **13**: p. 133–146.

15 Amonic, R.S., A.T.K. Cockett, P.H. Lorhan, and J.C. Thompson. Hyperbaric oxygen therapy in chronic hemorrhagic shock. *JAMA*, 1969. **208**: p. 2051–2054.

16 Meier, J., *et al.* Regional blood flow during hyperoxic haemodilution. *Clin Physiol Funct Imaging*, 2005. **25**(3): p. 158–165.

17 Sukhotnik, I., *et al.* Divergent effects of oxygen therapy in four models of uncontrolled hemorrhagic shock. *Shock*, 2002. **18**(3): p. 277–284.

18 Habler, O., *et al.* Hyperoxia in extreme hemodilution. *Eur Surg Res*, 2002. **34**(1–2): p. 181–187.

19 Neubauer, B., *et al.* Cardiac output changes during hyperbaric hyperoxia. *Int Arch Occup Environ Health*, 2001. **74**(2): p. 119–122.

20 Knighton, D.R., B. Halliday, and T.K. Hunt. Oxygen as an antibiotic. A comparison of the effects of inspired oxygen concentration and antibiotic administration on in vivo bacterial clearance. *Arch Surg*, 1986. **121**(2): p. 191–195.

21 Jaeger, K., B. Juttner, and W. Franko. Hyperbaric oxygen therapy—options and limitations. *Anasthesiol Intensivmed Notfallmed Schmerzther*, 2002. **37**(1): p. 38–42.

22 Tin, W. Oxygen therapy: 50 years of uncertainty. *Pediatrics*, 2002. **110**: p. 615–616.

23 Lambertsen, C.J., *et al.* Oxygen toxicity; effects in man of oxygen inhalation at 1 and 3.5 atmospheres upon blood gas transport, cerebral circulation and cerebral metabolism. *J Appl Physiol*, 1953. **5**(9): p. 471–486.

24 Clark, J.M. and C.J. Lambertsen. Pulmonary oxygen toxicity: a review. *Pharmacol Rev*, 1971. **23**(2): p. 37–133.

25 Greensmith, J.E. Hyperbaric oxygen reverses organ dysfunction in severe anemia. *Anesthesiology*, 2000. **93**(4): p. 1149–1152.

26 Bassett, B.E. and B.P. Bennett. Introduction to the physical and physiological bases of hyperbaric therapy. In Davis, J.C. and T.K. Hunt (eds.) *Hyperbaric Oxygen Therapy*. Undersea Medical Society, Betheseda, 1977. p. 20.

27 Tibbles, P.M. and J.S. Edelsberg. Hyperbaric-oxygen therapy. *N Engl J Med*, 1996. **334**(25): p. 1642–1648.

28 Hancock, D.L. Hyperbaric oxygen therapy. *Am J Anesthesiol*, 1997. **24**: p. 297–307.

29 Bateman, N.T. and R.M. Leach. ABC of oxygen. Acute oxygen therapy. *BMJ*, 1998. **317**(7161): p. 798–801.

30 Varvinski, A.M. and S. Hunt. Acute oxygen treatment. *Update Anesth*, 2000. **12**: Article 3.

31 Dobson, M.B. Oxygen concentrators for district hospitals. *Update Anesth*, 1999. **10**: Article 11.

32 Bouak, F. Lightweight portable hyperbaric chambers. *Technical Memorandum DRDC Toronto TM 2003–157*. Defence R&D Canada—Toronto, 2003.

33 Shimada, H., *et al*. Immediate application of hyperbaric oxygen therapy using a newly devised transportable chamber. *Am J Emerg Med*, 1996. **14**(4): p. 412–415.

34 Jay, G.D., *et al*. Portable hyperbaric oxygen therapy in the emergency department with the modified Gamow bag. *Ann Emerg Med*, 1995. **26**(6): p. 707–711.

35 Matos, L.A. Hyperbaric medicine. In Civetta, J.M., R.W. Taylor, and R. Kirby (eds.) *Critical Care*. Lippincott-Raven, Philadelphia, 1997. p. 777–785.

36 Leifer, G. Hyperbaric oxygen therapy. *Am J Nurs*, 2001. **101**(8): p. 26–34; quiz 34–35.

37 Sauerstoffüberdrucktherapie (Hyperbare Oxygenationstherapie; HOT). In Wiemann, K. (ed.) *MSD-Manual der Diagnostik und Therapie* 5th edn. Urban u. Fischer, Munich, 1993. p. 3228–3236.

38 Strelow, H. Die hyperbare Medizin—Möglichkeiten und Grenzen der Sauerstoff-Überdrucktherapie: 8. Folge: Komplikationen und Grenzen der OHP. *Die Schwester/Der Pfleger*, 1986. **25**: p. 96–101.

39 Suttner, S., *et al*. The influence of allogeneic red blood cell transfusion compared with 100% oxygen ventilation on systemic oxygen transport and skeletal muscle oxygen tension after cardiac surgery. *Anesth Analg*, 2004. **99**(1): p. 2–11.

40 Meier, J., *et al*. Hyperoxic ventilation enables hemodilution beyond the critical myocardial hemoglobin concentration. *Eur J Med Res*, 2005. **10**(11): p. 462–468.

41 Meier, J., *et al*. Hyperoxic ventilation reduces 6-hour mortality at the critical hemoglobin concentration. *Anesthesiology*, 2004. **100**(1): p. 70–76.

42 Meier, J., *et al*. Hyperoxic ventilation reduces six-hour mortality after partial fluid resuscitation from hemorrhagic shock. *Shock*, 2004. **22**(3): p. 240–247.

43 Weiskopf, R.B., *et al*. Oxygen reverses deficits of cognitive function and memory and increased heart rate induced by acute severe isovolemic anemia. *Anesthesiology*, 2002. **96**(4): p. 871–877.

44 McLoughlin, P.L., T.M. Cope, and J.C. Harrison. Hyperbaric oxygen therapy in the management of severe acute anaemia in a Jehovah's Witness. *Anaesthesia*, 1999. **54**(9): p. 891–895.

45 Hart, G.B., *et al*. Hyperbaric oxygen in exceptional acute blood-loss anemia. *J Hyperb Med*, 1987. **2**: p. 205–210.

46 Hart, G.B. Exceptional blood loss anemia. Treatment with hyperbaric oxygen. *JAMA*, 1974. **228**(8): p. 1028–1029.

47 Van Meter, K.W. A systematic review of the application of hyperbaric oxygen in the treatment of severe anemia: an evidence-based approach. *Undersea Hyperb Med*, 2005. **32**(1): p. 61–83.

48 Hart, G.B., *et al*. Amelioration of sickle cell crises with intensive hyperbaric oxygen. *J Hyperb Med*, 1991. **6**: p. 75–85.

49 Mychaskiw, G., II, *et al*. In vitro effects of hyperbaric oxygen on sickle cell morphology. *J Clin Anesth*, 2001. **13**(4): p. 255–258.

11 Preparation of the patient for surgery

The outcome of a patient's surgery is likely to be more favorable if suitable preparations are made. Once a specific goal has been established—in our case improving the outcome of treatment by appropriate blood management—advance preparation is required. Preoperative planning is essential to reducing or avoiding allogeneic blood transfusions.

Objectives of this chapter

1 Review how to take a history and perform a physical examination while focusing on avoiding donor blood transfusions.
2 Be able to calculate a patient's blood volume and allowable blood loss.
3 Practice how to draw up a plan of care.
4 Know how to prepare patients with commonly encountered diseases for surgery in a blood management program.

Definitions

Preparation: The English words for "preparation" or "to prepare" have their roots in the Latin words "paratus" and "preparo." These words mean "prepared," "ready," "equipped," and "skilled." Closely related is the word "apparatus" meaning not only "equipment" but also "exertion" and "effort." Another Latin word rendered "prepared" is promptus. It means "ready at hand." It also denotes persons who are prepared, resolute, or prompt. The full scope of the word "preparation" therefore means to be ready, to have the needed equipment, to be skilled,

and to be prompt in taking action. Preparation also means exertion and effort.

The algorithm

This chapter gives an overview of how to prepare a patient for surgery in a blood management program. Reference is frequently made to other chapters of this book. Help is given on how to integrate the various drugs and methods that have been explained into a whole treatment concept. The following algorithm (Fig. 11.1) is discussed step by step. Practice using this algorithm even if patients initially present for minor surgery only. Internalize the lines of the algorithm so that you always think along these lines. In time, even patients presenting as complex cases will be easy to prepare.

Step 1. History and physical examination

It has been said that taking a good history and performing a physical examination are 90% of the diagnosis [1]. In fact, it could also be said that it constitutes 90% of a patient's blood management. A skilled history and physical examination are the basis for preparing the patient, surgery, equipment, and the surgeon. A thorough preoperative workup serves to identify the problems unique to the patient and helps spot potential obstacles to transfusion-free therapy. The first step in the algorithm is therefore to take a focused history and perform a physical examination [2].

Take a focused history

A health-care provider surely needs no explanation of how to take a history. There are, of course, different styles,

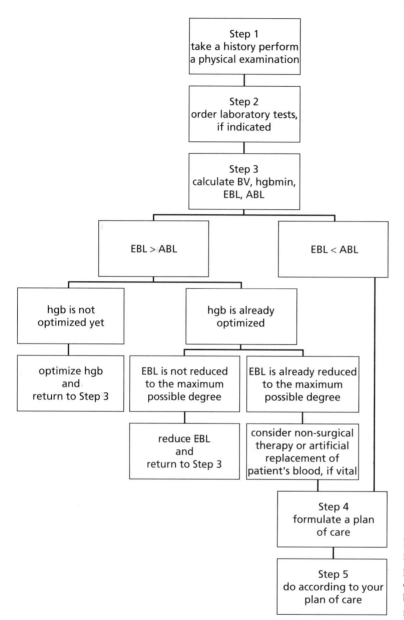

Fig 11.1 Algorithm: preparing a patient for surgery in a blood management program. BV, blood volume; EBL, expected blood loss; ABL, allowable blood loss; hgb, hemoglobin; hgbmin, minimally tolerable hemoglobin.

each with advantages and disadvantages. No matter how history taking is structured, all the information needed has to be obtained in as convenient a manner as possible. A systematic approach to history taking makes it easier and helps avoid overlooking important issues. Some suggestions as to what to include in the history, in the style you prefer, are given below. The facets of the patient's history relevant to blood management are also included.

Practice tip

As a reminder of what information needs to be gathered from a patient in preparation for surgery, a form can be developed. This may be used to record the findings of the history-taking and the physical examination as well as the required preparations (e.g., workup of anemia, availability of equipment). Such a sheet can be kept in the patient's file where it is available for any necessary review.

Begin as usual with the patient's demographic data. This will provide the first pieces of the puzzle that finally constitute the individual picture the patient presents. Interestingly, there are a number of studies that use demographic data to predict the likelihood of a patient receiving a transfusion.

• Age: Tolerance of anemia is age-dependent. Young children tolerate anemia much better than the elderly. There are also age-dependent differences in the probability of the patient presenting with morbidities relevant to blood management. Increasing age itself is a significant predictor for transfusions [3, 4].

• Gender: There are differences between genders relevant to blood management. Women are more likely to get transfusions than men [3–5]. They have a lower average red blood cell count and are prone to regular blood loss via menses and childbirth. Both may precipitate iron loss and deficiency. Hormonal differences between genders exist and account, at least partially, for the different hemoglobin levels. The decision of what therapy to use for anemia may also be influenced by the gender of the patient (e.g., whether to use recombinant human erythropoietin (rHuEPO) or androgens for the therapy of renal anemia).

• Weight and height: To calculate drug dosage, blood volumes, and allowable blood loss, note the patient's height and weight. Patients' size may also provide indications as to whether they are usually considered transfusion candidates. Low body weight and a small size are predictors for transfusions in some procedures [3, 4], while obesity contributes to the risk of getting transfusions in other surgeries [6].

• Race, ethic background, religion, and a long-term stay abroad are also relevant. Some types of anemia and coagulation disorders are more common in certain races. For instance, there is a high prevalence of factor XI deficiency in Ashkenazic Jews. Inhabitants of Mediterranean regions often suffer from anemia due to favism. The nutritional status may also be affected by the background of the patient, influenced by the manner of life and food permitted or prohibited by religion.

Areas of special interest: in analogy to chief complaint

While taking the history of a patient in their care, most health-care providers would proceed by first inquiring about the chief complaint. The same procedure is used for patients whose blood management is the responsibility of the health-care provider. In addition to inquiring about the condition that brought the patient to the office,

continue asking about the five main patient-related obstacles to transfusion-free therapy, namely, anemia, hemostatic disturbances, medical conditions that may increase perioperative blood loss, obstacles to surgical hemostasis, and factors that decrease anemia tolerance. These issues should be evaluated in detail. The following questions and hints serve as a reminder of what to ask for.

First, some simple questions help elucidate a possible *history of anemia*. Has the patient been anemic in the past? How did the anemia manifest itself? What was the reason for the anemia? When did it occur and how long did it last? What treatment was used and did the treatment help? Has the patient ever received transfusions of red blood cell concentrates? Why was the transfusion given? Were there any side effects? Who treated the patient? The latter is important because the patient may not know the details of the anemia and it might be useful to ask the patient's former health-care provider for medical records. Patients may be heterozygous for an inherited anemia that may manifest itself only under severe (surgical) stress, drugs, and disease, and the patient may as yet be unaware of any such problem. A family history may help identify such inherited disorders.

Often, the patient is unaware of whether he is or ever has been anemic. Therefore, ask for signs and symptoms that may indicate anemia. Moderate or severe anemia produces symptoms such as decreased exercise tolerance, dyspnea, palpitations, headache, dizziness, vertigo, fainting, anorexia, nausea, intolerance to cold, amenorrhea, menorrhagia, loss of libido, and impotence. In persons with atherosclerosis, symptoms of angina pectoris or intermittent claudication may be more easily provoked than previously. Also, difficulty swallowing (Plummer Vinson Syndrome) and eating of indigestible items such as earth, paper, etc. (Pica) may be indicative of anemia. Patients with such symptoms should raise your index of suspicion; further evaluation is needed.

Second, assessment of the patient's bleeding history is the most sensitive way to identify patients with impaired hemostasis and those at increased risk for perioperative hemorrhage [7]. Continue with the history and inquire about a *history of coagulation problems*. First, ask directly about any known coagulation disorder. Has the patient ever had a problem with hemostasis? How was this manifest? What was the reason for the disorder? When did it occur and how long did it last? What treatment was used and did the treatment help? Has the patient ever received a transfusion of coagulation products? If so, for what reason and did the transfusion achieve the desired goal? And once again, who treated the patient?

Occasionally, patients are unaware of impaired coagulation. Therefore, ask directly about signs of hemorrhage obvious to a layman (e.g., Do you bleed or bruise easily?). In cases of injury or surgical intervention, ask about prolonged hemorrhage or a return of bleeding either immediately following or some hours after the insult. Minor cuts and dental extractions may serve as examples of hemostatic challenges. Bleeding disorders may be disguised if there has been no previous surgical challenge but there are subtle signs that should arouse suspicion. A defect in hemostasis is suspected when spontaneous hemorrhage occurs or when hemorrhage exceeds the amount expected after injury. Nose bleeds, especially bilateral ones, gums that bleed more than 3 minutes after teeth brushing, easy bruising, bleeding after cuts all occur if hemostasis is impaired. Ask about the sites of bleeding, timing in relation to the insult, duration, and frequency. Also, ask about the severity of hemorrhage, e.g., by comparing the size of a bruise with a coin (bigger or smaller than one known coin). Often, however, the only sign of a coagulation disorder is a heavy menses. A substantial proportion of women with menorrhagia and a normal pelvis examination have an inherited bleeding disorder [8]. To standardize questioning about a possible history of bleeding disorders it has been proposed that patients fill out a supplementary questionnaire before they see their health-care provider. Table 11.1 gives examples of questions for such a questionnaire [7, 9].

It is easy to determine whether a clotting problem is more related to defects or deficiencies in the platelets or to

Table 11.1 Questions to be used in a screening questionnaire to evaluate the patient's hemostatic system.

Have you ever suffered from prolonged bleeding?

Do you develop bruises or "black spots" without being able to remember when or how you injured yourself?

What was the longest time you bled after having a tooth pulled? Did bleeding ever start again after it had stopped?

Was it hard to stop the bleeding?

Have you ever bled excessively after surgery or during labor?

Have you ever bled from the gums or nose without any apparent reason?

In your opinion, do you bleed excessively during menstruation?

Within the past 5 years have you ever had a medical problem requiring a doctor's care? Do you have any disorders of the liver or kidneys?

What medications have you taken during the last 14 days?

Has any blood relative ever had a problem with unusual bruising or bleeding?

Have you or a blood relative ever had transfusions?

clotting factors. In platelet disorders bleeding occurs right after the injury and occurs mainly in the skin and mucosa. If the problem is mainly fibrin clot formation (as in factor deficiencies) hemorrhage occurs some time, even hours, after initial injury. It tends to affect deep tissue and the joints.

Third, medical conditions associated with increased perioperative blood loss should be identified. The association between liver diseases and impaired coagulation is well established. Renal failure leading to uremia is also known to impair hemostasis, lead to anemia and perioperative bleeding complications, and increase the likelihood of the patient being transfused. Patients with musculoskeletal disorders often seem to have impaired hemostasis potentially leading to increased perioperative blood loss. This has been described for patients with scoliosis and various types of muscular dystrophy [10, 11]. Patients with thyroid diseases may also occasionally have impaired hemostasis [12].

Fourth, what should also be of interest are *obstacles to surgical hemostasis.* The surgeon's main aim is to operate well and cause the least possible blood loss. However, there are some conditions that make this a challenge. What are they? Clearly, a procedure differs depending on whether it is being done for the first time in the patient or if it is a repeat procedure in the same patient. Reoperations tend to cause greater blood loss and have a higher transfusion rate than first-time procedures [13]. Vascular supply may be altered by a previous procedure done in the same area as the proposed operation. Ask explicitly about previous surgery. Prior infection in the area of the operation may cause abnormalities. For example, after pelvic inflammation, adhesions may make patients more prone to bleeding after further surgery. Congenital alterations in anatomy may equally be a cause for unusual blood supply and should prompt further evaluation.

Fifth, the general condition of the patient is what determines how well anemia is tolerated.

Review of systems with respect to blood management

A review of systems is a systematic way to take a history while using body systems as a guideline. Go through the systems from head to toe and double-check any complaint that may have been forgotten. While not directly related to anemia and hemostasis, disturbances in almost every part of the body can have an impact on blood management. To determine the lowest acceptable hemoglobin level find out about the patient's comorbidities.

Neurology: A history of stroke may indicate arteriosclerosis that may decrease the patient's ability to tolerate anemia. Syncope may be a sign for anemia.

The *lung* is essential for oxygenation and diseases of the lung may impair this process. Lung diseases such as chronic obstructive pulmonary disease may also increase the likelihood of the patient getting transfused [13]. Do not forget to ask if the patient suffers from shortness of breath, asthma, chest pain, bloody sputum, or any lung diseases.

Cardiovascular system: While healthy hearts often tolerate very low hemoglobin levels, hearts suffering from coronary artery disease do not tolerate anemia to the same extent. Symptoms such as ankle edema, claudication, angina pectoris, orthopnea, paroxysmal nocturnal dyspnea, dyspnea on exertion, palpitations, dizziness, etc. may all be indicators for heart (or vascular) disease.

Urogenital tract: The kidneys are the site of manufacture for erythropoietin and kidney failure may lead to anemia. The urinary tract and the female genitalia are sites where bleeding may be visible in coagulopathy, e.g., via hematuria. As a natural form of blood loss, menstruation can also cause anemia.

Gastrointestinal tract: Occult bleeding in the gastrointestinal tract may lead to anemia. A history of peptic ulcers and gastritis indicates that the patient is prone to a recurrence of such in the perisurgical period. Further, blood loss via the gastrointestinal tract can often be prevented by prudent intervention. Worm infestations are often found in tropical countries and precipitate blood loss and vitamin deficiency with consequent anemia. Ask about the appearance of the stool. Is it dark indicating bleeding in the gastrointestinal tract? Are there indicators for worm infestations? Is there any hematemesis, melena, or abdominal pain? As part of the gastrointestinal tract the liver is essential since coagulation factors and albumin are synthesized here and may be diminished if the liver is diseased. Diabetes mellitus, another disorder related to the gastrointestinal tract, is often accompanied by silent cardiovascular disease.

Skin and connective tissues: Signs of autoimmune disorders often present with skin changes. Bones and joints may be the sites of chronic disorders such as rheumatism. Diseases of the connective tissues may indirectly indicate anemia of chronic disease or hematological derangements due to autoimmune processes. In rheumatic patients, cardiopulmonary disease due to serosa involvement must not be overlooked.

General: Malignancies and infections often cause anemia, therefore it is beneficial to look for their signs. Ask about any recent weight loss, night sweats, fever, shivers, rashes, lumps or masses. The nutritional status of the patient is also of concern because this affects hematopoiesis, synthesis of factors involved in hemostasis, and the patient's general condition. A lack of vitamins K and C may cause coagulopathy. A deficiency in B vitamins and iron can cause anemia. Both under- or malnutrition decrease the patient's ability to tolerate anemia, heal wounds, synthesize clotting factors, etc.

Closely related to nutrition are allergies, which should be asked for explicitly. They may cause loss of red cells and platelets. Some foods and drugs may cause hemolysis, as in favism, and should be, therefore, avoided.

The drugs taken by patients may cause all kinds of hindrances to optimal blood management. Some drugs may cause anemia either by inducing bleeding (nonsteroidal antirheumatic drugs (NSAR), coumadin), causing hemolysis, or suppressing erythropoiesis (chemotherapeutics). Other drugs may cause coagulopathies. This may be the desired effect, such as in the case of heparin and aspirin, or they may cause coagulopathies as a side effect. Long-term antibiosis damages the intestinal flora, which normally synthesize vitamin K. If such is lacking, coagulopathies result. If aspirin or nonsteroidal antirheumatic drugs are taken, occult blood loss via the gastrointestinal tract may occur, causing anemia and iron deficiency.

It is therefore very important to have a complete list of drugs taken currently and in the recent past. This should also include nonprescription drugs, nutritional supplements, and so-called alternative medicines. A patient may not readily report on all drugs, especially if he fears the doctor would disapprove or because of the general perception that such drugs are harmless. Asking specifically for all drugs helps obtain a complete drug list.

Perform a physical examination

After having taking a history, continue with the physical examination of the patient. Look for hints that support and supplement the information already obtained.

In particular, look for signs of anemia. Pallor is the leading sign of anemia. It is most obvious on mucous membranes, conjunctivae, and nail beds. An icterus may also be indicative of anemia since it may be caused by hemolysis. A maxillary overgrowth is associated with chronic hemolytic anemia. Decubital ulcers are often associated with anemia [14]. Tachycardia is sometimes present, especially when anemia is accompanied by hypovolemia.

Further, look for signs of coagulation disorders. Ecchymoses and large deeper hematomas are signs of impaired humoral hemostasis. Petechiae are suspect for a defect or deficiency of platelets or a problem with the vessel wall.

Multiple small red spots on the lips (dilated capillaries), as found in hereditary hemorrhagic teleangiactasia, bleed easily when traumatized. Patients with this disease frequently have nose bleeds and bleed from the gastrointestinal tract. Indirectly related to coagulation disorders are signs of a liver disease, which may cause clotting factor deficiencies. Spider angioma, palmar erythema, dilated veins on the abdomen (caput medusae), light pink or silver colored nails, a bright, shiny, red tongue, and glossy lips are indicators for liver disease that should be evaluated further.

Signs of infections and chronic illness (e.g., rheumatic arthritis) should also be noted since such conditions may cause anemia, impair coagulation, and influence the overall condition of the patient. Hypersplenism is especially suspect since thrombocytopenia and anemia are often present. Especially before surgery in the elderly, assessment of the nutritional and volume status is mandatory. Perform the physical examination as usual keeping in mind all the symptoms related to the patient's blood management.

Step 2. Laboratory and other tests

The second step in our algorithm is to order tests as indicated. Judicious use of laboratory tests adds to the evaluation. However, care must be taken to avoid undue preoperative iatrogenic blood loss. As shown in Chapter 12, blood loss caused by phlebotomy may be significant and may even lead to transfusions in certain patient populations. Therefore, diagnostic phlebotomy needs to be restricted. There is no such thing as a standing order for patients in general. Order laboratory tests only if they provide potentially valuable information that will influence the treatment. Now that history taking is complete and the physical examination has been concluded it is easy to determine which laboratory values are needed. Based on the findings decide now which tests are most likely to contribute to the therapy.

Preoperative workup of anemia

The hemoglobin value is of central importance to the patient's blood management. In contrast to other laboratory studies, a hemoglobin level should be obtained routinely

for all patients unless patients present for minor surgery with little blood loss. However, if there are indications of cardiovascular or renal disease, a malignancy, diabetes mellitus, aspirin or nonsteroidal antirheumatic drug use, or full anticoagulation, a hemoglobin value should be obtained even in patients with only minimal expected blood loss. To reduce iatrogenic blood loss and to speed up the medical workup, a fingerstick hemoglobin can be obtained in the office on the patient's first visit. In areas where laboratory workup is beyond patients' means or otherwise unavailable, the Haemoglobin Color Scale [15] recommended by the World Health Organization (WHO) can aid in estimating patients' hemoglobin.

Once it has been established that the patient is anemic, the reason for the anemia must be found. The algorithm developed by the Society for the Advancement of Blood Management (Fig. 11.2) guides through the anemia workup. A systematic search for the cause of anemia can be performed based on a complete blood count, preferably done more than 30 days before elective surgery.

Preoperative workup of impaired clotting

It is tempting to rely on global coagulation laboratory tests to screen for the risk of intra- and postoperative hemorrhage. Unfortunately, there is no such laboratory test that can predict this. The most common bleeding disorders cannot be detected with Quick, international normalized ratio (INR), activated partial thromboplastin time (aPTT), template bleeding time, and platelet count [16–21]. However, this is no reason to despair. A detailed history has already been taken and a physical examination has been performed. These are the most important steps in determining whether the patient is at risk for a coagulation problem or not. If the history and physical examination are negative in this respect, then it is very unlikely that the patient has a coagulation disorder [7]. "Patients without historical risk factors or physical findings suggestive of an increased bleeding risk are unlikely to have congenital or acquired coagulopathies that will result in increased postoperative bleeding and do not require testing" [22].

Laboratory testing is warranted for patients with a positive history of coagulation disorder or physical findings suggesting such. If the underlying disorder is already known, then laboratory testing is straightforward. Refer to Table 11.2 for the indicated tests [23].

If a thorough coagulation history of the patient is unobtainable, a set of coagulation tests may be indicated if the patient is about to undergo surgery with potential major

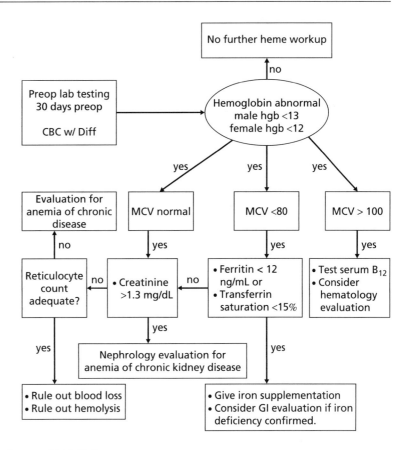

No further heme workup

Preop lab testing
30 days preop

CBC w/ Diff

Hemoglobin abnormal
male hgb <13
female hgb <12

no

yes   yes   yes

Evaluation for
anemia of chronic
disease

MCV normal

MCV <80

MCV > 100

no   yes   yes   yes

Reticulocyte
count
adequate?

no

• Creatinine
 >1.3 mg/dL

no

• Ferritin < 12
 ng/mL or
• Transferrin
 saturation <15%

• Test serum B$_{12}$
• Consider
 hematology
 evaluation

yes

yes

Nephrology evaluation for
anemia of chronic kidney disease

yes

yes

• Rule out blood loss
• Rule out hemolysis

• Give iron supplementation
• Consider GI evaluation if iron
 deficiency confirmed.

Fig 11.2 Clinical care pathway for identification and evaluation of anemia in elective surgical patients.

Table 11.2 Laboratory tests in relation to a known or highly likely coagulation disorder.

Known or probable cause of coagulation disorder	Indicated tests
Dysfibrinogenemia	Fibrinogen level
Factor VII deficiency	Factor VII
Hemophilia A	Factor VIIIc
Hemophilia B	Factor IX
Factor XI deficiency	aPTT, Factor XI
Factor XIII deficiency	Factor XIII
Von Willebrand's disease	von Willebrand factor antigen, ristocetin cofactor, factor VIII activity
Patient with liver disease	Platelet count, Quick, aPTT, fibrinogen, hematocrit (possibly factors II, V, VII, IX, X, protein C, protein S, antithrombin III)
Patients with kidney disease	Quick, aPTT, platelet count, hematocrit, global platelet function test

aPTT, activated partial thromboplastin time.

blood loss. It has been suggested that Quick, aPTT, fibrinogen, platelet count, and a global platelet function test [24] be used.

If the history and physical examination reveal a bleeding disorder and there is no obvious underlying disease, start with a set of global coagulation tests. For instance, use the combination of Quick, aPTT, fibrinogen, von Willebrand factor test(s), factor XII, platelet count, and a global test for platelet function [24]. Depending on the results of the tests, refer to Table 11.3 to follow up on the patient. If diagnosis of the bleeding disorder is not straightforward or if the tests suggested are unavailable at the institution, consider sending the patient to a specialist, if available.

Preoperative workup of accompanying disorders

Preoperative blood tests other than for hemoglobin level and coagulation profile are seldom recommended if neither the history nor physical examination give sound

Table 11.3 Follow-up of patients with a pathologic coagulation test result.

Pathologic test	Differential diagnosis	Further tests to confirm diagnosis
Quick	Vitamin K deficiency or therapy with vitamin K antagonist (factor V normal)	Factors II, V, VII, X, fibrinogen
	Factor synthesis in liver disturbed or loss of coagulation factors (factor V reduced)	
	Congenital deficiency of factors II, V, VII, IX, X, hypo- or dysfibrinogenemia	
aPTT	First: measure thrombin time	
	If thrombin time is prolonged: heparin effect	
	If thrombin time is normal: factor deficiency of factors V, VIII, IX, XI, XII (also in vitamin K deficiency due to lack of factor IX)	
	Autoimmune diseases causing inhibitors	
	Factor XII deficiency does not cause increased blood loss during or after surgery	Thrombin time, factors V, VIII, IX, XI, XII
Von Willebrand test(s)	Congenital or acquired deficiency (e.g., drug-induced)	
Factor XIII assay	Acquired or congenital factor XIII deficiency	
Platelet count	Pseudothrombocytopenia drug-related thrombocytopenia, hypersplenism, bone marrow diseases	Repeat platelet count to check for pseudothrombocytopenia, ultrasound of spleen, antiplatelet antibodies
Global platelet function test		Platelet aggregation tests

aPTT, activated partial thromboplastin time.

reason to believe something is wrong. In certain situations, creatinine, glucose, and a pregnancy test are recommended. But a full-fledged laboratory workup is not recommended routinely and should be avoided to reduce unnecessary preoperative blood loss.

Since tolerance of anemia depends on the ability of the heart to compensate for decreased red cell mass by increasing cardiac output, the heart should also be focused on in the workup. However, an electrocardiogram and imaging for screening of a heart disease is of little value if the history and the physical exam do not suggest a problem. An electrocardiogram has been recommended for patients with a cardiovascular disease, hypertension, or diabetes. If a normal electrocardiogram has been obtained within the last 6 months and there is no reason to assume the onset of a new disease or worsening of a known one, no new electrocardiogram needs to be written. A chest x-ray is also not indicated in all patients presenting for surgery. It may be done in patients with known respiratory or cardiovascular disease. If there has not been an intervening clinical event, a chest radiograph taken during the previous year usually suffices. If indicated for coronary artery disease, cardiac revascularization should be done well before elec-

tive surgery with expected major blood loss. To test who is eligible for this procedure, the history and possibly a stress test are crucial. Valvular diseases are also best identified before surgery so that special monitoring of such patients can be prepared. Cardiac arrythmias are not usually a direct cause of perioperative morbidity. They are rather a marker for an underlying disease. If present, reason their should be looked for; look especially for silent heart disease.

Step 3. Some mathematics

Now the history has been taken, a physical examination has been performed, and all the results of the tests ordered have been obtained. Everything reasonably possible has been done to elucidate the patient's key problems. As the third step in the algorithm, calculate with the variables found in the workup. Four things are particularly important: the expected blood loss of the patient's proposed procedure, the patient's blood or red cell volume, the minimum tolerable hemoglobin or hematocrit, and the allowable blood loss.

Expected blood loss

To prepare the patient anticipate how much blood loss can be reasonably expected. The literature abounds with reports about average blood losses for a specific surgery [25–28]. Average blood losses for a given procedure vary greatly [29]. Therefore, a blood manager must obtain estimates of average blood losses for a given procedure performed at his own institution. Since the blood loss entailed in a certain procedure depends greatly on the skills of the surgeon, it is not only important to know *what* procedure will be done, but also *who* will do it. Do not hesitate to ask the surgeon for the expected blood loss.

Surgeons should be able to give an estimate of the expected blood loss. Estimating the blood loss for a certain surgical procedure is difficult and is typically underestimated. Collecting blood in graduated containers, measuring the amount of lavage fluids, and weighing sponges and drapes help, but it is still difficult because losses by evaporation and blood lost on the floor are not easy to estimate.

There are also methods to calculate how much blood a patient loses based on the average amount of blood usually transfused. Models to estimate blood loss are based on one, two, or three variables (uni-, bi-, trivariate) [30]. For the univariate analysis, units of blood transfused to all patients undergoing a certain procedure are recorded over a period of time. Then a calculation is made of how many units are needed so that in 80–90% of cases enough blood is available to fill the perceived need. In a bivariate analysis, the units of blood transfused to patients with certain admission hematocrits are used to predict further needs of patients with the same admission hematocrit. In a trivariate analysis, the patient's blood and red cell volumes are used as the third variable. To estimate red cell loss during surgery and the following 5 days use an equation such as is shown below:

Estimated RBC loss (mL of RBCs)

$$= \text{BV} \times (\text{Hct before surgery} - \text{Hct day 5 postop})$$
$$+ \text{mL of RBC transfused,}$$

where RBC, red blood cells; Hct, hematocrit; BV, blood volume.

In addition to variables involving the surgeon, patient variables also influence perioperative blood loss and thus use of donor blood. As shown above, smaller patients, females, and the elderly are at higher risk for transfusion than larger patients, males and the young. Low preoperative hemoglobin is a predictor for transfusions. Apart from those general characteristics, procedure-specific variables may influence blood loss and subsequent transfusions. Consider cardiac surgery as an example. It has been shown that cardiac patients undergoing heart surgery who are smokers, insulin-dependent diabetics with circulatory or renal manifestations or who present with a new episode of myocardial infarction have a higher risk for transfusions than other patients. Patients who have undergone reoperations or emergency surgery, who have had a heart catheterization during the same hospitalization, who have been on cardiac bypass at low body temperature for longer periods and who have had a low-dose heparin regime have greater blood losses than other patients. The number of bypass grafts is a predictor for transfusions as well [3, 31–34]. Other surgeries have other risk factors for bleeding. The amount of blood loss in burn patients depends on the area of burns to be excised [35]. The amount of blood loss in patients undergoing hip replacement depends on the way the prosthesis is fixed [36]. The presence of metastasis in surgery for colorectal cancer is associated with a higher likelihood for transfusions [37]. And the size of a liver resection is also a predictor for the transfusion rate [38]. Such points must also be kept in mind when estimating the expected blood loss.

Estimate the blood volume of the patient

There are many methods that can be used to estimate a person's blood volume (Table 11.4). For our purposes we assume that a male has 66 mL of blood per kilogram ideal

Table 11.4 Methods to estimate the blood volume of a patient.

EBV men [l] $= (3.29 \times (\text{BSA [m}^2])) - 1.229)$
EBV women [l] $= (3.47 \times (\text{BSA [m}^2])) - 1.954)$

EBV men $= 2740 \text{ mL/m}^2 \text{ BSA}$
EBV women $= 2370 \text{ mL/m}^2 \text{ BSA}$

EBV [mL] $= (\text{factor for gender}) \times \text{body weight [kg]}$
Factor for men: 66 mL/kg; factor for women: 60 mL/kg
   (according to the American Association of Blood Banks)

Allen's formulas
EBV men [L] $= (0.417 \times ((\text{height [m]})^3))$
$\qquad\qquad + (0.0450 \times (\text{weight [kg]})) - 0.030$
EBV women [L] $= (0.414 \times ((\text{height [m]})^3))$
$\qquad\qquad + (0.0328 \times (\text{weight [kg]})) - 0.030$

Note: Blood volume based on lean body mass tends to be more accurate than that based on actual body weight.
EBV, estimated blood volume; BSA, body surface area.
Source: The Medical Algorithm Project (www.medal.org).

body weight and a female has 60 mL of blood per kilogram ideal body weight.

Minimum tolerable hemoglobin

Unfortunately, there is no simple calculation for the minimum tolerable hemoglobin level. To set a reasonable limit use the information from the history based on clinical judgment. A child or a healthy youth easily tolerates a hemoglobin of 5 mg/dL or less while a sickly, elderly person may experience problems if the hemoglobin drops below 9 g/dL. Taking into consideration what comorbidities exist and how historical patient populations with a certain comorbidity were able to handle anemia serves as guideline. Determining a minimum tolerable hemoglobin is an aid to estimate the patient's risk of receiving transfusions and is a help in taking appropriate transfusion avoidance measures. The minimum tolerable hemoglobin level thus determined must not, however, be confused with a transfusion trigger.

Allowable blood loss

Finally, calculate how much blood loss the patient can reasonably tolerate. Use the following equation:

Allowable RBC loss = (blood volume × Hct$_{actual}$)

−(blood volume × minimum tolerable hematocrit)

(To convert hemoglobin to hematocrit, multiply by 3. A hemoglobin of 10 mg/dL equals a hematocrit of about 30%.)

Step 4. The plan of care

After completing the first three steps of the algorithm, all the information needed is available. It is now time to tailor an individual treatment concept for the patient. Having a detailed plan of care is the basis for successful blood management [39, 40], the lack of a plan may result in disaster [41].

Take a sheet of paper and begin by listing the key features of the patient and make an inventory of all obstacles to blood management, e.g., relevant drugs, malnutrition, comorbidities. This will be the problem list. A brief glance at the list will show whether care of the patient can be continued or whether support is needed. An experienced colleague may be asked to assist if there are only a limited number of problems for which help is needed. If a case is anything other than simple and straightforward, a multidisciplinary approach to the patient's blood management is likely the way to go. A decision-making and planning team including the patient, surgeon, anesthesiologist, hematologist, and transfusion specialist need to develop the plan of care [42].

Since the patient's problems have already been listed, it should be easy to handle them one at a time and find the appropriate treatment. As a team decide how to handle the problems. Determine not only the treatment but also set therapy goals and time limits for reevaluation and arrange for consultations with specialists if such are indicated.

How much preparation and how much blood conservation is needed depend a great deal on the expected blood loss and allowable blood loss. Understandably, less preparation is needed for a young, healthy adult undergoing a procedure with an expected blood loss of only 50 mL. On the other hand, if expected blood loss greatly exceeds the allowable blood loss or if the patient does not have sufficient reserves to compensate for blood loss, preparations will be more extensive.

If the allowable blood loss is greater than the expected blood loss, proceed as usual with preparation. However, if the expected blood loss exceeds the allowable blood loss, more intensive preparation is needed. The hematocrit is the strongest predictor for perioperative transfusions [3, 43]. Patients with high-normal or slightly supranormal hematocrits are less likely to receive transfusions than anemic patients. Therefore, first plan how to increase the patient's hematocrit. In any case, therapy of any bleeding disorder should also have high priority in the plan of care.

Once the patient's hemoglobin level has been optimized, a new calculation is warranted. If the estimated blood loss still exceeds the allowable blood loss, measures to reduce estimated blood loss should be added to the treatment concept. In some cases it may be prudent to prepare for surgery by reducing the volume of tissue to be operated on. Tumors can be downstaged by chemotherapeutic pretreatment or radiation therapy. In hypervascular tumors or organs that present a high risk of bleeding, vessels can be electively embolized [44, 45]. Surgical and anesthetic measures to reduce blood loss should be included in the plan as well as methods using autologous blood. Decisions about the method of surgical cutting, the use of a cell salvaging device and hemodilution should be made. Several treatment options can be combined to gain the desired effect. The blood-saving effects add up.

Procedures with expected major blood loss may at times be staged. Staged procedures (also called planned reoperation) are performed by dividing the surgery into two or more steps performed one at a time at intervals. This allows the patient to recover from the blood loss experienced in one surgical step giving him time to recuperate before the next step of the procedure is performed. Proper care and especially suitably adapted alimentation facilitate the recovery. The total blood loss (and the complications) of all steps of the procedure combined may even be less than the blood loss of the same procedure performed in one step [46].

The duration of surgery is directly related to amounts transfused [47]. Measures to shorten the operating time also reduce patients' exposure to allogeneic blood. Two instead of one surgeon or other reasonable increases in team size can shorten the duration of surgery.

In recent years, computer-based planning has been advocated by some specialists. The basis for such planning is usually imaging of the area under consideration. A spiral CT (computerized tomography) scan or an MRI (magnet resonance imaging) provides details of the patient's anatomy. Data are fed into a computer that give a three-dimensional image. The surgeon can study the blood supply and use a simulation program to try different approaches to surgery. It is not clear whether this rather sophisticated method will help avoid transfusions, but it is an interesting approach to the planning of complicated procedures.

At times reducing the estimated blood loss below the allowable blood loss may seem difficult. In such a case, continue developing the plan of care by reevaluating the method for the planned surgical intervention. Often there is more than one surgical approach to the treatment of the patient. The procedure chosen may be modified or replaced by another method. The decision on the surgical method is an important step in reducing blood loss. At times, minimally invasive techniques are superior to traditional procedures with respect to minimizing blood loss. Occasionally, expected blood loss may still exceed allowable blood loss. Under such circumstances it may be wise to consider other treatment for the patient rather than a surgical procedure. Radiation therapy may offer as good a prognosis as surgery. Chemotherapy and interventional radiology may be reasonable alternatives in cases when it seems there are no methods available that avoid allogeneic transfusions. By taking a broader look at the therapeutic options open to patients, successful therapy may still be possible without resorting to allogeneic transfusions.

While pondering over which procedure to recommend to the patient, think also about possible emergencies that may complicate treatment. This anticipatory, provident approach to surgery leads to questions such as "What

preparations need to be taken to handle such emergencies?" The plan of care should include the equipment actually needed as well as equipment to handle emergencies. If there is any uncertainty about caring for emergencies alone, having a colleague as a backup is helpful.

Once decision-making has advanced to the stage where a certain manner of treatment has been decided on, put the plans down in writing. Record:
• How the patient's medical problems are to be treated, e.g., coagulation problems
• How to optimize the hemoglobin level
• What surgery is to be done and how it will be prepared
• What measures will be taken to reduce blood loss
• What emergencies can be expected and how they will be dealt with.
Also, list all the additional personnel, items, and drugs needed.

While trying to formulate a plan of care it may become clear that items are missing in the institution or that insufficient capability, willingness, and experience are available to take care of the patient. Equipment may also be lacking. It may not be possible to handle a potential emergency correctly. Pride on the part of the surgeon in such a situation may endanger the life of the patient. The patient's fair chance of a favorable outcome may be forfeited by insistence on taking care of the patient although another doctor may be in a much better position to do so. In such a situation, transferal of the patient is the only ethically and medically correct decision. So as to be prepared to transfer a patient, gather information about other physicians and centers where patients could be transferred.

An example of a plan of care

> ### The case
>
> A 46-year-old white woman who has lived in South Africa all her life comes and asks to have a large myoma removed from her uterus. She has been experiencing back pain and progredient menorrhagia for 3 years. Exams in the gynecologist's office strongly suggest this is due to the myoma. The patient would rather not have a total abdominal hysterectomy but agrees if it is the only way to avert a life-threatening situation. The patient should be scheduled for elective surgery.

Step 1 (46-year-old white female, 75 kg, 180 cm)

The workup of the patient reveals the following:

Present complaint: progredient back pain, began 3 years ago; heavy menses for 3 years; apart from this the patient feels a little tired and weak, but has no other complaints

History related to blood management:

Anemia: no known prior anemia; feels a little weak, sports difficult because of dyspnea

Coagulation: no easy bruising, no nose bleeds, birth uneventful, no exaggerated bleeding after surgery, heavy menses for about 3 years

Systemic data:

Allergies: penicillin (rash)

Habits: non-smoker all her life, occasional moderate alcohol use

Medicines: occasionally takes aspirin for migraine (never more than 1500 mg/day, last dose 3 days ago)

Past medical history: normal childhood diseases without complications

Open appendectomy age 13 (uneventful)

Spontaneous birth of two healthy girls

Hepatitis A at 21 after trip through Bangladesh, uncomplicated recovery

History of pelvic inflammation; treated with antibiotics 3 years ago

Family history: unremarkable

Social history: married for 26 years, two healthy daughters (20 and 22 years), secretary

Review of systems:

General: no recent weight changes, no fever, no lumps, no bleeding other than menstruation, no rashes

Respiratory: occasional shortness of breath, slight dyspnea on exertion

Cardiovascular: no edema, no orthopnea, no angina pectoris, occasional palpitations

Gastrointestinal: bowel movement once per day, no blood, no melena, no heartburn

Genitourinary: compare present complaint; urine: no urinary frequency, normal color

CNS: migraine about four times per year (reacts well to aspirin), dizziness, one syncope 1 year ago, patient did not consult a doctor

Physical examination: no acute distress, alert and oriented × 3, good general and nutritional condition, pale

Vital signs: heart rate 110 beats per minute, blood pressure 100/70 mm Hg, temperature 36.6°C, respiration rate 22/minute

Head: unremarkable, no icterus

Lungs: thorax within normal limits, lungs clear

Cardiovascular system: good capillary refill, pulses all ++, on auscultation systolic 2/6 heart murmur, punctum maximum Erb, otherwise heart rhythmic

Abdomen: bowel sounds normal, abdomen soft, no tenderness, no masses, scars unremarkable, liver and spleen within normal limits, rectal unremarkable

Genital: enlarged uterus with bulky surface, painful examination

Skin: no rashes, pale, no hematoma, no petechiae, and no ecchymoses, no lumps, normal turgor

Step 2: tests

The history and the physical examination suggest the following problems:

Blood loss anemia with subsequent iron loss due to menorrhagia, possible coagulation disorder

The stepwise workup gives the following results:

Hematocrit 0.23, hemoglobin 7.5 g/dL

Transferrin saturation: 10%; ferritin: 50

Coagulation tests normal, platelets 250 gpt

Step 3: calculations

Estimated blood volume: 4.5 l (75 kg × 60 mL/kg); = 900 mL red cell mass

Expected blood loss: 500 mL

Minimum hematocrit: 0.18

Allowable blood loss: about 450 mL; allowable RBC loss: 90 mL

Step 4: plan of care

A 46-year-old white female, 75 kg, 180 cm (EBL: 500 mL; Hct minimal: 0.18; ABL: 450 mL)

Problem list:

(a) Existing: (1) anemia; (2) ongoing blood loss

(b) Potential: (3) bleeding due to myoma and surgery; (4) possible total abdominal hysterectomy; (5) possibility of adhesions may increase blood loss to 1000 mL

Surgical procedure: open myomectomy, possibly a total abdominal hysterectomy

Preparation

Ad 1: iron po 325 mg tid cum 100 mg vitamin C; multivitamin cum folate and vitamin B_{12}; reevaluation in 3 weeks, possibly EPO, target hemoglobin >13 g/dL

Ad 2: see gynecologist for hormonal therapy to suppress menses

Ad 3: use cell saver if blood loss is excessive; colleague as backup

To do list:

Check cell saver availability

Inform Dr J. Doe about the need for help and arrange surgery on a date when he is available.

Step 5. Preparation

Prepare the patient

Treating adverse conditions

PREOPERATIVE ANEMIA AND POLYCYTHEMIA

Preoperative anemia is a strong predictor for perioperative transfusions [3, 13]. A considerable proportion of patients presenting for surgery with anemia develop it during hospitalization while waiting for surgery [48]. Blood sampling, recent angiography and other invasive procedures, and the effect of drugs may be the cause. It is imperative in blood management to optimize hemoglobin preoperatively and avoid further blood loss. Conditions causing anemia, such as infection, inflammation, and malignancies, should be under control whenever possible. Using rHuEPO and hematinics as described in Chapters 3 and 4, anemia can be treated properly and the recommendations given in Chapter 12 will help prevent iatrogenic anemia.

Some patient populations are prone to preoperative transfusions. Among such are patients with sickle cell disease, a genetic disorder that presents with a sickle-shaped hemoglobin (HbS) in red cells that aggregates when deoxygenized and cause rigidity of the red cells. This results in hemolytic anemia and in tissue injury due to vasoocclusive diseases. Sickling of the hemoglobin and vasoocclusive crises can be caused by surgery and anesthesia and occur when pain, hypoxia, hypoperfusion, acidosis, dehydratation, and hypothermia are present. Based on clinical observations, preoperative transfusions have been recommended to prevent venoocclusion by dilution of HbS and to treat anemia. However, Dix [49] states "Recent studies have demonstrated that aggressive preoperative transfusion therapy is not beneficial over a more conservative approach." To prevent unnecessary exposure to donor blood in patients with sickle cell disease, the need to avoid the above-mentioned factors (hypoxia, hypoperfusion, etc.) is self-evident. Hydroxyurea, an antineoplastic agent that increases fetal hemoglobin, improves anemia in sickle cell

patients. It is used alternatively to reduce patient exposure to donor blood. Other promising therapies include butyrate compounds, clotrimazole, magnesium supplementation, poloxamer 188, antiadhesion agents, anticoagulant approaches, fructose 1–6 diphosphate, and nitric oxide [50]. Preoperatively, hydroxyurea or another suitable therapy should be initiated to increase the safety margin for patients with sickle cell disease. Close cooperation between the patient, his hematologist, and the surgeon is needed to choose the best available preparation method for surgery.

Patients with polycythemia have a high risk of perisurgical hemorrhage. Untoward effects are also due to hyperviscosity. Treatment before surgery is preferable. Phlebotomies, hydroxyurea, radioactive phosphorus, interferon, anagrelide, and antiplatelet medications are all used and choice is the subject of debate. No matter what treatment approach is used, elective surgery should be postponed until the red cell and platelet counts are normalized. In an emergency, phlebotomy is the treatment of choice.

COAGULATION DISORDERS

Functional hemostatic processes are vital for minimum blood loss. Preoperative optimizing of the patient's capability for hemostasis includes treatment as well as prevention of coagulation disorders.

Treat coagulopathies Now that the patient workup has been completed the cause of any bleeding disorder should be apparent. It should now be easy to treat such appropriately.

Von Willebrand's disease is a relatively common inherited bleeding disorder. Desmopressin is the treatment of choice in most patients. In selected cases, a factor concentrate may be indicated. Cryoprecipitate would work as well but is no longer recommended due to the risks involved [42].

Hemophilia A and B are inherited coagulation disorders with well-defined defects. Even if no major bleeding episodes have occurred so far, surgery may be a trigger sufficient to cause excessive intra- and postoperative bleeding if treatment is absent. The treatment typically is administration of desmopressin or replacement of the missing coagulation factor. For the latter, a variety of products are available, both derived from human blood and recombinant products. Keeping the kinetics of the factors in mind, replacement therapy is best started just prior to surgery

Table 11.5 Monitoring and reversal of common anticoagulants.

Agent	Coumarin and derivatives	Unfractionated heparin	Low-molecular-weight heparin	Fondaparinux Pentasaccharide	Danaparoid	Hirudin	Lepirudin	Bivalirudin	Argatroban
Mode of action	Antagonism of vitamin K	Binds to AT III for indirect thrombin inhibition	Activates to AT III to inhibit FIIa and FXa	Binds to AT to neutralize FXa	Inhibits F Xa and to lesser degree FIIa	Direct thrombin inhibitor	Direct thrombin inhibitor, almost irreversible	Thrombin inhibitor, reversible	Direct thrombin inhibitor
Monitoring	INR, Quick	aPTT, platelet count for HIT detection	Anti-Xa-test	May be not needed	Anti-Xa-activity	aPTT thrombin time, ecarin clotting time	aPTT [76] thrombin time, ecarin clotting time	ACT	aPTT
Reversal	Prothrombin complex concentrate, FEIBA, rHuFVIIa [60, 61], vitamin K	Specific antidote; protamine sulfate; consider: PEG-modified protamine heparinase I, certain peptides	Protamine reverses about 60% of anti-Xa activity	No specific antidote; try RFVIIa	No specific antidote; protamine reverses slightly; certain peptides	Dialysis with specialized equipment	Dialysis with specialized equipment	Case report: mix of hemodialysis, modified ul-trafiltration, rFVIIa, FFP, Cryo-ppt	

Note: The "Reversal" column lists not only well-established methods of reversal of anticoagulants or treatment of anticoagulant-induced bleeding, but also therapies whose

and is continued until wound healing has progressed sufficiently. Refer to Chapters 7, 8, and 19 for details.

Chronic renal failure causes a uremic bleeding disorder characterized by thrombocytopathy, anemia, and vessel wall abnormalities [51]. If there is still time left for preparation, anemia should be corrected. Patients with end-stage renal disease should be intensively dialyzed on the day before surgery. If the patient is dialyzed on the day of surgery it may be prudent to wait at least 12 hours to be sure dialysis heparin is metabolized to avoid excessive bleeding during surgery [52, 53]. Peritoneal dialysis seems to be superior to conventional dialysis in reducing bleeding risk. To further treat uremic coagulopathy, desmopressin, conjugated estrogens or low-dose transdermal estrogens can be used. Cryoprecipitate may also be administered in selected cases [23].

Patients whose coagulopathy is due to an underlying liver disease may present with a multifactoral bleeding disorder comprising thrombocytopathy and thrombocytopenia, lack of plasmatic coagulation factors, and accelerated fibrinolysis. Depending on the leading coagulation problem, antifibrinolytics, factor concentrates, or conjugated estrogens may be indicated [54].

Some patients with dysproteinemias, (and) myeloproliferative syndromes (…) clearly have excessive bleeding that appears to be caused by abnormal platelet function. In these patients, bleeding symptoms usually respond to appropriate therapy, such as plasmapheresis, cytoreductive therapy (and) intensive dialysis.... [55]

Thrombocytopenia in patients with rheumatic or other autoimmune diseases is often caused by increased platelet destruction. In this situation, platelet transfusions are usually not helpful. Steroids, danazol, intravenous immunoglobulin, or splenectomy are treatment options that should be considered before surgery.

Manage anticoagulation Therapeutic anticoagulation is a common treatment for a variety of disorders. When patients under anticoagulation present for surgery, anticoagulation drugs may increase the surgical blood loss [56, 57]. Whenever safely possible, these should be substituted using an agent that is easily reversible, stopped, or antagonized. The risk of thrombosis or embolism may increase when medications for anticoagulation are stopped and this should be taken into consideration. Weighing the competing risks of thromboembolism and bleeding is therefore prudent. Skilful surgery may avoid major bleeding complications even in anticoagulated patients.

Vitamin K antagonism is a common treatment principle to induce anticoagulation. In elective surgery, time can be planned until the effect of vitamin K antagonists wears off. Vitamin K administration speeds up this process. Emergency reversal is at times indicated. If patients are at significant risk of developing embolic complications when anticoagulation is interrupted, oral anticoagulation should be stopped temporarily for the briefest of intervals to perform surgery. Perioperatively, such patients on vitamin K antagonists should be treated with

Melagatgran	Ximelagatran	Abciximab	Eptifibatide	Tirofiban	Ticlopidine	Clopidogrel	Dipyridamole	Aspirin	Flurbiprofen
Direct thrombin inhibitor	Direct thrombin inhibitor	Blocks GPIIb/IIIa receptor of platelets	GPIIb/IIIa inhibitor	GPIIb/IIIa inhibitor	Irreversible blockage of platelet ADP receptor	Irreversible blockage of platelet ADP receptor		Thromboxane inhibition	Thromboxane inhibition
May be not needed	May be not needed	Hemodyne analysis, modified TEG				Specific platelet function tests (aggregometry or platelet count ratio) using ADP as an activator, platelet count	Platelet function assay		
	Chromogenic substrate (Chromozym), FEIBA, rFVIIa		Desmopressin	Dialysis, possibly desmopressin or rFVIIa, fibrinogen/cryo-ppt	Desmopressin, fibrinogen/cryo-ppt		Aprotinin, desmopressin, rFVIIa, plasmapherese		Desmopressin, Aprotinin

value is not yet fully understood. If the surgeon plans treating an anticoagulated patient, please refer to the literature for indication and dosages of the proposed agents.

full-dose heparin instead of vitamin K antagonists. This permits emergency reversal with protamine if bleeding occurs.

Another common anticoagulant is aspirin, an antiplatelet agent. It has been documented as a reason for an increased risk of perisurgical bleeding and increased use of transfusion [56], although this effect has not been demonstrated in other studies. The antiplatelet effect of aspirin is pronounced if the patient has taken other anticoagulants, has a preexisting problem with hemostasis, or if alcohol is taken concurrently [53]. Since aspirin irreversibly inhibits thromboxane synthesis in platelets, it is best stopped several days before surgery and the surgeon should wait until functional platelets are produced.

Nowadays many other anticoagulants are used in clinical practice. Table 11.5 provides an overview of the existing drugs and potential reversal methods if such become necessary [58–79].

Avoid pharmacologic coagulopathies Many drugs are not used for anticoagulation but nevertheless affect hemostasis (Table 11.6) [53, 80, 81]. Whether all such drug effects translate into increased perioperative bleeding has not yet been determined. However, if at all possible, such pharmacologically induced coagulopathies should be avoided. Often it is possible to switch from one drug to another or to stop the drug altogether. Drug-induced coagulopathies can be antidoted occasionally.

CARDIOPULMONARY AND GENERAL CONDITION
In coronary artery disease, the ability to increase the cardiac output is impaired, thus limiting the patient's ability to tolerate anemia. It is important to avoid cardiac ischemia. Perioperative analgesia, anxiolytic medications, normothermia, judicious beta-blockade, and close monitoring for cardiac events are recommended [82]. If

Table 11.6 Examples of drugs and herbs that can cause coagulopathies and may increase perioperative blood loss.

Nonsteroidal anti-inflammatory drugs
Penicillin
Some cephalosporins such as cefotaxime, moxalactam
Quinidine
Alteplase
Protamine
Nifedipine
Nitroglycerine
Paroxetine, fluvoxamine (vitamin C)
High-dose vitamin C
Valproate
St John's wort
Ginger
Garlic
Certain hydroxyethyl starches (desmopressin)
Propofol

Note: The agents in parenthesis may be used to counteract pharmacological coagulopathies.

the patient has had beta-blockers before surgery, such should be continued to prevent withdrawal, which may otherwise cause ischemia. The perioperative risk for ischemia can also be reduced by preoperative coronary revascularization.

There are several measures available to optimize patients' pulmonary function prior to surgery. Smokers should stop smoking at least 8 weeks before surgery. Incentive spirometry before and after surgery should be encouraged in patients with pulmonary problems. Medical therapy is at times indicated, such as bronchodilators for wheezing, and beta-agonists and atropine analogs in patients with asthma and chronic obstructive pulmonary disease.

A number of conditions can adversely affect anemia tolerance and counteract efforts to lower the patient's use of donor blood. Efforts should be taken to optimize the patient's condition preoperatively.

Optimizing the surgical field

In certain situations it seems prudent to optimize the surgical field. There are several methods for reducing the surgical field, for example, reducing the size of a tumor by preoperative chemotherapy or radiation. The vascularity of the surgical field can also be reduced. Preoperative embolization for primary tumors and metastases as well as for whole organs can reduce perfusion and thus blood loss [83–85]. Pharmacological therapy may be equally effective in selected cases. For instance, finasteride given before benign prostate hyperplasia operations reduces angiogenesis in the prostate and reduces bleeding and transfusions in patients [86–88].

Patient education

By definition, blood management is patient centered. This means that at all times the patient is the center of all efforts. It is crucial, therefore, to actively include him in the preparations for surgery or any other treatment. This is essential for a good patient–doctor relationship and improves patient compliance. The patient can do much to reduce exposure to donor blood. All patients should be advised not to take drugs on their own initiative. Help patients understand that a single aspirin for a headache or menstrual discomfort can increase blood loss. Sound habits such as healthy nutrition, sufficient sleep, and abstinence of noxae are very basic but improve patients' general condition. Moderate physical exercise may improve not only the overall condition of the patient but may also treat anemia [89]. An information booklet may be handed to the patient detailing the planned blood management procedures. It may also include a summary of what the patient can do during the treatment and perisurgical period. Such a booklet may remind the patient of the need to adhere to the prescribed schedule of therapy.

Prepare the equipment

Hours before the battle of Waterloo, Napoleon Bonaparte told his generals: "This affair will be no more serious than eating one's breakfast." Shortly thereafter, however, he was proven wrong. It was raining. The raindrops rendered the weapons useless, made the roads muddy and impassable for war wagons, blocked the vision of the combatants, and left the soldiers soaked to the skin. The battle at Waterloo was lost, at least in part, because proper, water-proof equipment was lacking. Something as insignificant as raindrops stopped Napoleon. Experience gained in years of campaigning was rendered useless due to the presence of rain. This drives home an important point. The most sophisticated equipment is of little use if it is damaged or unavailable. Therefore, make sure all devices and drugs are handy before surgery. When it starts pouring and vision is obscured, equipment must be readily available to master the situation. Always prepare the equipment and have the needed drugs available to ensure the patient does not meet his Waterloo.

Preparation should not only involve getting ready for the intended procedure. Emergency equipment should also be made ready. One suggestion is to prepare an emergency tray with all that is needed to treat sudden massive bleeding [90]. The contents of such a tray can be tailored to the specialty and skills of the surgeon. It may contain tourniquets, tamponade materials, catheters to block vessels, special clamps, glues, mashes, balloons, etc. It may also contain copies of algorithms that guide through the management of emergent or heavy bleeding [91]. Having such a tray ready saves time in an emergency and may reduce the total blood loss.

Be prepared

The duration of a surgical procedure influences the degree of blood loss. Independent of other factors, long operation times increase blood loss. However, speeding up a procedure at the expense of quality does not reduce blood loss either. Rehearsing the procedure before going to the operating theater is wise, because this helps the surgeon have the steps of the planned procedure fresh in mind. This may not only shorten the duration of the procedure but also improve the quality of the operation, both of which reduce blood loss.

Key points

• Algorithm for preparation of a patient for surgery
1 Take a thorough history and perform a physical examination, paying special attention to obstacles to transfusion avoidance and matters pertaining to blood management; Review test results already available
2 Order labs and other tests if such are clearly indicated but beware of iatrogenic blood loss
3 Based on the findings of #1 and #2, calculate the allowable blood loss, blood volumes, and determine the lowest tolerable hematocrit.
4 Formulate a plan of care (with a timetable). It should include the allowable blood loss and the expected blood loss. Record:
○ How the patient's medical problems will be treated, e.g., coagulation problems
○ How to optimize the hemoglobin level
○ What surgery is to be done and what preparations are necessary
○ What measures will be taken to reduce blood loss
○ What emergencies can be expected and how such will be dealt with.
  Further, list all additional personnel, items, and drugs required.
5 Prepare the patient and the equipment, and make personal preparation in accord with the plan of care.

Questions for review

• Which steps are vital to prepare a patient for surgery in a blood management program?
• How do drugs influence the blood management of patients?
• What measures need to be taken to work up a patient with anemia and with a coagulopathy?
• What preparations are required for surgery in a blood management program?

Suggestions for further research

Compile a list of drugs that have an impact on surgical blood loss.
List laboratory tests of coagulation and evaluate their value as predictors for surgical blood loss.

Exercises and practice cases

Answer the following questions:
• A patient does not complain of any signs of a bleeding disorder. During the physical examination petechiae and a splenomegaly are found. Which laboratory tests should be ordered for the patient?
• Last week, a patient presented with a Quick of 28. He was treated with appropriate doses of vitamin K. Today, he presents with a Quick of 35. What needs to be done?
• A female patient complains of heavy menstrual bleeding although no obvious anatomic pathology is found in a gynecologic exam. Otherwise, she is healthy. Her Quick is 114%, her aPTT is 24 seconds, her platelet count is 250, and her hematocrit is 28. What tests should be ordered?
• A male patient presents for elective hip replacement. He is scheduled for surgery in 3 weeks. On questioning, he states that he usually takes up to 2.5 g of aspirin per day about once a week for tension headache. Otherwise he is healthy. What tests should be ordered?

Introduce Miss B to a colleague. Discuss in a multidisciplinary fashion how her treatment should be continued and write a plan of care for Miss B.

Miss B is 70 years old; she has been sent by her family doctor for bilateral hip replacement. She suffers from a long-standing arthrosis. She has never had an operation before.

Miss B lives alone on the third floor of an apartment building and has increasing difficulty climbing stairs. Her friend Millie used to have the same trouble. Once she got artificial joints, the patient says, she was again able to go for extended walks in the park. Miss B wants to join her friend and asks for the same procedure.

Among other information the letter from Miss B's doctor contains the following:
Her height is 1.60 m and weight 55 kg
Miss B takes the following drugs:
  • Cordarone tablets 200 mg per os 1-0-0-0
  • Coumarin tablets 3 mg per os depending on the INR
  • Ibuprofen tablets 400 mg per os 1-1-1-1
Current laboratory test results:

Table 11.7 Proposal for emergency hemorrhage equipment used in obstetrics and gynecology.

Drugs/glues	Equipment	Plastinated emergency information	Remarks
Tranexamic acid, desmopressin, conjugated estrogens, aprotinin, oxytocin, ergot derivative, prostaglandin analogues (Carboprost, Misoprostol), anticoagulant for cell salvage (heparin, citrate), vasopressin and glues for enhancement of packing, other topical hemostatics (gelatin, collagen, etc.)	packing (5-yard roll), balloon device for uterine tamponade (Foley, Sengstaken- Blakemore), straight (10 cm) eyed-needles and large curved eyed-needles for use with No. 1 suture, 3 Heaney vaginal retractors, 4 sponge forceps, container and suction for cell salvage	diagrams + instructions for the various types of compression sutures and tamponade techniques; Algorithm for nonblood management of postpartum hemorrhage, phone number of radiology dept. (embolization), pharmacy (rhFVIIa), dosage and indications for mentioned drugs	Determine storage time, sterilization, responsible persons, intervals of checks, training

Hematocrit 0.30; hemoglobin 10 g/dL (red cell indices: mean corpuscular volume and mean corpuscular hemoglobin content decreased); leukocytes 8000; platelets 250000; electrolyte profile, liver, and kidney panel unremarkable.

Experience shows that implanting a single artificial hip joint causes the loss of 1000 mL of whole blood.

What is the allowable blood loss for patients with the following characteristics:

- 66 kg male with a minimum tolerable hematocrit of 20 and a current hematocrit of 45
- 100 kg male with a minimum tolerable hematocrit of 30 and a current hematocrit of 33
- 40 kg female with a minimum tolerable hematocrit of 25 and a current hematocrit of 37.

Homework

Take a focused history of three surgical patients in the hospital; be sure to get all the data needed for the patients' blood management.

Go to the hospital laboratory and find out whether platelet function tests are available. If so, obtain more information on them.

Find out what the three most common congenital and three most common acquired bleeding disorders are in your field of practice.

Following the example of Table 11.7, draw up a list of contents for an emergency hemorrhage tray or chart for at least one of the following departments: Emergency department (acute trauma care), gastroenterology, urology, operating room for unexpected major bleeding, pediatrics, ENT, any other you prefer.

References

1 Drager, L.F., *et al*. Impact of clinical experience on quantification of clinical signs at physical examination. *J Intern Med*, 2003. **254**(3): p. 257–263.

2 Keating, E.M. Preoperative evaluation and methods to reduce blood use in orthopedic surgery. *Anesthesiol Clin North America*, 2005. **23**(2): p. 305–313, vi–vii.

3 Scott, B.H., *et al*. Blood use in patients undergoing coronary artery bypass surgery: impact of cardiopulmonary bypass pump, hematocrit, gender, age, and body weight. *Anesth Analg*, 2003. **97**(4): p. 958–963, table of contents.

4 Khanna, M.P., P.C. Hebert, and D.A. Fergusson. Review of the clinical practice literature on patient characteristics associated with perioperative allogeneic red blood cell transfusion. *Transfus Med Rev*, 2003. **17**(2): p. 110–119.

5 Scott, B.H., F.C. Seifert, and P.S. Glass. Does gender influence resource utilization in patients undergoing off-pump coronary artery bypass surgery? *J Cardiothorac Vasc Anesth*, 2003. **17**(3): p. 346–351.

6 Tzilinis, A., A.M. Lofman, and C.D. Tzarnas. Transfusion requirements for TRAM flap postmastectomy breast reconstruction. *Ann Plast Surg*, 2003. **50**(6): p. 623–627.

7 Koscielny, J., *et al*. A practical concept for preoperative identification of patients with impaired primary hemostasis. *Clin Appl Thromb Hemost*, 2004. **10**(3): p. 195–204.

8 Kadir, R.A., *et al*. Frequency of inherited bleeding disorders in women with menorrhagia. *Lancet*, 1998. **351**(9101): p. 485–489.

9 Rapaport, S.I. Preoperative hemostatic evaluation: which tests, if any? *Blood*, 1983. **61**(2): p. 229–231.

10 Saito, T., *et al*. Coagulation and fibrinolysis disorder in muscular dystrophy. *Muscle Nerve*, 2001. **24**(3): p. 399–402.

11 Noordeen, M.H., *et al*. Blood loss in Duchenne muscular dystrophy: vascular smooth muscle dysfunction? *J Pediatr Orthop B*, 1999. **8**(3): p. 212–215.

12 Franchini, M. Hemostasis and thyroid diseases revisited. *J Endocrinol Invest*, 2004. **27**(9): p. 886–892.

13 Ouattara, A., *et al*. Identification of risk factors for allogeneic transfusion in cardiac surgery from an observational study. *Ann Fr Anesth Reanim*, 2003. **22**(4): p. 278–283.

14 Bergquist, S. and R. Frantz. Pressure ulcers in community-based older adults receiving home health care. Prevalence, incidence, and associated risk factors. *Adv Wound Care*, 1999. **12**(7): p. 339–351.

15 Dobson, M. World Health Organization Haemoglobin Colour Scale: a practical answer to a vital need. *Anesthesia*, 2002. **15**: Article 18.

16 Asaf, T., *et al*. The need for routine pre-operative coagulation screening tests (prothrombin time PT/partial thromboplastin time PTT) for healthy children undergoing elective tonsillectomy and/or adenoidectomy. *Int J Pediatr Otorhinolaryngol*, 2001. **61**(3): p. 217–222.

17 Gewirtz, A.S., K. Kottke-Marchant, and M.L. Miller. The preoperative bleeding time test: assessing its clinical usefulness. *Cleve Clin J Med*, 1995. **62**(6): p. 379–382.

18 Gewirtz, A.S., M.L. Miller, and T.F. Keys. The clinical usefulness of the preoperative bleeding time. *Arch Pathol Lab Med*, 1996. **120**(4): p. 353–356.

19 Peterson, P., *et al*. The preoperative bleeding time test lacks clinical benefit: College of American Pathologists' and American Society of Clinical Pathologists' position article. *Arch Surg*, 1998. **133**(2): p. 134–139.

20 Zwack, G.C. and C.S. Derkay. The utility of preoperative hemostatic assessment in adenotonsillectomy. *Int J Pediatr Otorhinolaryngol*, 1997. **39**(1): p. 67–76.

21 Derkay, C.S. A cost-effective approach for preoperative hemostatic assessment in children undergoing adenotonsillectomy. *Arch Otolaryngol Head Neck Surg*, 2000. **126**(5): p. 688.

22 Eckman, M.H., *et al*. Screening for the risk for bleeding or thrombosis. *Ann Intern Med*, 2003. **138**(3): p. W15–W24.

23 DeLoughery, T.G. Management of bleeding with uremia and liver disease. *Curr Opin Hematol*, 1999. **6**(5): p. 329–333.

24 Dempfle, C.E. Perioperative Gerinnungsdiagnostik. *Anaesthesist*, 2005. **54**: p. 167–177.

25 Hu, S.S. Blood loss in adult spinal surgery. *Eur Spine J*, 2004. **13**(Suppl 1): p. S3–S5.

26 Senthil Kumar, G., O.A. Von Arx, and J.L. Pozo. Rate of blood loss over 48 hours following total knee replacement. *Knee*, 2005. **12**(4): p. 307–309.

27 Yuasa, T., *et al*. Intraoperative blood loss during living donor liver transplantation: an analysis of 635 recipients at a single center. *Transfusion*, 2005. **45**(6): p. 879–884.

28 Cushner, F.D., *et al*. Blood loss and transfusion rates in bilateral total knee arthroplasty. *J Knee Surg*, 2005. **18**(2): p. 102–107.

29 Surgenor, D.M., *et al*. The specific hospital significantly affects red cell and component transfusion practice in coronary artery bypass graft surgery: a study of five hospitals. *Transfusion*, 1998. **38**(2): p. 122–134.

30 NATA. *TAB: Transfusion Medicine and Alternatives to Blood Transfusion*. 2000. Edition. Available on http://www.nataonline.com/CONNATTex2.php3.

31 Surgenor, D.M., *et al*. Determinants of red cell, platelet, plasma, and cryoprecipitate transfusions during coronary artery bypass graft surgery: the Collaborative Hospital Transfusion Study. *Transfusion*, 1996. **36**(6): p. 521–532.

32 Despotis, G.J., *et al*. Factors associated with excessive postoperative blood loss and hemostatic transfusion requirements: a multivariate analysis in cardiac surgical patients. *Anesth Analg*, 1996. **82**(1): p. 13–21.

33 Parr, K.G., *et al*. Multivariate predictors of blood product use in cardiac surgery. *J Cardiothorac Vasc Anesth*, 2003. **17**(2): p. 176–181.

34 Moskowitz, D.M., *et al*. Predictors of transfusion requirements for cardiac surgical procedures at a blood conservation center. *Ann Thorac Surg*, 2004. **77**(2): p. 626–634.

35 Criswell, K.K. and R.L. Gamelli. Establishing transfusion needs in burn patients. *Am J Surg*, 2005. **189**(3): p. 324–326.

36 Grosflam, J.M., *et al*. Predictors of blood loss during total hip replacement surgery. *Arthritis Care Res*, 1995. **8**(3): p. 167–173.

37 Nilsson, K.R., *et al*. Preoperative predictors of blood transfusion in colorectal cancer surgery. *J Gastrointest Surg*, 2002. **6**(5): p. 753–762.

38 Mariette, D., *et al*. Preoperative predictors of blood transfusion in liver resection for tumor. *Am J Surg*, 1997. **173**(4): p. 275–279.

39 Hunt, P.S. Bleeding ulcer: timing and technique in surgical management. *Aust N Z J Surg*, 1986. **56**(1): p. 25–30.

40 Forest, R.J., *et al*. Repair of hypoplastic left heart syndrome of a 4.25-kg Jehovah's Witness. *Perfusion*, 2002. **17**(3): p. 221–225.

41 Lawry, K., J. Slomka, and J. Goldfarb. What went wrong: multiple perspectives on an adolescent's decision to refuse blood transfusions. *Clin Pediatr (Phila)*, 1996. **35**(6): p. 317–321.

42 Bolan, C.D., M.E. Rick, and D.W. Polly, Jr. Transfusion medicine management for reconstructive spinal repair in a patient with von Willebrand's disease and a history of heavy surgical bleeding. *Spine*, 2001. **26**(23): p. E552–E556.

43 de Andrade, J.R., *et al*. Baseline hemoglobin as a predictor of risk of transfusion and response to Epoetin alfa in orthopedic surgery patients. *Am J Orthop*, 1996. **25**(8): p. 533–542.

44 Hansen, M.E. and S. Kadir. Elective and emergency embolotherapy in children and adolescents. Efficacy and safety. *Radiologe*, 1990. **30**(7): p. 331–336.

45 Chou, M.M., *et al.* Internal iliac artery embolization before hysterectomy for placenta accreta. *J Vasc Interv Radiol*, 2003. **14**(9, Pt 1): p. 1195–1199.

46 Tsirikos, A.I., *et al.* Comparison of one-stage versus two-stage anteroposterior spinal fusion in pediatric patients with cerebral palsy and neuromuscular scoliosis. *Spine*, 2003. **28**(12): p. 1300–1305.

47 Matin, S.F., *et al.* Evaluation of age and comorbidity as risk factors after laparoscopic urological surgery. *J Urol*, 2003. **170**(4, Pt 1): p. 1115–1120.

48 Karski, J.M., *et al.* Etiology of preoperative anemia in patients undergoing scheduled cardiac surgery. *Can J Anaesth*, 1999. **46**(10): p. 979–982.

49 Dix, H.M. New advances in the treatment of sickle cell disease: focus on perioperative significance. *AANA J*, 2001. **69**(4): p. 281–286.

50 Mankad, V.N. Exciting new treatment approaches for pathyphysiologic mechanisms of sickle cell disease. *Pediatr Pathol Mol Med*, 2001. **20**(1): p. 1–13.

51 Weigert, A.L. and A.I. Schafer. Uremic bleeding: pathogenesis and therapy. *Am J Med Sci*, 1998. **316**(2): p. 94–104.

52 Krishnan, M. Preoperative care of patients with kidney disease. *Am Fam Physician*, 2002. **66**(8): p. 1471–1476, 1379.

53 George, J.N. and S.J. Shattil. The clinical importance of acquired abnormalities of platelet function. *N Engl J Med*, 1991. **324**(1): p. 27–39.

54 Chou, R. and T.G. DeLoughery. Recurrent thromboembolic disease following splenectomy for pyruvate kinase deficiency. *Am J Hematol*, 2001. **67**(3): p. 197–199.

55 Papers to Appear in Forthcoming Issues. *Gynecol Oncol*, 1998. **68**(2): p. 218.

56 Ferraris, V.A., *et al.* Preoperative aspirin ingestion increases operative blood loss after coronary artery bypass grafting. *Ann Thorac Surg*, 1988. **45**(1): p. 71–74.

57 Chu, M.W., *et al.* Does clopidogrel increase blood loss following coronary artery bypass surgery? *Ann Thorac Surg*, 2004. **78**(5): p. 1536–1541.

58 Kessler, C.M. Current and future challenges of antithrombotic agents and anticoagulants: strategies for reversal of hemorrhagic complications. *Semin Hematol*, 2004. **41**(1, Suppl 1): p. 44–50.

59 van Aart, L., *et al.* Individualized dosing regimen for prothrombin complex concentrate more effective than standard treatment in the reversal of oral anticoagulant therapy: an open, prospective randomized controlled trial. *Thromb Res*, September 20, 2005.

60 Levi, M., N.R. Bijsterveld, and T.T. Keller. Recombinant factor VIIa as an antidote for anticoagulant treatment. *Semin Hematol*, 2004. **41**(1, Suppl 1): p. 65–69.

61 Freeman, W.D., *et al.* Recombinant factor VIIa for rapid reversal of warfarin anticoagulation in acute intracranial hemorrhage. *Mayo Clin Proc*, 2004. **79**(12): p. 1495–1500.

62 Hanslik, T. and J. Prinseau. The use of vitamin K in patients on anticoagulant therapy: a practical guide. *Am J Cardiovasc Drugs*, 2004. **4**(1): p. 43–55.

63 Baker, R.I., *et al.* Warfarin reversal: consensus guidelines, on behalf of the Australasian Society of Thrombosis and Haemostasis. *Med J Aust*, 2004. **181**(9): p. 492–497.

64 Chang, L.C., *et al.* PEG-modified protamine with improved pharmacological/pharmaceutical properties as a potential protamine substitute: synthesis and in vitro evaluation. *Bioconjug Chem*, 2005. **16**(1): p. 147–155.

65 Stafford-Smith, M., *et al.* Efficacy and safety of heparinase I versus protamine in patients undergoing coronary artery bypass grafting with and without cardiopulmonary bypass. *Anesthesiology*, 2005. **103**(2): p. 229–240.

66 Schick, B.P., *et al.* Novel design of peptides to reverse the anticoagulant activities of heparin and other glycosaminoglycans. *Thromb Haemost*, 2001. **85**(3): p. 482–487.

67 Warkentin, T.E. and M.A. Crowther. Reversing anticoagulants both old and new. *Can J Anaesth*, 2002. **49**(6): p. S11–S25.

68 Stratmann, G., *et al.* Reversal of direct thrombin inhibition after cardiopulmonary bypass in a patient with heparin-induced thrombocytopenia. *Anesth Analg*, 2004. **98**(6): p. 1635–1639, table of contents.

69 Bodendiek, I., *et al.* Chromogenic substrate as antidote against the thrombin inhibitor Melagatran. *Hamostaseologie*, 2003. **23**(2): p. 97–98.

70 Elg, M., S. Carlsson, and D. Gustafsson. Effect of activated prothrombin complex concentrate or recombinant factor VIIa on the bleeding time and thrombus formation during anticoagulation with a direct thrombin inhibitor. *Thromb Res*, 2001. **101**(3): p. 145–157.

71 Reiter, R.A., *et al.* Desmopressin antagonizes the in vitro platelet dysfunction induced by GPIIb/IIIa inhibitors and aspirin. *Blood*, 2003. **102**(13): p. 4594–4599.

72 Li, Y.F., F.A. Spencer, and R.C. Becker. Comparative efficacy of fibrinogen and platelet supplementation on the in vitro reversibility of competitive glycoprotein IIb/IIIa (alphaIIb/beta3) receptor-directed platelet inhibition. *Am Heart J*, 2001. **142**(2): p. 204–210.

73 Akowuah, E., *et al.* Comparison of two strategies for the management of antiplatelet therapy during urgent surgery. *Ann Thorac Surg*, 2005. **80**(1): p. 149–152.

74 Nacul, F.E., *et al.* Massive nasal bleeding and hemodynamic instability associated with clopidogrel. *Pharm World Sci*, 2004. **26**(1): p. 6–7.

75 Samama, M.M., *et al.* Biochemistry and clinical pharmacology of new anticoagulant agents. *Pathophysiol Haemost Thromb*, 2002. **32**(5–6): p. 218–224.

76 Lubenow, N. and A. Greinacher. Drugs for the prevention and treatment of thrombosis in patients with heparin-induced thrombocytopenia. *Am J Cardiovasc Drugs*, 2001. **1**(6): p. 429–443.

77 Dyke, C.M., *et al.* Preemptive use of bivalirudin for urgent on-pump coronary artery bypass grafting in patients with potential heparin-induced thrombocytopenia. *Ann Thorac Surg*, 2005. **80**(1): p. 299–303.

78 Greilich, P.E., *et al.* Near-site monitoring of the antiplatelet drug abciximab using the Hemodyne analyzer and modified thrombelastograph. *J Cardiothorac Vasc Anesth*, 1999. **13**(1): p. 58–64.

79 Tanaka, K.A., *et al.* Clopidogrel (Plavix) and cardiac surgical patients: implications for platelet function monitoring and postoperative bleeding. *Platelets*, 2004. **15**(5): p. 325–332.

80 Tielens, J.A. Vitamin C for paroxetine- and fluvoxamine-associated bleeding. *Am J Psychiatry*, 1997. **154**(6): p. 883–884.

81 Winter, S.L., *et al.* Perioperative blood loss: the effect of valproate. *Pediatr Neurol*, 1996. **15**(1): p. 19–22.

82 Nierman, E. and K. Zakrzewski. Recognition and management of preoperative risk. *Rheum Dis Clin North Am*, 1999. **25**(3): p. 585–622.

83 Wirbel, R.J., *et al.* Preoperative embolization in spinal and pelvic metastases. *J Orthop Sci*, 2005. **10**(3): p. 253–257.

84 Chatziioannou, A.N., *et al.* Preoperative embolization of bone metastases from renal cell carcinoma. *Eur Radiol*, 2000. **10**(4): p. 593–596.

85 Layalle, I., *et al.* Arterial embolization of bone metastases: is it worthwhile? *J Belge Radiol*, 1998. **81**(5): p. 223–225.

86 Li, G.H., *et al.* Effect of finasteride on intraoperative bleeding and irrigating fluid absorption during transurethral resection of prostate: a quantitative study. *Zhejiang Da Xue Xue Bao Yi Xue Ban*, 2004. **33**(3): p. 258–260.

87 Hagerty, J.A., *et al.* Pretreatment with finasteride decreases perioperative bleeding associated with transurethral resection of the prostate. *Urology*, 2000. **55**(5): p. 684–689.

88 Crea, G., *et al.* Pre-surgical finasteride therapy in patients treated endoscopically for benign prostatic hyperplasia. *Urol Int*, 2005. **74**(1): p. 51–53.

89 Dimeo, F., *et al.* Endurance exercise and the production of growth hormone and haematopoietic factors in patients with anaemia. *Br J Sports Med*, 2004. **38**(6): p. e37.

90 Baskett, T.F. Surgical management of severe obstetric hemorrhage: experience with an obstetric hemorrhage equipment tray. *J Obstet Gynaecol Can*, 2004. **26**(9): p. 805–808.

12 Iatrogenic blood loss

A number of patients are transfused after they developed anemia or a coagulopathy, due to surgery or trauma with major blood loss or due to an underlying medical condition. However, there is another group of patients who, although not belonging to the above, are transfused anyway. Many of these patients lost blood as a result of medical interventions. A series of small iatrogenic blood losses can add up resulting in patients becoming anemic. This chapter will address seven of the major causes of such iatrogenic blood loss and describe methods that minimize these losses.

Objectives of this chapter

1 List different ways in which a medical caregiver causes blood loss.
2 Describe methods how iatrogenic blood loss is minimized.
3 Explain the vital role of minimizing iatrogenic blood loss in a comprehensive blood management program.

Definitions

Iatrogenic blood loss: The word "iatrogenic" stems from the word "iatros" which is Greek and means "physician," and "genesis," which means "origin" or "cause." "Iatrogenic" therefore means "caused by a physician." All blood losses that are, directly or indirectly, caused by a physician's intervention are summarized under the phrase "iatrogenic blood loss." Actually, iatrogenic blood loss is not caused by physicians only. Every member of the care team can cause blood loss. In turn, every member of the medical care team can also help to reduce iatrogenic blood loss.

Causes of iatrogenic blood loss

You may ask: "How can a physician (or any medical caregiver) be the culprit?" and, "What ways are there to cause iatrogenic blood loss?" Well, almost everything a medical team does has the potential to cause blood loss. Not only have the surgeons caused blood loss by their operation. No, every specialty can cause blood loss—directly or indirectly. Blood loss may be caused simply by the fact that a patient has to see a physician. The patient may be so stressed by the very thought of seeing a doctor that he develops a stress ulcer and bleeds internally. Patients prescribed bed rest soon show a lowered red cell count. Many diagnostic procedures cause blood loss. Some of them to such an extent that physicians are moved to transfuse. Also, many therapeutic interventions cause blood loss. This holds true for drug therapy as well as for more invasive approaches, such as dialysis and other forms of extracorporeal circulation (ECC). Nevertheless, all of these interventions can be adapted so that iatrogenic blood loss is minimized.

Problem 1: phlebotomy—laboratory testing causes blood loss

Blood loss by phlebotomy is not a new phenomenon. For ages, phlebotomy in the form of blood letting was a legitimate "cure" for all kinds of ailments, including anemia. While beneficial in selected cases, phlebotomy to the extent of blood letting more often than not harmed the patient, even resulting in his death. Blood losses by today's phlebotomists are more subtle, yet clearly detectable as well. They have a great impact on patient care and also on transfusion practice. Since laboratory results are an important tool to achieve a diagnosis and to guide medical care, a certain amount of blood usually is required to get the needed information. However, a great quantity of blood drawn for laboratory testing is drawn needlessly. One major problem is that laboratories are drawn without good reason, drawn too often, or drawn despite not being indicated. Some members of the care team ordering blood tests are not aware of the significance of the results obtained. Often, laboratory results do not influence patient's care at all. So, what is the point of obtaining them?

Table 12.1 Average phlebotomy-induced blood loss in critically ill patients.

Reporting country	Setting	Average phlebotomy-induced blood loss
United States	Cardiothoracic ICU	Avg. 377 mL/day
United States	General surgical ICU	Avg. 240 mL/ day
United States	Medical surgical ICU	Avg. 41.5 mL/day
Great Britain	First day in ICU	Avg. 85.3 mL/day
Great Britain	Following days	Avg. 66.1 mL/day
Europe	Medical ICUs	Avg. 41.1 mL/day

ICU, intensive care unit; Avg., average.

Another problem with phlebotomy is that excessive blood volumes are drawn. A study in a neonatal intensive care unit (ICU), for instance, indicated that almost 20% of the blood drawn was not needed in the laboratory to perform the requested tests [1].

When blood is drawn from indwelling arterial or venous lines, a certain amount of blood ("dead space volume") is withdrawn to clear the line, before the actual phlebotomy volume is drawn. This is done in order to reduce the mixing of the catheter flushing solution with the blood sample. The drawn dead space volume is usually discarded. Depending on local custom, the discarded volume differs between 2 and 10 mL per blood draw [2].

The total daily amount of blood drawn for laboratory tests differs, depending on the pathology and the length of stay. Sicker patients experience more blood loss than those less sick, placing the sicker patients at higher risk for anemia. Table 12.1 demonstrates how substantial the total daily amounts of blood drawn from one patient can be [2].

Possible solution: reduction of phlebotomy-induced blood loss

Strategies to reduce phlebotomy-induced blood loss exist and are usually employed in patients at high risk for anemia, such as neonates, pediatric patients, the critically ill, and patients for whom transfusions are not an option.

Reduction of the amount of phlebotomy

Reducing the amount of blood for phlebotomy starts with the plain avoidance of unnecessary phlebotomy. Thoughtless ordering of a variety of parameters does not contribute

to your value as a caregiver, nor does it help your patient. Ask yourself: What would change in the care of the patient if I do or do not have the result? If there is no clear indication for a blood test, it is most probably not indicated and a waste of blood and money. Standing orders ("Mr. Miller is going to have his liver function test every other day, no matter what") should be reconsidered and in many instances eliminated.

When you know what laboratory values are needed, think whether batching the requests is possible. One specimen is often sufficient to obtain several values at a time. Then, make sure that you know how much blood is needed to perform the requested tests. Phlebotomy overdraw can be substantial. Especially in small children, small amounts of blood, drawn unnecessarily, matter. Collection tubes with fill lines should help in this regard [1]. Drawing the blood up to the fill line prevents overdraw, either caused by drawing too much blood for one sample or by drawing blood for the same test twice. The latter may be the case when insufficient blood is drawn into the container resulting in a wrong mixing ratio of blood and the additive provided in the container (e.g., anticoagulant). In this case, blood has to be drawn again, resulting in unnecessary blood loss.

Patients at high risk for anemia will probably benefit from further means to reduce blood draws. The use of neonatal tubes, with a smaller fill volume, reduces blood loss and at the same time provides the needed results (Table 12.2). A switch from adult to pediatric-sized tubes may reduce the diagnostic blood loss by over 40% [3]. A more blood-saving method is microsampling. Only few microliters of blood are needed to obtain required information, e.g., 150 µL for blood gases, electrolytes, hemoglobin and hematocrit, and the blood sugar. Devices for point-of-care testing [4] often require only small blood volumes. Some point-of-care devices are even able

Table 12.2 Phlebotomy volumes of commercially available blood tubes.

	Regular	Pediatric	Neonatal/ microsampling
Hematology	3.5–9 mL	2.6–3.0	
Serology	4.9–10 mL	2–2.7 mL	250 µL–1 mL
Coagulation	4–10 mL	2.9–3.0 mL	
Blood sugar	2.6–3.0 mL		20–50 µL (or less)
Sedimentation rate	2 mL		
Blood gases	1–3 mL		100–500 µL

to return the drawn blood directly back to the patient after it has been analyzed [5]. In areas where rather expensive point-of-care devices are not available, color scales may help to obtain fairly accurate laboratory results, using only one drop of the patient's blood [6, 7].

Keeping track of the amount of phlebotomy of individual patients is especially helpful in high-risk patients (neonates, severely anemic). It sensitizes the members of the personnel (physicians, nurses, phlebotomists, laboratory technicians) to take greatest care in their efforts of blood conservation. Therefore, it may be beneficial to mark such high-risk patients, to alert personnel to be especially careful. Having every member of the care team who orders or executes phlebotomy sign a special sheet may also be of help, especially in the initial phase of establishing blood saving techniques.

> ### Practice tip
>
> Place a sheet of paper next to all patients in the ICU and have all persons who draw blood list the total volume of blood drawn. After the patient leaves the unit, add all losses up and present them to the health-care team for discussion.

Reduction and elimination of discard volume

Dead space volume drawn before obtaining the blood sample is usually discarded. It was shown that a volume of only twice the catheter dead space is sufficient to gain the required accuracy of the drawn laboratory values [8]. Whatever goes beyond this volume is a wasted resource.

To avoid discard volume as a source of iatrogenic blood loss altogether, several methods are used. The simplest one is probably just to return the sterile dead space volume once the blood sample is drawn. Discard volume is completely eliminated when a passive extracorporeal arteriovenous backflow is used [9]. For this technique, a double-stopcock-system connects the central line and the arterial line. When the appropriate stopcocks are opened, blood from the arterial line flows back, through the tubing, toward the venous line. The blood is allowed to flow a certain distance (which equals the usual discard volume) past a sampling port. Then, the blood sample is drawn through the sampling port and the blood is directed back to the patient.

Additionally, special systems, using a reservoir that is meant to be included in an arterial line, are available for the withdrawal of dead space volume and subsequent retrans-

fusion. Adapting arterial blood draws, by using a closed system, reduces the blood loss by about 50% [10].

Replacement of phlebotomy by "bloodless" monitoring

Another way to eliminate the need for blood draws is the use of methods that deliver the needed information without a blood draw. Some values (e.g., pH, partial pressure of carbon dioxide (PCO_2), partial pressure of oxygen (PO_2), arterial oxygen saturation (SaO_2), bicarbonate, base excess) can be obtained, with satisfying accuracy, using indwelling measuring catheters with photochemical sensors [11]. The catheter can either be inserted into an ECC [11] or directly into the vascular system [12]. Photochemical sensors can be placed intravascular for continuous measurement, or extravascular for on-demand-measurement. To obtain some blood values, direct contact between blood and a measuring device is not always necessary. Skin sensors may be placed on patients who are at high risk for iatrogenic blood loss. The sensors measure the partial pressures of carbon dioxide and oxygen in the blood and the blood glucose level through the skin, obviating the need for serial blood draws.

Education

Educating members of the team on techniques for reducing unnecessary blood loss, e.g., ordering only essential blood tests, exercising the greatest care in infants, practicing drawing blood samples into syringes, etc., may also help. While studies to evaluate the effect of education on the appropriate use of phlebotomy did not show a significant change in practice, the introduction of mandatory policies and guidelines for laboratory use did.

Problem 2: resting patients lose blood

Even patients who do nothing at all may lose blood. One reason for this is that inactivity and bed rest elicit physiological responses that lead to anemia [13]. Another problem of bed-resting patients may be the development of decubital ulcers, leading to so-called "pressure sore anemia" [14]. Anemia due to decubital ulcers is characterized by mild to moderate anemia with low serum iron and normal or increased ferritin in combination with hypoproteinemia and hypoalbuminemia. Anemia probably develops because of the chronic inflammatory state caused by the presence of pressure ulcers.

Possible solution: keep them moving

Since the blood count of resting patients may gradually decrease, unnecessary bed rest in hospitalized patients should be avoided. There is no evidence that ambulation of patients decreases their transfusion exposure, but there is some evidence that it reduces postoperative pneumonia, length of stay in the hospital, and psychological changes [15]. Moderate physical training has been shown to reduce anemia [16–18]. The reasons for this phenomenon are not clear. One hypothesis is that exercise increases hormones that stimulate erythropoiesis and leucopoiesis. Growth hormones, granulocyte colony-stimulating factor (G-CSF), and a variety of other cytokines are produced during exercise. Besides, cytokines, which are typically produced in an inflammatory state and inhibit hematopoiesis (e.g., interleukin 6), seem to diminish during exercise [19, 20].

Whatever the reason, exercise may ameliorate anemia, and you can use this effect to the good of your patient. Educate the patient and his family that moderate exercise is very beneficial. Also, you may be able to prescribe a regimen of physical therapy. This may be especially beneficial for patients with chronic anemia (such as dialysis patients). These patients should be advised to exercise regularly. If you see a dialysis patient, in order to plan elective surgery, this may be a good time to start him on an exercise program. Certain types of anemia react very well to exercise. Through an exercise routine, the blood levels of preoperative anemia patients can be optimized. Thirty minutes per day of interval training, on a stationary ergometer, for 3 weeks, may be sufficient for a substantial improvement of the patient's blood count. Patients who experience prolonged periods of chemotherapy-induced anemia may start with moderate exercise immediately after chemotherapy. If it is not possible for the patient to get out of bed, exercise in the supine position, using a "bed bike" or cycling in the air, may be recommended. Most of your medical and surgical patients will benefit from being mobilized as early as possible. Adequate pain management, nutrition, and a schedule for mobilization and exercise may support the patient compliance to your prescribed program [16–19].

Pressure ulcers, which can develop during bed rest, contribute to anemia as well. Diligent nursing staff know how to avoid the development of such sores. If they are already present, appropriate therapy is warranted. Pressure sore anemia needs to be taken seriously. Iron therapy is said to be useless. Instead, it has been recommended to treat serum protein alterations, prescribing a diet rich in protein and calories [21]. Both anemia and hypoproteinemia disappear after the pressure ulcers heal.

Problem 3: stressed patients lose blood

Not only resting patients suffer from iatrogenic blood loss and anemia. Stressed patients share the same fate, but due to completely different underlying mechanisms. Critically ill patients regularly (40–100%) develop alterations in the mucosa of the gastrointestinal tract. This may contribute to the development of stress "ulcers" in the gastrointestinal tract. Up to 90% of ventilated patients admitted to an ICU suffer from stress ulcers on the 3rd day of their stay [22, 23]. These may lead to occult gastrointestinal hemorrhage. About 1–2% of the patients even experience severe hemorrhage, leading to blood transfusion [24]. Such blood loss is aggravated by anticoagulant use and the presence of coagulation disturbances.

While all pediatric and adult patients may develop stress ulcers, there are a variety of conditions that obviously predispose patients to stress ulcers. The classical conditions are head and brain trauma, major burns, emergency or major surgery, major trauma, shock, coagulopathies, mechanical ventilation for more than 2 days, therapy with drugs that may cause ulcers, and a history of gastrointestinal ulcers.

Possible solution: ulcus prophylaxis

Stress ulcer prophylaxis is an integral part of a strategy to avoid iatrogenic blood loss. The first and most important method is to attempt to maintain adequate mucosal perfusion. Unfortunately, specific measures to do so are limited. Maintaining sufficient cardiac output and giving sufficient amounts of oxygen enhance the mucosal integrity, forming the basis for ulcer prophylaxis.

A simple measure, yet often overlooked, to protect the integrity of the mucosal lining in the gastrointestinal tract is enteral feeding. This is thought to be due to the neutralizing effect on the acid in the stomach as well as the nutritional effect of the food on the mucosa. Patients should be asked to eat. If this is not possible, tube feeding has the same effect.

If enteral feeding is not possible, or the patient is at high risk of developing stress ulcers, medical prophylaxis is indicated. Histamine-2-receptor antagonist therapy aims at reducing the gastric acid levels in the stomach. It was shown to decrease incidences of gastrointestinal hemorrhage. There is a trend toward decreased hemorrhage when antacids are used for the same purpose (compared with no therapy). Sucralfate may be as effective in reducing hemorrhage as gastric pH-altering drugs. Advantages of sucralfate include a lower rate of pneumonia and mortality, as well as lower costs [25]. Proton pump inhibitors may be even more effective than Histamine-2-receptor-2-antagonists. They reduce transfusions in patients with ulcer hemorrhage and effectively decrease rebleeding [26].

Problem 4: diagnostic interventions cause blood loss

Diagnostic and therapeutic interventions, at times, cause blood loss. Among them are the placement of arterial and central lines as well as interventions such as tracheostomy [27] and angiography.

The impact of blood loss caused by the insertion of a central line is obvious when an untrained individual performs the insertion. Often, blood flows back freely, pouring out on to the drapes and is lost. Quantifying such blood losses is difficult. One study on iatrogenic blood loss mentioned the insertion of arterial and central venous catheters as source of blood loss, but did not determine the amount of blood lost [28]. Though the magnitude of blood loss is not clearly defined, obtaining vascular access and a variety of other procedures doubtless cause blood loss.

Also, the presence of arterial lines causes blood loss. This happens when blood is drawn freely using this easy access to the patient's blood [29].

Possible solution: practice

A certain amount of skill is needed to obtain vascular access. It seems that unskilled health-care providers, such as beginners, lose, on average, more blood than skilled persons. In patients at high risk of anemia, a skilled health-care provider may be more appropriate for the placement of the lines than a beginner.

Also, the choice of technique to obtain vascular access may influence the amount of blood lost during the procedure. Inserting an arterial line in open Seldinger's technique causes more blood loss than the same procedure performed in modified Seldinger's technique (closed system) or by direct cannulation. Slight changes in the method of using the guide wire also promise to reduce blood loss. One article describes this as follows [30]: "The method entails inserting the guide wire through a previously created side hole in a standard 5 ml plastic syringe. The problems

of needle dislodgement, air embolism and blood loss are virtually eliminated with this technique." The use of valves in the introducer sheaths for large vascular catheters may help reduce blood loss as well [31].

Another way to minimize blood loss that is associated with placed arterial or central venous lines is to remove them soon as possible. This will also reduce access to the patient's blood [29].

The method with which some interventions are performed can result in more or less average blood loss. Tracheostomy, for instance, can be performed as a conventional surgical procedure or as a percutaneous dilatational tracheostomy. The latter was shown to have a lower peri- and postoperative blood loss than the conventional approach. The reason may be that "following percutaneous placement, the stoma fits snugly around the tracheostomy tube. This lack of dead space conceivably serves to . . . tamponade bleeding vessels" [27]. There are also different methods for the insertion of a permanent pacemaker, some of which cause less blood loss than others [32].

Problem 5: medications may cause blood loss

Medications may cause blood loss by many different mechanisms. Over-anticoagulation may contribute to the blood loss, as well as side effects of medications given during hospitalization. Commonly encountered mechanisms that increase iatrogenic blood loss include the following, as outlined in Table 12.3.

Possible solution: "medica mente, non medicamente"

Since medications have the potential to increase iatrogenic blood loss, care must be taken in their choice. If the patient's comorbidities reveal a "sensitivity," allergy or intolerance to drugs, such medications should be avoided, if possible.

If anticoagulation is required, judicious use of the drugs is warranted. For several anticoagulants, monitoring is prudent, and should be employed to prevent over-anticoagulation, which may lead to undue blood loss. When a patient is at high risk of hemorrhage, for instance, when he has a very low platelet count, anticoagulation may not be the wisest choice. Thrombosis prophylaxis may be more appropriate using nondrug methods such

Table 12.3 Drug effects that may increase iatrogenic blood loss.

Examples of drugs	Effect
Aspirin and other nonsteroidal antirheumatic drugs, glucocorticoids	(Occult) gastrointestinal hemorrhage
Heparin, aspirin, heart glycosides, thyrostatics, Histamine-2-receptor-antagonists	Thrombocytopenia
Metamizol, allopurinol, indapamide	Agranulocytosis or aplastic anemia
Chloramphenicol, cis-platinum and other chemotherapeutics, gold derivatives, neuroleptics, pyrimethamine	Blunted hematopoiesis
Some cephalosporins	Toxic changes in the blood count, e.g., leucopenia, thrombocytopenia
Ajamlin, L-asparaginase, carbamazepine, rifampicin, thiazides, rapid infusion of hypotonic solutions	Hemolysis
High-dose penicillins, aspirin, valproic acid, serotonin antagonists	Impairment of coagulation

as inflatable pressure stockings or, in selected cases, the placement of a Greenfield filter.

Other drug regimens, which may alter the patient's blood, may also be amendable for adaptation. Chemotherapy can be varied to reduce the impact it has on hematopoiesis. Antibiotics can be chosen so as not to unnecessarily aggravate coagulopathy. Hemolysis, due to hypotonic solutions and other medications is also preventable. It goes beyond the scope of this chapter to engage in an in-depth discussion of all possible effects of drugs on blood loss. Just a little hint: a short look into a reference book is often tremendously helpful.

Problem 6: blood loss caused by ECC

Patients with end-stage renal failure, patients undergoing open heart surgery, patients with potentially reversible heart or lung failure all have something in common: they have a good chance of needing therapy that includes an ECC, such as hemodialysis, cardiopulmonary bypass, ventricular assist devices, or extracorporeal membrane oxygenation. The basic principle of an ECC is the same,

regardless of the specific purpose of the device. All these devices have the potential to cause iatrogenic blood loss. Additionally, other devices being introduced in the blood stream of a patient (such as intra-aortic balloon pumps, ventricular assist devices, and prosthetic heart valves) may cause iatrogenic hemolysis [33].

ECC is a nonphysiological approach to blood circulation that takes its toll on the blood. The blood in the ECC comes into contact with air and foreign surfaces, and the shear stress within the blood increases. Furthermore, the flow pattern in the circulation changes from a pulsatile to a nonpulsatile flow. All of this leads to alterations of the corpuscular elements of the blood, the activation of coagulation and complement cascade, and the activation and adherence of a variety of other blood proteins. As a result, red cells hemolyze, platelets are activated and change in number, shape, and functionality, the clotting ability is disturbed, and blood proteins are reduced in the circulation.

Anticoagulation is needed for the successful use of ECC. However, it contributes to blood losses and allogeneic transfusions. Over-, as well as under-anticoagulation may lead to intra- and postoperative coagulopathies and unnecessary blood loss. If the patient is exposed to excess amounts of an anticoagulant, he may hemorrhage due to the action of the anticoagulant. If he is not sufficiently anticoagulated, his clotting factors and platelets are activated and used up during the ECC, leaving the patient with lower levels of available clotting potential after ECC. This also leads to coagulopathies. Besides, reversal of anticoagulation in excess of the present anticoagulant may also add to coagulopathies.

Other factors, directly or indirectly related to the use of an ECC, influence the magnitude of iatrogenic blood loss as well. Blood remaining in the tubing, after discontinuation of the procedure, adds to the blood loss. Also, coagulopathy induced by anticoagulation and patient-specific factors (e.g., a disturbed erythropoiesis in renal insufficiency) contribute to the fact that patients requiring an ECC are at higher risk for anemia than other patients. According to a study, daily blood loss in patients requiring dialysis or hemofiltration in an ICU was 5.8 times higher than the blood loss in intensive care patients, not requiring such therapy [28].

Possible solution: minimizing blood loss due to ECC

The use of an ECC inevitably causes blood loss. Happily, the extent of these changes depends on a variety of factors, most of which can be altered to reduce the effect of the ECC on the blood.

In former times, patients on an ECC, such as the cardiopulmonary bypass, were transfused with a lot of blood. Even the ECC was primed with donor blood. Today, this is obsolete in most instances. Primes of crystalloid solutions are sufficient to start the pump. This leads to hemodilution. While hemodilution is a benefit to patients undergoing hypothermia and who experience the accompanying increase in blood viscosity, some patients may not benefit. In such instances, retrograde autologous priming is a method that reduces the hemodiluting effect of the ECC. The use of autologous blood to prime the circuit reduces not only hemodilution but also the patient's exposure to transfusions [34]. It maintains higher intraoperative hemoglobin levels. Since it does not require extra disposables, retrograde autologous priming is a very inexpensive technique [35]. Several techniques for retrograde autologous priming have been advocated. Basically, the circuit is partially primed with asanguinous fluids such as crystalloids. The patient's own blood, draining from the venous tube, is used to further fill the circuit.

Preoperative normovolemic hemodilution and blood component pheresis

Since the contact of blood with the ECC causes a variety of changes, one method to avoid this is to take some blood out of the patient's circulation before the ECC is initiated. Such procedures are performed mainly in connection with the ECC initiated prior to cardiac surgery. Acute normovolemic hemodilution and the fractionation of whole blood for platelet-rich and platelet-poor plasma are methods to spare blood contact with the ECC.

Platelet anesthesia

The term "platelet anesthesia" refers to a concept that is still in the experimental stage. It is a strategy to minimize platelet activation and adhesion during the period the blood is circulating via ECC (usually during cardiopulmonary bypass). Short-acting platelet inhibitors are used during the ECC period, which temporarily inhibit platelet activation and adhesion. When the action of the inhibitor wears off after the end of the ECC, a larger number of functionally adequate platelets are still available. This is thought to reduce postoperative blood loss and normalize in vitro coagulation parameters.

Several drugs can be used to achieve platelet anesthesia. Phosphodiesterase inhibitors, such as dipyridamole,

have been used. However, the action of the drugs is not quickly reversible after the end of the ECC. Prostanoids, such as prostacyclin, are also used, but cause severe hypotension. More promising drugs are glycoprotein IIb/IIIa membrane receptor inhibitors (e.g., ticlopidine, tirofiban) or the direct thrombin inhibitor argatroban. It remains to be seen whether the concept of platelet anesthesia can effectively reduce transfusions.

Adaptation of the extracorporeal circuit

Technical details of the ECC influence the magnitude of the changes in the blood components.

Blood contact with artificial surfaces leads to activation of humoral and cellular elements of the blood. The contact activation or its effects can be reduced by using the different methods. The most common approach is the coating of tubing and other surfaces with heparin. The benefits of the heparinization of surfaces include fewer alterations to the blood as well as a reduced need for systemic anticoagulation. In turn, blood loss may be reduced. This was shown in some, but not all, studies. Allogeneic transfusions were shown to be reduced with the use of heparinized circuits as well [36]. Further benefit may be added by a leukocyte filter in the ECC. This filter may reduce the effects of activated leukocytes in the patient. It has been theorized that the reduction of activated leukocytes may also reduce coagulation disturbances after ECC [36].

The choice of an appropriate oxygenator, in ECCs used to oxygenate the blood is also important. It has an impact on the denaturation of blood proteins and the change in the amount, function, and structure of blood cells. In general, membrane oxygenators tend to influence in vitro markers of protein activation and blood cell alterations less than bubble oxygenators (the latter ones have a larger blood-surface interface). In vivo, membrane oxygenators seem to be superior to bubble oxygenators in patients undergoing long perfusion periods. During shorter perfusion times, in vivo experiments did not show a reduction in blood loss with membrane oxygenators [37].

Minimized extracorporeal circulation (MECC) for heart surgery may also reduce iatrogenic blood loss and is associated with a low transfusion rate [38]. An MECC consists of a heparin-coated tubing system with a pump and oxygenator. A venous reservoir and a vent are not included. The priming volume is much lower than in conventional extracorporeal circuits (ca. 450 mL instead of about 1500 mL [38]. For very small children, the cardiopulmonary bypass system can be minimized so that the priming volume is as low as 130–160 mL [39]. Minimized extracorporeal circuits were shown to cause higher hemoglobin levels and decreased hemolysis when compared to the conventional ECC, in patients undergoing a heart surgery [40]. Minimized extracorporeal circuits are helpful when performing heart surgery on small children, without exposure to allogeneic blood [39].

Retransfusion of blood left in the ECC

Blood left in the tubing after termination of the ECC would be wasted if not given back to the patient. There are different ways to return the remaining blood to the patient. It can just be reinfused or it can be processed and then given back. Blood can be centrifuged using a cell saver or it can be hemoconcentrated with a filter. The use of the centrifuge removes platelets and plasma components, giving back mainly the concentrated red cells. It has the advantage that heparin is not given back to the patient. In contrast, ultrafiltration and the return of unprocessed blood return heparin to the patient, but also preserve plasma components and platelets [41]. Ultrafiltrated blood may be more hemolyzed than unprocessed blood, but the hemoconcentration achieved by ultrafiltration prevents the return of large amounts of fluids [42]. The right choice of method to return residual blood after ECC seems to have an impact on the red cell mass, the degree of hemodilution, the extend of coagulopathy, and the patient's exposure to allogeneic blood.

Monitoring and reversal of anticoagulation

Since inadequate heparinization as well as excessive or insufficient reversal of heparin may cause coagulopathies and blood loss, anticoagulation calls for close monitoring. The individual patient's response to heparin, is variable. A variety of laboratory values and tests are instrumental in monitoring anticoagulation. Among them are thrombin time, prothrombin time (PT), activated partial thromboplastin time (aPTT), activated coagulation time (ACT), and heparin concentration monitoring as well as the use of the thrombelastogram. However, no single one of the mentioned tests is able to monitor anticoagulation reliably. The combination of two or more tests seems to increase the reliability when the clinical picture is added to the assessment (e.g., ACT and heparin concentration). Some studies demonstrated a reduced blood product use when appropriate monitoring techniques were employed [43].

Appropriate reversal of anticoagulation also contributes to a reduced blood loss and reduced exposure of the pa-

tient to allogeneic transfusions. The preferred antidote for heparin is protamine. Protamine is positively charged and binds to the negatively charged heparin whereby it neutralizes the anticoagulant effect of heparin. Excess of a protamine, however, also impairs coagulation and reduces the platelet count. Since protamine can cause such abnormalities itself, it is beneficial to use only the amount required to neutralize the heparin. To this effect, monitoring methods for anticoagulation were proposed. It remains to be seen whether these prove effective to reduce postoperative coagulopathies and patient's exposure to allogeneic transfusions. The best method to avoid undue protamine use is still the appropriate use of heparin.

Problem 7: timing influences blood loss

In some instances, elapsing time causes blood loss. If a patient bleeds, immediate intervention to prevent further blood loss is mandatory. Blood loss likens a bucket with a hole. To keep it filled, you can pour in more fluid (in our case, transfusing blood), or you can fix it by closing the hole. If hemorrhaging patients are not treated immediately, blood loss increases. All blood loss that can potentially be stopped is, strictly speaking, iatrogenic blood loss.

On the other hand, rushing an unprepared patient into a surgical or medical intervention, although he is not prepared for it, may also increase blood loss and may increase his likelihood to receive allogeneic transfusions.

Possible solution: carpe diem

Time is a precious commodity, especially for patients who bleed. Achieving timely hemostasis must be of uppermost importance in a blood management program. This should be reflected in the way trauma and other surgical and medical teams prepare for bleeding patients. Up-to-date algorithms for hemorrhage, appropriate training, trauma drills, and equipment readily available and fully functional contribute to minimize the time that elapses until definite hemostasis is achieved. Depending on the severity of the ongoing blood loss, diagnostic measures should be expedited. Such rapid treatment of patients not only reduces blood loss and subsequent transfusion exposure, but may even improve survival rates. This has been shown for different kinds of hemorrhage, such as early endoscopy in gastrointestinal hemorrhage [44] and trauma patients. Similarly, patients who develop anemia or coagulopathy in a more gradual fashion also benefit from early recognition and asanguinous treatment of their condition. This is especially true for patients who develop anemia while suffering from cardiovascular disease or renal insufficiency [45]. Waiting under "transfusion protection" for a possible spontaneous resolution of bleeding is futile and dangerous. A "wait and see attitude" definitely does not have a place in the therapy of an acutely hemorrhaging patient.

In contrast, elapsing time may also be beneficial. It provides a patient with the opportunity to recover from blood loss. Patients who underwent angiography, for instance, may need surgery. If this surgery can be postponed safely for some days, the time may be sufficient for hematopoiesis to synthesize blood components lost during the diagnostic procedure [46]. Another example where allowing time may be beneficial is cord clamping after delivery of a baby. Waiting just 30–120 seconds before the cord is clamped increases the hematocrit of the baby and reduces its transfusion exposure [47]. Early cord clamping would result in blood loss for the baby.

The role of iatrogenic blood loss in blood management

After discussing common sources of iatrogenic blood loss, you may ask yourself: "Does iatrogenic blood loss really matter?", "Does it have an impact on the use of transfusions?", and "Does avoiding such small and probably insignificant blood losses enhance patient care, reduce the patients exposure to allogeneic transfusions, or improve the outcome?"

Unquestionably, medical personnel cause substantial blood losses in their patients. Among them, phlebotomy is the most extensively studied example. It seems that there is a substantial overdraw of blood for laboratory testing. In the United States, hospitals caring for adults draw 2.5–10 times more blood for standard laboratory panels than pediatric hospitals [48]. A study performed in Great Britain showed that attempts to reduce the blood loss stemming from phlebotomy were rare. In adult ICUs, only 18.4% returned the dead space volume and only 9.3% used pediatric tubes. In contrast, pediatric ICUs return their dead space volume in 67% of cases [49]. This demonstrates that there is still great room for improvement. Diagnostic blood loss is a major determinant of anemia in adult and neonatal ICUs, accounting for substantial amounts of transfused blood [1, 50]. In fact, in the ICU setting, the total amount of diagnostic blood loss is a significant predictor of allogeneic transfusion [28]. As shown above, comprehensive blood management effectively reduces phlebotomy-induced blood loss [51, 52] and such attempts reduce the patient's exposure to allogeneic transfusions [5, 53].

Apart from phlebotomy, there are many other items under the control of a medical care team that affect the blood count of a patient. In many instances, attention to detail helps to avoid unnecessary blood loss [7, 54, 55]. Even if there are not many randomized controlled studies demonstrating that attention to every one of the above-mentioned details translates into reduction of transfusions given or in improvement of outcome, it appears that this is a reasonable recommendation.

Key points

• Blood loss occurs directly and indirectly by the work of medical caregivers, e.g., due to
  ○ Diagnostic phlebotomy
  ○ Bed rest
  ○ Occult gastrointestinal hemorrhage and stress ulcers
  ○ Invasive monitoring (arterial lines, etc.)
  ○ Drugs including anticoagulants
  ○ Extracorporeal circulation
  ○ Unnecessarily wasting time while the patient bleeds
  ○ Blunted erythropoiesis due to iatrogenic malnutrition
• Iatrogenic blood loss accounts for increased use of transfusions.
• Iatrogenic blood loss and with it the development of iatrogenic anemia and coagulopathy can be minimized.
• Ways to minimize iatrogenic blood loss include:
  ○ Reduction of the frequency of phlebotomy and the volume of blood drawn
  ○ Return of dead space volume
  ○ Ulcer prophylaxis
  ○ Attention to details in diagnostic or therapeutic interventions, including the choice of a skilled practitioner and choice of a suitable technique
  ○ Judicious use of drugs, including anticoagulants
  ○ Adaptation of procedures involving an ECC
  ○ Expedited hemostasis in all hemorrhaging patients

Questions for review

• What can be done to reduce blood loss induced by phlebotomy?

- What diagnostic procedures are available that reduce iatrogenic blood loss?
- How can ECC be adapted to minimize blood loss?
- Does timing play a role in avoiding iatrogenic blood loss?
- How do sports influence iatrogenic blood loss?

Suggestions for further research

What different methods are available for autologous retrograde priming of a cardiopulmonary bypass? (compare: http://perfline.com/textbook/local/rap/rap.html)

What is the suggested effect of leukocytes in the development of coagulopathies after ECCs and how is this affected by the use of leukocyte filtration during ECC?

How does thrombelastography work and how do the tracings change with changes in amount and functionality of plasmatic clotting factors, platelets, red cells, and decrease in temperature?

Exercises and practice cases

A 65-year-old diabetic man is admitted to the ICU with a pneumonia and partial respiratory insufficiency. His weight is 70 kg, his height is 170 cm, his initial hematocrit is 0.34. He is monitored with a central venous catheter and an arterial line.

Use the following information to estimate the blood loss he suffers during his stay in the ICU.

All blood draws are taken from the central line, except the ones for the blood cultures, which are taken directly from the vein. Before a blood sample is drawn into the sampling tubes from the central line, 10 mL of the blood is discarded. Before blood is drawn from the arterial line, 5 mL of the blood is discarded. The blood tubes used are the standard tubes in the ICU with the following volumes: hematology 9 mL, serology 10 mL, coagulation profile 10 mL, blood glucose levels 3 mL, erythrocyte sedimentation rate 2 mL, blood gases 2 mL, blood cultures 10 mL each for aerobic, anaerobic, and fungal cultures.

The order "ICU complete" means complete blood count with differential, erythrocyte sedimentation rate, blood glucose level, Quick, aPTT, D-dimer, troponin, C-reactive protein, sodium, potassium, calcium, chloride, lactate, liver panel, and kidney panel.

The order "ICU small" means complete blood count, blood glucose level, Quick, aPTT, C-reactive protein, sodium, potassium, calcium, and chloride.

Since the hospital laboratory is small, some blood is sent to specialized laboratories. One blood sample is sent for serology of HIV and hepatitis, another sample is sent to determine the procalcitonin (PCT).

On the first day, intensive diagnosis is made. Therefore, the attending physician orders: "ICU complete, blood cultures now and in 2 hours, blood glucose levels ×5, PCT, HIV/hepatitis serology, central venous oxygen saturation every 6 hours, arterial blood gases every 6 hours."

On the second and on the following days, the attending physician orders: "ICU small, blood glucose levels ×5, central venous oxygen saturation every 6 hours, arterial blood gases every 6 hours."

Homework

- Practice giving back the dead space volume when you draw blood the next time.
- Check the volumes for the blood tubes you currently use. Implore whether there are alternative tubes with smaller volumes.

References

1 Lin, J.C., *et al.* Phlebotomy overdraw in the neonatal intensive care nursery. *Pediatrics*, 2000. **106**(2): p. E19.

2 Fowler, R.A. and M. Berenson. Blood conservation in the intensive care unit. *Crit Care Med*, 2003. **31**(12, Suppl): p. S715–S720.

3 Smoller, B.R., M.S. Kruskall, and G.L. Horowitz. Reducing adult phlebotomy blood loss with the use of pediatric-sized blood collection tubes. *Am J Clin Pathol*, 1989. **91**(6): p. 701–703.

4 Guiliano K.K., *et al.* Blood analysis at the point of care: issues in application for use in critically ill patients. *AACN Clin Issues*, 2002. **13**(2): p. 204–220.

5 Widness, J.A., *et al.* Reduction in red blood cell transfusions among preterm infants: results of a randomized trial with an in-line blood gas and chemistry monitor. *Pediatrics*, 2005. **115**(5): p. 1299–1306.

6 Lewis, S.M., G.J. Stott, and K.J. Wynn. An inexpensive and reliable new haemoglobin colour scale for assessing anaemia. *J Clin Pathol*, 1998. **51**(1): p. 21–24.

7 Lewis, J.E. A simple technique for anticipating and managing secondary puncture site hemorrhage during laparoscopic surgery. A report of two cases. *J Reprod Med*, 1995. **40**(10): p. 729–730.

8 Rickard, C.M., *et al.* A discard volume of twice the dead space ensures clinically accurate arterial blood gases and electrolytes

and prevents unnecessary blood loss. *Crit Care Med*, 2003. **31**(6): p. 1654–1658.

9 Weiss, M., *et al.* Evaluation of a simple method for minimizing iatrogenic blood loss from discard volumes in critically ill newborns and children. *Intensive Care Med*, 2001. **27**(6): p. 1064–1072.

10 Gleason, E., S. Grossman, and C. Campbell. Minimizing diagnostic blood loss in critically ill patients. *Am J Crit Care*, 1992. **1**(1): p. 85–90.

11 Rais-Bahrami, K., *et al.* Continuous blood gas monitoring using an in-dwelling optode method: comparison to intermittent arterial blood gas sampling in ECMO patients. *J Perinatol*, 2002. **22**(6): p. 472–474.

12 Meyers, P.A., *et al.* Clinical validation of a continuous intravascular neonatal blood gas sensor introduced through an umbilical artery catheter. *Respir Care*, 2002. **47**(6): p. 682–687.

13 Krasnoff, J. and P. Painter. The physiological consequences of bed rest and inactivity. *Adv Ren Replace Ther*, 1999. **6**(2): p. 124–132.

14 Turba, R.M., V.L. Lewis, and D. Green. Pressure sore anemia: response to erythropoietin. *Arch Phys Med Rehabil*, 1992. **73**(5): p. 498–500.

15 Kamel, H.K., *et al.* Time to ambulation after hip fracture surgery: relation to hospitalization outcomes. *J Gerontol A Biol Sci Med Sci*, 2003. **58**(11): p. 1042–1045.

16 Goldberg, A.P., *et al.* Exercise training reduces coronary risk and effectively rehabilitates hemodialysis patients. *Nephron*, 1986. **42**(4): p. 311–316.

17 Hagberg, J.M., *et al.* Exercise training improves hypertension in hemodialysis patients. *Am J Nephrol*, 1983. **3**(4): p. 209–212.

18 Dimeo, F., *et al.* Effects of aerobic exercise on the physical performance and incidence of treatment-related complications after high-dose chemotherapy. *Blood*, 1997. **90**(9): p. 3390–3394.

19 Dimeo, F., *et al.* Endurance exercise and the production of growth hormone and haematopoietic factors in patients with anaemia. *Br J Sports Med*, 2004. **38**(6): p. e37.

20 Dimeo, F.C., *et al.* Effect of aerobic exercise and relaxation training on fatigue and physical performance of cancer patients after surgery. A randomised controlled trial. *Support Care Cancer*, 2004. **12**(11): p. 774–779.

21 Fuoco, U., *et al.* Anaemia and serum protein alteration in patients with pressure ulcers. *Spinal Cord*, 1997. **35**(1): p. 58–60.

22 Raynard, B. and G. Nitenberg. Is prevention of upper digestive system hemorrhage in intensive care necessary? *Schweiz Med Wochenschr*, 1999. **129**(43): p. 1605–1612.

23 Eddleston, J.M., *et al.* Prospective endoscopic study of stress erosions and ulcers in critically ill adult patients treated with either sucralfate or placebo. *Crit Care Med*, 1994. **22**(12): p. 1949–1954.

24 Marino, P.L. *Das ICU Buch. Praktische Intensivmedizin*, 2nd edn. Urban und Schwarzenberg, München, Wien, Baltimore, 1999.

25 Cook, D. J., *et al.* Stress ulcer prophylaxis in critically ill patients. Resolving discordant meta-analyses. *JAMA*, 1996. **275**(4): p. 308–314.

26 Leontiadis, G.I., V.K. Sharma, and C.W. Howden. Systematic review and meta-analysis: proton-pump inhibitor treatment for ulcer bleeding reduces transfusion requirements and hospital stay – results from the Cochrane Collaboration. *Aliment Pharmacol Ther*, 2005. **22**(3): p. 169–174.

27 Freeman, B.D., *et al.* A meta-analysis of prospective trials comparing percutaneous and surgical tracheostomy in critically ill patients. *Chest*, 2000. **118**(5): p. 1412–1418.

28 von Ahsen, N., *et al.* Important role of nondiagnostic blood loss and blunted erythropoietic response in the anemia of medical intensive care patients. *Crit Care Med*, 1999. **27**(12): p. 2630–2639.

29 Smoller, B.R. and M.S. Kruskall. Phlebotomy for diagnostic laboratory tests in adults. Pattern of use and effect on transfusion requirements. *N Engl J Med*, 1986. **314**(19): p. 1233–1235.

30 Kiell, C., S. Curtas, and M.M. Meguid. Refinement of central venous cannulation technique. *Nutrition*, 1989. **5**(1): p. 37–38.

31 Vesely, T.M., A.G. Fazzaro, and D. Gherardini. Preliminary evaluation of a valved introducer sheath for the insertion of tunneled hemodialysis catheters. *Semin Dial*, 2004. **17**(1): p. 65–68.

32 Liu, K.S., *et al.* Permanent cardiac pacing through the right supraclavicular subclavian vein approach. *Can J Cardiol*, 2003. **19**(9): p. 1005–1008.

33 Scharte, M. and M.P. Fink. Red blood cell physiology in critical illness. *Crit Care Med*, 2003. **31**(12, Suppl): p. S651–S657.

34 Zelinka, E.S., *et al.* Retrograde autologous prime with shortened bypass circuits decreases blood transfusion in high-risk coronary artery surgery patients. *J Extra Corpor Technol*, 2004. **36**(4): p. 343–347.

35 Saxena, P., N. Saxena, A. Jain, and V.K. Sharma. Intraoperative autologous blood donation and retrograde autologous priming for cardiopulmonary bypass: a safe and effective technique for blood conservation. *Ann Card Anaesth*, 2003. **6**: p. 47–51.

36 Martens, S., *et al.* Heparin coating of the extracorporeal circuit combined with leukocyte filtration reduces coagulation activity, blood loss and blood product substitution. *Int J Artif Organs*, 2001. **24**(7): p. 484–488.

37 Spiess, B.D., *et al. Perioperative Transfusion Medicine*. Williams and Williams, Baltimore, 1998.

38 Remadi, J.P., *et al.* Clinical experience with the mini-extracorporeal circulation system: an evolution or a revolution? *Ann Thorac Surg*, 2004. **77**(6): p. 2172–2175; discussion 2176.

39 Ando, M., Y. Takahashi, and N. Suzuki. Open heart surgery for small children without homologous blood transfusion by using remote pump head system. *Ann Thorac Surg*, 2004. **78**(5): p. 1717–1722.

40 Vaislic, C., *et al.* Totally minimized extracorporeal circulation: an important benefit for coronary artery bypass grafting in Jehovah's Witnesses. *Heart Surg Forum*, 2003. **6**(5): p. 307–310.

41 Boldt, J., *et al.* Acute preoperative plasmapheresis and established blood conservation techniques. *Ann Thorac Surg*, 1990. **50**(1): p. 62–68.

42 Smigla, G.R., *et al.* An ultrafiltration technique for directly reinfusing residual cardiopulmonary bypass blood. *J Extra Corpor Technol*, 2004. **36**(3): p. 231–234.

43 Despotis, G.J., *et al.* The impact of heparin concentration and activated clotting time monitoring on blood conservation. A prospective, randomized evaluation in patients undergoing cardiac operation. *J Thorac Cardiovasc Surg*, 1995. **110**(1): p. 46–54.

44 Spiegel, B.M., N.B. Vakil, and J.J. Ofman. Endoscopy for acute nonvariceal upper gastrointestinal tract hemorrhage: is sooner better? A systematic review. *Arch Intern Med*, 2001. **161**(11): p. 1393–1404.

45 McCullough, P.A. and N.E. Lepor. The deadly triangle of anemia, renal insufficiency, and cardiovascular disease: implications for prognosis and treatment. *Rev Cardiovasc Med*, 2005. **6**(1): p. 1–10.

46 Karski, J.M., *et al.* Etiology of preoperative anemia in patients undergoing scheduled cardiac surgery. *Can J Anaesth*, 1999. **46**(10): p. 979–982.

47 Rabe, H., G. Reynolds, and J. Diaz-Rossello. Early versus delayed umbilical cord clamping in preterm infants. *Cochrane Database Syst Rev*, 2004. (4): p. CD003248.

48 Hicks, J.M. Excessive blood drawing for laboratory tests. *N Engl J Med*, 1999. **340**(21): p. 1690.

49 O'Hare, D. and R.J. Chilvers. Arterial blood sampling practices in intensive care units in England and Wales. *Anaesthesia*, 2001. **56**(6): p. 568–571.

50 Corwin, H.L., K.C. Parsonnet, and A. Gettinger. RBC transfusion in the ICU. Is there a reason? *Chest*, 1995. **108**(3): p. 767–771.

51 MacIsaac, C.M., *et al.* The influence of a blood conserving device on anaemia in intensive care patients. *Anaesth Intensive Care*, 2003. **31**(6): p. 653–657.

52 Dech, Z.F. and N.L. Szaflarski. Nursing strategies to minimize blood loss associated with phlebotomy. *AACN Clin Issues*, 1996. **7**(2): p. 277–287.

53 Madan, A., *et al.* Reduction in red blood cell transfusions using a bedside analyzer in extremely low birth weight infants. *J Perinatol*, 2005. **25**(1): p. 21–25.

54 Enk, D., *et al.* Nasotracheal intubation: a simple and effective technique to reduce nasopharyngeal trauma and tube contamination. *Anesth Analg*, 2002. **95**(5): p. 1432–1436, table of contents.

55 Singer, A.J., *et al.* Comparison of nasal tampons for the treatment of epistaxis in the emergency department: a randomized controlled trial. *Ann Emerg Med*, 2005. **45**(2): p. 134–139.

13 The physics of hemostasis

Sufficient hemostasis is vital to reduce the number of allogeneic transfusions. A basic knowledge of the methods is essential to enable a blood manager to critically appraise the potential value of the various available methods to prevent or stop surgical or post-trauma hemorrhage. Therefore, this chapter explores some of the physical methods used during surgery to achieve hemostasis, their indications, contraindications, and value to reduce blood loss.

Objectives of this chapter

1 Relate the basic principles of surgical cutting and hemostasis.
2 Explore alternatives to a scalpel.
3 Learn about surgical maneuvers to reduce blood loss.

Definitions

Cautery: The word cautery is derived from the Greek word "causis" meaning "to burn" or the Latin word "cauterium" for "searing iron." Cautery means the act of coagulating blood and destroying tissue with a hot iron, by freezing, or by a caustic agent. The term cautery is also used for the instrument used to perform cauterization. *Electrocautery* means cauterization (cutting or hemostasis) is achieved by bringing an electrically heated metal instrument into contact with the tissue.

Diathermy: The word diathermy is derived from the Greek "dia" for "through" and "thermos" for "heat." Diathermy means the generation of heat in the tissue by means of electrical current. Medical diathermy is used for the therapeutical heating of tissue. Surgical diathermy (synonymous with *electrosurgery*) means the localized heating of tissue for cutting and hemostasis (*electrocoagulation*) by absorption of a high-frequency electric current.

Desiccatio: Coagulation resulting in dehydrated cells. Desiccation is sometimes used synonymously with fulguration.

Thermal knife: Refers to any surgical cutting device that uses heat as the acting physical principle for cutting.

Surgical coagulation: The disruption of tissue by physical means to form an amorphous residuum. With respect to blood vessels, two forms are distinguished:

- *Obliterative* coagulation occurs by direct electrode contact with or electrical arching to the tissue. Vessel walls shrink and the lumen is occluded by contracted tissue and thrombosis. It is the best method for vessels below 1 mm diameter.
- *Coaptive* coagulation occurs by mechanically apposing the edges of the vessel with a hemostat or forceps and current applied to the hemostat. The adventitia of the vessel is destroyed, the muscular layer shrinks, and the intima fuses.

A brief look at history

Surgical cutting and attempts to achieve hemostasis are not new. Ayurvedic medicine, which claims to be about 6000 years old, mentions the use of sharp bamboo splinters for surgical cutting. In early human history, all kinds of knives were used as scalpels, the use of which was not without problems. Hemorrhage and death occurred as a result of injury or surgical interventions. King Hammurabi of Babylon (1955–1912 BC) therefore introduced laws that dealt with surgical cutting. Hammurabi's Code contains a paragraph dealing with the surgeon who uses a bronze knife (scalpel) for wound care: "If a physician makes a wound and cures a freeman, he shall receive ten pieces of silver (. . .). However it is decreed that if a physician treats a patient 'with a metal knife for a severe wound and has caused the man to die—his hands shall be cut off'" (Code of Hammurabi) [1]. This decree puts much emphasis on the proper use of a scalpel and achieving hemostasis, and imposes a severe penalty on the physician who was unfortunate enough as to lose a surgical patient.

As testified to by ancient papyri, such as the Edwin Smith Papyrus (circa 1600 BC) and the Eber Papyrus (circa 1500 BC), the ancient Egyptians used the sharp blade of a papyrus reed as the equivalent of a scalpel. They also used scalpels, which they heated, thus becoming the precursors of the modern hemostatic scalpel. Attempts to achieve hemostasis included cautery and tamponade with linen. The Edwin Smith Papyrus also makes the first mention of sutures for wound care.

Greek physicians, among them Hippocrates (466–377 BC), tapped Egyptian medical wisdom. Hippocrates recommended the use of compressive bandages. About 700–800 BC, Homer's "Iliad" reports detailed means of surgical hemostasis for wounds.

The Romans learned from the Greeks. The Roman Celsus reported the use of a hemostatic forceps [2]. Galen (AD 131–201), one of the most influential physicians in the Roman world, got sufficient training in wound care and trauma surgery while working with gladiators. Galen's most important contribution to surgery is the first mention of ligature of vessels to halt bleeding. In turn, Paul of Aegina (sixth century AD) was the first to recommend ligature of blood vessels *before* a surgical procedure in the wound (extraction of an arrow).

In the Islamic realm, the physician Al-Razi (AD 841–926) was famous for his work. He used silk sutures and alcohol for hemostasis. The Persian physician Avicenna (Ibn-Cina) (AD 980–1037) described vessel ligature in his work "Canon."

During the Middle Ages (circa AD 400–1400), in the Christian world, some clergymen, who were able to read and had access to old writings, often worked as surgeons. However, in AD 1131, the Council of Reims issued a papal decree forbidding clerics to do surgical work. For a long time, the edict: "Ecclesia abhorrent a sanguine!" (Church abhors blood!) proved to be a death-blow to surgery. It meant that lettered men were no longer allowed to practice surgery. Important knowledge was lost, e.g., the knowledge about ligature of blood vessels. Unlettered laymen, e.g., barbers, were now in charge of wound care. They were unable to read the old authors and consequently could not benefit from the knowledge accumulated by their ancestors.

Guy de Chauliac (AD 1300–1368), one of the most influential surgeons of the fourteenth and fifteenth centuries, revived surgical hemostasis and as shown in his surgical text book (*Collectorium cyrurgie*, AD 1363) he considered hemostasis to be a central issue of surgery. He built on the work of Al-Zahrawi (circa AD 930–1013) who practiced near Cordoba and used special cotton, cautery and ligaturing of blood vessels to achieve hemostasis. Guy de Chauliac quoted Al-Zahrawi over 200 times. De Chauliac's writings remained influential in Europe until the publications of Ambrose Paré in the sixteenth century.

The French-man Ambroise Paré (AD 1510–1590), originally a barber, advanced to become a surgeon on the battle field. Using traditional methods such as treating wounds with hot oil and the searing iron to stop bleeding, he observed in AD 1537, during a battle in Italy, that— because of a lack of oil—"untreated" soldiers did better than those treated with hot oil. Paré stopped the use of hot oil and the searing iron for wound care and hemostasis. Instead, he re-invented ligature of vessels and used it for amputations [3].

About AD 1700, a new technique for hemostasis appeared—the tourniquet [4]. Pelet coined the actual term "tourniquet" in 1718. The use of a tourniquet was accompanied by Esmarch's limb exsanguination technique in 1873. In 1904, Cushing developed a pneumatic tourniquet [5], similar to the one used today.

The nineteenth century brought a drastic change in surgical cutting and hemostasis. In 1854, the surgeon Albrecht Theodor Middeldorpf published a monograph on galvanocautery. He described a platinum wire that was caused to glow by connecting it to an electrical battery [6]. Although not his invention, Middeldorpf was the first to develop galvanocautery into a usable surgical method. This was one of the earliest uses of electrical current for surgery. Modern surgical diathermy with high-frequency alternating current was introduced in 1909 by the dermatologist Franz Nagelschmidt from Berlin [6]. The electrosurgical instrument, introduced by W. T. Bovie and H. Cushing in 1928, became such a ubiquitous instrument that even today's surgeons refer to their electrosurgical knife as "The Bovie." At the time of invention, the explosive anesthetics made electrosurgery a hazardous undertaking. It was therefore not widely used. In the 1950s and 1960, nonexplosive anesthetics were introduced. This accelerated the spread of electrosurgery into the operating room.

Finally, the twentieth century brought the advent of countless machines and equipment for surgical cutting and concomitant hemostasis. As early as the 1920s, Irving Langmuir worked with the flow of highly ionized gases in a closed atmosphere. He laid the groundwork for the surgical use of plasma. Experiments with plasma as a surgical cutting tool started in the 1960s. Already in 1976, Russian scientists reported about the clinical use of a plasma scalpel. The argon plasma coagulator was finally invented by Dr Jerome Canady; he applied for the U.S. patent in July 1991 and it was granted in May 1993. In 1960, the first laser was built and it was used shortly thereafter in surgery. The microwave tissue coagulator was introduced by Tabuse in 1979 [7]. In 1982, Papachristou reported on the first use of a water jet in surgery. The Filipino surgeon Wilmo Orejola invented the harmonic scalpel that was introduced commercially in 1993. Many more cutting and coagulation methods have been invented or modified since.

Basics of surgical techniques

The amount of blood loss during surgery has a profound impact on morbidity and mortality. In fact, patient outcome is determined more by intraoperative blood loss than by the preoperative hemoglobin level [8]. Although inadvisable in elective surgery, patients with low hemoglobin levels can even safely undergo surgery if precautions are taken to minimize blood loss. Therefore, learning how to operate without causing unnecessary blood loss is a major contribution to improved patient outcome. Obviously, it is the surgeon who is often responsible for the decision to transfuse or not. To fulfill this important role, the surgeon must demonstrate expertise in reducing whatever blood loss is reducible.

Before surgery, some basic issues should be kept in mind: the choice of surgeon, the choice of surgical technique, and excellence in surgical performance. The surgeon needs to consider his own expertise, skills, and experience. In seriously ill patients, where substantial minimization of blood loss is needed, an experienced surgeon may be more suitable for the patient than another with limited experience. Referral to another surgeon seems to be appropriate in situations where blood loss is a predominant issue. Fast, but not careless, hands are needed. Accurate hemostasis and the speed to achieve it are crucial. The choice of an appropriate surgeon is therefore the first and most vital step in the reduction of blood loss and minimizing amounts transfused.

The choice of surgical technique or surgical access reportedly influences the amount of blood lost as well as that transfused. Some surgical techniques provide better hemostasis than other approaches to the same problem. For example, modified methods for aortic surgery translates into reduced blood loss and reduced transfusion exposure. Minor changes in the surgical technique—the addition of some strategically placed sutures—reduce blood loss [9]. Access to the surgical site is variable.

Transabdominal access is most widely accepted in treatment of infrarenal abdominal aortic aneurysms. This approach may cause significant intraoperative loss of fluid and may be accompanied by high transfusion rates. An alternative approach is the minimal access procedure, which may be as good as the transperitoneal approach, causes less physiologic disturbance and reduces postoperative morbidity in well-elected cases. The minimal access approach may significantly reduce the intraoperative replacement of fluid and blood.

Another basic of "bloodless" surgery is expert surgical craftsmanship. Long before transfusions became en vogue, surgeons realized that hemostasis is a sine qua non of professional patient care. This is mirrored in the principles of Dr Halsted who formulated the "Tenets of Halsted," namely:
1 Gentle tissue handling
2 Aseptic technique
3 Sharp anatomic dissection of tissues
4 Careful hemostasis (using fine, nonirritating suture material in minimal amounts)
5 Obliteration of dead space in the wound
6 Avoidance of tension
7 Importance of rest

Although partially controversial, these tenets are the basis for modern surgical craftsmanship [10]. They also form the basis of surgical transfusion avoidance. Certain aspects, derived from Halsted's tenets, deserve special consideration when it comes to surgical transfusion avoidance [11]:
1 *Attention to detail*: Any bleeding, major or minor, needs to be stopped. Even small losses add up constituting major bleeding if left unattended.
2 *Partial dissection*: Incising a portion of a wound, achieving hemostasis and continuing with another portion.
3 *Avoid stripping*: Stripping of fat layer off fascia makes identification of layers easier for closure, but increases blood loss.
4 *Anatomical dissection*: Cutting along anatomic, avascular planes requires a thorough knowledge of anatomy. It reduces uncontrolled vessel injury.
5 *Gentle tissue handling*: A "rip and tear" approach to surgery increases tissue damage and blood loss and should be avoided.

As adjuncts to surgical craftsmanship, there are many surgical devices that are able to reduce incisional blood loss. However, reduction of blood loss is more a result of the surgeon's skill than of the use of sophisticated equipment. Nevertheless, in the hands of a gifted surgeon, such devices can be employed beneficially. No surgeon can master every method and not every method suits all surgeons. It is better to master a limited number of techniques that fit the procedures performed than to have a whole array of gadgets without really mastering any in particular.

Surgical tools: Cold steel & Co.

The ideal cutting device combines a number of different characteristics [12]. It can cut at least as well as a scalpel and coagulate at least as well as monopolar electrosurgery while causing minimal tissue injury, producing little or no smoke to obscure the visual field, and posing no danger either to the patient or personnel. No special patient preparation is needed, and surgeons can handle it without special training. It also incurs no great costs. It is easily perceived that this is the "ideal," as yet nonexistent method. Every cutting method has its advantages and disadvantages that make it suitable for one procedure or another. It is up to the surgeon to determine from the equipment available which is best suited for the case.

Scalpel

The oldest means of cutting still in use is the scalpel. Despite the overwhelming flood of surgical instruments, the scalpel has kept its prominent position. Its universal availability, independence of electricity, and low cost make it the method of choice in many surgical interventions.

A plain scalpel is most frequently used for the skin incision. It gives a clean cut which is associated with a small scar and relatively rare wound infections. Only in selected circumstances, e.g., in patients who have a coagulopathy or who will receive anticoagulation during surgery, a method may be preferred that provides cutting and hemostasis simultaneously from the first incision [13].

Heat in surgery

Heat transferred to tissue can either benefit or harm the patient. Knowledge of the basic characteristics and effects of heat in tissue helps to get the best out of equipment that uses heat for surgery while minimizing the associated risks.

Heat can be transferred to and within tissue by conduction (increased molecular energy that occurs with increased temperatures), convection (through movement of matter, e.g., blood), and radiation (which is not so important here). Distribution of heat in tissue will increase tissue temperature and cause changes in the tissue. The extent of such changes not only depends on the temperature, but also on the time the tissue is influenced by the temperature, and on the characteristics of the tissue itself. The extent to which tissue is perfused also influences the effect of the heat. Blood flow diverts heat away from the site of thermal injury (i.e., cutting or coagulation).

Heat alters tissue elements in a temperature-dependent fashion. Proteins coagulate at about 60°C. Tissue temperatures between 60 and 80°C cause shrinkage of Type I collagen that occurs in the walls of blood vessels, airways, and bile ducts. Collagen shrinkage closes the lumen and seals the vessel. Cellular changes occur up to 100°C. Cell wall and membrane damage as well as DNA denaturation and enzyme deactivation occur. Above 100°C, the water content of the tissue vaporizes and the remains of the cells pyrolyse (i.e., the primary structure of the compound dissociates). Temperatures from 300 to 400°C are needed to pyrolyse triglycerides and about 600°C to pyrolyse proteins.

Surgical methods that use heat to cut are often used to achieve coagulation; hemostasis is provided simultaneously with cutting. It is also possible to either cut or coagulate exclusively. Cutting and coagulating both cause some degree of tissue damage. If the heat is decreased, so is the effect on hemostasis.

Exposure of tissue to thermal energy for cutting or coagulation also has some clinical effects. Epithelium migration and wound healing are delayed. The average width of a scar is greater than that which develops after a scalpel incision. Wounds made with a thermal knife are less resistant to bacterial infection than those made with "cold steel."

Thermocoagulator

The thermocoagulator (hot-jet coagulator) uses a stream of hot air to coagulate bleeding surfaces. Temperatures of up to 500°C develop at the tip of the instrument. The tip can be held just above the bleeding tissue to coagulate the tissue surface [14].

Electrical current for surgery

Two basic methods to use electrical current, each with many variations, have been introduced into surgery: electrocautery and electrosurgery (= diathermy or "cold caustic"). In electrocautery, a metal applicator is heated by means of an electrical current. The cautery effect is restricted to the site where heat is transferred from the metal to the tissue. No current enters the patient's body. In electrosurgery, heat is created at the metal–tissue interface through tissue–current interactions.

Depending on the frequency, electrical currents affect tissue in a distinct way. If tissue is exposed to up to 3000 Hz, nerves and muscles are stimulated in a dose-dependent fashion. Between 3000 and 5000 Hz, a plateau is reached. At currents between 5000 and 10,000 Hz, neuromuscular effects decrease. At frequencies of more than 10,000 Hz, neuromuscular reaction no longer occurs. At this point, body tissue works as an electrical conduction path. Conduction is limited by the tissue resistance to the flow of current (also called impedance). Resistance can be expressed as follows:

Resistance = Resistivity × (Length/Area)

Resistivity, the biological impedance (ohm cm), depends on tissue characteristics and on the frequency of the electrical current. The larger the area in which the current spreads, the lower the resistance to a specific electrical current will be. Applied to surgical cutting, this means the smaller the area touched by the electrode, the hotter the tissue. The small active electrode in the wound touches a small area of tissue. There is a high current density. If this high current meets the resistance of the tissue, heat develops as the current has to struggle against the resistance of the tissue. The tissue is heated locally. As the current spreads throughout the body, however, there is a large mass of tissue (i.e., a larger surface area) and no significant heating occurs. The current leaves the body (in monopolar surgery) by way of a grounding pad, which has a large surface area. Again, no significant heat develops at this large exit for the current.

The degree of coagulation and the speed or depth of cutting with electrical current depend on the power delivered. Power is the product of current squared by the resistance. This means that, if the current is doubled, four times the heat occurs in the tissue. The higher the power, the faster and deeper the cutting and it will cause more coagulation and tissue damage. The mode of operation, cutting, or coagulation, depends also on the waveform of the current:

- strictly cutting, no coagulation: undamped continuous sinus wave
- coagulation, no cutting: damped, intermittent sinus wave
- combined, cutting and coagulation: interrupted sinus wave.

Method 1. Electrocautery: the hemostatic scalpel

A hemostatic scalpel unit consists of a controller, a handle, and a disposable scalpel blade similar to a conventional scalpel blade [15]. The blade consists of various metal layers. Between the layers there is an electrical microcircuit that heats the blade. The blade temperature range is adjustable from 110 to 270°C. Skin is usually incised at a temperature of 110°C and vessels with a diameter of up to 2 mm are sealed at temperatures between 210 and 270°C. When the scalpel blade touches the tissue, hemostasis is achieved by direct transmission of heat to the tissue. Since no electrical current is transmitted into the tissue there is no interference with electrically powered monitoring. Muscles do not contract or fibrillate.

A variation of electrocautery was introduced in 1994. A procedure termed "muscle fragment welding" uses electrocautery through a rectum muscle fragment. A piece of muscle is applied to the bleeding area and then cautery forms a coagulum out of the muscle fragment. This provides hemostasis that seems to be immediate and permanent. Rectus muscle fragment welding is an effective and practical method of controlling presacral and other hemorrhage [16, 17].

Method 2. Electrosurgery

In electrosurgery, a closed electrical circuit is created of which the patient is part. Alternating high-frequency current travels through tissue. This causes ionized molecules in the tissue to oscillate and the tissue heats up (up to 300°C). A pure cutting current produces a small line of tissue destruction at the edges of the incision. The upper layer consists of carbon particles, beneath is a layer of desiccated or coagulated tissue. The current also desiccates the tissues, forms scars, and produces smoke.

Surgical diathermy has three adjustable variables: (1) power, (2) frequency (which provides the choice between coagulation and cutting), and (3) polarity (monopole vs. bipole, referring to the distance between the electrical poles).

In monopolar electrosurgery ("The Bovie"), the active electrode is in the wound. The current returns to the large return electrode which is placed elsewhere on the patient, far away from the active electrode. The current flows through the patient. Heat develops in the tissue around the active electrode.

An instrument for bipolar electrosurgery looks like a pair of forceps, one arm being the active electrode, the other the return electrode. The active and the return electrode are only millimeters apart. Both are in the wound. The current flows through the tissue that is grasped between the forceps and coagulation takes place. Cutting is not possible in bipolar electrosurgery.

While electrosurgery is very safe, some hazards must be kept in mind and measures taken to prevent them. Current follows the path of least resistance. In monopolar surgery, this may cause problems, namely, electrical burns in the area of the return electrode or any area by means of which the patient is grounded by (grounding injury). Since the electrical current flows directly through the body, pacemakers and monitoring may be disturbed and cardiac arrhythmias induced. Some disadvantages are shared alike by bipolar and monopolar electrosurgery. While there is no longer any danger of explosion from anesthetic gases, other gases still pose a hazard. Bowel gases (methane, hydrogen) are explosive and can cause injury if they come into contact with electrosurgical equipment. Electrosurgery also generates smoke, delays healing, and may promote infection.

Electrosurgery is used in almost all kinds of procedures. It is especially practical for surgery in densely vascularized areas. However, it is relatively ineffective in treating areas of diffuse or heavy bleeding and cumbersome if used to treat a broad bleeding surface. Sticking of tissue debris to the active electrode is a further disadvantage. A scratch pad helps to rid the blade of charcoaled tissue.

When vessels are coagulated in electrosurgery, the desired effects are a change in color (tanning) and retraction of the tissue. A typical popping sound is heard when tissue is cauterized, leaving a charcoal coating. Overzealous use of the device creates unnecessary tissue damage [12].

Variations in the use of electrical current in surgery

Saline-enhanced thermal sealing

The underlying principle of saline-enhanced thermal sealing is a combination of electrosurgery with a cooling flow of saline applied directly at the tip of the active electrode. When connected to a conventional electrosurgical generator, set at 40–140 W, the tip of the device transmits electrical energy to the tissue. This energy heats the tissue (as in normal electrosurgery). The continuous flow of saline (4–8 mL/min) reduces the heat developing in the tissue. The tissue temperature is kept below 100°C. This prevents desiccation, eschar, smoke, and sticking of tissue debris to the electrode [18].

Different types of devices allow for either monopolar or bipolar use of saline-enhanced thermal sealing. The monopolar device, called "floating ball", uses continuous infusion of saline through the tip of a ballpoint-pen-like device. A similar device can be used in bipolar mode. A bipolar device (sealing forceps, resembling an endoscopic stapler) is also available. During operation, tissue is grasped in the forceps which are activated until tissue adjacent to the forceps blanches.

Indications for saline-enhanced thermal sealing include lung surgery where the technique not only provides hemostasis but also aerostasis. The technique may be used in trauma surgery (splenic and hepatic lacerations), for partial nephrectomy and radical prostatectomy as well as laparoscopic myomectomy [19].

Electrothermal bipolar vessel sealer

Electrothermal bipolar vessel sealing [20] uses a combination of pressure and radiofrequency to achieve hemostasis. A generator senses the density of the tissue held between a forceps-like device and adjusts the energy delivered. It employs high currents (4 A) and low voltage (<200 V) bipolar radiofrequency. The high current fuses collagen and elastin and forms a plastic-like sealed zone. This produces a permanent and translucent seal that obliterates the vessel lumen.

Electrothermal bipolar vessel sealing is usable for vessel diameters of 1–7 mm and for bundles of tissue. It takes 2–5 seconds to seal a vessel. Heat sidespread is less than 2 mm. Electrothermal bipolar vessel sealing is a suitable measure for hemostasis in tight and deep spaces. It saves time compared to hemostasis by suture ligature. It has been shown to be usable in a wide variety of laparoscopic and open surgeries, such as hemorrhoidectomy [21], hepatectomy [22], hysterectomy [23, 24], splenectomy, prostatectomy, cystectomy, and nephrectomy [25].

Microwaves in surgery

That microwaves are used to heat and cook food is well known. They can also be used to heat tissue, making microwaves suitable for surgical use in the form of microwave coagulation.

Microwave coagulation

Microwaves are generated at a frequency of 2450 MHz. The energy is transmitted from a generator through a cable to

Table 13.1 Examples of lasers in medicine.

Ruby laser	Visible wavelength, pulsed mode	Remarks
Argon laser	Blue-green light, therefore strongly influenced by the tissue color, preferentially absorbed by red tissues	Most suitable for coagulation, due to the wavelength being readily absorbed by hemoglobin, used to (endoscopically) photocoagulate gastrointestinal bleeding
Neodymium: YAG laser (neodymium: yttrium–aluminium garnet laser)	Invisible, near infrared beam, relatively independent of tissue color, most powerful surgical laser (up to 100 W)	High initial costs, stringent safety requirements
CO_2 laser	Invisible, far infrared beam, completely independent of tissue color	Vaporizes skin/tissue for cutting or coagulation. Cuts if in focus, coagulates if defocused

a handle, which holds a needle probe. Probes of varying lengths are inserted into the tissue and are activated at 60 W for 30 seconds to coagulate the tissue. A further 15 seconds are allowed for dissociation of tissue from the probe. Five to eight millimeters away from the original site, the probe is reinserted into the tissue, and the procedure is repeated, thus coagulating the intended cut line piece by piece. Afterward, the tissue is dissected using a normal scalpel or scissors. Because the tissue is sealed before it is cut, bleeding should not occur. If bleeding does occur, however, the vessels are difficult to ligate using regular sutures, because coagulated tissue is brittle. In such a case, gentle handling, careful suturing, and the use of glue provide the needed hemostasis.

The technique can be used for partial nephrectomy. It is also used for controlling parenchymal bleeding in other solid vascular organs, such as liver and spleen [26, 27].

Light in surgery

Similar to electrical current, light can be used for cutting. It interacts with tissue and can heat it. Targeted light in the form of lasers is usable for surgery.

Infrared contact coagulator

The infrared contact coagulator uses a beam of infrared light in order to coagulate bleeding surfaces. A halogen light beam is modified by various optical devices (reflectors, quartzes) and can be targeted at the site of bleeding. Using this means, bleeding in the spleen, liver, kidney, lungs, or in cancer sites can be stopped [28–31].

Laser

LASER is an acronym standing for Light Amplification by Stimulated Emission of Radiation (Table 13.1). Light is an electromagnetic wave that is generated by atomic processes. Laser light is generated when an atom with a high energy state is struck by a photon of a precise frequency. This results in the emission of two photons of the same frequency and direction. These photons stimulate others so that the light is amplified exponentially in a manner similar to a chain reaction. The resulting light is monochromatic (of the same color and thus, wavelength) and the beam can be focused on a very small spot.

When light touches tissue, it can either be reflected, travel through the tissue, or be absorbed. Absorbed light heats up tissue. Light that is not absorbed travels through deeper tissue layers and does not create the energy density needed for tissue vaporization.

Absorption of light in the visible electromagnetic range is influenced by the color of the tissue. Nonpigmented tissue does not absorb much light energy. However, if wavelengths longer than 1 μm are used, the absorption becomes independent of the tissue color. The longer the wave, the more independent the absorption becomes in relation to tissue color.

Laser can be used in two different ways. Firstly, it can be used as a heat source for an instrument. The instrument heats up and upon contact of the instrument with the tissue, the tissue is coagulated. This is equivalent to electrocauterization. Secondly, the laser can be directed right into tissue where it heats up the tissue to achieve the effects described above [32].

One of the inherent problems of laser surgery is fluid. If fluids impede the laser, its cutting ability is diminished substantially.

The use of lasers is associated with complications and calls for stringent safety measures. Laser can easily perforate tissue, e.g., the bowel, and hemorrhage may occur. CO_2 gas, when absorbed (e.g., from the gastrointestinal tract), can cause respiratory distress [33]. Laser beams or reflections (e.g., on metal instruments in the wound) may cause eye and skin lesions. Spectacles need to be worn. Fire and explosion may result if unsuitable materials are exposed to the beam, e.g., drapes, clothing (unless kept moist), plastics, flammable anesthetics, and skin preparations.

Lasers have been used in a variety of clinical settings. Depending on how they are used, they can increase or decrease blood loss [34–38].

Lightning

Plasma (not to be confused with blood plasma) is a partially ionized hot gas. It is generated by creating an electrical arc between two electrodes and then passing a gas (e.g., argon, helium) between them under high pressure. The electrical energy is converted to heat in the gas, causing the gas to become extremely hot. The heat frees electrons from the atoms of the gas (partial ionization). After the gas leaves the electrical field it cools down and the free electrons recombine with the atoms, releasing a photon.

Plasma scalpel

If a hot plasma stream is directed against tissue, it can be used for cutting [39]. A fine, hot gas jet (3000°C) delivered from a nozzle performs the cutting. Some energy diffuses through the edges of the incision so that the tissue is also coagulated. When the plasma stream is used for cutting, the handle is placed directly on the tissue. For coagulation, the handle is held 1–2 cm above the tissue. The jet of hot gas clears both the tissue of blood and coagulates at the same time. The tip of the handle can even be submerged in fluid and it still works. As it cuts, the plasma scalpel effectively cauterizes blood vessels up to 3 mm in diameter [40].

Argon beam coagulation

Argon is a colorless, odorless, inert gas that does not support combustion. It is readily available and inexpensive. At room temperature, ionized argon gas transmits electrical current. It can therefore be used to transfer electricity to tissue.

An argon beam coagulator (= argon plasma coagulator) has a pen-like handle that emits a gentle coaxial flow of argon gas at room temperature. This gas blows away blood and debris to optimize visualization. When the tip of the nozzle is within 1 cm of the tissue surface, radiofrequency energy is transferred through the stream to the tissue. Electrical energy is "sprayed," "painting" the surface of the bleeding tissue. The beam leaves a 1–2 mm eschar (consisting of small consolidated coagulated blood vessels) firmly attached to the tissue surface by which hemostasis is provided. There is no contact between any metal or nozzle and the tissue. Therefore, less tissue adhesion occurs, less tissue damage results, and no debris sticks to the electrode.

Argon beam coagulation has been used for a wide range of procedures, in particular, in liver and spleen, head an neck surgery, and urological surgery (kidneys, bladder, in irradiated area, prostate) [41–44]. It can also be used for endoscopic application. The argon beam coagulator is not made to cut but is suitable for use in areas where diffuse bleeding occurs. It is especially helpful in coagulating bleeding from the surface of parenchymal organs.

Kinetic energy in surgery

Water jet

Water that has been put under pressure and then focused into a small jet has long been used to cut metal. The same principle can be used to cut tissue in surgery. Water is delivered under pressure through a variety of nozzle sizes. Both the diameter of the nozzle and the water pressure have an effect on the amount of blood lost, the speed of dissection, and the degree of tissue necrosis. No thermal damage occurs in surrounding tissue.

Hepatic surgery is the classical indication for a water jet. Liver parenchyma are washed away by high-pressure water, leaving vessels and nerves intact. The exposed intrahepatic vessels stand out clearly for accurate ligation or coagulation. Apart from use in liver surgery [45, 46], a water jet can be used for other types of tissue, such as the kidney [47], the brain [48], and the gastrointestinal tract. It can even be used in laparoscopy [49].

High-frequency water jet

A variation of the water jet combines the properties of a water jet and of electrosurgery. A high-frequency electrical current is applied to the water stream and current is transmitted to the patient. Using this combination, cutting and coagulation can be combined [50] so that smaller vessels are coagulated and larger ones remain for separate ligation.

Vibration for surgical cutting

Vibration can cause tissue damage. If harnessed, vibration can be used for surgical interventions. Mechanical energy is transferred to the tissue and cavitational bubbles result from pressure differentials causing vacuolization in the cells. The vacuoles expand and collapse leading finally to fragmentation of tissue. The rate of cavitational activity is proportionate to the water content of the cells. Soft, fleshy tissue with a high-water content is fragmented readily.

Two cutting methods use vibrations as their acting principle: the ultrasonic scalpel and the cavitron ultrasonic surgical aspirator (CUSA).

Ultrasonic scalpel (harmonic scalpel)

The harmonic scalpel uses ultrasound technology facilitating both cutting and coagulation. An ultrasound generator creates a natural harmonic frequency of 55.5 kHz [29]. The acoustic wave sets the tip in vibration, causing cavitational fragmentation and cutting rather than electrical coagulation. An ultrasonic scalpel provides a focused area of dissection with excellent hemostasis. Since the tip vibrates, it becomes warm. The temperatures that develop (50–100°C) are lower than those used in electrosurgery or by lasers. Coagulation occurs as a result of protein denaturation when the vibrating blade sticks to proteins, forming a coagulum that seals small vessels. When the effect is prolonged, secondary heat is produced that seals larger vessels. If increased hemostasis is desired, the cutting speed is reduced.

The harmonic scalpel has distinct advantages. Much less heat is transferred into the tissue, causing less tissue damage and smoke. There is no risk of injury to adjacent tissue through heat or electrical energy. Since smoke does not develop, the harmonic scalpel can be used favorably in laparoscopy [51]. A harmonic scalpel also functions in liquids, which makes it useful for cutting submerged tissue.

Cavitron ultrasonic surgical aspirator

The CUSA is a dissecting tool that consists of a hollow titanium tip, vibrating along its length at 23 or 36 kHz. The excursion of the tip (amplitude) is set to remove tissue within a 1–2 mm radius. Tissue damage is confined to an area of about 25–50 μm surrounding the tip, with minimal thermal injury and protein denaturation.

The CUSA simultaneously unites three functions: ultrasonic fragmentation, irrigation, and aspiration. The irrigant helps to emulsify tissue and cools the shaft and tip of the tool, which may become warm with extended use. Aspiration through the center of the unit removes dissected tissue and any debris or blood.

The rate of cavitational activity is proportionate to the water content of the cells, i.e., soft, fleshy tissue with high-water content is fragmented more readily than other tissue. Therefore, different types of tissue fragment at different rates, with the result that dissection can be performed leaving blood vessels, ureters, and connective tissue skeletonized and intact.

The CUSA has been used in neurosurgery, general and oncologic surgery, heart surgery, and in gynecology for open as well as for laparoscopic procedures [52].

The impact of surgical cutting on blood loss

Several studies compared cutting devices and their contribution to a reduction of blood loss and allogeneic transfusion exposure [24, 27, 36, 45, 46, 52–55]. The essence of the studies is that many of the above-described methods for cutting reduce blood loss when compared to the conventional scalpel [13, 55]. Some of these studies are listed in Table 13.2.

The use of laser can either increase or decrease blood loss, depending on the type of laser used. Carbon dioxide laser incisions are reported to be less bloody than scalpel or electrosurgical incisions. During other interventions, incisional blood loss was increased when compared with the scalpel or even electrosurgery [35].

Comparisons between what is thought to be standard (scalpel, suture, and electrocautery) and newer techniques demonstrate the superiority of the new techniques for certain indications. An argon beam coagulator reduces blood loss drastically, even when severe hemorrhage occurs, and reduces the risk of postoperative hemorrhage [42, 44]. In comparison with steel and electrosurgical scalpels, plasma surgery reduced bleeding [40].

Table 13.2 Comparison of different cutting devices with regard to occurring blood loss.

Compared methods	Intervention	Blood loss	Source
Water jet vs. tissue fracture	Liver resection	1386 vs. 2450 mL	Baer *et al.* [45]
Ligasure vs. conventional ligation	Prostatectomy	569 mL vs. 685 mL	Daskalopoulos *et al.* [53]
Ligasure vs. conventional ligation	Cystectomy	637 mL vs. 744 mL	Daskalopoulos *et al.* [53]
CUSA vs. tissue fracture	Liver resection	Lobectomies: 685 mL vs. significantly lower (?) segmentectomies: 540 mL vs. significantly lower (?)	Fasulo *et al.* [52]
Electrocautery vs. scalpel	Mastectomy	134 mL vs. 331 mL	Kurtz and Frost [54]
Electrosurgical bipole vessel sealer vs. suture	Vaginal hysterectomy	68 mL (range 20–200) vs. 126 mL (range 25–600)	Levy and Emery [24]
Electrocautery vs. scalpel	Mastectomy	352 vs. 507 mL	Miller *et al.* [55]
Jet-cutter vs. CUSA	Liver resection	18.4 mL/cm^2 vs. 34.4 mL/cm^2	Rau *et al.* [46]
Contact neodymium yttrium–aluminum–garnet laser scalpel vs. scalpel	Mastectomy	149 vs. 421 mL	Wyman and Rogers [36]
Microwave vs. conventional hepatectomy	Hepatectomy in tumor with liver cirrhosis	215 ± 189 mL vs. 652 ± 1008 mL	Zhou *et al.* [27]

Methods to achieve hemostasis and to avoid undue blood loss

Apart from the sophisticated equipment available for cutting and coagulation, there are also many manual or low-cost measures to stop bleeding or to reduce blood loss. The methods involve selectively occluding vessels, applying pressure on whole organs and bleeding surfaces, or lowering hemostatic pressure in vessels leading to the surgical field.

Selective occlusion of vessels—externally and internally

Classical methods: sutures and clips

Bleeding from injured vessels can be stopped by ligation with a suture. This is an efficient yet tedious and time-consuming task. Metal or plastic clips are available to make vessel ligation easier. Clips are easily placed and staplers help to reach even deep vessels. However, staplers are expensive, clips can dislodge. The use of sutures as well as clips for hemostasis leaves foreign material in the body. Nevertheless, sutures and clips are still the mainstay of hemostasis in many surgical interventions.

Vascular maneuvers

One of the most feared operative hazards during the work on parenchymal organs is hemorrhage. Ligation of vessels supplying certain organs may help to reduce blood loss.

The liver is a delicate organ and bleeds easily. About 20–30% of the cardiac output flow through the liver. During hepatic surgery, blood loss is almost invariably high, unless specific techniques are used to prevent and stop bleeding. It is not surprising that there have been described many different variations of occlusion of liver vessels. Stopping such blood flow prevents excessive hemorrhage during dissection of the parenchyma. Examples are as follows:

- *Pringle maneuver* (pedicle ligation technique): For the Pringle maneuver (Pringle 1908), a soft clamp—or better, a banding, or just the fingers—are used to temporarily occlude the portal triad. By means of this maneuver, the arterial and portal vein inflow to the liver is stopped, but the back flow from the hepatic veins is still active.
- For *total vascular exclusion*, the vena cava is isolated above and below the liver and occluded. Additionally, the portal vein and hepatic artery are occluded. This technique provides the best possible vascular control. It is used for large tumors close to the vena cava. A severe side effect may be significant hemodynamic derangement.

- *Selective hepatic vascular exclusion*: To control inflow and outflow only to major hepatic veins, without occlusion of the caval blood flow, hemihepatic vascular clamping and occlusion of the corresponding hepatic vein or clamping of the hepatic pedicle with occlusion of the three hepatic veins is possible. It is much more effective than the Pringle maneuver for controlling intraoperative bleeding (prevention of backflow bleeding), and it may be associated with better postoperative liver function and shorter hospital stay [56]. Another advantage is that the caval blood flow is not interrupted, avoiding grave hemodynamic changes. But this method is much more sophisticated to use and needs an experienced team of surgeons.
- *Makuuchi's maneuver* [57] (hemihepatic vascular clamping): During this procedure, vascular clamping selectively interrupts the arterial and venous inflow to the right or left hemi liver. This avoids both splanchnic blood stasis and ischemia or ischemia-reperfusion injury to the whole liver. The negative aspect is that bleeding of the resection plane cannot be completely avoided.

Temporary clamping of vessels may do some damage to them. It may lead to clamp trauma, meaning intimal denudation and medial arterial wall damage. This may lead to postoperative stenosis and spasm of the vessels. Occlusion of vessels leading to the liver may also lead to ischemic damage of the organ. Ischemic and reperfusion damage is usually negligible when surgical time is kept short [58]. Nevertheless, transient elevations in hepatic enzymes may be seen, but such do not result in increased morbidity when compared to control groups. Patients with cirrhotic and fatty livers may experience more damage since they do not tolerate ischemia as well. To prolong the tolerable ischemia time, several modifications have been proposed. Ischemic preconditioning of the liver is one of them. Another is intermittent inflow occlusion. Good results were observed when the vessel occlusion was released every 5–20 minutes. Some concerns have been voiced regarding frequent reperfusion periods, which may be worse than only one reperfusion period. Intermittent release of the vessel occlusion may not be necessary since ischemic injury is usually not a problem. A third method to reduce ischemic damage is cooling of the liver. Fortner and colleagues described this technique for the first time in 1974. Such cooling is only necessary when long periods of liver ischemia are expected, e.g., in liver transplant procedures.

Liver surgery is not the only surgery in which vascular occlusion is beneficial. The kidney, spleen, uterus, and other organs can be handled similarly [59].

Endovascular grafts

Occluding vessel walls from within while preserving blood flow through this vessel is the principle behind endovascular grafts. Via vessel puncture, a wire is inserted in a vessel and is guided under radiological control to the damaged part of the vessel. There, a graft is applied through the vessel puncture to tape the vessel wall from within. It is used to stop or prevent surgical or traumatic hemorrhage and has been advocated for a variety of indications [60]. If life-threatening hemorrhage occurs from a large, yet hard to reach or entirely inaccessible vessel (such as the retro-hepatic inferior vena cava), an endoluminal stent-graft can be used to manage the bleeding [61]. It can also be used as a blood-conserving, alternative approach to repair of an abdominal aortic aneurysm [62] or for the treatment of aortobronchial or other vessel fistulae.

Embolization

Another way to occlude vessels from within is embolization. Via a catheter inserted through a fitting vessel, the vessel can be occluded. This can be performed to occlude a vessel temporarily or permanently. A great variety of embolizing agents have been proposed, among them contrast media like lipiodol, sclerosing agents, cyanoacrylate, various particulate substances, or coils.

Embolization can be used in emergency situations to treat bleeding in the brain, the nose (epistaxis), uterus, bladder [63], liver [64], spleen [65], gastrointestinal tract (e.g., peptic ulcers), chest wall, pelvic fractures [66], extremities, etc. However, care must be taken that necessary surgical interventions are not delayed. This may lead to further unnecessary blood loss.

Nonbleeding vessels can be prophylactically embolized to prevent major blood loss during surgery or to prevent rebleeding. This has been described for a variety of cancer and metastatic surgeries [67], myoma resection of the uterus [68], uterine bleeding expected during delivery when mothers have errant placentation [69], and for gastrointestinal bleeding [70]. It is also possible to simply place catheters for embolization preoperatively, and then proceed with the surgery and if major blood loss should occur, the vessels can be embolized through catheters that are already correctly placed.

Also, embolization can be employed as an alternative to surgery. Such has been described for the therapy of uterine fibroids or for tumors and metastases. This may prevent the blood loss which would have been associated with surgery.

Tourniquet

A more indirect way to achieve temporary vascular occlusion, mainly of the extremities, is the use of a tourniquet. This results in an almost bloodless surgical field. In this instance, occlusion is gentler than direct vessel clamping. A tourniquet minimizes the amount of vessel dissection required and improves visualization and mobilization of vessels in the surgical field. It avoids trauma of vessels associated with temporary clamping. Using a tourniquet also prevents postoperative stenosis and spasms of vessels which would occur if vessels were clamped.

Before a tourniquet is applied, the limb should be protected by soft cotton padding. Heparin may be given in a dose of 100 mg/kg i.v. 3–5 minutes before the tourniquet is inflated with the intention of prolonging the safe ischemic interval. Limb elevation for 1–2 minutes before inflation of the tourniquet is also beneficial to reduce the amount of blood in the extremity. Proper wrapping with a rubber bandage (Esmarch) just before tourniquet inflation is crucial to completely exsanguinate the extremity. If there is still oozing after application of a tourniquet, usually poor exsanguination is the cause, not inadequate pressure of the tourniquet. Esmarch bandage techniques should not be used in patients with infected wounds (to prevent dissemination of bacteria) and in patients with deep vein thrombosis.

A pneumatic tourniquet can be inflated with a predetermined pressure [5]. The pressure used for inflation depends on the limb circumference, systolic blood pressure, tourniquet width, limb shape, cuff design, and vascular status of the limb. The optimal pressure should be kept as low as possible. As a rule of thumb, arterial occlusion pressure plus 50 mm Hg is recommended. About 140–320 mm Hg is used. Wide cuffs require less pressure than narrower cuffs and reduce the potential for damage to underlying nerves and muscles.

The complications of tourniquet are nerve compression and ischemic muscle damage. A complete nerve conduction block develops from 15 to 45 minutes after inflation of tourniquet and is restored within 30 minutes after deflation, given that the total tourniquet time does not exceed 2 hours. By the same token, ischemia times of less than 2 hours do not seem to cause lasting muscle damage. The metabolism of the muscle recovers within 20 minutes after deflation of the cuff. Tourniquet times of more than 2 hours may be associated with irreversible changes of nerve and muscle tissues. The "safe" ischemic interval can be prolonged by the use of heparin.

A full-blown "post tourniquet syndrome" consists of tissue edema, muscle weakness without paralysis, stiffness, and dysesthesia with pain or numbness. The syndrome usually resolves within 1 week, though the recovery period may be prolonged. Complications associated with tourniquets can be avoided if two tourniquets are applied simultaneously and inflated alternately. Placing good padding beneath the tourniquet is also important to prevent any fluids running under the tourniquet. Cooling the extremity of the limb may prolong the safe ischemia time.

Some surgeons favor release of the tourniquet before the wound is closed. They argue that this enables them to visualize vessels that bleed after tourniquet release and the vessels can be ligated or cauterized before the wound is closed. Others release the tourniquet only after the wound is closed and compressive bandages are applied. As studies for knee arthroplasty demonstrated, the latter approach leads to reduced total blood loss [71].

A tourniquet is used mainly on limbs, such as in localized endarteriectomy, arteriovenous fistula creation, joint replacement, and many other procedures that potentially lead to heavy hemorrhaging from the limbs. Tourniquets, however, can not only be applied to extremities, but also to whole organs. Uterine bleeding, for instance, can be treated temporarily by application of a tourniquet around the cervix [72].

Compression

Manual wound compression

Direct manual compression of bleeding wounds, arteries leading to the wound or of whole organs are recognized techniques for first aid [73]. It helps prevent exsanguination and wins some time until complete hemostasis is achievable. Manual compression is also helpful in the surgical setting. It may prevent hematoma formation, permits clotting or for the initiation of other hemostatic measures.

Traditionally, manual compression is applied directly over the area of an injured vessel, such as after vessel puncture, especially after arterial puncture. Manual compression of the aorta is also often a lifesaver and can be used for uterine bleeding, ruptured aortic aneurysm [74], or for any injury below a compressible aortic area, e.g., in massive pelvic hemorrhage. Such compression may bridge the time until a patient can be taken to a facility where definite hemostasis can be achieved.

Whole organs can also be compressed to prevent exsanguination. The liver is compressible when the abdomen is open. The uterus can be compressed in an open abdomen as well as from the outside. Uterine massage may also help to reduce bleeding when the patient suffers from postpartal atonic hemorrhage [75].

Compressive bandaging

The use of compressive bandaging is often preferred over extended manual compression since it frees the hands of the health-care provider to continue administering further care. It also increases the comfort of the patient. Compressive bandages are applied in emergencies, as well as in the perioperative period, to achieve temporary hemostasis at the site of injury. A prerequisite is that bandaging of the bleeding wound is possible. This may be difficult at some locations. Elastic adhesive bandages may broaden the spectrum of wounds which can be bandaged while applying compression [73]. Addition of hemostatic agents to the bandage may further add to its hemostatic value [76, 77].

Packing

Direct control of bleeding is the most desirable choice. However, in some instances this is not possible. Diffuse bleeding ("oozing") may make surgical hemostasis difficult or impossible. Topical hemostasis may be achieved with glues, mesh, argon beam, etc., or by correcting an underlying coagulation defect intraoperatively. At times, hemostasis cannot be achieved by these measures. Hemodynamic stabilization as well as the correction of any underlying coagulopathy is required beforehand. Packing the wound or the bleeding body cavity with sterile towels and tamponades slows the bleeding and allows time to correct the coagulopathy (hypothermia, acidosis, and preexisting coagulopathy) by reversing the underlying cause.

Abdominal packing is a lifesaving technique for temporary control of severe injury. It is used in the pelvic area and for liver and spleen lacerations [78]. Control of bleeding from the abdominal cavity can be achieved by applying controlled pressure with several large abdominal packs. It is also possible to apply packs in organ-specific techniques (early abdominal packing). The packing must exert enough pressure to tamponade the bleeding, but must not stop blood flow through the organ. Skin is closed lightly or by interposing surgical mesh to give room for expansion—to prevent increased intra-abdominal pressure leading to respiratory and perfusion problems. Packing is usually removed 48–72 hours later in the operating room. But

also after 7–10 days of packing, no increased infection rate has been observed.

Immediate failures of packs are substantially due to bleeding, especially in "underpacking." A problem of abdominal packing is increased intra-abdominal pressure (overpacking) with respiratory and renal complications, abdominal compartment syndrome, even leading to multiorgan failure.

Mesh wrap

Since intra-abdominal packing increases intra-abdominal pressure and the complication rate, it has been proposed that a damaged organ be selectively compressed rather than compressing the whole abdomen. An absorbable mesh tailored to a lacerated organ can be applied (Fig. 13.1) instead of the usual packing with surgical

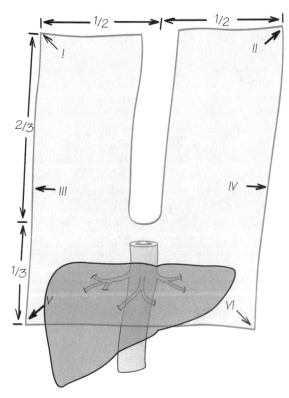

Fig 13.1 Mesh graft for liver lacerations. The mesh is wrapped around the liver and sutured together along the line made by points I–II and V–VI, respectively. Point I is sutured to V and II to VI; then, beginning from point III, the mesh is closed by suturing from III to the point where I and V unite. The same is done with the opposite side.

towels. Pressure is applied to the organ by varying the tension applied while suturing the mesh around the organ. Tamponade is self-contained and does not impair the flow through the vessels leading to the organ. Intra-abdominal pressure is not increased by this method. It is not necessary to reopen the abdomen. Mesh wraps are applied around the liver [79], the kidney, and the spleen [80].

Balloon tamponade

Self-made or commercially available balloons are a very valuable adjunct to achieving hemostasis in a great variety of settings.

Hepatic injuries are associated with high morbidity and mortality. Many techniques have been devised to stem bleeding. Balloon tamponade is among the armamentarium of the surgeon and is especially helpful when the injury is near the hilus of the liver, when the caudate lobus is involved or when central wounds are present. The technique of balloon tamponade is easy and is described as follows: "The balloon tamponade is accomplished by the use of a 1×12-inch Penrose drain and a 16-French red rubber Robinson catheter. One end of the Penrose drain is ligated with a 2-0 silk suture. The red rubber catheter is placed into the open end of the Penrose, and this end is then ligated with a second 2-0 silk suture, making it air and water tight. This is then passed through the wound, allowing 2–3 cm on each side. The Penrose drain is inflated with sterile normal saline, using an Asepto syringe (gastrographin may be added to make it radio-opaque). The amount of inflation depends on the size of the defect. Normal saline is added until it is clear that tamponage has been achieved" [81]. The balloon inflation time can be between 24 hours and 10 days.

Various balloons specifically designed to stop hemorrhaging are on the market [82–84]. The Sengstaken–Blakemore tube was designed for use in bleeding esophageal varices. The tube has two inflatable balloons, a round one at the distal end and a cone-shaped one in the middle. With the balloons deflated, the tube is inserted into the stomach and the distal balloon is inflated in the stomach. Then the tube is drawn back until the inflated balloon reaches the cardia and increased resistance to withdrawal of the tube is encountered. At that point, the second balloon is inflated. It is now situated in the esophagus and compresses the bleeding varices. The tube is kept under slight tension until the balloon is inflated. After about 12 hours, the balloon is deflated and after

12 more hours, the tube can be gently removed. Bleeding should have stopped by then.

A similar device is the Linton–Nachlas tube. It has only one balloon which is pear-shaped and is situated at the distal end of the tube. The tube is inserted into the stomach, the balloon is inflated, and the tube is pulled back slightly until it meets the resistance of the cardia. Since the balloon is pear-shaped, it fits well into the cardia and compresses bleeding at that point. The Linton tube is mainly used for Mallory–Weiss-tears.

Foley catheters are simple, safe, and effective tools to stop hemorrhage in a wide variety of settings and are also usable in emergencies. Many different bleeding sites can be compressed by the balloons of such catheters. Examples are the retropubic space [85], the prostatic urethra after transurethral resection of the prostate, the cervix [86], the nonpregnant, pregnant or postpartum uterus [87, 88], the nasopharynx [89], the nose in epistaxis [90], colon [91], neck and supraclavicular fossae [92], in bleeding from extraperitoneal pelvic bullet tracks [93], rectum [94], maxillofacial wounds [95], and liver [96]. Foley catheter tamponade has even been employed in unusual situations such as in intercostal hemorrhage in preterm infants [97] and penetrating left ventricular wounds [98]. The catheter can be filled with saline. The balloon may be deflated after a few hours to check whether bleeding has stopped. If this is not so, the catheter can be blocked again by reinjecting saline. Radio-opaque fluid may also be used instead of saline. This permits radiological control of the position of the balloon.

Use of drains

The use and misuse of drains in surgery is an ongoing topic in medical literature. There are not many evidence-based indications for drains. However, drains can increase postoperative blood loss [99, 100].

Complete avoidance of wound drainage is sometimes favored over the use of drains. When blood or other fluids collect in a closed wound cavity, they cause compression and may reduce further blood loss. At times, suction drains are clamped for a certain period after surgery to achieve the same compressive effect, e.g., after knee replacement.

An advanced method of drain use is retrograde infusion of saline into the wound. After knee arthroplasty, about 50 mL saline is injected via the suction drain. When surgery is finished and compressive bandages are applied, saline is infused. To enhance the effect of the saline infusion, a low concentration of epinephrine (1:200000) can be added (at times together with an antibiotic) [101]. After the saline is injected, the drain is clamped and left for a few hours, after which it is unclamped and then suctioned in the routine fashion. Clamp times vary from 1 to 24 hours.

Drain clamping effectively reduces postoperative bleeding after total knee replacement. The hemostatic effect is enhanced by the use of epinephrine in saline when compared with saline alone [102].

Positioning

Appropriate positioning of the patient prior to surgery sometimes improves hemostasis and access to vessels. A lateral position, for instance, may support the surgeon in performing a splenectomy [51]. Elevating the area operated on reduces perfusion in the surgical area and blood loss. Such elevation can easily be accomplished by adjusting the position of the operating table or by using pillows. For more details of intraoperative positioning, please refer to Chapter 14.

Positioning is also important in the postsurgical period. After knee surgery, tension on the wound can be increased by positioning the leg appropriately. This tension aids in hemostasis and decreases blood loss. A pillow to flex both hip and knee joints in a 90° angle helps. The position should be maintained for 24 hours after surgery. Elevation of the knee reduces postoperative hyperemia in the wound and the anatomic dead space within the knee. There are also mechanical components that partially compress the flow in the popliteal vessels [103].

Key points

• Low intraoperative blood loss facilitates surgery in anemic patients.
• The faster appropriate hemostasis is achieved, the better the patient outcome.
• Even the most sophisticated equipment is useful only if the surgeon is capable and willing to avoid any undue blood loss.
• The choice of an appropriate hemostatic device can reduce intraoperative blood loss and transfusions.
• Pay attention to the "tenets of bloodless surgery":

(1) Attention to detail, (2) Partial dissection, (3) Avoid stripping, (4) Anatomical dissection, (5) Gentle tissue handling.

Questions for review

• What are the Halstedian principles?
• What devices are there to make a surgical incision? How do they work? What are the benefits and down-sides of each of the methods?
• How can vessels be occluded to provide hemostasis?
• What are the means to exert compression on a bleeding wound?
• How do drains influence blood loss?

Suggestions for further research

What are safety measures taken in an operating room to prevent hazards potentially caused by surgical methods to cut?
What maintenance measures are required to keep the technical means to make a surgical incision and to stop bleeding functioning?

Exercises and practice cases

With the following exercises, practice skills required for hemostasis and increase your ability to improvise:
• Imagine you are the first on the site of a car accident and the patient is bleeding heavily from his knee; jot down 5 ways to stop the bleeding.
• Gather all the materials needed to make a balloon tamponade as described in the chapter.
• Take a piece of tissue and tailor it to fit around a lacerated liver. Then suture it accordingly.

Homework

For the following devices, research their availability in your home hospital. List its manufacturer and their contact information, the departments where they are used, and the persons who are trained in their use. Record your findings in your address book in the Appendix E.

Scalpel, thermocoagulator, hemostatic scalpel, electrosurgery (mono- + bipolar), saline-enhanced thermal sealing, electrothermal bipolar vessel sealing, microwave coagulation, infrared contact coagulator, laser, plasma scalpel, argon beam coagulation, water jet, high-frequency water jet, harmonic scalpel, cavitron ultrasonic surgical aspirator (CUSA), sutures, clips, endovascular grafting, tourniquets (pneumatic, manual), Bandages, nonadhesive vs. adhesive, packing with towels, absorbable mesh, foley catheter, Sengstaken–Blakemore tube, Linton–Nachlas tube, drains + epinephrine, pillows for positioning.

References

1 Goodrich, J.T. *History of Spine Surgery in the Ancient and Medieval Worlds.* http://www.medscape.com/viewarticle/468452? rss Volume.

2 Sachs, M., M. Auth, and A. Encke. Historical development of surgical instruments exemplified by hemostatic forceps. *World J Surg*, 1998. **22**(5): p. 499–504.

3 Dröge C, V.T.B. *Ambrose Pare. Biographisches-Bibliographisches Kirchenlexikon*, Volume, http://www.bautz.de/bbkl/p/Pare.shtml. 1993.

4 Ruisinger, M.M. Da hilft nur noch die Säge! Die Amputation im 18. Jahrhundert. Institut für Geschichte der Medizin, Erlangen-Nürnberg. Available at: http://www.gesch .med.unierlangen.de/messer/ausstell/amput/t_amp18.htm. Accessed June 11, 2006.

5 Snyder, S.O., Jr. The pneumatic tourniquet: a useful adjunct in lower extremity distal bypass. *Semin Vasc Surg*, 1997. **10**(1): p. 31–33.

6 Sachs, M.S.H. Aus der Geschichte des chirurgischen Instrumentariums: 7. Das erste elektorchirurgische Instrumentarium: Galvanokauter und elektrische Schneideschlinge (1854). *Zentralbl Chir*, 1998. **123**: p. 950–954.

7 Naito, S., *et al.* Application of microwave tissue coagulator in partial nephrectomy for renal cell carcinoma. *J Urol*, 1998. **159**(3): p. 960–962.

8 Spence, R.K., *et al.* Is hemoglobin level alone a reliable predictor of outcome in the severely anemic surgical patient? *Am Surg*, 1992. **58**(2): p. 92–95.

9 Pratali, S., *et al.* Improving hemostasis during replacement of the ascending aorta and aortic valve with a composite graft. *Tex Heart Inst J*, 2000. **27**(3): p. 246–249.

10 Guis, J.A. *Fundamentals of General Surgery*, 2nd edn. Yearbook Medical Publishers, Chicago. 1962. p. 27.

11 Spence, R.K., *et al.* Transfusion and surgery. *Curr Probl Surg*, 1993. **30**(12): p. 1103–1180.

12 Amaral, J.F. Laparoscopic cholecystectomy in 200 consecutive patients using an ultrasonically activated scalpel. *Surg Laparosc Endosc*, 1995. **5**(4): p. 255–262.

13 Glover, J.L., P.J. Bendick, and W.J. Link. The use of thermal knives in surgery: electrosurgery, lasers, plasma scalpel. *Curr Probl Surg*, 1978. **15**(1): p. 1–78.

14 Aagaard, J., B.G. Skov, and E. Hjelms. An experimental study of hot air thermocoagulation in cardiac surgery. *Eur J Cardiothorac Surg*, 1991. **5**(10): p. 546–548.

15 Pilnik, S. and F. Steichen. The use of the hemostatic scalpel in operations upon the breast. *Surg Gynecol Obstet*, 1986. **162**(6): p. 589–591.

16 Ayuste, E., Jr. and M.F. Roxas. Validating the use of rectus muscle fragment welding to control presacral bleeding during rectal mobilization. *Asian J Surg*, 2004. **27**(1): p. 18–21.

17 Xu, J. and J. Lin. Control of presacral hemorrhage with electrocautery through a muscle fragment pressed on the bleeding vein. *J Am Coll Surg*, 1994. **179**(3): p. 351–352.

18 Yim, A.P., *et al.* A new technological approach to nonanatomical pulmonary resection: saline enhanced thermal sealing. *Ann Thorac Surg*, 2002. **74**(5): p. 1671–1676.

19 Pearson M, *et al.* Saline enhanced thermal sealing of tissue: Potential for bloodless surgery. *Min Invas Ther Allied Technol*, 2002. **11**(5/6): p. 265–270.

20 Belli, G., *et al.* Pancreaticoduodenectomy in portal hypertension: use of the Ligasure. *J Hepatobiliary Pancreat Surg*, 2003. **10**(3): p. 215–217.

21 Chung, Y.C. and H.J. Wu. Clinical experience of sutureless closed hemorrhoidectomy with LigaSure. *Dis Colon Rectum*, 2003. **46**(1): p. 87–92.

22 Horgan, P.G. A novel technique for parenchymal division during hepatectomy. *Am J Surg*, 2001. **181**(3): p. 236–237.

23 Tamussino, K., *et al.* Electrosurgical bipolar vessel sealing for radical abdominal hysterectomy. *Gynecol Oncol*, 2005. **96**(2): p. 320–322.

24 Levy, B. and L. Emery. Randomized trial of suture versus electrosurgical bipolar vessel sealing in vaginal hysterectomy. *Obstet Gynecol*, 2003. **102**(1): p. 147–151.

25 Crawford, E.D. Use of the LigaSure vessel sealing system in urologic cancer surgery. *Grand Rounds Urol*, 1999. **1**: p. 10–17.

26 Lau, W.Y., *et al.* Microwave tissue coagulator in liver resection for cirrhotic patients. *Aust N Z J Surg*, 1992. **62**(7): p. 576–581.

27 Zhou, X.D., *et al.* Microwave surgery in the treatment of hepatocellular carcinoma. *Semin Surg Oncol*, 1993. **9**(4): p. 318–322.

28 Angerpointner, T.A., *et al.* Infrared-contact coagulation of parenchymatous organs—report of three cases. *Z Kinderchir*, 1983. **38**(5): p. 356–358.

29 Angerpointner, T.A., K.L. Lauterjung, and A. Hoffecker. Haemostasis in injuries of parenchymatous organs by infrared contact coagulation. *Prog Pediatr Surg*, 1990. **25**: p. 32–38.

30 Hofstetter, A., *et al.* The infrared contact coagulator for hemostasis in the renal parenchyma (author's transl). *MMW Munch Med Wochenschr*, 1976. **118**(47): p. 1537–1540.

31 Welter, H., *et al.* Hemostasis in the liver, lungs, and spleen using an infra-red contact coagulator. *Zentralbl Chir*, 1980. **105**(2): p. 94–101.

32 van Melick, H.H., G.E. van Venrooij, and T.A. Boon. Laser prostatectomy in patients on anticoagulant therapy or with bleeding disorders. *J Urol*, 2003. **170**(5): p. 1851–1855.

33 Dwyer, R. The history of gastrointestinal endoscopic laser hemostasis and management. *Endoscopy*, 1986. **18**(Suppl 1): p. 10–13.

34 Corbitt, J.D., Jr. Laparoscopic cholecystectomy: laser versus electrosurgery. *Surg Laparosc Endosc*, 1991. **1**(2): p. 85–88.

35 Pearlman, N.W., *et al.* A prospective study of incisional time, blood loss, pain, and healing with carbon dioxide laser, scalpel, and electrosurgery. *Arch Surg*, 1991. **126**(8): p. 1018–1020.

36 Wyman, A. and K. Rogers. Randomized trial of laser scalpel for modified radical mastectomy. *Br J Surg*, 1993. **80**(7): p. 871–873.

37 Wyman, A. and K. Rogers. Radical breast surgery with a contact Nd: YAG laser scalpel. *Eur J Surg Oncol*, 1992. **18**(4): p. 322–326.

38 Wyman, A., *et al.* Preliminary evaluation of a new high power diode laser. *Lasers Surg Med*, 1992. **12**(5): p. 506–509.

39 Link, W.J., F.P. Incropera, and J.L. Glover. The plasma scalpel. *Med Prog Technol*, 1976. **4**(3): p. 123–131.

40 Link, W.J., F.P. Incropera, and J.L. Glover. A plasma scalpel: comparison of tissue damage and wound healing with electrosurgical and steel scalpels. *Arch Surg*, 1976. **111**(4): p. 392–397.

41 Khan, K., *et al.* Argon plasma coagulation: clinical experience in pediatric patients. *Gastrointest Endosc*, 2003. **57**(1): p. 110–112.

42 Quinlan, D.M., M.J. Naslund, and C.B. Brendler. Application of argon beam coagulation in urological surgery. *J Urol*, 1992. **147**(2): p. 410–412.

43 Rolachon, A., E. Papillon, and J. Fournet. Is argon plasma coagulation an efficient treatment for digestive system vascular malformation and radiation proctitis? *Gastroenterol Clin Biol*, 2000. **24**(12): p. 1205–1210.

44 Ward, P.H., D.J. Castro, and S. Ward. A significant new contribution to radical head and neck surgery. The argon beam coagulator as an effective means of limiting blood loss. *Arch Otolaryngol Head Neck Surg*, 1989. **115**(8): p. 921–923.

45 Baer, H.U., *et al.* Hepatic resection using a water jet dissector. *HPB Surg*, 1993. **6**(3): p. 189–196; discussion 196–198.

46 Rau, H.G., *et al.* Liver resection with the water jet: conventional and laparoscopic surgery. *Chirurg*, 1996. **67**(5): p. 546–551.

47 Basting, R.F., N. Djakovic, and P. Widmann. Use of water jet resection in organ-sparing kidney surgery. *J Endourol*, 2000. **14**(6): p. 501–505.

48 Oertel, J., M.R. Gaab, and J. Piek. Waterjet resection of brain metastases—first clinical results with 10 patients. *Eur J Surg Oncol*, 2003. **29**(4): p. 407–414.

49 Shekarriz, H., *et al.* Hydro-Jet-assisted laparoscopic cholecystectomy: a prospective randomized clinical study. *Surgery*, 2003. **133**(6): p. 635–640.

50 Rau, H.G., *et al.* Jet-cutting supported by high frequency current: new technique for hepatic surgery. *World J Surg*, 1997. **21**(3): p. 254–259; discussion 259–260.

51 Rothenberg, S.S. Laparoscopic splenectomy using the harmonic scalpel. *J Laparoendosc Surg*, 1996. **6**(Suppl 1): p. S61–S63.

52 Fasulo, F., *et al.* Cavitron ultrasonic surgical aspirator (CUSA) in liver resection. *Int Surg*, 1992. **77**(1): p. 64–66.

53 Daskalopoulos, G., *et al.* Electrothermal bipolar coagulation for radical prostatectomies and cystectomies: a preliminary case-controlled study. *Int Urol Nephrol*, 2004. **36**(2): p. 181–185.

54 Kurtz, S.B. and D.B. Frost. A comparison of two surgical techniques for performing mastectomy. *Eur J Surg Oncol*, 1995. **21**(2): p. 143–145.

55 Miller, E., *et al.* Scalpel versus electrocautery in modified radical mastectomy. *Am Surg*, 1988. **54**(5): p. 284–286.

56 Smyrniotis, V.E., *et al.* Selective hepatic vascular exclusion versus Pringle maneuver in major liver resections: prospective study. *World J Surg*, 2003. **27**(7): p. 765–769.

57 Makuuchi, M., *et al.* Safety of hemihepatic vascular occlusion during resection of the liver. *Surg Gynecol Obstet*, 1987. **164**(2): p. 155–158.

58 Quan, D. and W.J. Wall. The safety of continuous hepatic inflow occlusion during major liver resection. *Liver Transpl Surg*, 1996. **2**(2): p. 99–104.

59 Kwawukume, E.Y. and T.S. Ghosh. Extraperitoneal hypogastric artery ligation in control of intractable haemorrhage from advanced carcinoma of cervix and choriocarcinoma. *East Afr Med J*, 1996. **73**(2): p. 147–148.

60 Erzurum, V.Z., *et al.* Inferior vena cava endograft to control surgically inaccessible hemorrhage. *J Vasc Surg*, 2003. **38**(6): p. 1437–1439.

61 Weiss, V.J. and E.L. Chaikof. Endovascular treatment of vascular injuries. *Surg Clin North Am*, 1999. **79**(3): p. 653–665.

62 Kapma, M.R., *et al.* Endovascular treatment of acute abdominal aortic aneurysm with a bifurcated stent graft. *Eur J Vasc Endovasc Surg*, 2005. **29**(5): p. 510–515.

63 Gine, E., *et al.* Successful treatment of severe hemorrhagic cystitis after hemopoietic cell transplantation by selective embolization of the vesical arteries. *Bone Marrow Transplant*, 2003. **31**(10): p. 923–925.

64 MacKenzie, S., *et al.* Recent experiences with a multidisciplinary approach to complex hepatic trauma. *Injury*, 2004. **35**(9): p. 869–877.

65 Liu, P.P., *et al.* Use of splenic artery embolization as an adjunct to nonsurgical management of blunt splenic injury. *J Trauma*, 2004. **56**(4): p. 768–772; discussion 773.

66 Kimbrell, B.J., *et al.* Angiographic embolization for pelvic fractures in older patients. *Arch Surg*, 2004. **139**(7): p. 728–732; discussion 732–733.

67 Wirbel, R.J., *et al.* Preoperative embolization in spinal and pelvic metastases. *J Orthop Sci*, 2005. **10**(3): p. 253–257.

68 Ngeh, N., *et al.* Pre-myomectomy uterine artery embolisation minimises operative blood loss. *BJOG*, 2004. **111**(10): p. 1139–1140.

69 Weinstein, A., *et al.* Conservative management of placenta previa percreta in a Jehovah's Witness. *Obstet Gynecol*, 2005. **105**(5, Pt 2): p. 1247–1250.

70 Tesdal, I.K., *et al.* Transjugular intrahepatic portosystemic shunts: adjunctive embolotherapy of gastroesophageal collateral vessels in the prevention of variceal rebleeding. *Radiology*, 2005. **236**(1): p. 360–367.

71 Jorn, L.P., A. Lindstrand, and S. Toksvig-Larsen. Tourniquet release for hemostasis increases bleeding. A randomized study of 77 knee replacements. *Acta Orthop Scand*, 1999. **70**(3): p. 265–267.

72 Ikeda, T., *et al.* Tourniquet technique prevents profuse blood loss in placenta accreta cesarean section. *J Obstet Gynaecol Res*, 2005. **31**(1): p. 27–31.

73 Naimer, S.A., N. Anat, and G. Katif. Evaluation of techniques for treating the bleeding wound. *Injury*, 2004. **35**(10): p. 974–979.

74 Kin, N., *et al.* External manual compression of the abdominal aorta to control hemorrhage from a ruptured aneurysm. *J Anesth*, 2002. **16**(2): p. 164–166.

75 Diagnosis and management of postpartum hemorrhage. ACOG technical bulletin number 143—July 1990. *Int J Gynaecol Obstet*, 1991. **36**(2): p. 159–163.

76 Vournakis, J.N., *et al.* The RDH bandage: hemostasis and survival in a lethal aortotomy hemorrhage model. *J Surg Res*, 2003. **113**(1): p. 1–5.

77 Poretti, F., *et al.* Chitosan pads vs. manual compression to control bleeding sites after transbrachial arterial catheterization in a randomized trial. *ROFO*, 2005. **177**(9): p. 1260–1266.

78 Shen, G.K. and W. Rappaport. Control of nonhepatic intraabdominal hemorrhage with temporary packing. *Surg Gynecol Obstet*, 1992. **174**(5): p. 411–413.

79 Stevens, S.L., K.I. Maull, and B.L. Enderson. Total hepatic mesh wrap for hemostasis. *Surg Gynecol Obstet*, 1992. **175**(2): p. 181–182.

80 Leemans, R. and J.B. van Mourik. A new surgical, splenic salvage technique: the Vicryl net. *Neth J Surg*, 1987. **39**(6): p. 197–198.

81 Seligman, J.Y. and M. Egan. Balloon tamponade: an alternative in the treatment of liver trauma. *Am Surg*, 1997. **63**(11): p. 1022–1023.

82 Burcharth, F. and J. Malmstrom. Experiences with the Linton–Nachlas and the Sengstaken–Blakemore tubes for bleeding esophageal varices. *Surg Gynecol Obstet*, 1976. **142**(4): p. 529–531.

83 Panes, J., *et al.* Efficacy of balloon tamponade in treatment of bleeding gastric and esophageal varices. Results in 151 consecutive episodes. *Dig Dis Sci*, 1988. **33**(4): p. 454–459.

84 Teres, J., *et al.* Esophageal tamponade for bleeding varices. Controlled trial between the Sengstaken–Blakemore tube and the Linton–Nachlas tube. *Gastroenterology*, 1978. **75**(4): p. 566–569.

85 Aungst, M. and M. Wagner. Foley balloon to tamponade bleeding in the retropubic space. *Obstet Gynecol*, 2003. **102**(5, Pt 1): p. 1037–1038.

86 Bowen, L.W. and J.H. Beeson. Use of a large Foley catheter balloon to control postpartum hemorrhage resulting from a low placental implantation. A report of two cases. *J Reprod Med*, 1985. **30**(8): p. 623–625.

87 Garcia Leon, F., *et al.* Current state of uterine tamponade with Foley catheter in intractable bleeding. *Ginecol Obstet Mex*, 1998. **66**: p. 483–485.

88 Marcovici, I. and B. Scoccia. Postpartum hemorrhage and intrauterine balloon tamponade. A report of three cases. *J Reprod Med*, 1999. **44**(2): p. 122–126.

89 de Figueiredo, D.G. and F.F. de Carvalho. Balloon tamponade of the pharynx in transnasophenoidal operations: technical note. *Neurosurgery*, 1981. **8**(5): p. 567–568.

90 Wurtele, P. How I do it: emergency nasal packing using an umbilical cord clamp to secure a Foley catheter for posterior epistaxis. *J Otolaryngol*, 1996. **25**(1): p. 46–47.

91 Ganchrow, M.I. and T.L. Facelle. Control of hemorrhage from a mucous fistula with Foley catheter tamponade. *Dis Colon Rectum*, 1992. **35**(10): p. 1001–1002.

92 Gilroy, D., *et al.* Control of life-threatening haemorrhage from the neck: a new indication for balloon tamponade. *Injury*, 1992. **23**(8): p. 557–559.

93 Gonzalez, R.P., *et al.* A method for management of extraperitoneal pelvic bleeding secondary to penetrating trauma. *J Trauma*, 1997. **43**(2): p. 338–341.

94 Khan, S.A., *et al.* Hemorrhoidal bleeding following transrectal prostatic biopsy. Etiology and management. *Dis Colon Rectum*, 1982. **25**(8): p. 817–819.

95 Shuker, S. The management of hemorrhage from severe missile injuries using Foley catheter balloon tamponade. *J Oral Maxillofac Surg*, 1989. **47**(6): p. 646–648.

96 Thomas, S.V., S.A. Dulchavsky, and L.N. Diebel. Balloon tamponade for liver injuries: case report. *J Trauma*, 1993. **34**(3): p. 448–449.

97 McElroy, S.J., J.B. Pietsch, and J. Reese. Foley catheter tamponade of intercostal hemorrhage in preterm infants. *J Pediatr*, 2004. **145**(2): p. 241.

98 McQuillan, R.F., T. McCormack, and M.C. Neligan. Penetrating left ventricular stab wound: a method of control during resuscitation and prior to repair. *Injury*, 1981. **13**(1): p. 63–65.

99 Parker, M.J., C.P. Roberts, and D. Hay. Closed suction drainage for hip and knee arthroplasty. A meta-analysis. *J Bone Joint Surg Am*, 2004. **86-A**(6): p. 1146–1152.

100 Walmsley, P.J., *et al.* A prospective, randomised, controlled trial of the use of drains in total hip arthroplasty. *J Bone Joint Surg Br*, 2005. **87**(10): p. 1397–1401.

101 Yamada, K., *et al.* Comparison between 1-hour and 24-hour drain clamping using diluted epinephrine solution after total knee arthroplasty. *J Arthroplasty*, 2001. **16**(4): p. 458–462.

102 Ryu, J., *et al.* The postoperative drain-clamping method for hemostasis in total knee arthroplasty. Reducing postoperative bleeding in total knee arthroplasty. *Bull Hosp Jt Dis*, 1997. **56**(4): p. 251–254.

103 Timlin, M., *et al.* The 90/90 pillow reduces blood loss after knee arthroplasty: a prospective randomized case control study. *J Arthroplasty*, 2003. **18**(6): p. 765–768.

14 Anesthesia—more than sleeping

The anesthetist plays an important role in the perioperative blood management of patients. His work is not just inducing hypnosis, relaxation, and pain control, but also includes many facets of blood management. This includes preparing the patient for surgery, reducing blood loss during surgery, and caring for the patient after surgery. This chapter will outline some of the basic methods which an anesthetist can use to reduce his patient's blood loss and to enhance his outcome.

Objectives of this chapter

1 Explain the role of an anesthetist in a blood management team.
2 Identify a variety of methods an anesthetist can use to reduce blood loss.
3 Describe the impact of these measures on the overall blood management of the patient.

Definitions

Anesthesiology: The medical specialty of preparing patients for anesthesia, rendering patients insensitive for painful surgical, obstetrical, diagnostic and other therapeutic procedures, and monitoring, maintaining or restoring homeostasis in perioperative and critically ill patients.

The anesthetist in a blood management team

Anesthetists are vital for a blood management team. They should be included in the planning team for a patient's procedure right from the beginning. Anesthetists contribute to the success of the team with their experience in preparing patients for surgery. Also, the various intraoperative and postoperative activities they perform, as well as their knowledge of the therapy of severely sick patients, are of great benefit for the team.

Preoperatively, anesthetists are in a good position to coordinate the optimization of the patient's condition. In many hospitals around the world, the anesthetist meets with the patient well before surgery. He is therefore in a good position to detect obstacles to optimal blood management at an early stage. This is due to an initial assessment of the patient performed during the preoperative visit of the anesthetist. Typically, anesthetists aim at optimizing the cardiopulmonary function of the patient. They might also be able to assess the hematological status of the patient and may resolve any derangements (coagulopathy or anemia) if they are present. In cooperation with the surgeon, he can adapt anticoagulatory regimens, change drug regimens if necessary and initiate specialist consultations when needed. The best anesthetic procedure can be chosen. Besides, logistical decisions can be made by the anesthetists, e.g., ordering drugs or special monitoring or cell salvage devices for use in the operating room.

Intraoperatively, the anesthetist is responsible for the well-being of the patient. This includes not only administering anesthesia, but also monitoring the cardiopulmonary and hematological status, administration of fluids and drugs, performing autologous transfusion, and stabilizing the cardiopulmonary condition of the patient. The anesthetist cooperates closely with the surgical team to position the patient.

Postoperatively, the anesthetist is responsible for the care of the patient in the recovery room and sometimes even for some time after the patient has returned to the ward. There, he can oversee the return of autologous blood, administer further drugs, and continue monitoring the patient.

In the intensive care unit and the emergency room, anesthetists often care for severely sick patients. Such patients are often eligible for blood management measures. As such, they benefit also from the anesthetists expertise in the various aspects of blood management.

All this shows that it is vital for a blood management team to include anesthetists right from the beginning of patient care. Besides, it demonstrates that all anesthetists should be aware of the immense role they can play in blood management and should therefore educate themselves continually to keep pace with modern blood management rather than limping behind on the crutches of outdated transfusion therapy.

Specific intraoperative anesthetic measures to reduce blood loss

Positioning

Before surgery starts, the patient is usually positioned to meet the needs of the surgery. Positioning allows a good view of the body part being operated on. It also allows for comfortable access to the surgical site and minimizes the risk of nerve damage and compression damage due to a certain position. Another aspect of positioning is its ability to reduce blood loss. For many types of surgery, there are different positions that are suitable for the intended operation. Some of them may increase blood loss, while others decrease it. The choice of a patient's position must take reduction of blood loss into consideration.

Some basic mechanisms explain how blood loss can be influenced by the position of the patient. To a certain extent, the position of a patient determines the perfusion of the body. Blood flow and pressure in different vascular sections vary with the position of the patient. In the venous system, the blood pressure is determined by hydrostatic pressure (as determined by hydration status and position) and by transmural pressure. When the patient stands, approximately 500–800 mL of blood follow gravity and is found in the depending parts of the body. This effect is reversed when the patient is brought into the supine position. In arteries, the blood flow and pressure is much less dependent on volume and position. Arterial blood pressure is actively regulated by humoral factors (e.g., epinephrine) and neurovegetative reflex mechanisms. The global blood pressure is maintained by reflex mechanisms that also react to changes in posture so that perfusion pressure of vital organs is maintained.

Surgical positions affect blood pressure and flow. When a patient is positioned on his abdomen, blood is squeezed into the extremities and the venous return flow is hindered. The preload and the cardiac output are reduced. Besides, when the vena cava is compressed, blood pressure therein

rises [1] and blood flows increasingly through anastomoses found peri- and intravertebrally. This increases the perfusion of the spinal region.

When the patient is positioned with his legs positioned higher than his head (Trendelenburg position, lithotomy position), blood returns readily to the trunk and preload increases. In this position, normally baroreceptor reflexes are elicited, and blood pressure increases, but cardiac output decreases. On the other hand, when the patient's feet are positioned below the level of the head (reverse Trendelenburg position, sitting position), venous return is decreased. When the patient's legs and hips are flexed, the venous return flow is hindered even further. Again, this decreases preload and cardiac output. However, if baroreceptors are intact, peripheral vascular resistance increases and blood pressure returns near to normal.

These physiological reactions of the body in response to a change in position can be used effectively to reduce blood loss. It must be taken into consideration through, that reflex mechanisms that would allow a hemodynamic response to the position may be blunted by anesthetics.

Two basic principles should guide the preoperative positioning of the patient.
• First principle: Elevate the surgical field.

If possible, the surgical field should be elevated above the heart level. This decreases the perfusion pressure in the vessels of the surgical area. Some examples may illustrate this. For prostatectomy, a patient can be kept at a 25–30% Trendelenburg position to reduce blood loss [2]. Orthognathic procedures can be performed in the head-up position to reduce blood loss [3]. Patients for intracranial surgery can often be positioned in sitting posture. Sitting up of the patient seems to be associated with a reduced blood loss and lesser transfusions when compared with horizontal positioning [4].
• Second principle: Do not compress venous drainage of the surgical field.

This means that unnecessary flexion of the extremities should be avoided. Besides, the patient's body or positioning tools should not be placed so as to compress venous plexus or other main routes of venous drainage. Here are some examples: In head surgery, the head should not be turned to one side or the other in order not to hinder venous drainage of the surgical field. If the patient is positioned supine for abdominal surgery, compression of the vena cava should be avoided and pressure should be taken from the cava. This is easily accomplished by slightly rotating the operating table to the left. When the patient is in the prone position, e.g., for spinal or other back surgery,

Table 14.1 Positions proposed to reduce blood loss in spinal surgery.

Positions without frames	Positions with frames
Use of chest rolls	Canadian frame (Hastings 1969)
Kneeling position (Ecker 1949)	Relton-Hall frame (1969)
Mohammedan praying position (Lipton 1950)	Andrews frame
Knee–chest position (Tarlov 1967)	Wilson bank
Tuck position (Wayne 1967)	Jackson table
	Cloward surgical saddle Heffington frame

Remarks in parentheses: Person who was attributed to have it described first.

pressure should be taken from the abdomen and especially the vena cava. This can be done by supporting the hips and the shoulders with pillows or other devices (frames) (Table 14.1). The blood can now follow gravity and collects in the abdomen, rather than in the surgical area [1]. Blood loss decreases [5].

Intraoperative positioning may also serve purposes that are only tangentially associated with reducing blood loss. Liver resection may be performed in 15° head-down position. This may seem contrary to the principle of positioning patients with elevated surgical fields. However, when liver surgery is performed in controlled hypotension tilting the head down may improve renal perfusion and aid in maintaining a marginal urine output during surgery [6]. Thus, this position may allow for reduction of blood loss by means of the reduced systemic blood pressure without unduly compromising renal perfusion.

Using certain positions may indeed reduce blood loss. However, care must be taken that nerves are not injured, eyes not unduly compressed, and joints not overly flexed, being especially detrimental for patients with joint replacement or joint diseases. As well, an overly flexed position may cause vascular compression and myolysis with resulting renal failure. Therefore, care must be taken that the chosen position is attained carefully and points of pressure must be padded.

The patient's posture not only influences intraoperative blood loss, but may also be important in the postoperative period. In the recovery room, patients can be positioned to reduce blood loss from a variety of sites. The same basic principles of intraoperative positioning apply here as well.

After knee surgery, the leg can be elevated in the hip (35° flexion) and kept straight in the knee or the knee (70–90°) and the hip (90°) can be flexed. Both measures seem to reduce blood loss significantly [7].

Controlled hypotension

Surgical bleeding is a result of many factors, ranging from the number and size of dissected blood vessels, the time until bleeding vessels are closed, the coagulation profile of the patient, and the blood pressure in the opened blood vessels. Reducing the latter—in the form of controlled hypotension—is a simple and effective means to reduce blood loss.

The concept of controlled hypotension (also called induced hypotension or deliberate hypotension) means purposely reducing the blood pressure during surgery in which major blood loss is expected. This translates into reduced hydrostatic pressure in the vessels in the wound and leads to the reduction of blood loss. This kind of hypotension is typically induced by reducing the peripheral vascular resistance. The aim is to maintain the cardiac output despite reduced blood pressure.

It is not only a low blood pressure that reduces blood flow to the wound. Blood flow is also a result of the cardiac output. If cardiac output is very high, blood flow can be increased despite the pressure being low. It has been claimed that the cardiac output (and especially the heart rate) needs to be normalized in order to reduce blood loss. Otherwise, controlled hypotension was thought to be ineffective [8]. However, it has also been claimed that despite an increased cardiac output, hypotension has reduced blood loss [9].

While low blood pressure may be beneficial to reduce blood loss, too low may also be detrimental. A basic understanding of the pathophysiology of hypotension is needed to practice this safely. Hypotension may be divided in two groups, the first being induced by volume or blood loss. This results in vasoconstriction and in a reduced cardiac output with low blood flow. This reduction in blood flow reduces the blood pressure and causes hypotension. This kind of hypotension may be detrimental since it may result in ischemic complications. The second kind of hypotension is caused by vasodilatation and results in a compensatory increased cardiac output. The latter form of hypotension does not pose such a high risk for ischemia as the first one.

Practically speaking, there are three ways to induce controlled hypotension: fluid restriction, vasodialating drugs, and regional anesthesia. Restricting fluid administration

Table 14.2 Agents for induction of controlled hypotension.

Agent	Group/mechanism of action	Remarks
Adenosine	Endogenous purine analogue	Potent vasodilator, acts more on arteries then on veins, very short half life, continuous infusion required
Esmolol	Beta-receptor blocker, negative inotrope, vasodilatation	Rapid acting
Nitroprusside	Direct vasodilatation, forms nitric oxide	Cave: cyanide poisoning may occur in prolonged use, relaxes arterial and venous smooth muscles
Nitroglycerin	Smooth muscle relaxation, forms nitric oxide	Venous dilatation more pronounced than arterial dilatation
Trimetaphan	Ganglion blocker, direct smooth muscle relaxation	Arterial and venous dilatation, decreases cardiac output
Nicardipine	Calcium channel blocker, negative inotrope, vasodilatation	Rapid acting
Fenoldopam	Dopamine D1 receptor agonist	May preserve renal and splanchnic perfusion in hypotension
Prostaglandin E1 (PGE1)	Vasodilator	Mechanism of action mainly unknown
Labetalol	Sympathetic receptor blocker (alpha 1, beta 1, beta 2)	Lowers blood pressure without reflex tachycardia
Isoflurane, desflurane	Inhalational anesthetics	Arterial dilatation more pronounced than venous dilatation
Propofol	Intravenous anesthetic	
Morphine	Opioid	Arterial and venous pressure decrease (histamine release, vascular tone reduced)
Fentanyl, Remifentanil	Opioids	

may also contribute to hypotension. This seems to be effective for selected patients undergoing procedures with a limited duration. However, restricting volume infusion during surgery only to induce hypotension comes with the increased risk of regional ischemia. Therefore, fluid restriction is usually not an option. This is especially true when a procedure is expected to be prolonged and/or severe blood loss is anticipated.

The second way to induce hypotension is more practical. It uses drugs to induce vasodilatation. A variety of agents have been proposed for this purpose [10–12] (Table 14.2). It has not yet been determined which drug is best for a given situation. Some of the drugs primarily reduce venous pressure, while others predominantly the arterial pressure. A common way to induce hypotension is by using anesthetics, such as gases (desflurane, sevoflurane, and isoflurane), which induce mainly vasodilatation. Intravenous anesthetics (propofol or thiopental) also induce hypotension but mainly by reducing cardiac output, a less desirable effect. High-dose fentanyl (30 mcg/kg) has

been used for induction of controlled hypotension [13]. Remifentanil is also usable to induce hypotension and may be easily titrated. Another group of drugs are those not used for anesthesia but for the sole purpose of inducing hypotension [14]. Table 14.2 shows some of the drugs that have been used for induction and maintenance of hypotension.

The third way to induce hypotension resorts to regional or epidural anesthesia of which induces vasodilatation in the anesthetized parts of the body by reducing sympathetic activity. The required degree of hypotension is achievable with a combination of bolus or continuous epidural infusion, possibly with a vasopressor to counteract any overshooting hypotension [15]. Epidural anesthesia combines the blood-saving properties of regional anesthesia with those of controlled hypotension.

Controlled hypotension is a very old and time-proven technique. When only moderate degrees of hypotension are used (80–90 mm Hg systolic), it is very safe for the majority of patients. However, there are some patients who may experience side effects and therefore need to be excluded from (marked) hypotension. Patient selection is therefore essential. Patients who have an impaired vascular response (as in untreated hypertension, atherosclerosis, or diabetes mellitus) or those who are susceptible to ischemia (severe ischemic heart or brain disease) may not undergo hypotension or at least not to the same degree as healthy patients. However, it may actually be possible to use mild hypotensive anesthesia in some of these patients as well.

In surgery using hypotensive anesthesia, a goal must be set. On the one hand, the blood pressure must be reduced to an extent that blood loss decreases; on the other hand, perfusion of vital organs must be maintained. Controlled hypotension is usually targeted to a certain mean arterial or systolic pressure. Different levels of hypotension have been described: mild hypotension with a mean arterial pressure of 70–80 mm Hg, moderate hypotension with a mean arterial pressure of 55–70 mm Hg, and marked hypotension with mean arterial pressure of 45–55 mm Hg. In other instances, the central venous pressure, rather than the mean arterial pressure is used as a guide. This is the case in liver surgery since blood loss during such procedures depends more on the central venous rather than on the arterial blood pressure. Low central venous pressure, e.g., of not more than 5 mm Hg, may be a reasonable goal to reduce blood loss in liver surgery [6, 16, 17].

Intraoperative monitoring also contributes to the safety of controlled hypotension. For safe monitoring of controlled hypotension, a continuous arterial blood pressure reading is desirable. Signs of hypoperfusion and cardiac impairment must be recognized (serum lactate, acidosis, reduced urine output, ST-segment changes, and arrythmia on the EKG). If the pulse oximeter does not show a reading, systemic hypoperfusion may have developed. For some indications, such as spinal surgery, evoked EEG potentials are used to monitor the progress of surgery. These may also be used to monitor hypovolemia. When latency or amplitude of the potentials increases, hypotension may be the cause and should be abandoned. When anemia reaches below a certain hematocrit level, controlled hypotension should be abandoned [18].

When the above-mentioned precautions are taken, side effects are extremely rare. When they occur, then they are usually the result of regional hypoperfusion. Rare occasions of myocardial ischemia or infarction have been reported. A very rare, yet much feared, complication of controlled hypotension is ischemic optic neuropathy, resulting in postoperative blindness. This has been described in cardiac surgery patients who were severely anemic and recently also in patients having received spinal surgery, especially when performed in prone position. Although it is not proven that hypotension is the cause for this blindness, it seems to contribute to its development.

Controlled hypotension is usable for many surgeries, such as joint arthroplasty [19], spinal surgery [18], prostatectomy [20], cystectomy [21], burn surgery, orthognathic surgery [22], and gynecological surgery. It may be used in adults as well as in children. Studies report reductions of blood loss of about 50% compared to that of the control group. In addition, reductions of transfusion volume have been reported to range from 20 to 83% [9].

Hypotensive anesthesia is most useful when combined with other measures, such as cell salvage, surgical techniques for hemostasis, and anesthetic measures to reduce blood loss. While somewhat controversial, controlled hypotension has also been successfully used in combination with moderate acute normovolemic hemodilution [23]. Hypotensive anesthesia may be a suitable measure for reducing of blood loss when other blood-sparing techniques are deemed contraindicated, e.g., in infected prosthesis after hip replacement.

Warming

The human body was designed to work best at 37°C. This is particularly true of the many enzymatic reactions that are vital for health, including those participating in the clotting process. Additionally, the platelet count in peripheral blood is higher in normothermic individuals compared with hypothermic patients. When a patient becomes hypothermic, he develops a profound, yet reversible hemostatic defect. This is caused by platelet dysfunction (platelet thromboxane A2 and glycoprotein IB decrease). The humoral clotting factor activity is reduced. Fibrinolysis is increased [24]. It comes as no surprise that blood loss increases when patients get cold. Patients who are at special risk of becoming chilled are those undergoing surgery. A marked reduction of the core temperature can already be seen after induction of general anesthesia. This is due to a redistribution of cold blood from the periphery to the core, as well as reduced metabolic heat production during anesthesia. In addition, infusing fluids at room temperature reduces the core temperature. And during surgery, the patient loses even more heat in the cold environment of the operating room.

It was shown that patients with lower than optimal body temperature lose more blood. Therefore, in an attempt to reduce blood loss, an anesthetist needs to keep his patients warm. Several methods have been described.

Patients should be covered with warm blankets at arrival in the preoperative holding area or in the operating room. They should be actively warmed for about 30 minutes before induction of anesthesia. This process is called pre-warming. The idea behind this procedure is that patients who are actively warmed to have warm extremities do not suffer from a drop of their core temperature when anesthesia causes a redistribution of blood flow. This prevents the aforementioned drop of core temperature. In addition to prewarming, all fluids given to the patient need to be warmed. Also, ambient air temperature can be increased.

By warming the patient, considerable reductions in blood loss as well as in transfusion of allogeneic blood products have been described in gastrointestinal [25] as well as in orthopedic surgery [26, 27]. The reduction of blood loss ranged from 20 to 25%.

Choice of ventilation patterns and blood loss

How a patient is ventilated influences the amount of blood lost during surgery. Essentially, two mechanisms have been postulated: changes of intravascular pressure and reflex vasoconstriction or vasodilatation induced by ventilation.

Mechanical ventilation with positive pressure, typically used during general anesthesia, has profound hemodynamic effects. These effects are pronounced when large tidal volumes are used as well as during the application of positive end-expiratory pressure (PEEP). Due to the resulting increase in intrathoracic pressure, the pressure in intrathoracic vessels increases. When the patient is in the prone position, an increased intra-abdominal pressure may add to increased pressure that results from high pressure ventilation. The venous return is reduced. This may lead to increased venous bleeding (especially in caval anastomoses).

Ventilation of the patient influences the level of blood gases. When a patient is hypoventilated, that is, hypercapnic and/or hypoxic, sympathetic stimulation and other reflex mechanisms change the vascular tone. The systemic arterial pressure rises. On the contrary, when a patient is hyperventilated, only intracranial (intact) vessels constrict, while vessels in the periphery dilate. Such effects can be used to a certain extent to reduce blood loss.

Adjusting ventilatory patterns in order to reduce blood loss have been attempted. It has been established that ventilation with high pressures during hepatic surgery contributes to an increased blood loss. Therefore, it may be wise to reduce the PEEP or to avoid it entirely during phases of surgery where blood loss from the liver usually occurs. It has also been proposed that the use of increased PEEP in postoperative cardiac patients may reduce blood loss. However, this seems not to be the case [28]. It was also proposed to use spontaneous ventilation during general anesthesia in order to reduce blood loss, since spontaneous ventilation does not increase blood pressures as in general anesthesia with mechanical ventilation [29].

As a general rule, normoxia and normocapnia using normoventilation should be achieved during anesthesia. Hypoventilation must be avoided. When local anesthesia is used together with sedation, care must be taken that the level of sedation does not induce hypoventilation. This would lead to hypercapnia with resulting increased blood loss. In contrast, under certain circumstances, mild hyperventilation may theoretically aid in reducing blood loss. Since hyperventilation causes vasoconstriction in certain areas of the body, such as the brain and the uterus, it may be used to reduce blood loss during surgery on these body parts. However, a study on patients receiving uterine evacuation did not confirm these theoretical advantages of hyperventilation [30].

Choice of drugs

Anesthetics exert a variety of effects which may contribute to the amount of blood lost during surgery. Generally, anesthesia must be deep enough to prevent sympathetic stimulation in reaction to surgical activities. Such stimulation would increase the blood pressure and with it the blood loss.

As was shown decades ago, blood loss varies with the chosen drugs. See Table 14.3 for measurements made during uterine evacuation [30].

The reasons for the differences in blood loss in relation to the chosen anesthetic drug are not clear. One reason may be that many anesthetics impair coagulation [31].

Table 14.3 Blood loss in relation to the chosen anesthetic regimen for uterine evacuation.

Drug regime	Blood loss in mL
1% halothane	283
0.5% halothane + 75% nitrous oxide	169
0.5% halothane + 75% nitrous oxide + thiopental + meperidine	286
5% fluroxene	233
80% nitrous oxide + thiopental + meperidine	58
Paracervical block with 1% lidocaine	25

Halothane seems to be the most potent platelet inhibitor compared with other inhalational agents. Sevoflurane also seems to have clinically important inhibitory actions on platelets, while this seems not to be true for isoflurane and desflurane. The inhibitory effects of inhalational agents on platelets seem to last 1–6 hours postoperatively. Nitrous oxide also seems to have inhibitory effects on coagulation, but its role is controversial. Propofol, in clinically used doses also inhibits platelets, while barbiturates and benzodiazepines do not seem to do this. There are no data available whether etomidate or ketamine affect bleeding. Opioids, clonidine, and muscle relaxants also seem not to affect clotting ability. Local anesthetics exert an antithrombotic effect and inhibit platelets, but only in higher than clinically used concentrations. Many of the drugs used as anesthetic adjuvants also impair coagulation, among them starch and dextrane solutions as well as a variety of antibiotics. Avoiding such platelet inhibitors may be clinically significant when patients have reduced levels or an impaired function of platelets and in patients where hemostasis is critical.

Timing of fluid administration

Restrictive fluid administration before surgical hemostasis is achieved may contribute to the reduction of blood loss. When fluids are used cautiously until hemostasis is achieved, the intravascular pressure is not as high as it would be with liberal fluid administration, and hemostasis may be easier to achieve in the not so intensely distended veins. After the major bleeding is controlled, normovolemia must be established [2, 6].

Choice of anesthetic procedure

The choice of the anesthetic given affects the perisurgical blood loss. In general, regional anesthesia seems to reduce blood loss when compared with general anesthesia. This was studied mainly for epidural and spinal anesthesia, but occasionally also in plexus anesthesia [32]. Initially, it was thought that spinal and epidural anesthesia reduce blood loss, since they induce arterial hypotension. This may be the case. However, patients who receive epidural anesthesia but who are kept normotensive during surgery lose less blood than with general anesthesia. Other mechanisms may, therefore, play a role in epidural anesthesia. Peripheral venous blood pressure is also reduced, resulting in a reduced oozing from the wound. This effect is observable intraoperatively and may also extend into the postoperative period. Spontaneous ventilation, which does not

increase the pressure in the vena cava (as does mechanical ventilation), has been implicated as a reason for the reduced blood loss.

The reduction of blood loss during epidural anesthesia has been demonstrated in a variety of procedures, among them gynecological, urological [33], and orthopedic [29]. For knee replacement, hypotensive epidural anesthesia without tourniquet use reduces total blood loss even more than spinal anesthesia with tourniquet [34]. Even in spinal surgery, epidural anesthesia in combination with general anesthesia reduces blood loss. However, this effect is seen mainly in procedures performed on the lumbar, but not the thoracic spine [35]. When comparing epidural with general anesthesia for elective Cesarean section for placenta previa, transfusions were reduced in the epidural group [36]. In contrast, epidural anesthesia seems not to reduce intraoperative blood loss in gastrointestinal surgery [37].

Key points

• The anesthetist contributes many facets to the blood management of a patient. This includes preoperative measures, intra- and postoperative reductions of blood loss and the care of the critically ill or severely injured. He is therefore best involved with the planning of procedures from the time the patient present himself for evaluation.
• There are a variety of anesthetic methods that reduce blood losses, including
  ○ Positioning intra- and postoperatively
  ○ Controlled hypotension
  ○ Warming of the patient
  ○ Choice of ventilation patterns
  ○ Choice of drugs
  ○ Timing of fluid administration
  ○ Choice of anesthetic procedure
• When appropriate, different methods can be combined to enhance their blood-sparing effects.

Questions for review

• Why is it important to warm the patient before induction of anesthesia?
• How does the choice of the anesthetic procedure affect blood loss?
• Which two basic principles aimed at reducing blood loss underlie the positioning of patients?
• By what mechanisms do anesthetic agents influence intraoperative blood loss?

• What monitoring methods may be useful for patients undergoing controlled hypotension? What are you looking for during the monitoring? What would prompt you to abandon controlled hypotension?

Suggestions for further research

What drugs used for controlled hypotension are most suitable for different types of surgery, e.g., spinal surgery, Cesarean section, prostatectomy? What drugs should not be used for these types of surgery and why?

Exercises and practice cases

Obtain a description for the mentioned positions according to Table 14.1 and use a friend to practice. After that, have him position you in these positions and note where pressure points exist and what positions are most comfortable or most uncomfortable.

What positions may be appropriate for the blood management of patients undergoing the following surgeries:
• Radical cystectomy
• Resection of a meningioma in the posterior fossa
• Resection of a meningioma in the spinal canal at level T10
• Gastrectomy
• Right total hip replacement
• Shunt revision on the right forearm of a dialysis patient

Homework

Check whether there are positioning aids available for patients undergoing spinal surgery.

What fluid warming devices are available? What devices for warming the patient are there? When are they used?

References

1 Lee, T.C., L.C. Yang, and H.J. Chen. Effect of patient position and hypotensive anesthesia on inferior vena caval pressure. *Spine*, 1998. **23**(8): p. 941–947; discussion 947–948.

2 Schostak, M., *et al.* New perioperative management reduces bleeding in radical retropubic prostatectomy. *BJU Int*, 2005. **96**(3): p. 316–319.

3 Rohling, R.G., *et al.* Alternative methods for reduction of blood loss during elective orthognathic surgery. *Int J Adult Orthodon Orthognath Surg*, 1999. **14**(1): p. 77–82.

4 Orliaguet, G.A., *et al.* Is the sitting or the prone position best for surgery for posterior fossa tumours in children? *Paediatr Anaesth*, 2001. **11**(5): p. 541–547.

5 Nelson, C.L. and H.J. Fontenot. Ten strategies to reduce blood loss in orthopedic surgery. *Am J Surg*, 1995. **170**(6A, Suppl): p. 64S–68S.

6 Melendez, J.A., *et al.* Perioperative outcomes of major hepatic resections under low central venous pressure anesthesia: blood loss, blood transfusion, and the risk of postoperative renal dysfunction. *J Am Coll Surg*, 1998. **187**(6): p. 620–625.

7 Ong, S.M. and G.J. Taylor. Can knee position save blood following total knee replacement? *Knee*, 2003. **10**(1): p. 81–85.

8 Phillips, W.A. and R.N. Hensinger. Control of blood loss during scoliosis surgery. *Clin Orthop Relat Res*, 1988. **229**: p. 88–93.

9 Sollevi, A. Hypotensive anesthesia and blood loss. *Acta Anaesthesiol Scand Suppl*, 1988. **89**: p. 39–43.

10 Lustik, S.J., *et al.* Nicardipine versus nitroprusside for deliberate hypotension during idiopathic scoliosis repair. *J Clin Anesth*, 2004. **16**(1): p. 25–33.

11 Yoshida, K., *et al.* Autologous blood transfusion and hypotensive anesthesia for rotational acetabular osteotomy. *Nagoya J Med Sci*, 1998. **61**(3–4): p. 131–135.

12 Sum, D.C., P.C. Chung, and W.C. Chen. Deliberate hypotensive anesthesia with labetalol in reconstructive surgery for scoliosis. *Acta Anaesthesiol Sin*, 1996. **34**(4): p. 203–207.

13 Purdham, R.S. Reduced blood loss with hemodynamic stability during controlled hypotensive anesthesia for LeFort I maxillary osteotomy using high-dose fentanyl: a retrospective study. *CRNA*, 1996. **7**(1): p. 33–46.

14 Testa, L.D. and J.D. Tobias, Pharmacologic drugs for controlled hypotension. *J Clin Anesth*, 1995. **7**(4): p. 326–337.

15 Kiss, H., *et al.* Epinephrine-augmented hypotensive epidural anesthesia replaces tourniquet use in total knee replacement. *Clin Orthop Relat Res*, 2005. **436**: p. 184–189.

16 Jones, R.M., C.E. Moulton, and K.J. Hardy. Central venous pressure and its effect on blood loss during liver resection. *Br J Surg*, 1998. **85**(8): p. 1058–1060.

17 Massicotte, L., *et al.* Effect of low central venous pressure and phlebotomy on blood product transfusion requirements during liver transplantations. *Liver Transpl*, 2006. **12**(1): p. 117–123.

18 Dutton, R.P. Controlled hypotension for spinal surgery. *Eur Spine J*, 2004. **13**(Suppl 1): p. S66–S71.

19 Qvist, T.F., P. Skovsted, and M. Bredgaard Sorensen. Moderate hypotensive anaesthesia for reduction of blood loss during total hip replacement. *Acta Anaesthesiol Scand*, 1982. **26**(4): p. 351–353.

20 Boldt, J., *et al.* Acute normovolaemic haemodilution vs controlled hypotension for reducing the use of allogeneic blood

in patients undergoing radical prostatectomy. *Br J Anaesth*, 1999. **82**(2): p. 170–174.

21 Ahlering, T.E., J.B. Henderson, and D.G. Skinner. Controlled hypotensive anesthesia to reduce blood loss in radical cystectomy for bladder cancer. *J Urol*, 1983. **129**(5): p. 953–954.

22 Lessard, M.R., *et al.* Isoflurane-induced hypotension in orthognathic surgery. *Anesth Analg*, 1989. **69**(3): p. 379–383.

23 Suttner, S.W., *et al.* Cerebral effects and blood sparing efficiency of sodium nitroprusside-induced hypotension alone and in combination with acute normovolaemic haemodilution. *Br J Anaesth*, 2001. **87**(5): p. 699–705.

24 Michelson, A.D., *et al.* Reversible inhibition of human platelet activation by hypothermia in vivo and in vitro. *Thromb Haemost*, 1994. **71**(5): p. 633–640.

25 Bock, M., *et al.* Effects of preinduction and intraoperative warming during major laparotomy. *Br J Anaesth*, 1998. **80**(2): p. 159–163.

26 Winkler, M., *et al.* Aggressive warming reduces blood loss during hip arthroplasty. *Anesth Analg*, 2000. **91**(4): p. 978–984.

27 Schmied, H., *et al.* Mild hypothermia increases blood loss and transfusion requirements during total hip arthroplasty. *Lancet*, 1996. **347**(8997): p. 289–292.

28 Ruel, M.A. and F.D. Rubens. Non-pharmacological strategies for blood conservation in cardiac surgery. *Can J Anaesth*, 2001. **48**(4, Suppl): p. S13–S23.

29 Modig, J. and G. Karlstrom. Intra- and post-operative blood loss and haemodynamics in total hip replacement when performed under lumbar epidural versus general anaesthesia. *Eur J Anaesthesiol*, 1987. **4**(5): p. 345–355.

30 Cullen, B.F., A.J. Margolis, and E.I. Eger. The effects of anesthesia and pulmonary ventilation on blood loss during elective therapeutic abortion. *Anesthesiology*, 1970. **32**(2): p. 108–113.

31 Kozek-Langenecker, S.A. The effects of drugs used in anaesthesia on platelet membrane receptors and on platelet function. *Curr Drug Targets*, 2002. **3**(3): p. 247–258.

32 Tetzlaff, J.E., H.J. Yoon, and J. Brems. Interscalene brachial plexus block for shoulder surgery. *Reg Anesth*, 1994. **19**(5): p. 339–343.

33 Shir, Y., *et al.* Intraoperative blood loss during radical retropubic prostatectomy: epidural versus general anesthesia. *Urology*, 1995. **45**(6): p. 993–999.

34 Juelsgaard, P., *et al.* Hypotensive epidural anesthesia in total knee replacement without tourniquet: reduced blood loss and transfusion. *Reg Anesth Pain Med*, 2001. **26**(2): p. 105–110.

35 Kakiuchi, M. Reduction of blood loss during spinal surgery by epidural blockade under normotensive general anesthesia. *Spine*, 1997. **22**(8): p. 889–894.

36 Hong, J.Y., *et al.* Comparison of general and epidural anesthesia in elective cesarean section for placenta previa totalis: maternal hemodynamics, blood loss and neonatal outcome. *Int J Obstet Anesth*, 2003. **12**(1): p. 12–16.

37 Fotiadis, R.J., *et al.* Epidural analgesia in gastrointestinal surgery. *Br J Surg*, 2004. **91**(7): p. 828–841.

15 The use of autologous blood

When thinking about ways to avoid allogeneic transfusion, the first thing that comes to mind is the use of the patient's own blood. Autologous immunotherapy, autologous stem cell use, and placental blood harvest from umbilical cords are just a few examples of a nearly endless list of methods using autologous blood. This chapter, however, will take a closer look at the more common forms of autologous blood use, namely preoperative autologous donation, hemodilution, and the use of perioperative apheresis.

Objectives of this chapter

1 Review how autologous blood can be used.
2 Learn how acute normovolemic hemodilution and its modifications are performed.
3 Compare acute normovolemic hemodilution and preoperative autologous donation as to their clinically important features.

Definitions

Autologous blood transfusion: It is the transfusion of blood in which donor and recipient are identical.
Preoperative autologous donation (PAD): It is the collection of the patient's own blood before an anticipated procedure. Blood is stored in a blood bank until surgery and is transfused as deemed necessary.
Hemodilution: It is the dilution of blood.
  • *Acute hypervolemic hemodilution (AHH)*: It is the intravascular dilution of the patient's blood components by infusion of acellular fluids to attain and maintain hypervolemia during surgery, with the intent to increase the allowable blood loss.
  • *Acute normovolemic hemodilution (ANH)*: It is a form of intraoperative autologous donation, during which the hemoglobin concentration is reduced by drawing blood and simultaneously replacing the drawn volume with acellular fluid. Blood is kept outside the body and is

retransfused as needed, ideally after surgical hemostasis is achieved.
Plasma-/platelet-sequestration: It is the selective pre- or intraoperative withdrawal of plasma or platelet-rich plasma (PRP) by apheresis. The goal is to harvest autologous blood products for intra- or postoperative use.

A brief look at history

To turn the patient into his own blood bank is not a new idea. But it was not before storage of blood became feasible that preoperative autologous donation began its way into transfusion practice. Fantus, who founded the first blood bank in the United States, proposed preoperative autologous donation. This was in 1937 [1]. Initially, the use of autologous blood was advocated mainly for patients with rare blood groups. Technology was not as advanced as today and liquid storage times were restricted to about 3 weeks. It was in the mid-1980s that preoperative autologous donation received wider acceptance. The AIDS crisis awoke physicians as well as the informed public and they called for safer blood. One of the answers was preoperative autologous donation. Autologous donation programs mushroomed. During the 1980s, the volume of autologous blood donations increased by more than 17 times (in the United States) [2]. Today, the use of preoperative autologous donation is rather heterogeneous. Some institutions use it excessively while others rarely recommend it to their patients.

Apart from preoperative autologous donation, there is another way to use the patient's own blood. It is acute normovolemic hemodilution. The German physician Konrad Messmer first advocated intentional hemodilution. In the late 1960s [3] he reported about deliberately making patients anemic and in the 1970s he reported on his clinical experiences [4]. In the beginning, ANH was used for patients undergoing cardiac surgery with cardiopulmonary bypass and hypothermic arrest to reduce blood viscosity and post-bypass bleeding by infusing fresh blood after coming off the bypass apparatus. Although hemodilution was initially described as a therapeutic measure to reduce exposure to allogeneic blood transfusion, it can be used for much more. Parallel to the development of ANH, background research on hemodilution provided a better understanding of the physiology of hemodilution, anemia tolerance, and adaptation to volume and red cell loss. All of those research areas now provide a basis for reasonable blood management.

As time went by, PAD and ANH were modified. Plateletpheresis, as a blood bank technology, was first used in 1968 [5]. In the late 1980s, this technology was transferred into the operating rooms, and intraoperative plateletpheresis was introduced into clinical practice [6]. The first relevant clinical trials on intraoperative plateletpheresis were published by Giordano in 1988 [7]. Since then, this method underwent further evaluation and modifications.

Preoperative autologous donation

The preoperative collection of autologous blood, its storage and retransfusion during surgery with major blood loss was shown to reduce allogeneic transfusions in different procedures, such as cardiac, orthopedic, and pediatric surgeries. Therefore, it is used in procedures in which blood needs to be typed and cross-matched, namely in all procedures with an anticipated blood loss of 1000 mL or more. In some countries, physicians are even required by law to inform patients about the possibility of autologous donation before procedures with anticipated major blood loss. Let us have a closer look at this technique.

Who is eligible and who not?

PAD is a relatively safe procedure. Therefore, eligibility is hardly limited by age and weight of the patient. Children and older persons may be equally fit for donation. Even pregnancy is not a contraindication for PAD. When contemplating the eligibility of a patient for PAD, one should keep in mind that a patient who is eligible for elective surgery with anticipated major blood loss is most probably also able to donate autologous blood.

There are, however, limits to the ability to donate preoperatively. The American Association of Blood Banks (AABBs) does not permit preoperative donation in cases where the hematocrit of the patient is less than 33%. Similar thresholds are valid in countries not governed by the AABBs.

According to guidelines of the Swiss Red Cross, patients with cardiovascular disease requiring heart surgery are, per se, not eligible for PAD. However, studies were able to demonstrate that selected patients with cardiovascular risk factors can donate autologous blood with an acceptably low rate of side effects [8]. No sound scientific data is available about contraindications for autologous donations. What is considered a contraindication is often determined by the head of the donor center or the responsible person in the hospital. Many sick patients donate their own blood without relevant adverse effects. Sicker patients, however, have a higher incidence of adverse reactions. Contraindications for PAD generally agreed upon are the following conditions: a recent myocardial infarction, chronic heart failure, aortic stenosis, transitory ischemic attack, arrythmias, hypertension, and instable angina pectoris. Patients with bacteremia or suspected bacteremia (diarrhea or in patients with a leukocytosis) are not fit for donations since bacteremia increases the risk for bacterial contamination of the stored blood. For practical reasons, patients with inappropriate venous access also cannot donate blood.

How it works

The basis for a well-organized PAD program is a functioning administrative system. It coordinates the needs of the patient and the hospital or physician. It keeps track of the units donated and reduces the risk of clerical error. Patients are screened for eligibility and unnecessary donations preferably are prevented. PAD can only be performed within the framework of such an administrative system.

As with every procedure performed on a patient, informed consent must be obtained. The patient should know about the general risks of blood donation (e.g., hematoma, infection, fainting, nausea, etc.). Additionally, risks unique to the patient need to be considered. This may be true for the effects of waiting for surgery while donating blood in contrast to having surgery soon. Since there is the general perception among patients that autologous blood is completely safe, inherent risks need to be discussed with the patient. Also, the patient needs to be informed about possible storage problems, technical problems with getting the donated units in time and that autologous blood is no guarantee not to be transfused with allogeneic blood. Where applicable, the patient needs to know that his blood is tested for infections and that he and his physician will be informed in case any results are positive.

Blood is collected in donor centers or hospitals. Whole blood can be stored or red cell concentrates are made out of the collected blood. If the latter is the case, plasma may be given together with the red cell unit, discarded or used for manufacturing plasma fractions. After collection, the units may be tested for HIV, HBV, HCV, and syphilis. ABO and rhesus type are determined as well.

Advance deposit of a patient's blood for elective surgery needs to be scheduled far enough in advance to permit collection and storage of sufficient amounts of blood. It usually begins 3–5 weeks before scheduled surgery. Usually, 2–4 units, i.e., 1–2 L are drawn. On each occasion, approximately 500 mL of blood are collected. Patients with more than 50 kg body weight usually donate 500 mL of blood in one session; patients with less than 50 kg body weight donate smaller volumes. The volume collected should not be more than 10% of the patient's estimated blood volume. One donation per week is usually scheduled, although more aggressive donation schedules are possible. In theory, donations every 3 days are feasible. The last donation takes place not later than 48–72 hours before surgery. This is to allow for the equilibration of blood volume.

Increasing the time interval between blood collection and surgery results in an increase in red cell mass regenerated and thereby increases the efficacy and cost-efficiency of PAD. Under normal storage conditions (units of red cells are stored at refrigerator temperature of 4°C); units of harvested blood can be stored up to 6 weeks (42 days). Countries differ with regard to the time blood products are stored. Whole autologous blood may be stored for about 35 days; autologous red cell concentrates for 42–49 days. However, storage lesions occur soon after the start of storage and increase with time.

Another way of blood storage is cryopreservation which is the storage of blood in a frozen state. It is very expensive, but may provide blood products that have a much longer shelf life than the usual product stored as a liquid. It may be stored for up to 10 years. Preparation procedures are needed to prevent red cells from severe damage. And before retransfusion, deglycerolization is needed. This prolongs the time until the units are ready. The freezing process makes the red cells more prone to damage than other conservation methods. Cryopreservation is not usually performed. Only in special circumstances, such as polysensitized patients with a complex antibody spectrum or patients with very rare blood groups are in line for this procedure. Cryopreservation is performed only in a few specialized centers. Some consider cryopreservation as a suitable means of collecting blood for catastrophes with a high rate of blood product transfusions, but this is currently not much more than a vision.

A word on the retransfusion of PAD blood: The physician's perception that autologous blood hardly has side effects often causes unnecessary transfusions. Often, the blood is transfused only because it is available or just not to disappoint the patient. Other concerns are the wastage of the unused blood. The blood is rather transfused than discarded. It is reasonable, however, to destroy units of blood if there is no good reason for transfusion, since the risk of even this autologous blood does not justify transfusion just because blood is available.

If it is deemed necessary to transfuse during a surgical procedure, intraoperatively collected blood should be given first. If this does not meet the perceived needs of the patient, it was recommended that the youngest PAD unit should be transfused first, since this unit most probably has the least storage lesions.

Advantages and disadvantages

The guidelines of donor centers often set a certain hematocrit as a prerequisite for autologous donation. However, quite a few patients already have anemia prior to scheduled autologous donation. Other patients are left anemic after blood collection. Patients in both groups would not be able to donate blood at all, or the amount collected would be reduced. To gain a reasonable amount of autologous blood, patients can be treated. One unit of donated blood contains about 450 mg of iron and lowers the hemoglobin level about 1 g/dL. Therefore, iron therapy is recommended for patients prior to blood donation. Another idea is to treat donating patients with erythropoietin [9, 10]. Giving erythropoietin and iron substantially increases a patient's ability to donate the large amount of blood. Economic considerations preclude the routine use of erythropoietin in many parts of the world.

The use of one's own predonated blood substantially reduces the risk of contracting one of the transfusion-transmitted diseases, especially the risk of viral infections such as hepatitis B and C as well as HIV. It also reduces immunologically mediated hemolytic, febrile, and allergic reactions. Potentially, PAD may reduce postoperative risk of bacterial infection and cancer recurrence, since the effects of immunomodulation are fewer than that of allogeneic blood transfusion. However, while PAD reduces the patient's exposure to allogeneic blood, it increases the total amount of blood transfused [11]. This may add unnecessary problems, since autologous, yet stored blood also has hazards, including the effects of storage lesions on the immune system and on oxygen delivery capacities.

Occasionally, another theoretical benefit is cited when it comes to PAD—the stimulation of erythropoiesis. Aggressive blood donation indeed stimulates erythropoiesis—

if the patient is not iron-depleted. In practice, however, aggressive donation is prevented by the limitations donor centers set—namely that patients are eligible for donation only if they have a hematocrit of more than 33%. Additionally, many patients are iron-depleted. The benefit of stimulated erythropoiesis is therefore of limited value. On the contrary, up to 50% of the patients donating blood arrive anemic for surgery.

A series of disadvantages of PAD need to be considered as well. PAD itself is a relatively safe procedure. Nevertheless, concerns were expressed about the safety of PAD, especially in sicker or older patients. Mild side effects like diaphoresis, light-headedness, and nausea occur in about 1–3% of all donors. Studies reported an incidence of 1–2% of severe reactions during PAD in patients with high risks, e.g., myocardial infarction, angina, and death [12].

It takes several weeks until autologous blood units harvested by PAD are available. During this time, the condition of the patient may worsen. Cardiac patients, cancer patients, and patients with aortic aneurysms may be eligible for PAD. But there is still the risk of the condition progressing or even death due to the deferral of the procedure. Also, the patient may be anxious about the surgical procedure and the time waiting for surgery may be a heavy burden.

Preoperative autologous donation shares several disadvantages with allogeneic blood. One main concern is the quality of the autologous blood. Since it is stored, it undergoes the same deterioration as allogeneic blood and has the same storage lesions. Improper storage as well as microbial contamination cannot be excluded. Due to mislabeling and administrative errors, incompatibility reactions are possible with the same consequences as allogeneic blood.

Preoperative autologous donation is only possible for elective surgeries. The limited storage time may cause problems. Patients may get sicker, or other causes for deferral of the surgical procedure may render the donation schedule invalid. Meanwhile, donated units may pass their shelf life and become out of date. Only a few donor centers consider frozen storage in this case. Otherwise, the blood has to be discarded.

Pregnancy is another issue to consider. There is an overall transfusion rate of 1–2% of all deliveries. The risk of bleeding is increased in placenta previa, Cesarean section, and a history of postpartum hemorrhage. The frequency of side effects of PAD for the mother is similar to the effects of other autologous donors. The fetus, however, may be more affected by anemia, hypovolemia, and hypotension. Labor may be induced by the process of donation.

Prevalent anemia in pregnancy may preclude donation of considerable amounts of blood.

PAD is a very expensive method to procure autologous blood. Patients have to dedicate time and travel expenses. The blood bank has to engage trained personnel to perform PAD. Also, the blood requires special handling and special labeling ("autologous blood"). The blood is stored as a leukocyte-depleted unit, whole blood, or following separation into blood components. Different institutions test the blood for diseases and determine blood groups, also increasing the costs. All these factors contribute to the costs of PAD. Studies, which did not take into consideration that there is a cost-reduction by the prevention of adverse effects related to allogeneic transfusions, demonstrated that PAD is more expensive than allogeneic blood. Adding to the average costs is the high discard rate for unused PAD blood which is about 30–50%. "Crossover," that is, the transfusion of unused autologous blood in allogeneic recipients, was proposed to increase cost-efficacy of PAD. It remains controversial. Many autologous donors do not meet the criteria for donors set by the American FDA. Crossover is not permitted in several countries.

Hemodilution

There are different kinds of hemodilution—normovolemic and hypervolemic. The idea behind both techniques is to dilute the patient's blood so that—if blood is shed during surgery—less blood components are lost per milliliter blood loss.

Acute hypervolemic hemodilution

The technique of AHH is not as widespread as ANH, a technique that will be described later. Studies suggested that AHH and ANH are equally effective in reducing a patient's exposure to donor blood and incur similar costs. Since there are, to date, not enough data about the use and safety of this technique, we will simply give the basics about AHH and will not further dwell on it.

How it works

Acute hypervolemic hemodilution is performed by infusing considerable amounts of crystalloids or colloids [13]. It dilutes the patient's red cells within his body by temporarily expanding the blood volume, increasing the allowable blood loss. A target hematocrit is aimed at, e.g., 25%. During surgery, less blood cells are lost per milliliter of shed blood. The technique requires a patient who can tolerate hypervolemia. To prevent excessive increase in blood pressure, the vasodialating effect of anesthetic drugs is used [14].

Early literature sources recommend an infusion volume of 20 mL/kg of body weight. However, considerably higher volumes were used in other groups of patients. Kumar and colleagues [14] proposed an equation to calculate the amount of volume expansion required to achieve a particular target hematocrit. The volume to be added is calculated as follows:

$$\text{Volume} = \text{EBV} \times [(H_0 - H_f)/H_f]$$
$$\times \text{ expansion factor for intravenous fluid,}$$

where EBV is the estimated blood volume of the patient; H_0 is the preoperative hematocrit; H_f is the final, post-dilutional hematocrit (target); and expansion factor describes the ability of the fluid, used for hemodilution, to expand the plasma volume of the patient, e.g., a fluid with a volume effect of 80% would have an expansion factor of $100/80 = 1.25$.

During surgery, hypervolemia is sustained by further volume infusion as needed. Crystalloid as well as colloid solutions were used for AHH. To keep the patient hypervolemic during the whole surgical procedure, it is prudent to choose a fluid that has an intravascular residence time that is similar to the time of surgery.

Practice tip

Acute hypervolemic hemodilution is a good starter for an anesthesiologist who would like to practice blood management. Infusing 500–1000 mL of prewarmed hydroxyethyl starch in patients who will experience major blood loss is a simple, safe, and effective method to reduce blood loss.

Advantages and disadvantages

Hypervolemia causes changes in hemodynamics. The blood pressure of the patient may increase. It was reported that such changes revert quickly due to decreased systemic vascular resistance and decreased blood viscosity. Care must be taken in patients with cardiac and autonomous nervous system disorders, where the ability to perform the compensatory adjustments for AHH may be impaired. Intact renal function is crucial to excrete the excessive volume.

Overall, AHH is simple and can be performed at low cost. It deserves, therefore, more attention. If further proof demonstrates the safety and efficacy of AHH, it is an attractive method to reduce the use of allogeneic transfusions [15].

Acute normovolemic hemodilution

Acute normovolemic hemodilution was shown to reduce red cell transfusions, as well as the use of other allogeneic blood products. Therefore, this technique is endorsed by the NIH Consensus Conference on Perioperative Red Blood Cell Transfusion and the American Society of Anesthesiologists.

Indications and eligibility

The classical indication for ANH is cardiac surgery to decrease blood viscosity during hypothermia. Another reason for its use is to save functional platelets and clotting factors for the time after cardiopulmonary bypass. There are many more indications for ANH. Basically, every major surgery with expected high blood loss (e.g., >1000 mL in adults) may be an indication for ANH. Besides cardiac surgery, ANH has been successfully used in orthopedic, gynecologic, urologic, and vascular surgery [15, 16]. All age groups have benefited from ANH—from neonates to adults and elderly persons.

A couple of conditions are relative contraindications for ANH. Among them are severe coronary artery stenosis, congestive heart failure, severe COPD (if oxygenation is severely impaired), hemoglobinopathies, coagulation disorders, poor renal function, severe aortic stenosis, instable angina pectoris, and major organ system failure. Anemia is only a relative contraindication. While some authors do not recommend performing ANH in patients with preoperative anemia, i.e., with a hematocrit of less than 33%, case reports show that it is possible to perform ANH also in patients with lower preoperative hematocrits [17].

How is it done?

Let us now learn how to perform this simple yet ingenious procedure [18]. Before you start, you have to calculate how much blood you can safely remove from your patient. You may want to use the following equation to calculate the tolerable blood loss [19].

$$\text{ABV} = \frac{\text{EBV} \times (H_0 - H_T)}{(H_0 + H_T)/2},$$

where ABV is the autologous blood volume to be withdrawn; H_0 is the prehemodilution hematocrit (zero time); H_T is the target hemoglobin; and EBV is the estimated blood volume of the patient.

It is a matter of knowledge and experience to define a reasonable target hemoglobin. Medical literature [19] defines different levels of hemodilution: mild (hematocrit 25–30%), moderate (hematocrit 20–24%), and profound/severe/extreme (hematocrit <20%). Some consider a target hematocrit of less than 20%, in the absence of hypothermia and cardiopulmonary bypass, too risky, since it is considered to impair oxygen delivery [19]. However, other authors use much lower target hemoglobins without unwanted side effects (e.g., in children for scoliosis surgery).

The patient receiving ANH needs at least one large-bore vascular access. Preferably, this is a central or arterial line. If this is not available, one or two peripheral venous accesses will do it as well. The vascular access is connected to a blood bag and blood drains by gravity. The blood collection bags contain an anticoagulant (citrate–phosphate–dextrose–adenosine = CPD-A). Occasional gentle rocking of the blood bag ensures that the anticoagulant and blood mix well. It takes about 10 minutes to harvest one unit. To make sure you have removed the correct volume, a scale may be useful to estimate the blood volume in the bag.

Blood collection is usually started after the introduction of anesthesia and before surgical blood loss occurs. The blood must be labeled with the patient's name and time of withdrawal and is stored at room temperature in the operation room. Six (to eight) hours are an accepted limit for storage at room temperature. If at all possible, blood is returned to the patient after major surgical blood loss has ceased. If needed, return of the collected blood has to start earlier, namely when the lowest acceptable hematocrit level is reached or when signs of hypoxia occur and none of the maneuvers described below reverse the patient's condition. Blood is returned in reverse order, namely the unit with the highest hematocrit and most clotting factors last. It is recommended not to use microfilters (40 μm) for retransfusion since they may damage the platelets.

The main issue of save hemodilution is the maintenance of normovolemia. Withdrawn blood is substituted with acellular fluids. Usually, the first liter of withdrawn blood is replaced by a colloid, e.g., hydroxyethyl starch, in a ratio of 1:1. The remaining volume is replaced by crystalloid solutions in a ratio of 1 L of blood to 3–4 L of crystalloid. Excess administration of fluids, prior to

withdrawal of blood, results in hypervolemic hemodilution and diminishes the benefits of withdrawing blood. Therefore, preoperative intravenous fluids should be limited to the necessary amount. In an adult, about half a liter of blood can be withdrawn without immediate replacement of blood volume (the same amount is taken without volume replacement during allogeneic blood donation without side effects). This provides a nearly undiluted first unit. If the patient is stable, normovolemia should first be established after the withdrawal of blood has commenced.

ANH is a very safe procedure, provided it is performed by experienced hands and monitored well. Routine EKG and pulse oximetry help to rule out any signs of impaired oxygen delivery. The analysis of respired gases, arterial and central venous blood pressure, arterial blood gases, and coagulation profiles may be necessary in selected cases. Regular hemoglobin checks are mandatory. On-site test kits are available to get immediate results with minimal blood wastage.

Troubleshooting

During ANH, platelets and clotting factors are removed. There is a theoretical risk of dilutional coagulopathy. Clinically, no increased bleeding occurs. Clotting factors, although diminished, usually remain in the physiological range. Additionally, there is a state of hypercoagulability that develops during stress, anesthesia, and surgical intervention. This hypercoagulability may be brought back toward normal by the use of ANH.

What if hypoxia occurs? You have made the patient anemic and anemia might have been increased by ongoing surgical blood loss. If surgical blood loss is over, you should return the blood of the patient. If surgical blood loss is not over yet, you can try some other things first before you give back the blood prematurely. These maneuvers may be able to bridge the time until surgical hemostasis is achieved. First, check factors that may be the cause for hypoxia. Above all, ask yourself: Is normovolemia maintained? If not, try volume substitution. Another way to increase the safety margin of your patient is oxygen therapy. The arterial oxygen content can be increased by ventilating the patient with 100% oxygen (hyperoxic ventilation). This enhances the amount of oxygen physically dissolved in the plasma. Intraoperative hemodilution may be extended beyond the transfusion trigger by simply giving 100% oxygen. Clinical trials were able to demonstrate that even signs of tissue hypoxia could be reversed by merely increasing the FiO_2. This simple maneuver helps to bridge the time until major blood loss is over and ANH blood can be returned [20]. Increasing the FiO_2 from 0.5 to 1.0 increases the arterial oxygen content about 2 mL/dL. This equals a hemoglobin increase of about 1–1.5 g/dL [21].

ANH has many advantages

The beauty of ANH lies in its almost universal range of application. It can be used virtually in every type of surgery and in a wide variety of patients with different ages, weights, and comorbidities. Septicemia is also not a contraindication. Patients for elective as well as emergency surgery can benefit from the advantages of ANH. Minimal preoperative planning is needed. Patients that decline PAD often agree with the use of ANH (Table 15.1).

ANH is a safe procedure. There is a detectable stress response in PAD, which makes this technique not suitable for relatively sick patients. Not so with ANH. It is

Table 15.1 Comparison of preoperative autologous donation (PAD) and acute normovolemic hemodilution (ANH).

	PAD	ANH
Costs	high	low
Applicable in emergencies	no	yes
Storage lesions	yes	minimal
Risk of clerical error	yes	no
Risk of bacterial transmission	yes	minimal
Risk of transfusion-transmitted diseases	no	no
Reduction of immunologically induced complications, such as febrile and allergic reactions, ABO-incompatibilities	yes	yes
Immunomodulation and subsequent bacterial infection and cancer recurrence	reduced	reduced
Eligibility of patients	only selected patients	almost all
Hemostatic properties of blood	lost	intact
Usable in patients with systemic infection	no	yes
Inconveniences for patient	high	none
Wastage of blood	30–50%	minimal

performed under general anesthesia, reducing the stress for the patient. Also, ANH is performed not somewhere outside in a donor center. It is performed under the supervision of an anesthetist. Close monitoring is possible under operating room conditions. ANH blood remains in the operating room near the patient. So, the risk of administrative/clerical error (wrong blood for the wrong patient) is reduced. Immediate transfusion is possible, since the blood is already in the operating room, ready for transfusion.

Problems induced by storage of blood are negligible. The storage time of the autologous units is so brief that deterioration of cells and clotting factors is minimal. What is transfused to the patient is fresh blood with functional platelets and clotting factors. Also, bacterial contamination of the blood is hardly of concern. There is not much time for growth of the germs. Since the blood is stored at room temperature, leukocytes are fresh and active and not hampered in their ability of phagocytosis, so that they can still act bactericidal.

ANH is the most inexpensive way to harvest autologous blood. There are no costs for storage and testing. It does not require the commitment of patient's time for travel and absence from work. Also, there is no additional personnel requirement since ANH is performed by personnel in the operating room. And, unlike PAD, wastage costs of unused blood do not usually incur, since most, if not all blood, is returned to the patient after surgery.

Several further benefits are reported regarding ANH. Since the procedure reduces the viscosity of blood and aggregability of red cells [22], better organ perfusion and improved tissue oxygenation results. After orthopedic surgery with ANH [23], a reduced incidence of deep vein thrombosis was reported. A decreased incidence of wound infections was observed after ANH as well [5].

To date, there is no consensus about the safety of ANH. Some authors criticize ANH because of the possibility of perioperative complications (such as myocardial ischemia, elevated lactate levels, and increased blood loss). Most studies, however, did not demonstrate increased perioperative complications [24]. A very sensitive field is heart surgery. It has been claimed that hemodilution is detrimental for cardiac patients. Recent findings contradict this claim. Actually, hemodilution may be beneficial. Patients with severe coronary artery disease or aortic stenosis benefited from hemodilution to a target hematocrit of 28% prior to surgery. It was shown that there was not only no indication of myocardial ischemia, but also lower levels of cardiac enzymes indicating myocardial compromise (troponin I, creatine kinase) when compared with patients without hemodilution. Besides, hemodiluted patients have a better stroke volume [25–27]. Moderate hemodilution (target hematocrit of 21–25%) may even improve renal function when compared to nonhemodiluted or severely hemodiluted patients [28, 29].

To maintain normovolemia, large amounts of fluids are needed. Peripheral edema and abnormal postoperative pulmonary function and wound healing may occur. Although rare, pulmonary edema was observed following ANH. Generalized edema is more pronounced if crystalloids alone were used, and less after the use of colloids. Peripheral edema resolves within 72 hours. Nevertheless, the benefits of ANH outweigh the problems of increased intravascular fluid.

Advanced use of ANH

Several modifications of ANH promise better results. Among them are augmented ANH (A-ANH^{TM}) and fractionation.

As we learned, ANH is the intentional exchange of blood for colloids or crystalloids with the intent to return the collected blood ideally after surgical blood loss is stopped. This means that the patient is made anemic before surgery starts and will get more anemic as surgical blood loss continues and is replaced by acellular fluids. The efficacy of this technique depends on how low the hematocrit can go before the individual critical hematocrit level is reached. During certain procedures, the surgical blood loss causes the development of anemia below the individually tolerable level. After making use of the above-mentioned maneuvers, return of the ANH blood is usually considered, sometimes followed by donor blood transfusion. A-ANH^{TM} is a method that seeks to avoid this. At the point where return of ANH blood is considered, an artificial oxygen carrier is infused. This oxygen carrier has the ability to deliver oxygen to the tissue and can bridge the time until definite surgical hemostasis is achieved. After that, the ANH blood can be given back and, theoretically, no donor blood is used [30].

A-ANH^{TM} is a safe procedure that can maintain tissue oxygenation and is efficacious in terms of avoiding allogeneic transfusion. The problem with this technique is that most countries do not have an artificial oxygen carrier that is available for A-ANH^{TM}. South Africa and Russia are among the few countries that can use the benefits of artificial oxygen carriers. Physicians in other countries cannot use this promising technique until further notice.

Classical ANH includes the withdrawal of whole blood for later retransfusion. Under certain circumstances, only a distinct component of blood is required intraoperatively to provide the patient with exactly what is needed. To do this, blood harvested by ANH can be fractionated, that is, divided into its components. Using modern cell saving devices, whole blood can be divided into three components: red cells, PPP (platelet-poor plasma), and PRP. Some physicians prefer giving back part of the plasma immediately to diminish the theoretical risk of bleeding; others use the components for a targeted transfusion therapy. As with other advanced methods of autologous transfusion therapy, fractionation needs further evaluation before it can be recommended for wider application [31].

Does ANH reduce exposure to donor blood?

Models of ANH show that it requires high blood loss, high initial hemoglobin value, and low target hemoglobin value to be effective. However, clinical studies show that ANH is able to spare patients from being given allogeneic transfusions [32–35]. A meta-analysis of Bryson *et al.* demonstrated clinical efficacy of ANH as well [36]. The blood conserving effect was obvious in studies where at least 1000 mL of ANH blood were removed. A method called low-volume acute normovolemic hemodilution, during which only 5–8 mL/kg blood are withdrawn, could not demonstrate significant reduction in perioperative donor blood use [24].

ANH is especially useful in conjunction with a comprehensive blood management program. A multi-modality-approach combines the benefit of different procedures and drugs to reduce a patient's exposure to donor blood. Preoperative application of erythropoietin and iron to patients with low initial hematocrit levels has improved the effectiveness of ANH.

Platelet- and plasmapheresis

Parallel to PAD and ANH, there are also methods to use autologous platelets and plasma selectively. Both, preoperative and intraoperative procurement methods are available, with similar advantages and disadvantages as described for PAD and ANH.

Intraoperative autologous plateletpheresis is used mainly in cardiac surgery. Heart surgery, with its related procedures, may lead to coagulopathy. Among many other reasons, a reduction in number and function of platelets due to damage caused by the extracorporeal circulation is considered an important factor for postoperative coagulopathy and subsequent increased platelet, plasma, and red cell transfusions. Perioperative plateletpheresis seeks to remove platelets from the patient's circulation before the blood is exposed to the stress of the cardiopulmonary bypass. This can be done either some days before surgery in the blood bank or directly after induction of anesthesia in the operating room.

Reasons similar to those advocating plateletpheresis also recommend plasmapheresis. Clotting factors can be kept functional when plasma is spared the effects of cardiopulmonary bypass. Plasmapheresis can be performed either preoperatively, in a blood bank, or it can be done directly in the operating room. As with PAD, autologous plasma can be stored for some time before surgery. When it is shock frozen, it can be kept for up to 2 years.

The technique of choice to obtain the autologous products is platelet- or plasmapheresis. Techniques used in the blood bank are similar to the ones used in the operating room. Apheresis techniques differ with regard to the way blood is drawn (gravity versus active), place of collection (in collection bags or directly in the centrifuge), form of the centrifuge, speed of the centrifuge (2000–6000 rotations per minute), and the rate with which the blood is withdrawn (60–100 mL/min).

Advantages and disadvantages

A single allogeneic platelet transfusion often means exposure to 6–8 donors. This is less than desirable. Understandably, the fewer units of allogeneic platelets used the better. Successful plateletpheresis, therefore, means a great contribution to reducing a patient's exposure to multiple donors. Studies were able to demonstrate several benefits of intraoperative allogeneic plateletpheresis, such as decreased postoperative bleeding, reduced blood bank use, enhanced hemostasis due to fresh platelets and clotting factors, reduced chest tube drainage after cardiac surgery, better pulmonary function in comparison with patients undergoing no platelet sequestration [6], shorter stay in the intensive care unit, and higher postoperative fibrinogen and antithrombin III levels.

Plateletpheresis can be performed in patients in whom ANH is not possible due to anemia. As with the blood harvested by ANH, intraoperative plateletpheresis provides fresh blood products without the storage lesions seen in allogeneic platelets.

Although it was shown that the quality of intraoperatively harvested platelets is superior to the quality of allogeneic platelets, concerns remain regarding the quality of the harvested units. Citrate, as part of the anticoagulant, may damage platelets. Centrifugation releases platelet granules. Red cells returned after platelet sequestration are more fragile due to processing and are prone to hemolysis during cardiopulmonary bypass. Nevertheless, the lesions encountered by the apheresis process are smaller than the combined lesions of blood bank apheresis and storage. That is why freshly harvested platelets are more effective than allogeneic platelets.

The procedure of intraoperative plateletpheresis is time consuming. Depending on the device used and the hemodynamic stability of the patient, it takes 30–80 minutes to harvest therapeutical quantities of PRP. To reduce operating room time, apheresis may be performed parallel to patient preparation.

The net effect of platelet- or plasmapheresis on blood management is not fully appreciated yet. It is a labor and equipment intensive procedure, without well-defined advantages regarding reduction of allogeneic transfusions. Future research will demonstrate whether such pheresis procedures should have a fixed place in blood management.

Key points

- Hemodilution is a simple, safe, convenient, and effective alternative to PAD.
- Maintaining normovolemia is imperative for successful hemodilution.
- ANH can replace PAD as an autologous blood procurement method.

Questions for review

- What are the advantages and disadvantages of preoperative autologous donation?
- What are the advantages and disadvantages of acute normovolemic hemodilution?
- Do we have to exclude patients with severe coronary artery stenosis from hemodilution? Why do you answer so?
- How is acute hypervolemic hemodilution performed?

Suggestions for further research

What monitoring tools may indicate tissue hypoxia under acute normovolemic hemodilution?

Homework

Find out where you can get blood bags for hemodilution and record the contact and other pertinent information in the address book in the Appendix E.

Exercises and practice cases

Calculate how much blood can be drawn for ANH in the following patients and draw conclusions about your results.

50 kg healthy female with a hemoglobin level of 16 g/dL
50 kg healthy female with a hemoglobin level of 13 g/dL
50 kg healthy female with a hemoglobin level of 10 g/dL
100 kg healthy male with a hemoglobin level of 16 g/dL
100 kg healthy male with a hemoglobin level of 13 g/dL
100 kg healthy male with a hemoglobin level of 10 g/dL

References

1 Fantus, B. Blood preservation. *JAMA*, 1937. **109**: p. 128–131.

2 Popovsky, M., *et al.* Preoperative autologous blood donation. In Spiess, B.D., *et al.* (eds.) *Perioperative Transfusion Medicine.* Williams and Wilkins, Baltimore, 1997.

3 Messmer, K., *et al.* Überleben von Hunden bei akuter Verminderung der O_2-Transportkapazität auf 2,8 g% Hämoglobin. *Pflügers Arch Physiol*, 1967. **297**: p. R48.

4 Bauer, H., *et al.* Autotransfusion through acute, preoperative hemodilution—1st clinical experiences. *Langenbecks Arch Chir*, 1974. (Suppl): p. 185–189.

5 Spiess B.D., *et al. Perioperative Transfusion Medicine.* Williams and Williams, Baltimore, 1998.

6 Christenson, J.T., *et al.* Plateletpheresis before redo CABG diminishes excessive blood transfusion. *Ann Thorac Surg*, 1996. **62**(5): p. 1373–1378; discussion 1378–1379.

7 Giordano, G.F., *et al.* Intraoperative autotransfusion in cardiac operations. Effect on intraoperative and postoperative transfusion requirements. *J Thorac Cardiovasc Surg*, 1988. **96**(3): p. 382–386.

8 Walpoth, B.H., F. Aregger, C. Imboden, E. Auckenthaler, U. Nydegger, and T. Carrel. Safety of preoperative autologous blood donations in cardiac surgery. *Infus Ther Transfus Med*, 2002. **29**: p. 160–162.

9 Tryba, M. Epoetin alfa plus autologous blood donation and normovolemic hemodilution in patients scheduled for orthopedic or vascular surgery. *Semin Hematol*, 1996. **33**(2, Suppl 2): p. 34–36; discussion 37–38.

10 Braga, M., *et al.* Evaluation of recombinant human erythropoietin to facilitate autologous blood donation before surgery in anaemic patients with cancer of the gastrointestinal tract. *Br J Surg*, 1995. **82**(12): p. 1637–1640.

11 Forgie, M.A., *et al.*, for International Study of Perioperative Transfusion (ISPOT) Investigators. Preoperative autologous donation decreases allogeneic transfusion but increases exposure to all red blood cell transfusion: results of a meta-analysis. *Arch Intern Med*, 1998. **158**(6): p. 610–616.

12 Monk, T.G. and L.T. Goodnough. Blood conservation strategies to minimize allogeneic blood use in urologic surgery. *Am J Surg*, 1995. **170**(6, A Suppl): p. 69S–73S.

13 Galli, C., *et al.* Optimized hemodilution with hydroxyethyl starch. A blood saving method in malocclusion operations. *Mund Kiefer Gesichtschir*, 2001. **5**(6): p. 353–356.

14 Kumar, R., I. Chakraborty, and R. Sehgal. A prospective randomized study comparing two techniques of perioperative blood conservation: isovolemic hemodilution and hypervolemic hemodilution. *Anesth Analg*, 2002. **95**(5): p. 1154–1161, table of contents.

15 Saricaoglu, F., *et al.* The effect of acute normovolemic hemodilution and acute hypervolemic hemodilution on coagulation and allogeneic transfusion. *Saudi Med J*, 2005. **26**(5): p. 792–798.

16 Terai, A., *et al.* Use of acute normovolemic hemodilution in patients undergoing radical prostatectomy. *Urology*, 2005. **65**(6): p. 1152–1156.

17 Rehm, M., *et al.* Four cases of radical hysterectomy with acute normovolemic hemodilution despite low preoperative hematocrit values. *Anesth Analg*, 2000. **90**(4): p. 852–855.

18 Monk, T.G. Acute normovolemic hemodilution. *Anesthesiol Clin North America*, 2005. **23**(2): p. 271–281, vi.

19 Kafer, E.R. and M.L. Colins. Acute intraoperative hemodilution and perioperative blood salvage. *ACNA*, 1990. **8**: p. 543–567.

20 Habler, O., *et al.* Hyperoxia in extreme hemodilution. *Eur Surg Res*, 2002. **34**(1–2): p. 181–187.

21 Meier, J., *et al.* Hyperoxic ventilation enables hemodilution beyond the critical myocardial hemoglobin concentration. *Eur J Med Res*, 2005. **10**(11): p. 462–468.

22 Gu, Y.J., *et al.* Influence of hemodilution of plasma proteins on erythrocyte aggregability: an in vivo study in patients undergoing cardiopulmonary bypass. *Clin Hemorheol Microcirc*, 2005. **33**(2): p. 95–107.

23 Vara Thorbeck, R., *et al.* Prevention of thromboembolic disease and post-transfusional complications using normovolemic hemodilution in arthroplasty surgery of the hip. *Rev Chir Orthop Reparatrice Appar Mot*, 1990. **76**(4): p. 267–271.

24 Casati, V., G. Speziali, C. D'Alessandro, C. Cianchi, M.A. Grasso, S. Spagnolo, and L. Sandrelli. Intraoperative low-volume acute normovolemic hemodilution in adult open-heart surgery. *Anesthesiology*, 2002. **97**: p. 367–373.

25 Licker, M., *et al.* Cardiovascular response to acute normovolemic hemodilution in patients with coronary artery diseases: assessment with transesophageal echocardiography. *Crit Care Med*, 2005. **33**(3): p. 591–597.

26 Licker, M., *et al.* Cardioprotective effects of acute normovolemic hemodilution in patients undergoing coronary artery bypass surgery. *Chest*, 2005. **128**(2): p. 838–847.

27 Licker, M., *et al.* Cardioprotective effects of acute isovolemic hemodilution in a rat model of transient coronary occlusion. *Crit Care Med*, 2005. **33**(10): p. 2302–2308.

28 Karkouti, K., *et al.* Hemodilution during cardiopulmonary bypass is an independent risk factor for acute renal failure in adult cardiac surgery. *J Thorac Cardiovasc Surg*, 2005. **129**(2): p. 391–400.

29 Habib, R.H., *et al.* Role of hemodilutional anemia and transfusion during cardiopulmonary bypass in renal injury after coronary revascularization: implications on operative outcome. *Crit Care Med*, 2005. **33**(8): p. 1749–1756.

30 Kemming, G., O. Habler, and B. Zwissler. Augmented acute normovolemic hemodilution (A-ANH(tm)) in cardiac and non-cardiac patients. *Anasthesiol Intensivmed Notfallmed Schmerzther*, 2001. **36**(Suppl 2): p. S107–S109.

31 Potter, P.S. Perioperative apheresis. *Transfusion*, 2004. **44**(12, Suppl): p. 54S–57S.

32 Johnson, L.B., J.S. Plotkin, and P.C. Kuo. Reduced transfusion requirements during major hepatic resection with use of intraoperative isovolemic hemodilution. *Am J Surg*, 1998. **176**(6): p. 608–611.

33 Habler, O., *et al.* Effects of standardized acute normovolemic hemodilution on intraoperative allogeneic blood transfusion in patients undergoing major maxillofacial surgery. *Int J Oral Maxillofac Surg*, 2004. **33**(5): p. 467–475.

34 Matot, I., *et al.* Effectiveness of acute normovolemic hemodilution to minimize allogeneic blood transfusion in major liver resections. *Anesthesiology*, 2002. **97**(4): p. 794–800.

35 Wong, J., *et al.* Vascular surgical society of Great Britain and Ireland: autologous transfusion reduces blood transfusion requirements in aortic surgery. *Br J Surg*, 1999. **86**(5): p. 698.

36 Bryson, G.L., A. Laupacis, and G.A. Wells. Does acute normovolemic hemodilution reduce perioperative allogeneic transfusion? A meta-analysis. The International Study of Perioperative Transfusion. *Anesth Analg*, 1998. **86**(1): p. 9–15.

16 Cell salvage

It is obvious that we must try and save water because we cannot survive without it, but it should be just as obvious for us to save every drop of a patient's life-sustaining blood. If a blood vessel is leaking, every effort should be made to catch the blood running out—the idea behind cell salvage.

Objectives of this chapter

1 List the minimum utensils needed for cell salvage.
2 Describe basic principles of modern cell salvage.
3 Discuss potential contraindications of cell salvage and explain methods how to overcome them.

Definitions

Cell salvage: It is a measure of autologous transfusion with reclamation and use of the patient's blood lost during and after surgery or trauma. Cell salvage can be categorized by the timing of blood collection (intra- or postoperative) and by the methods used to return the blood (direct cell salvage for unwashed blood, indirect cell salvage for washed blood).

A brief look at history

In 1818, Dr James Blundell was requested to visit a woman who was, as he wrote, "sinking under uterine hemorrhage." Before long and despite all efforts, she bled to death. Reflecting on the "melancholy scene" he encountered in this woman's case, Blundell considered transfusion as the possible salvation for her. To ascertain the feasibility of transferring blood, he constructed a device for some experiments with dogs. He bled dogs from the femoral artery, collected the blood in a funnel-shaped bowl and retransfused the blood by a syringe connected to the bottom of the bowl. He observed that his dogs survived and he subsequently recommended this procedure to be used on patients if the need may arise [1]. Although Blundell did not report any cases where he used autologous transfusions in humans, he is considered the father of autotransfusion. Besides, with his transfusion device he constructed one of the first cell savers.

More than 50 years later, William Highmore, also an English physician, visited a woman suffering from severe postpartum hemorrhage. On arrival in the house of the patient, Dr Highmore saw blood everywhere: in the bed, on the sheets, and also collected in a vessel. Furthermore, he saw his colleague struggle to stop the bleeding. Although the hemorrhage was finally stopped, the patient died only 1 hour after Dr Highmore's arrival. Reflecting on this experience, Dr Highmore imagined that—since blood was available, as seen by the collection in the vessel—an attempt should have been made to return the blood to the patient. In 1874, he resolved: "I commend this plan (to autotransfuse) to the notice of the profession, and have resolved to use it myself in the first case of haemorrhage that may occur in my practice" [2].

Despite the fact that the feasibility of autotransfusion was shown in animal studies and it was recommended as a potentially life-saving procedure, it took some time until the first report of human autotransfusion appeared in the medical literature. In 1886, John Duncan took care of a patient with a crushed leg. Since Duncan's patient had lost much of his blood and was moribund, Dr Duncan amputated the crushed leg and collected the blood in a bowl. Phosphate of soda was added to prevent rapid clotting, and the blood was diluted with distilled water. Afterwards, the patient's blood was returned to him. The patient survived without any reported adverse effects of the cell salvage. So, Dr Duncan became one of the first who reported his experiences in returning the patients own blood lost during surgery. In an article describing his methods, Dr Duncan wrote: "I have now performed it in a sufficient number of cases . . . to enable me to speak with confidence as to its safety and value" [3].

In 1914, J. Thies reported on a series of three women with ruptured ectopic pregnancies in whom he practiced cell salvage. He used a ladle to scoop blood out of the abdominal cavity. He filtered the blood through two layers of gauze, diluted it with saline, and returned it to the patient. The first patient received a transfusion of 1.5 L blood subcutaneously; the other two patients received it intravenously [4]. With his report, Dr Thies seemed to be the first to use cell salvage in gynecologic hemorrhage, the indication for which was advocated decades before [2].

Cell salvage was later performed in selected cases of splenectomy, neurosurgery, and trauma. Side effects of attempts to autotransfuse were rare even when crude early methods were used. How resilient patients seemed to be is evident when we consider a case series of Griswold and Ortner [5]. One hundred patients with thorax or abdominal trauma received cell salvaged blood. Among them, only one died due to cell salvage. It was reported that the patient had multiple perforations in his small intestine. The blood used for direct autotransfusion was contaminated with fecal matter, to the extent that the infusion needle had become plugged with feces. At autopsy, the patient had multiple emboli in his lung.

The advent of a sufficient and seemingly safe blood supply influenced physicians to abandon autotransfusion for a while. Some factors rekindled the interest in autotransfusion. Physicians taking care of patients who refused allogeneic blood for religious reasons looked to devise methods to use the patient's own blood. Another impetus for autotransfusion was blood shortages, e.g., during wars. The lack of blood in the Vietnam war urged Gerald Klebanoff, a surgeon of the US Air Force, to develop a simple device of a cell saver [6]. He used basically parts of a cardiopulmonary bypass equipment and assembled it. His idea was later marketed as the Bentley ATS 100. The system was widely used, but some safety concerns caused its withdrawal from the market. However, the experience with this system helped develop other systems that tried to eliminate the problems encountered with Klebanoff's invention [7].

In the late 1960s and early 1970s, the engineer Allen "Jack" Latham developed a new form of cell salvage [8]. He introduced the Latham bowl, which offered the opportunity to wash blood before it was retransfused. This eliminated some of the side effects of direct autotransfusion practiced thus far. Since then, the methods of washing blood have been refined and are still to be refined even more.

Introduction

Cell salvage is a smart means to regain otherwise lost autologous blood. Under certain circumstances, blood lost can be returned without any additional processing. This kind of cell salvage is called direct cell salvage and delivers unwashed blood back to the patient. In contrast, blood can be returned to the patient after being more or less extensively processed. The processing usually consists of several steps that wash red cells. This kind of cell salvage is called indirect cell salvage.

If blood is given in the intraoperative period, it is usually regained from the surgical field or from body cavities opened in the surgical procedure. Postoperative cell salvage draws blood from drains, e.g., from chest or mediastinal drains or such ones coming from operative sites at the spine or from large joints (hip, knee).

Depending on the timing, cell salvage can be performed either solely intraoperatively or solely postoperatively. Sometimes, the same cell-saving device is used intraoperatively and taken along with the patient for the postoperative period. Intra- and postoperative cell salvage can either be performed with or without blood processing.

Cell savers—from basic to sophisticated

There are a variety of methods and devices used for intra- or postoperative cell salvage—from very simple ones to high-tech apparatus. The following methods have been used successfully and can be employed. The choice of the method will largely depend on local circumstances, such as patient criteria, the specifics of the planned procedure, costs, personal preference, and legislation.

Method 1: The simplest technique of cell salvage is the one already used by Thies [4]. To imitate his technique, it was proposed to use a sterilized soup ladle and a funnel. Blood is scooped out of the wound and filtered through several layers of gauze into a funnel. Then, the blood is collected in a bottle. If blood bags rather than bottles are available, the funnel is connected to a rubber tubing. The tube is clamped at one side and the needle of the blood bag is inserted into this rubber tubing. The blood follows gravity into the bags (Fig. 16.1) [9, 10]. The container in which the blood is collected needs to contain an anticoagulant.

Method 2: If no cell saver is available, cell salvage can be performed by assembling some things that may be available even in areas with low-cost medicine. As an example, the following cell saver can be assembled (which is similar to the one originally proposed by Klebanoff [6]: Suction tips are connected to a roller head pump so that blood can be sucked from the surgical field into a defoaming cardiotomy reservoir. Via an inline blood

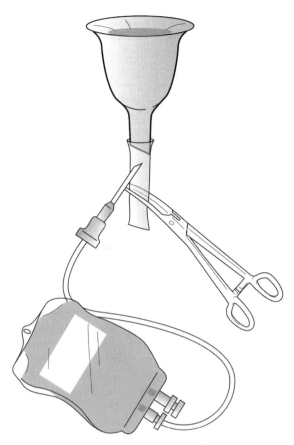

Fig 16.1 Use of blood bags for simple cell salvage.

filter, blood is collected into vacuum collection bags and is given back to the patient.

Using this self-made cell saver, the patient needs to be given an anticoagulant (typically heparin, 300 U/kg body weight) just prior to the expected blood loss. The cell saver system needs to be primed with an anticoagulant as well. Heparinization must be monitored closely and heparin is antagonized with protamine after the procedure. It is necessary to keep in mind that the returned blood contains heparin and reheparinizes the patient. The protamine dose needs to be adjusted accordingly. With this method, up to 23 units of blood have been reported to be given safely [11].

Method 3: If there is money to obtain a preassembled cell-saving device, many models are available to be chosen from. One low-cost alternative is a set that was designed for the use in developing countries [12]. It consists of several components, some of which are resterilizable, namely

- a blood reservoir bag with a double filter system and tubing,
- an electrically driven blood pump with a maximum suction pressure of 40 mm Hg,
- a 100 mL syringe and a collection bowl (for cases when there is electrical power failure).

The collection bowl is fitted with a funnel, which contains a filter and a transfusion tubing set. The pump, the syringe, and the collection bowl are resterilizable, while the reservoir bag, the filters, and the tubing are one-way materials.

Method 4: For direct postoperative cell salvage, specially designed containers are available which can be connected to the drain in the wound. The containers have a filter to remove debris coming from the wound. A port in the container can be spiked and the container can be hung above the patient to allow the collected blood to return to the patient via an intravenous line.

Method 5: Most developed countries with sufficient money in the health care system can use computerized blood washing devices. Blood is sucked from the field and mixed with an anticoagulant. The blood runs through a filter into a reservoir or a bowl and is processed (washed). Afterwards the washed blood is automatically transferred into blood bags where it is stored, ready to be given back (Fig. 16.2). The systems differ in the method used to wash blood.

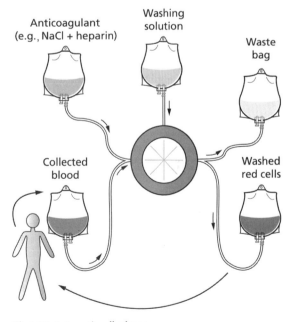

Fig 16.2 Automatic cell salvage.

How to wash blood

There are basically two different methods to wash blood—centrifugation and filtration. Centrifugation is most commonly used in commercially available cell salvage devices.

It is well known that blood constituents have different densities. Among other factors, this makes red cells sink to the bottom of a tube while other components stay above, a process called sedimentation. If sedimentation is complete, blood will stand in different layers. At the bottom, components with a high density settle, followed by components with lesser density. For blood, this means that the cells at the bottom of a vessel are red cells. Above, there is a small layer of platelets and leukocytes (called buffy coat), followed by a wide layer of platelet-poor plasma.

It is possible to speed up the separation of blood by density differences, namely by means of centrifugation. In a laboratory, blood is spun to be separated for further analysis. A very similar spinning process is used to separate red cells from other blood components in a cell saver, the so-called density gradient separation. During spinning, typically with 4400 or more rotations per minute [13], red cells are packed against the outer wall of the centrifuge bowl, while other, less dense components remain, more or less, in the center of the centrifuge. There are plasma, platelet remains, anticoagulant, cell debris, free hemoglobin, and other contaminants solved in the plasma phase. A washing solution is added. This solution dilutes the plasma supernatant, which is then removed from the centrifuge and discarded into a waste bag. After the washing process is finished, the red cell layer is pumped into blood bags and is ready for return to the patient.

Based on these simple principles, modern equipment washes blood either intermittently or continually.

Discontinuous, intermittent blood washing

The discontinuous washing method mostly uses a so-called Latham bowl. It looks like two bowls, a smaller one set into a bigger one. Both are turned around so that their undersides face upward. The inner bowl is stationary and holds an inlet and outlet port. The outer bowl rotates (Fig. 16.3). Another bowl for discontinuous washing uses a Baylor bowl (BRAT bowl). In comparison with the Latham bowl, it has vertical sides [13].

A wash procedure in a Latham bowl [14] consists of three separate steps: filling or priming, washing, and emptying. Blood is collected either directly from the surgical field or from the reservoir. Blood is pumped into the ro-

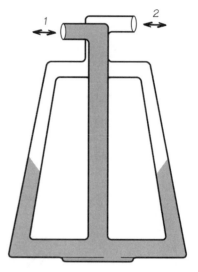

Fig 16.3 Latham bowl: (1) Port for blood (inlet and outlet); (2) Port for washing solution (inlet and outlet).

tating bowl. The centrifugal force drives the lighter supernatants medially and upward where they are removed from the outlet. The heavier red cells collect at the lateral walls of the centrifuge. When a certain red cell level is reached in the centrifuge, the filling phase ends and the washing phase begins. A washing solution, typically normal saline, enters the red cell layer at the wall of the outer bowl from below and circulates through the red cell layer. The solution washes away remaining debris. A minimum of three times the red cell volume is used to wash the red cells coming from relatively clean collection, such as from vessel injuries or from a cardiopulmonary bypass. A washing volume of as much as 10 times the bowl volume may be needed for contaminated blood from wounds or from wound drains. At any rate, at the end of the washing process, the washing solution used for the red cell layer should be clear. When the centrifuge—that is, the outer bowl—is stopped, the red cells are pumped out of the centrifuge.

Before an operator can start cell washing, a set of operational settings must be chosen. The first decision to be made is about the bowl size. A typical bowl holds 220–250 mL of fluid. To fill this with washable red cells, at least 500–750 mL of blood collected in the reservoir are needed. Bigger bowls, with a volume of 375 mL, are available for cases with rapid blood loss and smaller bowls, with volumes of about 125 mL, are available for smaller or slower blood losses.

Another decision must be made regarding the pump flow rate. This can be set from 25 to more than

1000 mL per minute and is chosen according to the rate of blood loss and according to the quality of the blood.

The quality of the finished autologous red cell concentrate, prepared by the Latham bowl, can partially be influenced by the operator [14]. Some parameters influencing the blood quality are adjustable, while others are set by predetermined wash programs.

The elimination of waste in a Latham bowl depends on three parameters:

(**a**) The *hematocrit prior to separation*: The lower the hematocrit in the blood needing washing, the better the elimination of solutes. The operator can influence this hematocrit by diluting the blood in the reservoir with additional saline.

(**b**) The *hematocrit inside the bowl after the filling phase*: The higher the hematocrit, the better the elimination of solutes. A desired hematocrit level is 50–70%. The hematocrit can be increased by reducing the inflow speed of blood that needs to be processed. Why? As we learned above, the fundamental principle of blood washing is sedimentation. The higher the, sedimentation rate the higher the density differences between the components and the higher the acceleration rate of a centrifuge. At a higher acceleration rate, the packing of the red cells is denser. The same is true with prolonged centrifugation. Transferred to the Latham bowl this means that with a lower inflow of blood it takes longer to fill the centrifuge. The increase in the length of the centrifugation period causes a higher hematocrit level in the bowl.

(**c**) The *amount of washing solution*: The more washing solution is used, the better the elimination of solutes. This, however, prolongs the washing process and reduces the amount of red cells finally recovered.

The quality of the processed blood is also influenced by parameters that are intrinsic to the system [14]. The design of the bowl determines where the washing solution enters the layer with red cells. Since the washing solution is also centrifuged, it follows the centrifugal force and is driven to the center of the bowl (since the density of saline or another washing solution is lower than the density of red cells and similar to the density of plasma). In turn, red cells at the wall of the bowl are not as thoroughly washed as red cells closer to the center of the bowl. Little design changes in the bowl can force the water to the outer parts of the bowl or can force the sedimented red cells to mix. Another way to improve the washing performance is to temporarily stop or at least slow down the centrifuge. This redistributes the content of the bowl and improves the elimination of the supernatant.

Unique to the Latham bowl is the "problem of the last bowl." If the remaining blood in the collection reservoir is not sufficient to fill the Latham bowl, the quality of the blood after being processed is inferior to the one of prior batches. The part-filled bowl does not reach high hematocrits after separation and the quality of the blood is inferior, since not the same degree of supernatant is eliminated. Attempts to solve the problem include to choose a small bowl to begin with, or to add the needed amount of red cells from the already washed portion in order to fill the bowl. Another attempt is to design the bowl to be adjustable to the volume. A membrane, instead of a rigid chamber wall, adjusts to the amount of blood that needs to be processed.

Continuous blood washing

For a continuous blood washing, blood is pumped from the collection reservoir into a special centrifuge chamber. This chamber looks like a double spiral (Fig. 16.4). Blood is pumped into the inner spiral of the rotating chamber. Centrifugal forces drive the red cells into the outer spiral of the chamber. On their way, they are washed by separately adding washing solution to the chamber. Lighter matter such as fat, washing solution with contaminants, and plasma components drift to the middle of the chamber and are pumped out from there. On its way through the spiral chamber, the red cell layer gets ever cleaner and denser. When a certain hematocrit is reached, washed red cells are pumped into the retransfusion bag while the chamber is still rotating. The continued rotation prevents contaminants being driven back into the red cell layer after the chamber is stopped. This would recontaminate the red cells.

In contrast to blood processing with the Latham bowl, the separation phase and the washing phase in the

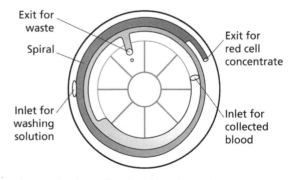

Fig 16.4 Continuous blood washing with a spiral bowl.

spiral-shaped chamber work continually. The quality of the blood is constant, no matter how much blood is processed and how high the hematocrit. The bowl size does not need to be chosen according to the expected blood loss. The maximum achievable hematocrit using the continuous system is higher than with the discontinuous system.

Filtration techniques

The second basic method of cell washing is filtration. The components of blood or a blood-containing solution have different sizes and each carrying a different electrical charge. This facilitates separation by the use of appropriate filters. For cell salvage, usually ultrafiltration is used. Blood is passed over a semipermeable membrane. The hydrostatic pressure of the fluid pushes smaller molecules through the fine pores of the membrane while the larger ones are left on the original side. Depending on the membrane, either all plasma is filtered leaving mainly red cells or only water with smaller solutes is filtered, preserving plasma proteins (fibrinogen, antithrombin, etc.) and platelets.

Ultrafiltration can be used as a means of hemoconcentration. This process has been traditionally used for renal failure patients to dialyze them. The method is nowadays increasingly used to concentrate the blood that remains at the end of a cardiopulmonary bypass [15]. The membrane is chosen so that most of the blood components can be given back to the patients, while only excess water and small molecular components (e.g., complement factors) are filtered out. This has helped to prevent fluid overload and reduces the systemic inflammatory reaction seen after extracorporeal circulation. It also helps to reduce patient's exposure to donor blood.

The process of ultrafiltration can also be used in a classical cell salvage device. Salvaged blood is suspended in a solution, which typically consists of normal saline with heparin for anticoagulation. It is mixed gently and thereby washed (vortex mixing). The blood is pumped through a membrane for filtration. The membrane is chosen so that most of the plasma is filtrated and only cellular components remain [16].

Blood quality after cell salvage

Unwashed blood

Unwashed blood contains whatever is found in the blood leaving the wound or body cavity. Enormous differences in the blood quality have been observed. Those differences depend partially on the flow (amount of blood collected over time), the method of blood collection, and the addition of anticoagulant. The use of substances like bone cement, glues, etc. and the area operated on (with much or less free fat) influence the final blood product.

With a high flow of blood and immediate return, intraoperatively collected blood contains most of the platelets and plasma coagulation factors. It was reported that even after a turnover of as much as about five times the blood volume of the patient, coagulation was sufficient at the end of surgery [17]. With prolonged blood procurement, platelet counts vary, ranging from near normal to almost zero. Platelets are usually morphologically and functionally altered, used up, or have formed microaggregates.

Blood collected postoperatively has generally lost its capability to coagulate. Contact with the wound defibrinizes the blood. But it still contains activated procoagulatory and fibrinolytic components, such as prothrombin fragments, fibrin split products, and soluble fibrin. Fibrin split products may impair the function of fibrin and of platelets.

Blood in a container for postoperative cell salvage has a comparatively low hematocrit. In studies, hemoglobin concentrations as low as 7–12 g/dL have been reported [18]. Intact red cells for retransfusion have a near normal survival rate entering the body. However, before red cells are ready for retransfusion, they may be damaged by processes in the wound or by the collection. This damage leads to an increased amount of free hemoglobin in the blood.

Complementary factors are activated by the process of blood collection. Leukocytes may be activated, leading to elevated cytokine levels in the blood. Especially interleukin 6, but also interleukin 1 and 8 as well as tumor necrosis factor alfa were found to be increased in wound blood [19]. Many other immunologically active ingredients have been found in the blood, such as leukotrienes, elastase, prostaglandins, and others.

Washed blood

Washing blood reduces and sometimes entirely eliminates contaminants found in blood after collection. These contaminants include the washing solution, almost the whole plasma fraction and many iatrogenically added substances (antibiotics, glues, and irrigants).

Fresh autologous red cells tolerate centrifugation well [20] so that the product, after processing can contain up to 80% of the lost red cells. Depending on the way the blood is processed, the hematocrit after washing lies between 52 and 80% [20]. Free hemoglobin, potassium, and protein are sufficiently reduced by the washing process. Washed blood essentially returns red cells, reconstituted in saline. The product does not contain sufficient plasma coagulation factors or platelets to assure coagulation.

Washing blood eliminates approximately 80–94% of all leukocytes, although there are cell savers that eliminate them only by 50%. Leukocytes are activated in the process of cell collecting and washing. Granulocytes, for instance, start their intrinsic functions when they are activated to a certain threshold. When this threshold is reached, changes in adhesion, migration, degranulation, and phagocytosis occur and the respiratory burst is initiated. This may result in epithelial damage also affecting pulmonary vessels. Respiratory distress syndromes have therefore been attributed to activated leukocytes retransfused with salvaged blood. Further research has shown that most probably related circumstances triggered the pulmonary problems. Leukocytes, although slightly altered, seem not to be activated to the extent compatible with serious pulmonary problems. Current literature does not support the notion that leukocytes need to be eliminated entirely and the use of a leukocyte depletion filter for the sole purpose of eliminating leukocytes seems not to be justified for autotransfusion [21].

Besides compounds naturally occurring in blood, other contaminants are also removed by the washing of blood. This also holds true for the added anticoagulant. Only a minimal heparin activity after correctly washing (0.3–0.5 U/mL) is observed. Also, hirudin derivates used for anticoagulation during cell salvage have been shown to be reduced to an insignificant level [22]. Thus, correctly washed blood does not contain anticoagulants that would impair clotting.

Fat is often present in wound blood during orthopedic surgery. It has been shown to cause fat embolism and related damage such as pulmonary damage due to toxic fatty acids. Damage of the pulmonary endothelium results in an increased permeability of the pulmonary vasculature. Cell savers using a discontinuous washing process reduce fat contents in the blood, but still have significant amounts of fat in the remaining blood. Some physicians therefore do not return the remaining 50 mL of processed blood as it contains the floating fat layer. Such blood waste may be tolerable in adults, but children do not easily tolerate such losses. Cell savers with a continuous washing system are better able to remove fat. Blood does not need to be wasted. In this regard, continuous washing is superior to its counterparts [23].

Advantages of cell salvage

Cell salvage is usable in emergency as well as in elective procedures. Several liters of blood can be salvaged intraoperatively—much more than with other methods of autologous donation. Large volumes of blood are available, even in patients with a rare blood type. Since cell salvage may be combined with other techniques of blood management, e.g., hemodilution [24], it considerably reduces the use of allogeneic transfusions. All techniques of cell salvage provide a fresh, autologous blood product. This intrinsically comes with certain advantages. The risk of transfusion-transmittable diseases and the risks of allergic or hemolytic reactions are small or eliminated.

Since blood recovered in a cell saver is fresh and near room temperature, red cells are viable, have a near-normal osmotic membrane stability (in contrast to stored homologous blood), and come with a potentially normal life span. Their level of 2.3-DPG is near normal [19]. This means that their oxygen carrying capacity is not different from that of the patient's circulating blood [25]. In contrast, red cells available through donations and after cold storage are nearly devoid of 2.3-DPG and have (at least temporarily) lost their ability to release oxygen to the tissue. Cerebral and cardiac functions—dependent on available oxygen extraction—are not impaired by fresh autologous cells as they are by transfused cells [25].

An important point is the outcome of patients undergoing cell salvage when compared with allogeneic transfusions. Unfortunately, there is not much data available to draw solid conclusions. However, there are some randomized controlled trials demonstrating significant lower infection rates after surgery with cell salvage when compared to their counterparts using donated red cells [26]. The reason for this finding may be the absence of immunosuppression encountered with allogeneic blood. Besides, immunosuppression associated with surgery and blood loss (reflected in a reduced frequency of natural killer cell precursors and decreased interferon gamma) can be reversed by transfusion of autologous salvaged blood, suggesting that cell saver blood contains immunostimulants [27]. In fact, it has been shown that the activity of neutrophils and the amount of natural killer cell precursors are enhanced [27, 28].

Some advantages of cell salvage are related to the method used. Unique to cell salvage providing unwashed blood is its simplicity. The device is simple to use, inexpensive, easy to handle, and rapidly available in emergency situations. This makes unwashed cell salvage especially applicable where health-care resources are limited or in mass disaster. Especially when large amounts of blood are collected in a relatively short time, e.g., during the time a surgical leak is detected until the patient is taken back to the operating room for revision, direct cell salvage is beneficial. When large amounts of blood are collectable from body cavities, e.g., from a drained hemothorax, direct retransfusion is also beneficial.

The primary advantage of cell salvage with a washing step is that activated clotting factors, free hemoglobin, and debris are removed. Computerized cell salvage markedly reduces the risk of embolism through a series of control steps, checks, valves, and sensors.

Practical considerations for cell salvage with a washing step

Before a cell salvage procedure is initiated, some basic considerations are warranted. First, the right technique and the right equipment need to be chosen. Since techniques provide different blood products with different properties, the right choice can make a difference. Factors like the procedure, comorbidities of the patient, the surgeon and the expected blood loss, cost issues, and the need for postoperative cell salvage need to be considered to make the right choice. Sensitive patients, such as children, require more care in the choice of a cell-saving device than other patient populations. Continuous cell salvage offers distinct advantages for the pediatric population. Such devices deliver a higher hematocrit after processing. Smaller blood volumes can be processed. A classic Latham bowl may need a refill with already washed blood. This may be difficult in small children since the blood may already have been given back to the patient with a small blood volume [29]. Therefore, continuous cell salvage is the recommended procedure in pediatrics.

Another thought should be given to the setup of the cell saver. If it is most probable that there is major blood loss, the cell saver is set up completely prior to surgery. In case the patient allows only a certain kind of cell salvage, the cell saver is set up accordingly, e.g., when it is necessary to prepare the cell saver to ascertain that blood sucked from the surgical field is in constant contact with the circulation of the patient. To this end, the blood bag is spiked with a saline-filled infusion system and the system is connected to the patient's circulation. When the patient does not insist on constant contact of the blood with the circulation and it is questionable whether much blood can be collected, some have chosen to set up the

cell saver only partially (so-called "stand-by cell salvage"). Only the suction and the collection reservoir are set up. If enough blood is collected, the remaining parts of the cell saver are assembled and the blood is processed. When not much blood is collected, expensive parts of the cell saver (e.g., the centrifuge) are not used. Another way to reduce costs with cell salvage is a modified approach. Smaller equipment is used for procedures with slow blood loss.

For extensive procedure, physicians often use two suction tubes: one for blood leading to the collection reservoir of the cell saver, and the other for "dirty business," e.g., irrigants, glues, and bone cement. To avoid undue blood damage, the suction tip should not suck at the blood–air interface and the suction has to be adjusted to the lowest functioning pressure.

The success of cell salvage depends on the amount of blood that can be collected and recovered for retransfusion. Typically, blood is sucked from the surgical site. Expeditious and thorough suction is needed to recover as much blood as possible. If necessary, the surgeon as well as the assistant can use a suction tip. To this end, the cell saver can be equipped with two, instead of one reservoir, with attached suction.

> **Practice tip**
>
> When a wound situated at the side of a patient is emptying its blood on the floor, plastic bags can be taped right below the wound so that the blood collects there and can be sucked out by the suction tip placed in the plastic bag.

Not all blood is collected by suction. Considerable amounts (about 1/3 of the total red cell recovery in one study) [30] of blood are taken up by sponges. Sponges and surgical towels soaked with blood can be rinsed in a bowl containing saline. After washing and wringing out of the towels, the blood is sucked into the cell saver, processed and reclaimed [25, 31].

If blood has collected in a body cavity and may be under pressure during surgical incision, it may flow out too rapidly to be collected entirely by suctioning. In such instances, a preincision drainage with a needle or similar equipment may be indicated to collect the blood. Or a small incision is made only and the peritoneum is "tented" to avoid spillage [10]. Afterward, the body cavity is opened in the intended manner, the remaining blood is collected and surgery continues.

Laparoscopically guided blood salvage is also possible. It is an option when the findings in the abdomen are unclear and chances are that the bleeding problem has either already resolved itself (e.g., in a small splenic tear) or it can be solved laparoscopically [31]. Laparoscopy often provides a very good view of the bleeding source, and the hemoperitoneum can be removed. Repeated examinations are possible easily. When compared with methods to achieve a nonsurgical management of a splenic tear, where patients wait under "transfusion protection" for the spontaneous stop of hemorrhage, an initial laparoscopic approach may reduce the use of allogeneic blood.

Collected blood needs to be labeled properly. It has to be indicated on the container that the blood is autologous. The name and birth date of the patient as well as the date and time of the start of blood procurement have to be noted on the blood bags or bottles.

Autologous blood needs to be given back in time since it is not stored in a cold environment and not under the usual safety precautions prescribed for blood storage. It is recommended that blood is given back only up to 6 hours after warm storage. This ensures the viability of blood cells and reduces bacterial contamination.

During the entire process of cell salvage and retransfusion, the patient needs to be monitored. This is usually not a problem during intraoperative cell salvage. If blood is returned postoperatively, monitoring must continue until all blood is given. Monitoring includes the patient (temperature, vital signs), the aspect of blood intended for return (clots?), and the amount of blood coming from drains. Excessive bleeding from the drain in the presence of normal coagulation parameters is indicative of a surgically solvable problem, not of a coagulopathy [32]. Changes induced by cell salvage need to be taken into consideration when it comes to postoperative monitoring. In unwashed blood, confusion may occur in the interpretation of results of the coagulation profiles.

Anticoagulation and filters

Anticoagulant: Blood coming slowly from a drained wound is usually defibrinated and not able to clot any more. Thus, the addition of an anticoagulant is usually not necessary. Only if brisk bleeding occurs and the contact time of the blood with the wound is not sufficient to defibrinize all the blood, clotting may occur. To prevent this, an anticoagulant may be added.

Intraoperative cell salvage with or without washing requires anticoagulation as well. Either the patient is anticoagulated (as in Method 2), or the collected blood is anticoagulated. Typically, heparin is used as anticoagulant when a cell-saving device calls for systemic anticoagulation. Heparin is also added to the collected blood in the cell saver. About 10000–100000 IU are added to 1 L saline (typically: 30000 IU/L) and the mixture is added in about equal amounts as blood is collected.

Another anticoagulant for cell salvage is citrate in the form of citrate–phosphate–dextrose (CPD) or citrate–phosphate–dextrose–adenine (CPD-A). One part of citrate is mixed with 7–8 parts of blood. Citrate chelates calcium and prevents so clotting. The dextrose in the citrate provides the substrate for glycolysis and preserves the metabolism in red cells. The chelating effect of citrate also protects platelets. Citrate is metabolized in the liver and should therefore be avoided in patients with grave liver damage. When calcium-containing solutions are used in the field, e.g., Ringer's solution for irrigation, CPD is also not ideal. In such patients, heparin is the anticoagulant of choice.

If a patient has a history of heparin-induced thrombocytopenia or there are other reasons not to give heparin, citrate, danaparoid or hirudin derivatives [22] are viable alternatives.

Filters: Blood filtration is recommended before cell saver blood is returned. The filter will eliminate gross debris. Typically, a standard blood filter of 170 μm is used. Since the centrifugation of blood may concentrate particular debris, a microaggregation filter (40–60 micron blood filter) is recommended for the return of the blood to add more safety.

Risks and side effects of cell salvage

The risks and side effects of cell salvage are dependent on the type of procedure, on the way blood is processed, and on the amount of blood returned. Three groups of problems can be encountered with cell salvage: equipment malfunction, operator error, and blood-related sequelae (contamination, quality of blood). Equipment and related problems as well as operator error were greatly reduced by microprocessor technology. Design refinements and the increased experience of cell saver users make cell salvage a safe procedure.

Air embolism was reported with some cell salvage devices. It has been attributed to infusion pumps attached directly to a reservoir and to pressure infusions applied to a retransfusion bag containing air. To avoid this, modern cell salvage devices do not transfuse directly from the centrifuge and have a system of air detection, which stops the system if air is introduced.

If citrate is used to anticoagulate blood, hypocalcemia may occur if much citrate is returned to the patient. Checking the calcium level and administration of calcium prevent this.

Andecdotal case reports describe a "salvaged blood syndrome" with multiple organ failure and consumption coagulopathy following autotransfusion [26]. Although it is known that cell salvage may cause a slight coagulopathy, especially after major blood turnover, there is no evidence that autotransfusion itself can cause this syndrome. A large review of over 36,000 cases did not provide evidence that the "salvaged blood syndrome" really is the result of autotransfusion. The incidence of coagulopathy was low (0.05%) and respiratory failure in combination with disseminated intravascular coagulation occurred in 18 cases only, all associated with major surgery. All patients had profound shock and received multiple transfusions. It is therefore most likely that associated problems, not the autotransfusion itself triggered the coagulopathy [33].

There are unique risks and side effects with unwashed and washed blood.

Unwashed blood

Febrile reactions have been reported after retransfusion of wound blood. They are dependent on the duration of blood collection. After 6 hours of collection, there are only 2% of febrile reactions. If the collection period was prolonged, more than 22% of the patients experienced febrile reactions [18]. Immunologic reactions, e.g., due to cytokines in the retransfused blood, and bacterial contamination are thought to be the reason for those reactions. The great majority of febrile reactions are mild and harmless.

Some case reports mention renal dysfunction after retransfusion of unwashed blood. This happens infrequently and in the presence of other risk factors. Some authors claim that free hemoglobin is the reason for the renal damage since hemoglobin is nephrotoxic and has the ability to scavenge nitric oxide causing microcirculatory disturbances. However, opponents of this theory claim that, once given, free hemoglobin is rapidly excreted by the kidneys. About 24 hours after retransfusion, hemoglobin levels are normal again. They add that normal amounts of free hemoglobin, found in unwashed blood, are safe. They say that restricting the infusion of unwashed blood to 15 mL/kg or 1 L in the adult seems to be without clinical consequences, since enough circulating haptoglobin is present to collect the free hemoglobin [19]. The real impact of free hemoglobin in the blood is still controversial although most authors agree that at least 1–2 L of

unwashed blood are usually well tolerated. If, despite this, renal damage occurs, markers of renal function should be assessed, autotransfusion is stopped, and intravenous hydration is increased.

Unwashed blood theoretically may introduce foreign materials into the circulation. Especially in orthopedics, bone fragments, fat, metal fragments from drills and saws, bone cement, and drugs may be infused. Although mostly a theoretical concern, washing of blood is preferred in such procedures.

If by-products of coagulation activation are retransfused, the patient may experience a mild, subclinical coagulopathy that returns to normal within 24 hours. It is questionable whether the induced coagulopathy is clinically relevant. Although unwashed blood is given back safely in the majority of cases, there are some case reports about massive coagulopathies associated with increased postoperative blood loss.

The risk–benefit ratio of unwashed cell salvage may not be favorable in some situations. There may be situations when a patient loses much blood during a relatively short time after surgery. Then, retransfusion in theory is effective. However, these are situations when a closer look at the patient is warranted. Is he coagulopathic or, more likely, does he need to be taken back to the operating room to have his surgical bleeding fixed? Such situations may make unwashed cell salvage effective, but may not be in the best interests of the patient. On the other hand, when postoperative blood loss is very slow, only small amounts of wound fluid with a low hematocrit will collect. If this is given back, the benefit to the patient regarding improvement of his hemoglobin level may be small and the amount of debris given back to him may be relatively high. Such extreme situations must be considered case by case to determine whether there is sufficient benefit to the patient, if the blood is returned.

Washed blood

The process of washing blood itself has an impact on the red cells and on the patient who later receives the blood. Normal saline is used for washing blood in the majority of cases. This has an effect on the product of cell salvage. Patients receiving the processed blood may develop a hyperchloremic metabolic acidosis and calcium, magnesium and proteins may decrease [34]. This is due to the presence of only sodium and chloride in the washing solution. Alternative washing solutions are under investigation [35]. They may prevent the drop in the pH and the electrolyte disturbances. This may be advantageous especially in surgery with major blood turnover.

Table 16.1 Examples of quality assurance parameters of cell salvage blood.

Quality marker	Cell salvage with washing step
Red cell recovery	>80%
Elimination of free hemoglobin	>90%; or <200 mg/dL
Hematocrit in autologous blood ready for retransfusion	>50%

Another concern with washed blood is the depletion of clotting factors and platelets that may lead to a coagulopathy. Dilutional coagulopathy, though, is infrequently observed in routine use of washed cell salvage [7].

While it is often claimed that the washing process eliminates all relevant contaminants, variations in this elimination process have been described. Free hemoglobin may be present in much higher levels than assumed and may lead to renal dysfunction [36]. It is therefore prudent to initiate a quality assurance process for cell salvage to make sure the blood quality is as expected (Table 16.1).

Concerns: how to overcome contraindications

There are concerns about the use of a cell saver in certain situations. These are when blood may be contaminated by bacteria, by tumor cells, or by amniotic fluids. Besides, some diseases have been considered a relative contraindication for cell salvage. However, with some adjustments made, cell salvage can be used in such situations as well.

Spread of bacterial contamination

Retransfusion of washed [37] and even unwashed blood with enteric contamination has been described [38]. Several outcome studies in trauma, colorectal, and gynecological surgery demonstrate the safety of cell washing and retransfusion also in such patients where the blood is known to be contaminated with bacteria. However, physicians are still hesitant to use cell salvage when they feel the blood could be contaminated with bacteria. Let us examine whether the concerns are always justified.

Well, it is a fact that most blood used for retransfusion after cell salvage is contaminated with bacteria. In a considerable proportion of cases (21–48% [39, 40]), even blood salvaged from "clean" surgical fields grows bacteria when cultured. However, upon retransfusion of this contaminated blood there seems to be no increased incidence of sepsis or other adverse effects for the patient. The bacteremia resulting from the infusion of such contaminated blood usually resolves spontaneously 24 hours after surgery. If infection occurs after surgery with autotransfusion, they are usually not related to cell salvage. The risk of complications due to infection seems to depend on other complicating factors (such as multiple injury) and not primarily on the contamination of blood. Usually, the kind of bacteria cultured in the salvaged blood does not correlate with the species cultured from the site of postoperative infection [40].

As of yet, bacterial contamination of blood collected for cell salvage, which is then washed, carries only a theoretical risk to the patient. Medical literature does not support the notion of avoidance of cell salvage on the grounds of bacterial contamination.

There are some measures that can be taken to reduce either the amount of bacterial contamination in the salvaged blood or to reduce bacteria that might have been collected. When a grossly contaminated area is encountered in the surgical field, e.g., the contents of an abscess, a second suction device should be used to drain the maximally bacteria-loaded material into a discard container. All other blood can be collected for cell salvage. Cell washing significantly reduces, but does not completely eliminate bacterial contamination. Leukocyte depletion filters may add to the safety of patients with gross bacterial contamination since they reduce the amount of bacteria infused [41]. Parenteral broad spectrum antibiotics are recommended for patients who receive cell salvaged blood [37]. Timing is important to avoid additional bacterial growth in the already collected blood. It is recommended to retransfuse blood within 6 hours after collection.

Contrasting cell salvage with allogeneic transfusion, one easily comes to the conclusion that there is a proven risk of bacterial infection with allogeneic transfusion, while there is only a theoretical risk of bacterial infection with salvaged autologous blood. It may be reasonable, therefore, to favor autologous cell salvage blood over allogeneic blood. Taking the above into account, you may want to join the author who wrote: "Even if sepsis is to occur, I have always maintained that it is better to have a live patient with a bacteremia than a dead patient with a sterile blood culture" [40].

Tumor cells

Oncological surgery often leads to massive blood loss. Nevertheless, allogeneic transfusions should be avoided in cancer patients since they adversely affect outcome.

Autotransfusion, as an alternative approach, can reduce the exposure of patients to donor blood. The question is whether autologous blood collected during oncologic surgery can be retransfused safely.

Malignant cells are often found in the blood circulation of cancer patient prior to surgery. As soon as the surgeon touches the tumor, many more cells are released into the circulation. It was shown that even salvaged blood contains viable, tumorigenic cells. Due to the theoretical concern of tumor spread by retransfusion of cancer cells, some practitioners refuse to use cell salvage in oncological surgery. However, this seems not to be justified, neither is there convincing proof in the literature that it is detrimental for the patient.

To address even these theoretical concerns, methods have been tested to reduce the amount of tumor cells in the blood returned to the patient. The process of washing the blood during cell salvage eliminates or destroys a considerable amount of tumor cells. Additional reduction of the tumor cell load in the blood is achievable by the use of leukocyte depletion filters. These two methods combined greatly reduce, but do not eliminate all tumor cells. However, some sources claim that the remaining tumor cells are not clonogenic [42]. Some authors prefer to add cytostatics to the cell salvage fluid to kill the tumor cells. But since the patient is then also exposed to the cytostatics, this method did not find widespread use. To finally damage all viable tumor cells, irradiation of salvaged blood with 50 Gray is used effectively [43]. Irradiation takes 6–15 minutes and the blood should be available for retransfusion within a reasonable time. The technique of blood irradiation obviously is costly and taps on valuable resources. Special blood bags are needed to prevent undue hemolysis, irradiation facilities need to be available as well as technicians trained and persons for the transfer of the blood to and from the operating room. Nevertheless, to date it seems to be the only method to completely inactivate tumor cells, whether this is important or not.

The theoretical risk of tumor spread by infusing blood with viable cells has not been confirmed in available studies [44]. We are therefore called upon to balance risks and benefits coming with transfusions in oncological surgery. M.J.G. Thomas, in a review entitled "Infected and malignant fields are an absolute contraindication to intraoperative cell salvage: fact or fiction?", finds a series of questions to help weigh the risks and benefits of cell salvage in oncological surgery. Ask yourself: "In what percentage of cases will cells have already been disseminated? Will dormant cells be awakened simply by surgery (*or by allo-geneic transfusion,* italics ours)? What effect does the skill of the surgeon contribute? Is intravascular spread . . . far less important than local deposits? Will reinfusing additional malignant cells negate the reduction in immunomodulation, achieved by the use of autologous blood?" [40]. After considering available facts, the mentioned author concluded: "However, on balance, it would appear that the use of filters, whether alone or in combination with irradiation, could produce a product that is as safe, if not safer, than allogeneic blood" [40].

Amniotic fluid embolism

Amniotic fluid is essentially an electrolyte solution. Toward the end of pregnancy, the fluid contains additional products, such as tissue factor, squamous cells and phospholipids (in the form of lamellar bodies resulting from lung maturation of the fetus), and fetal hemoglobin. Amniotic fluid can cause an amniotic embolism which is a rare, but potentially fatal complication of pregnancy. It develops with pulmonary hypertension, hypoxia, heart failure, and acute respiratory distress syndrome as well as disseminated intravascular coagulation and uterine atonia with massive hemorrhage. The pathophysiology of amniotic fluid embolism is poorly understood. Initially, emboli of fetal debris (e.g., squamous cells, vernix, mucin) have been thought to be the reason for the amniotic fluid embolism and tissue factor has been implicated as a reason for a disseminated intravascular coagulation. But fetal squamous cells are also commonly found in the circulation of patients in labor who do not develop the syndrome. Also, during a Cesarean section, parts of the amniotic fluid routinely enter the circulation of the mother without causing any unwanted effects. Recent findings suggest that amniotic fluid embolism is more akin to anaphylaxis. The term "anaphylactoid syndrome of pregnancy" has been suggested instead.

Amniotic fluid embolism usually occurs during labor but sometimes occurs during abortion, abdominal trauma, and amnioinfusion. Also, as regards cell salvage, there is a concern about causing amniotic embolism by the spread of amniotic contents into the circulation of the parturient. True, blood sucked into the cell saver reservoir contains many of the particles thought to be responsible for amniotic embolism. But, as of yet, there is no proof that blood collected during Cesarean section causes amniotic embolism [45].

Washing blood in a cell saver reduces many of the constituents of amniotic fluid. This also includes tissue factor. A further reduction of potentially offensive parts is achievable with certain leukocyte depletion filters. After cell washing and filtration, the amount of amniotic fluid constituents, such as lamellar bodies and squamous cells, are at least as low as in the mother's blood, if not lower.

Among constituents of amniotic fluid, only fetal hemoglobin increases in the mother's blood after returning the cell saver blood. Fetal hemoglobin naturally enters the mother's circulation during birth. This is without consequences unless there is an incompatibility of the blood groups leading to complications in further pregnancies. To avoid risks due to rhesus-incompatible blood, rhesus immunization of the mother is recommended. The dose of rhesus immunoglobulin should be calculated after the cell salvaged blood is returned, since the infused fetal hemoglobin can increase the needed dose of immunoglobulin.

Cell salvage and concomitant diseases

Cell salvage can be performed in patients with almost all comorbidities. While solid tumors cause some physicians to think twice before the blood is returned, malignancy of the hematopoietic system, such as leukemia and plasmacytoma, do not constitute a contraindication for cell salvage and special considerations are not needed.

Hereditary anemia, e.g., spherocytosis and thalassemia [46], are also deemed safe for autologous transfusion. Sickle cell anemia does not constitute a contraindication for cell salvage. Sickle cells typically develop when hemoglobin is deoxygenated and in an acidotic environment. However, in cell salvage, blood is in contact with air and therefore oxygenated. Besides, carbon dioxide dissolves in the salvaged blood that causes a "metabolic alkalosis." Thus, in theory, sickling of red cells in the cell salvage process is unlikely and it has been concluded that sickle cell anemia is therefore no contraindication for cell salvage [47]. In contrast, the washing process of a cell saver has been described in sickle cell patients to cause severe sickling in a blood smear obtained from the processed blood and the author concluded that sickle cell disease may be a contraindication to cell washing [48].

Cell salvage is actually the method of choice when it comes to blood conservation of patients with certain hematologic disorders. Predepositing of blood of patients with sickle cell anemia and spherocytosis is not recommended since the storage conditions (low pH, etc.) may lead to irreversible sickling in sickle cell disease and a dramatically shortened life span of spherocytes [47].

Indications for cell salvage

Autologous transfusions including cell salvage have been shown to reduce the use of allogeneic red cell transfusions [49, 50]. This is true for postoperative cell salvage [51, 52] as well as for intraoperative cell salvage. To make cell salvage effective, patients must be carefully selected. It has proven difficult to formulate universal criteria for patients most likely to benefit from cell salvage. In an emergency, a cell saver should be ready whenever significant blood loss is anticipated or possible. Current guidelines suggest the following criteria for cell salvage: adults who undergo surgery with an anticipated blood loss of more than 1000 mL, or the patient may lose more than 20% of his blood, patients undergoing procedures where more than 10% are transfused allogeneically in the perioperative period or where the mean transfusion rate is more than 1 unit. However, from the perspective of the good quality of fresh autologous blood as well as from the cost perspective, a cell saver may be indicated much earlier. Interestingly, it has been calculated that setting up a cell saver in the stand-by mode (using only suction and reservoir with anticoagulant), costs about the same as it does to type and cross-match 2 units of red cell concentrates [53].

Reports on successful cell salvage abound. One or the other method of cell salvage has been used in the following procedures:

- Major vascular surgery, e.g., aortic aneurysm repair
- Thoracic and cardiac surgery, e.g., coronary artery bypass surgery, valve replacement [50, 54]
- Neurosurgery [55], e.g., for spinal fusion, basilar aneurysms, tumors
- Orthopedic surgery [24, 56], e.g., for hip and knee arthroplasty, especially bilateral or reoperations, scoliosis surgery
- Transplantation, e.g., liver transplantation
- General surgery, e.g., for exploratory laparotomy with free fluids intraperitoneally, liver surgery
- Gynecologic and obstetric procedures, e.g., hysterectomy [57] and myomectomy, Cesarean section, especially in complicated placentation, ruptured ectopic pregnancy [58]
- Trauma management [17], e.g., hemothorax [59], abdominal trauma, spine surgery
- Plastic surgery [55, 60], e.g., in burn excision [61]
- Ear–nose–throat (ENT) surgery: major maxillofacial surgery

- Pediatric procedures, e.g., craniosynostosis correction [55], acetabuloplasty [62]

Key points

- Cell salvage can be performed intra- or postoperatively. Blood can either be directly given back or after a washing process. The quality of blood for direct return differs greatly from the quality of washed blood. Both types of cell salvage come with advantages and disadvantages.
- When life is at stake, there is no contraindication to proficient cell salvage. Relative contraindications have been cited but can be overcome by the following methods:
  ○ *Bacterial contamination*: cell washing, leukocyte depletion filtration, systemic broad spectrum antibiotics
  ○ *Contamination with tumor cells*: cell washing, leukocyte depletion filtration, adding cytostatics to the blood, irradiation
  ○ *Amniotic fluid contamination*: cell washing and leukocyte depletion filtration
- Cell salvage has many advantages, namely:
  ○ Provision of the patient's own blood. This means a low risk of disease transmission, clerical error, and immunological complications.
  ○ Reduced or eliminated the use of allogeneic blood products.
  ○ A blood product that contains viable, fresh red cells with a near-normal lifespan and ability to release oxygen to the tissue.
  ○ May reduce costs.
  ○ Improves outcome of patients.
  ○ Availability of compatible blood in elective as well as emergent surgery.

Questions for review

- What methods are available to perform cell salvage?
- From where does the blood come which is salvaged?
- What is the difference between cell salvage with washed and unwashed blood? How is the quality of the blood influenced?
- What are the contraindications of cell salvage? Can they be overcome and how?
- Which diseases need special consideration when it comes to cell salvage?
- Describe the different modes of anticoagulation of the salvaged blood.

Suggestions for further research

Find out whether there is a way to wash blood and still have major amounts of coagulation factors available?

Exercises and practice cases

Calculate how much blood you would get back from a cell saver that washes the following blood: After you have collected 1.5 L of blood with a hematocrit of 35, you diluted it with 1.5 L of anticoagulant containing solution. The cell saver concentrates red cells to a hematocrit of 70% and recovers 80% of the delivered red cells.

Homework

Ask a sales representative to demonstrate a cell saver. If possible, find representatives of a system that uses unwashed blood and a representative for a system for washed blood. Record the contact and other pertinent information in the address book in the Appendix E.

Find out where to get a leukocyte depletion filter to be used in connection with a cell saver.

Check whether there are any guidelines in your hospital that guide any kind of blood salvage. If there are, get a copy.

References

1 Blundell, J. Experiments on the transfusion of blood by the syringe. *Med Chir Trans*, 1818. **9**: p. 56–92.
2 Highmore, W. Practical remarks on an overlooked source of blood-supply for transfusion in post-partum haemorrhage suggested by a recent fatal case. *Lancet*, 1874. p. 89.
3 Duncan, J. On re-infusion of blood in primary and other amputations. *BMJ*, 1886. **1**: p. 192–193.
4 Thies, J. Zur Behandlung der Extrauteringravidität. *Zentralblatt für Gynäkologie*, 1914. **38**: p. 1191–1193.
5 Griswold, R.A. and A.B. Ortner. Use of autotransfusion in surgery of serous cavities. *Surg Gynecol Obstet*, 1943. **77**: p. 167–177.
6 Klebanoff, G. Early clinical experience with a disposable unit for the intraoperative salvage and reinfusion of blood loss (intraoperative autotransfusion). *Am J Surg*, 1970. **120**(6): p. 718–722.
7 Laub, G.W. and J.B. Riebman. Autotransfusion: methods and complications. In Lake, C.L. and Moore, R.A. (eds.) *Blood: Hemostasis, Transfusion, and Alternatives in the Perioperative*

Period. Lippincott Williams & Wilkins Publishers, USA, 1995. p. 381–394.

8 Catling, S.J., S. Williams, and A.M. Fielding. Cell salvage in obstetrics: an evaluation of the ability of cell salvage combined with leucocyte depletion filtration to remove amniotic fluid from operative blood loss at caesarean section. *Int J Obstet Anesth*, 1999. **8**(2): p. 79–84.

9 Whitehead, S.M. Using blood bags for autotransfusion. *Trop Doct*, 1982. **12**(4, Pt 1): p. 189.

10 Poeschl, U. Emergency autologous blood transfusion in ruptured ectopic pregnancy. *Anesthesia*, 1992. (2): Article 2.

11 Heimbecker, R.O. History of bloodless surgery in Canada: blood recycling in the operating room. In *The 73rd Annual Ontario Hospital Association Convention*, 1987.

12 Ovadje, O.O. An emergency auto-transfusion device designed for developing countries. *Intensive Care World*, 1991. **8**(2): p. 88–89.

13 Reeder, G.D. Autotransfusion theory of operation: a review of the physics and hematology. *Transfusion*, 2004. **44**(12, Suppl): p. 35S–39S.

14 Radvan, J., *et al.* Physical principles of autotransfusion systems. *AINS*, 2002. **37**(11): p. 689–696.

15 Eichert, I., *et al.* Cell saver, ultrafiltration and direct transfusion: comparative study of three blood processing techniques. *Thorac Cardiovasc Surg*, 2001. **49**(3): p. 149–152.

16 Shuhaiber, J.H. and S.M. Whitehead. The impact of introducing an autologous intraoperative transfusion device to a community hospital. *Ann Vasc Surg*, 2003. **17**(4): p. 424–429.

17 Heimbecker, R.O. Blood recycling eliminates need for blood. *CMAJ*, 1996. **155**(3): p. 275–276.

18 Waters, J.H., *et al.* Amniotic fluid removal during cell salvage in the cesarean section patient. *Anesthesiology*, 2000. **92**(6): p. 1531–1536.

19 Munoz, M., *et al.* Transfusion of post-operative shed blood: laboratory characteristics and clinical utility. *Eur Spine J*, 2004. **13**(Suppl 1): p. S107–S113.

20 Geiger, P., *et al.* New developments in autologous transfusion systems. *Anaesthesia*, 1998. **53**(Suppl 2): p. 32–35.

21 Innerhofer, P. and F.J. Wiedermann. Leucocyte activation through intra operative blood salvage. *AINS*, 2002. **37**(12): p. 738–740.

22 Marx, A., *et al.* Removal of lepirudin used as an anticoagulant in mechanical autotransfusion with Cell-Saver 5. *AINS*, 2001. **36**(3): p. 162–166.

23 Booke, M., *et al.* Fat elimination during intraoperative autotransfusion: an in vitro investigation. *Anesth Analg*, 1997. **85**(5): p. 959–962.

24 Borghi, B., *et al.* Autotransfusion in major orthopaedic surgery: experience with 1785 patients. *Br J Anaesth*, 1997. **79**(5): p. 662–664.

25 Ronai, A.K., J.J. Glass, and A.S. Shapiro. Improving autologous blood harvest: recovery of red cells from sponges and suction. *Anaesth Intensive Care*, 1987. **15**(4): p. 421–424.

26 Vanderlinde, E.S., J.M. Heal, and N. Blumberg. Autologous transfusion. *BMJ*, 2002. **324**(7340): p. 772–775.

27 Gharehbaghian, A., *et al.* Effect of autologous salvaged blood on postoperative natural killer cell precursor frequency. *Lancet*, 2004. **363**(9414): p. 1025–1030.

28 Iorwerth, A., *et al.* Neutrophil activity in total knee replacement: implications in preventing post-arthroplasty infection. *Knee*, 2003. **10**(1): p. 111–113.

29 Booke, M., *et al.* Intraoperative autotransfusion in small children: an in vitro investigation to study its feasibility. *Anesth Analg*, 1999. **88**(4): p. 763–765.

30 Haynes, S.L., *et al.* Does washing swabs increase the efficiency of red cell recovery by cell salvage in aortic surgery? *Vox Sang*, 2005. **88**(4): p. 244–248.

31 Smith, R.S., *et al.* Laparoscopically guided blood salvage and autotransfusion in splenic trauma: a case report. *J Trauma*, 1993. **34**(2): p. 313–314.

32 Halfman-Franey, M. and D.E. Berg. Recognition and management of bleeding following cardiac surgery. *Crit Care Nurs Clin North Am*, 1991. **3**(4): p. 675–689.

33 Tawes, R.L., Jr. and T.B. Duvall. Is the "salvaged-cell syndrome" myth or reality? *Am J Surg*, 1996. **172**(2): p. 172–174.

34 Halpern, N.A., *et al.* Cell saver autologous transfusion: metabolic consequences of washing blood with normal saline. *J Trauma*, 1996. **41**(3): p. 407–415.

35 Sumpelmann, R., *et al.* Massive transfusion of washed red blood cells: acid–base and electrolyth changes for different wash solutions. *AINS*, 2003. **38**(9): p. 587–593.

36 Klodell, C.T., *et al.* Does cell-saver blood administration and free hemoglobin load cause renal dysfunction? *Am Surg*, 2001. **67**(1): p. 44–47.

37 Timberlake, G.A. and N.E. McSwain, Jr. Autotransfusion of blood contaminated by enteric contents: a potentially lifesaving measure in the massively hemorrhaging trauma patient? *J Trauma*, 1988. **28**(6): p. 855–857.

38 Yamada, T., *et al.* Intraoperative blood salvage in abdominal simple total hysterectomy for uterine myoma. *Int J Gynaecol Obstet*, 1997. **59**(3): p. 233–236.

39 Kudo, H., *et al.* Cytological and bacteriological studies of intraoperative autologous blood in neurosurgery. *Surg Neurol*, 2004. **62**(3): p. 195–199; discussion 199–200.

40 Thomas, M.J. Infected and malignant fields are an absolute contraindication to intraoperative cell salvage: fact or fiction? *Transfus Med*, 1999. **9**(3): p. 269–278.

41 Waters, J.H., *et al.* Bacterial reduction by cell salvage washing and leukocyte depletion filtration. *Anesthesiology*, 2003. **99**(3): p. 652–655.

42 Konsgaard, U.E., *et al.* The efficacy of cell saver and leucocyte depletion filter for tumour cell removal. *Anesth Analg*, 1996. **82**: p. S244.

43 Hansen, E., V. Bechmann, and J. Altmeppen. Blood salvage in cancer surgery? *AINS*, 2001. **36**(Suppl 2): p. S128–S129.

44 Davis, M., *et al.* The use of cell salvage during radical retropubic prostatectomy: does it influence cancer recurrence? *BJU Int*, 2003. **91**(6): p. 474–476.

45 Rebarber, A., *et al.* The safety of intraoperative autologous blood collection and autotransfusion during cesarean section. *Am J Obstet Gynecol*, 1998. **179**(3, Pt 1): p. 715–720.

46 Waters, J.H., E. Lukauskiene, and M.E. Anderson. Intraoperative blood salvage during cesarean delivery in a patient with beta thalassemia intermedia. *Anesth Analg*, 2003. **97**(6): p. 1808–1809.

47 Dietrich, G.V. Autotransfusion in special procedure and diseases. *AINS*, 2002. **37**(12): p. 744–747.

48 Brajtbord, D., *et al.* Use of the cell saver in patients with sickle cell trait. *Anesthesiology*, 1989. **70**(5): p. 878–879.

49 Carless, P., *et al.* Autologous transfusion techniques: a systematic review of their efficacy. *Transfus Med*, 2004. **14**(2): p. 123–144.

50 Murphy, G.J., *et al.* Safety and efficacy of perioperative cell salvage and autotransfusion after coronary artery bypass grafting: a randomized trial. *Ann Thorac Surg*, 2004. **77**(5): p. 1553–1559.

51 Jones, H.W., *et al.* Postoperative autologous blood salvage drains—are they useful in primary uncemented hip and knee arthroplasty? A prospective study of 186 cases. *Acta Orthop Belg*, 2004. **70**(5): p. 466–473.

52 Steinberg, E.L., *et al.* Comparative analysis of the benefits of autotransfusion of blood by a shed blood collector after total knee replacement. *Arch Orthop Trauma Surg*, 2004. **124**(2): p. 114–118.

53 Waters, J.H. Indications and contraindications of cell salvage. *Transfusion*, 2004. **44**(12, Suppl): p. 40S–44S.

54 McGill, N., *et al.* Mechanical methods of reducing blood transfusion in cardiac surgery: randomised controlled trial. *BMJ*, 2002. **324**(7349): p. 1299.

55 Fearon, J.A. Reducing allogeneic blood transfusions during pediatric cranial vault surgical procedures: a prospective analysis of blood recycling. *Plast Reconstr Surg*, 2004. **113**(4): p. 1126–1130.

56 Borghi, B. and A. Casati, for The Rizzoli Study Group on Orthopaedic Anaesthesia. Incidence and risk factors for allogeneic blood transfusion during major joint replacement using an integrated autotransfusion regimen. *Eur J Anaesthesiol*, 2000. **17**(7): p. 411–417.

57 Braga, J., *et al.* Maternal and perinatal implications of the use of human recombinant erythropoietin. *Acta Obstet Gynecol Scand*, 1996. **75**(5): p. 449–443.

58 Yamada, T., *et al.* Intraoperative autologous blood transfusion for hemoperitoneum resulting from ectopic pregnancy or ovarian bleeding during laparoscopic surgery. *JSLS*, 2003. **7**(2): p. 97–100.

59 Sakamoto, K., *et al.* Autologous salvaged blood transfusion in spontaneous hemopneumothorax. *Ann Thorac Surg*, 2004. **78**(2): p. 705–707.

60 Giordano, G.F., *et al.* An analysis of 9918 consecutive perioperative autotransfusions. *Surg Gynecol Obstet*, 1993. **176**(2): p. 103–110.

61 Jeng, J.C., *et al.* Intraoperative blood salvage in excisional burn surgery: an analysis of yield, bacteriology, and inflammatory mediators. *J Burn Care Rehabil*, 1998. **19**(4): p. 305–311.

62 Nicolai, P., *et al.* Autologous transfusion in acetabuloplasty in children. *J Bone Joint Surg Br*, 2004. **86**(1): p. 110–112.

17 Blood banking

Clinicians committed to avoid allogeneic transfusions will probably have less frequent interactions with the blood bank than their colleagues who do not work toward the same goal. But it is the special knowledge that proficient blood managers have about the work of a blood bank that helps them reduce their transfusions, whenever possible. Besides, when the use of a blood product seems indicated, background knowledge about blood banking helps to facilitate the interaction of the clinician with the blood bank. Additionally, blood bankers often know certain details about their products and thus are a valuable source of information for a person committed to eliminate unjustified allogeneic transfusions. This is the reason why blood banking is included in a book that is committed to minimize the use of blood bank services.

Objectives of this chapter

1 Relate basic procedures to increase the safety of blood products.
2 Evaluate procedures of pathogen reduction in blood products.
3 Get an idea how blood is fractionated.

Definitions

Blood banking: It is the science of collecting, testing, processing, and storing blood for later use. Blood banks take care of the process of blood donation, of blood safety, and help to use blood properly.
Window period: It is the time for which a donor is potentially infectious but still displays negative serological test results [1].
Hemovigilance: It is the systematic monitoring and remedying of side effects and adverse incidents during the whole blood donation and transfusion process. According to the European Union Blood Directive definition, hemovigilance "shall mean a set of organised surveillance procedures relating to serious adverse or unexpected events or reactions in donors or recipients, and the epidemiological follow-up of donors" [2].

A brief look at history

In the early days, "blood transfusion" meant direct donor-to-patient contact without intermediate blood storage. When such direct blood transfers were performed, blood banks were neither available nor needed. The practice of drawing and storing human blood is a comparatively new science. Its basis was laid in 1901 when Karl Landsteiner, an Austrian physician, discovered the first human blood groups. Later, he devised methods for widespread use to determine the blood groups of collected blood. With the transfusion of blood group matched blood, transfusion did not lead to as many immediate deaths as before. This increase in transfusion safety spurred research in transfusion medicine. Major obstacles had to be overcome before the first blood bank could be founded.

In 1914, long-term anticoagulants were developed (e.g., by Richard Lewison) and tried in Europe. Two years later, Francis Rous and J.R. Turner introduced a citrate-glucose solution that permitted storage of blood for several days after collection. This allowed for blood to be stored for later transfusion. The discovery that blood can be stored for a period of time led to the establishment of the first blood "depot" by the British during World War I. These blood depots became the forerunners of modern blood banks.

Due to great advances in transfusion medicine, blood was used in the battlefield in World War I. The battlefield victims virtually provided a large-volume field test for transfusion. This test made it obvious that concerted efforts were needed in transfusion-related research as well as in providing sufficient amounts of donor blood.

After the First World War, Russia as one of the first countries perceived the need of an organized approach to transfusion medicine, an approach later called "blood bank." As a result of the great efforts of the Russian Dr Alexander

Bogdanov, Moscow saw the first institute of blood transfusion (now the National Research Center for Hematology of the Russian Academy of Medical Sciences) in 1926. It was the declared goal of the institute to strengthen the scientific basis of transfusions, to train physicians, and to prepare and sell blood products. Early beginnings were not easy. The building in which the institute was situated was in very bad shape and money was lacking. Also, the equipment the researchers could use was hardly sufficient to do their job. However, ingenuity helped to overcome even the fiercest problems and to obtain scientific results with obsolete methods. Bogdanov did not have the joy of leading the institute for long. He died in 1928 as a result of an experimental blood exchange with one of his students. Bogdanov was followed by other directors who continued his work. As early as 1930, a network of blood centers was developed throughout Russia, with the Moscow institute taking the lead. At that time, also cadaveric blood was stored for transfusion (by Yudin in 1934). The military was one of the users of the blood provided by the institute [3].

Few were aware of the immense work done by the Russians in the field of transfusion medicine when Dr Bernhard Fantus in 1937 came up with the concept of a blood bank in the Cook County hospital in Chicago [4]. He started a venture where blood was deposited and withdrawn and where credit was granted for times when much blood was transfused. Copying the financial world in its organizational approach, the term "blood bank" was coined. Within a few years, more blood banks were established in the United States.

While Chicago celebrated the first blood bank, the Russian institute continued its work. They did research in the field of blood preservatives and antibacterial agents, refined serum preparation, clarified the pathophysiology underlying transfusions and developed blood substitutes. All this was done with antiquated laboratory equipment and minimal financial means. Fighting these working conditions, the personnel at the Russian institute had to use sheer ingenuity to fill their large countries requests for transfusions [3].

Despite the existence of blood banks in some countries, not all parties in World War II used their service. Buddy transfusions were used on the front by British soldiers. Germans did not use donor blood, for fear of non-Aryan blood [5]. In contrast, the Americans used stored blood. The immense amount of blood transfused made them ask Dr Cohn to devise a method to use plasma more effectively. In turn, Dr Cohn and coworkers invented in the early 1940s a series of methods to fractionate plasma. They used ethyl alcohol and other compounds to divide plasma into different protein fractions—a process called fractionation down to this day [6, 7].

After the Second World War, the blood banking system spread throughout the world. Blood banking began growing rapidly, spurred on by physicians returning from war, who had seen transfusion therapy in action. Profit-making centers and nonprofit centers mushroomed. Many "bloody" surgical procedures evolved. With the backup of transfusions, surgeons' fears of extensive procedures were alleviated, and medicine made great advances.

The use of blood transfusions in civil life thus started only 60 years ago. The last six decades saw immense developments in blood banking techniques. In 1950, Carl Walter and W.P. Murphy, Jr., introduced the plastic bag for blood collection and storage. These plastic bags allowed freezing of blood, sterile handling, and lowered the risk of breakage of glass bottles [8]. In 1965, Judith Graham Pool identified a technique, now known as cryoprecipitation. Blood safety measures found their way into blood banking in the 1980s. Finally, 1999 saw the implementation of nucleic acid amplification testing. In parallel, the 1990s also saw the development of methods to alter blood products for special purposes (e.g., by altering blood group antigen expression on blood components). Blood products are becoming ever more specialized. In fact, some blood-derived products seem to be more akin to a drug than to blood. It remains to be seen who will take the lead in distributing those products—blood bank or pharmacy.

Blood donation

Donor recruitment

Donor recruitment is the first step in providing blood. Already at this basic step, transfusion safety comes into play. To reduce collection of blood from a donor population with a high incidence of transfusion-transmittable diseases (high-risk donors), recruitment of blood donors is targeted to low-risk groups. Volunteer nonremunerated blood donors from low-risk populations who regularly donate blood seem to be the safest source of blood. In contrast, donations from paid donors are less safe (Table 17.1). To avoid attracting persons who donate blood only for monetary reasons, donation incentives are kept minimal. However, many countries still have paid donors. In fact, source plasma for blood fractionation often comes from paid donors, even in countries where cellular components are donated solely by unpaid donors (Table 17.2).

Donor recruitment is usually initiated either by a commercial organization (e.g., manufacturers of clotting factor concentrates) or by charity organizations. Public

Table 17.1 Seroprevalence in blood donors in percent.

	High HDI	Medium HDI	Low HDI
HIV	0.0–0.8	0–9	0.3–14.0
HBV	0–7	0–30	0.1–70.0
HCV	0.0–1.2	0.0–13.1	0.0–9.2

High HDI for developed countries; medium and low HDI for developing countries.

HDI, human development index.

Source: WHO Global Data Base 2000–2001.

advertisements or adverts targeted to special groups (e.g., the employees or a certain company, college students) are released to recruit donors. Also, fostering the feeling in donors that they are providing a valuable service to society and fellow humans (rather than to the pocket of the manufacturer) serves as an incentive to donate, if possible, regularly.

Sometimes, a patient recruits his/her own donor (e.g., a friend or relative) for a directed or designated donation. The donated blood unit is given to this very patient. The public considers it safer to receive blood from a friend. However, peer pressure may urge the donor to donate. Besides, he/she may be embarrassed to tell about risky behavior (e.g., promiscuity) or other matters that may normally exclude a donor. Directed donations are thus not necessarily safer, perhaps even being less safe. Besides, when blood is donated by direct relatives of the patient, it has to be irradiated to prevent graft-versus-host diseases (GvHD). However, a directed donation may alleviate some fear in patients and have a positive psychological effect. Directed donation is recommended only for patients with rare blood groups or antibodies.

Table 17.2 Percentage of family/replacement or paid donors.

	High HDI	Medium HDI	Low HDI
Total donations	49.3 million	29.4 million	2.3 million
Voluntary, nonremunerated donors	94%	60%	33%
Family/replacement donors	4%	36%	64%
Paid donors	2%	4%	3%

High HDI for developed countries; medium and low HDI for developing countries.

HDI, human development index.

Other donation systems require family or replacement donors. The transfused patient or his/her family has to organize someone who donates blood equivalent to the amount the patient was transfused. Ideally, this is a family member. But often this is someone the family paid. Replacement donations are quite popular in developing countries where constant blood shortages are a problem. Patients who are to be transfused are required to bring someone with them who replaces the blood the patient receives. Such practices are discouraged by the WHO, since often such replacement donations are, in fact, masked paid donations. The patient or the relatives of the patient may pay a professional donor (someone who makes a living by selling his/her blood) to donate blood on behalf of the patient.

Another form of directed or designated blood donation is initiated by physicians for the purpose of "minimal exposure transfusion." The idea behind this practice is to limit the number of donor exposures to a patient. Minimal exposure transfusion has been favored based on the assumption that a decrease in transfusion-related infections or complications is achievable by such a transfusion strategy. A committed donor gives multiple units of blood over a period of time. A patient, typically a child, then receives the blood from only this donor. In case the child is very small and is transfused serially with only a small volume, one donation can be divided into several aliquots and is transfused over time, using the blood of the same donor [9].

Donor recruitment outside a "danger zone" is another way to reduce the likelihood for disease transmission. In the United Kingdom, for instance, plasma for the production of plasma products is imported from countries where there has not been bovine spongiform encephalopathy in cattle and the infection of the population with variant Creutzfeldt Jacob disease is not prevalent [10].

The process of blood donation

Blood can be donated by two distinct methods. Classical blood donation requires only a large-bore venous access. Whole blood drains by gravity into a container. When a certain amount of blood is donated, the blood is either stored or processed further, independent of the presence of the donor. The other kind of blood donation is an automated blood collection, called apheresis. The donor is submitted to an extracorporeal circulation. Blood is withdrawn from his/her vein, some blood components are separated automatically from the blood, and the remaining blood components are returned to the donor. A variety of products can be collected in this way, including plasma for fractionation or cellular components [11].

Blood is collected and stored either in glass bottles or in plastic bags. While glass bottles are still used in some parts of the world, they have been abandoned in many developed countries. Glass bottles can break easily and need to be opened to separate blood, leading to contamination. Plastic bags and systems of two to four bags in a connected closed system, sometimes with inline filters, are used often in developed countries. For red cells, plastic bags are used which contain emollients (plasticizers)—compounds that are afterward found in the donated blood. Platelets are collected in bags that do not contain such chemicals. The bags for platelets have a higher permeability for oxygen than those used for red cells.

Blood safety

Blood safety is a very controversial topic. Developed countries claim that their blood supply is "safer than ever." Incredible amounts of money are invested to detect tainted blood and to eliminate it from the donated blood pool. However, such interventions do not eliminate viral transmission completely. While developed countries invest a fortune into technology that will not provide the degree of blood safety the public is looking for (namely, no-risk blood), developing countries have a hard time to do even the most basic procedures of blood testing and storage [12]. Often, the blood cold chain cannot be upheld in such countries, let alone provide the WHO-recommended tests. Nevertheless, it is good to know about the manifold safety measures taken (or better, in many blood units—not taken).

The term *blood safety* is often used equivalently with avoidance of transfusion-transmittable diseases. This is understandable, since many infectious agents can be transfused by blood (compare Table A.1). The WHO estimates that worldwide, 5–10% of all HIV infections are caused by blood. And many more cases of hepatitis and other diseases are annually transferred by transfusion. Apart from transfusion-transmittable diseases, blood safety efforts also try to address some of the several other problems coming with allogeneic transfusions. This is possible by supporting clinicians to transfuse most appropriately, to avoid clerical errors, and to help in audits, and in other measures of quality assurance.

To assure a measure of blood safety, a series of "safety layers" [12] were devised. They include (1) donor education, (2) selection and deferral, (3) postdonation product quarantine, (4) a national vigilance system (with donor tracing and notification when instances of transmission are detected), and (5) procedures with the donated blood, namely, screening for some diseases and pathogen reduction. Each of these safety layers contributes another aspect to the overall risk minimization. However, all the mentioned safety layers refer to the reduction of the risk to transfuse blood carrying infectious agents. The measures are taken at the blood bank or at a national level. Some other measures of safety related to blood transfusions are taken at the clinical level in order to reduce the risk of giving the patient the wrong blood. However, the probably most important measures to reduce risks associated with blood transfusions have to be taken in the context of blood management. Only when a patient can be treated successfully without donor blood, transfusion-associated risks are really eliminated. The various expressions of immunomodulation, metabolic consequences of blood transfusion, and storage lesions cannot be totally eliminated by blood banks. Only clinicians who learn to treat patients without blood transfusions can really avoid risks associated with blood transfusions. Still, the safest transfusion is one that is made unnecessary and is thus not given.

However, as long as blood is transfused, safety measures are taken to reduce some risks to the patients.

Donor education

Most infectious transfusion-transmittable diseases are not, or cannot be, tested for at the present time. This underscores the importance of donors reporting any transmissible infections they have had or might have been exposed to in the past.

Donor education aims at informing the donors about the consequences of donating blood if there is a chance of having a disease. It motivates them to reveal relevant details of their health and lifestyle. It explains how to donate blood, alleviates fears about hurting oneself by the donation, and encourages regular unpaid donation. Besides, it asks the donors to report health problems becoming obvious after the donation. The WHO leaflet entitled "Safe blood starts with me: questions and answers about donating blood" is an example of donor education materials.

More details about the donor that need to be reported are listed in the so-called donor history questionnaires that must be administered on the date of donation. The questionnaire is usually filled in by the donor, with follow-up review by a trained donor historian.

Table 17.3 Examples of criteria for life-long donor exclusion (permanent deferral).

- HCV, HIV, HTLV-I/II-positive, hepatitis of unknown origin
- Homosexual and bisexual men, drug addicts, prostitutes, prisoners, immigrants with a high rate of infection of HCV, HIV, HTLV-I/II in their home country, alcoholism
- History of malaria, babesiosis, trypanosomiasis, leishmaniasis, syphilis, brucellosis, rickettsiosis, leprosy, recurrent fever, tularemia, osteomyelitis, malignant tumors (except cured basalioma and similar), therapy with human hypophysis hormone, human dura or cornea transplants, xenotransplants
- Suspicion of Creutzfeldt–Jakob disease
- Current salmonellosis chronic diseases when person endangers him-/herself or others by the donation

Donor selection and deferral

Based on donor education and the reviewed donor history questionnaire, donors with risks for having certain diseases are identified. This includes donors with a high-risk behavior and those with a travel history or a history of a disease or certain symptoms.

Donors with a hypothetical risk detected by a review of the donor history questionnaire may be deferred for the time being or indefinitely. There are different types of deferral. An *indefinite deferral* applies to a prospective donor who is unable to donate blood for someone else, as is ruled by current legislation. When legislation changes, the donor may be able to donate blood again. An example is a US-American donor who cannot donate blood since he/she has been in the United Kingdom for a certain period of time. A *permanent deferral* applies to a donor who will never be eligible to donate blood for someone else, e.g., one who is HIV positive (Table 17.3). A *temporary deferral* applies to a donor who is unable to donate blood for a limited period of time, e.g., after undergoing endoscopy (Table 17.4).

When a patient does not seem to have any risks requiring deferral, further investigation is needed to determine his/her physical fitness for donation. The criteria being body weight at least 50 kg, normal or near-normal blood pressure and pulse rate, hematocrit in females at least 38% and in males at least 40%, no signs of disease, no fever. Such criteria may identify a future donor of whole blood. These criteria are valid also for apheresis donors. Since apheresis includes an extracorporeal circulation in which the needed blood component is separated and the remaining components are given back, the donor must be especially fit and must fulfill further requirements.

Table 17.4 Examples of temporary deferral criteria.

- Persons are deferred for at least 12 mo if they had sexual contact with persons with an increased risk for hepatitis or HIV, prolonged travel to certain countries, rabies-shots after exposure, sera therapy of animal origin
- Persons are deferred for at least 6 mo after endoscopy, allogeneic organ transplants, blood transfusion, injury with blood contact of another person, after acupuncture, tattoos, body piercing
- Other deferral periods are valid after infectious diseases, vaccination with living vaccine, pregnancy and surgery, and a travel history

Postdonation product quarantine

When a donor presents with unclear symptoms after a donation, his/her blood is put under quarantine, if not already transfused. The length of postdonation quarantine depends on the maximum storage time for the product in question. Quarantine only makes sense when blood can still be used after it is ruled out whether the donor is sick or not. Since plasma can be stored in the frozen state for several months, it is sometimes kept frozen until the donor presents for a subsequent period of donation. If he/she is still healthy, the previous plasma unit is released for use.

National vigilance systems

As the number of facilities working in the blood banking business grows, countries typically take over the role of supervision. National vigilance systems are usually organized under the auspices of government representatives. Transfusionists, infectious disease scientists, laboratory specialists, blood bankers, clinicians, and members of the observed organizations usually share responsibilities. National vigilance systems organize ongoing surveillance programs for known and emerging infectious agents in the blood supply as well as take care of the reporting of transfusion-related hazards and the collection of incident reports. Transfusion policies and guidelines are established by such systems as well and are adapted to the current needs of the blood donation and transfusion system. Besides, research [13] and educational programs [14] are also organized by national vigilance systems. National vigilance systems sometimes include notification systems for instances when transfusion-transmittable diseases are detected. Donors are traced and their donated blood is withdrawn from the blood pool if it was not yet transfused.

About 30 years ago, only a minority of countries had such national vigilance systems. To change this precarious situation, the WHO proposed in 1975 (resolution WHA 28.72) to all countries to develop a national blood plan including functions, organization, and management of a national blood transfusion service. This service should establish national quality systems, guidelines for the operation of blood donation and use, staff training, and a system for monitoring and evaluation (national vigilance system). Despite the 30-year-long initiative of the WHO, currently only 35% of the member states of the United Nations have a national blood policy, legislation, and a responsible organization for blood safety [15]. More than half of all developing countries have no national policy and guidelines for transfusion at all.

Blood safety related to the donated blood

Screening

For a limited number of agents that can cause transfusion transmittable diseases, there is a screening test available. Such is used to screen blood. The WHO, speaking for the whole world, recommends testing all blood donations for HIV, HBV, and syphilis. Furthermore, it encourages including tests for HCV, Chagas disease, and malaria where appropriate and possible. Some countries decide to add other tests to the standard tests. HTLV and West Nile virus are tested for in some countries. When blood fractions are produced, some industries decide to also test for HAV and parvovirus B19. What blood is finally tested for depends largely on the country and on available means.

There are different methods to detect pathogens in blood. Formerly, unspecific disease markers were used to test blood. For instance, alanine aminotransferase (ALT, serum GPT) was routinely determined as a surrogate marker for "non-A, non-B hepatitis." Due to its low specificity and sensitivity it is no longer recommended. A more specific way to detect infections in blood is to test for pathogen-specific antibodies. These kinds of tests rely on the ability of the donor to develop antibodies that indicate the presence or absence of a pathogen. The most sensitive tests are nucleic acid amplification tests (NAT). They directly detect the genetic materials of viruses. One single copy of pathogen genome can be amplified by biotechnological means (PCR or TMA), and when present, detected. NAT can be performed in a single donor blood unit or in a pool of blood containing aliquots of many different units.

For some diseases, a variety of screening tests are available. For HIV, antibody tests for HIV 1 and 2 are feasible.

Additionally, NAT tests can be performed [1, 16]. Similarly, HBV and HCV can be detected by serological tests (antibodies to HBV surface antigen or HBV core antigen) as well as by NAT. Serological tests are commonly used to test for HTLV and syphilis (Venereal Disease Research Laboratory, treponema pallidum immobilization, treponema pallidum hemagglutination assay).

Pathogen reduction

Since an ever-wider variety of pathogens are found in the blood supply, with an anticipated increasing tendency, the perspective seems to be that testing for every single pathogen is not only expensive, but just impossible. This shows that blood always carries the risk to transmit a disease: Either the pathogen is not detected by screening, it is not screened for, or blood is mistakenly released although having tested positive. To increase the safety of blood, procedures to inactivate and eliminate pathogens in blood products were thus developed [17]. Pathogen inactivation happens by negating the viability of the pathogen in the blood product, but not by removing it. Pathogen elimination, in contrast, means to physically remove (major amounts of) the pathogen from blood. The latter can reduce the pathogen load in the blood, but does not kill the remaining pathogens.

Pathogen inactivation and elimination methods were originally introduced for use in plasma fractions. Also today, the use of many of the methods (Table 17.5) is still restricted to plasma and plasma products [1, 18, 19]. However, in recent times, selected methods of pathogen inactivation (viral, bacterial, protozoa) have been attempted in red cell or platelet concentrates. Molecules such as ethyleneimine and psoralen derivatives or amotosalen can be added, and they bind to DNA or RNA and prevent the growth of some pathogens [20]. Also, photochemical processes can be employed for that purpose [21].

Although pathogen elimination and inactivation may sound promising, they come with some disadvantage. The inactivation processes may introduce damaging, carcinogenic, or toxic agents into to product, may reduce the level of active clotting factors, and may need pooling of blood, the latter increasing the risk of viral transmission. The negative impact of pathogen elimination and inactivation techniques on product integrity may, in fact, be so severe that they probably cause more trouble than help prevent cases of disease transmission [18, 22]. Besides, the impact of the universal introduction of pathogen inactivation or elimination techniques to all blood products on the price of a unit of blood would be immense.

Table 17.5 Methods of pathogen elimination or inactivation.

Method	Description	Kills what and what not	Used for what kind of blood products
Pasteurization [PI]	Liquid plasma kept at 60°C for >10 h, with a stabilizer added or lyophilized protein kept at 50–70°C up to 144 h or at >80°C for 72 h	*Kills* a wide range of enveloped and nonenveloped viruses	
Steaming [PI]	10 h at 60°C at 1160 mbar		
Solvent–detergent (SD) [PI]	Alkyl phosphates and detergents added	*Kills* viruses with lipid envelopes; *does not kill* viruses without envelopes (e.g., HAV, parvovirus B19), bacteria, prions	Platelets, unfractionated and fractionated plasma (SD-FFP), tests in blood pools
Irradiation [PI]	With γ-rays or UV light		
Cold sterilization [PI]	β-Propiolactone and UV light		
Alcohol fractionation [PI]	Reduces viruses		
Leukocyte reduction [PE]	Filtration step in blood production process		
Nanofiltration [PE]	Filter retains viruses	E.g., parvovirus B19	
(Immunoaffinity) chromatography [PE]	Keeps only proteins back, reduces viruses		
Methylene blue (MB) activated by natural light (= phenothiazine color) [PI]	Binds to proteins and nucleic acids, activated by natural light, denaturalized bound molecules (may be cancerogenous)	*Kills* retroviruses, herpes viruses, West Nile virus (lipid enveloped viruses); *does not kill* intracellular viruses, bacteria, prions	MB-FFP, platelets; *not used* any more for coagulation proteins, not usable for red cells (light absorbed by red color), tests in single donor aliquots
Psoralen (S-59) with ultraviolet A (UVA)-light exposure [PI]		Inactivates HIV, HCV, bacteria, inactivates T-cells (GvHD)	S-59-UVA-FFP, platelet concentrates
Gentian violet [PI]	In endemic regions, parasite reduction for Chagas disease (cave: side effects)		

[PI], pathogen inactivation; [PE], pathogen elimination; FFP, fresh frozen plasma; GvHD, graft-versus-host disease.

Faults of the safety layers

The above-mentioned safety layers are all designed to increase the safety of the blood supply. However, there are major flaws in each of them. The detection and exclusion of donors at risk for diseases that are not screened for depends on the honest cooperation of the donor. When donors do not provide a complete history, donors may be counted eligible for donation when in fact they are not. This may indeed be the case when prospective donors are ashamed of their behavior or have other reasons not to report truthfully, resulting in a dangerous underreporting [23]. In many countries, donors are paid and often make a living on donating their blood. They are aware that they are not eligible for blood donation if they reveal a fact that may group them as a high-risk donor and are therefore reluctant to report certain facts relevant for donor selection.

Also, ever more sophisticated screening tests do not provide absolute safety. Tests are sometimes unreliable, particularly when staff is inadequately trained or when test kits are in short supply, as is frequently the case in developing countries. In fact, a recent report of WHO states that about one in five donations in developing countries is not sufficiently tested for viral agents [15].

For most of the agents transmittable by transfusion, there is no effective tool for donor screening and sometimes not even for testing, e.g., for babesiosis [24].

International traffic brings new agents not detected by conventional screening methods. The same is true of new, variant retroviruses. And even when tests are available, they are not universally applied. For instance, tests for HAV, HEV, parvovirus B19, Chagas disease, and malaria are not routinely used in the United States [1, 25]. In many African countries, blood is not tested for HCV, despite a high prevalence in the blood supply [26]. Serological tests performed in the window period and in immunosilent donors also do not detect present infections.

Pathogen inactivation and elimination as an alternative or addition to serological tests may take care of more pathogens than screening methods. However, it cannot be known with absolute confidence whether the employed methods eliminate or inactivate all pathogens. The action of the methods is tested with model pathogens that are thought to be representative for all other pathogens. This assumption, however, is probably not true. Another problem with pathogen inactivation is that even inactivated nucleic acid is able to integrate into the genome of the recipient and may cause cancer [27].

Blood storage

Whole blood can be stored for 6–8 hours at room temperature. After this time, it has to be transfused, processed and cooled (Table 17.6), or discarded. It is recommended either to cool down whole blood immediately or to keep blood at room temperature for 5–6 hours before it is fractionated. If blood is stored immediately after donation in cool condition, coagulation factors are preserved. However, if it is stored at room temperature for some hours after donation, bacteria that may have been in the blood

Table 17.6 Storage conditions of blood products.

Product	Storage condition	Maximum length of storage
Cryoprecipitate and fresh frozen plasma	−18 to −25°C<	3 mo
	≤25°C	24 mo
Granulocytes	No storage possible	
Platelets	20–24°C	5 days
Red cells	2–6°C	35–49 days, depending on legislation and additive

can be phagocyted by white cells. When blood is stored for more than 24 hours at room temperature, white cells disintegrate and bacteria are released again.

Bacterial contamination

Blood storage comes with two major disadvantages for the blood. First, it develops storage lesions, as discussed elsewhere in this book. Second, it can be contaminated with bacteria. Bacterial contamination of blood products poses serious threats to the blood supply. In fact, in developed countries, the risks through bacterial contamination are much greater than that of all transfusion-transmittable diseases taken together.

Red blood cells, since they are stored in a cold environment, are not likely to be significantly bacterially contaminated. Pathogens usually found in red cell concentrates can survive cold conditions and can multiply at lower temperature. *Yersinia enterocolica*, *Serratia*, and *Pseudomonas* are most commonly implicated pathogens. Up to 1:65,000 units were reported to contain *Y. enterocolica* [16]. The exact incidence of bacterial contamination in developed countries, however, is not known. Variations were observed and may be due to underrecognition, underreporting, and regional variation. When red cells contaminated with bacteria are transfused, the transfusion is often lethal.

More often, platelet concentrates are bacterially contaminated. Since they are stored at about 22°C, they provide ideal conditions for the multiplication of bacteria. Most often, platelet concentrates host skin germs, such as *Staphylococcus epidermidis* and *Staphylococcus aureus*, and *Streptococcus* spp. About 1 in 1000–3000 platelet units is bacterially contaminated [21, 28]. It is estimated that 1 in 4200 platelet transfusion events leads to septic complications. Pooled platelets carry a higher risk for bacterial contamination, since more phlebotomies are needed to collect the platelets [28, 29], with more chances of introducing bacteria into the final product.

As well, stored autologous blood may be bacterially contaminated. It is even more likely to be bacterially contaminated, since the autologous units are not tested as rigorously as donated units and are stored longer, with maximal chance for bacterial growth.

To prevent bacterial contamination, a thorough donor screening—to make sure that only healthy patients without bacteremia are donating—is the first step. Then, a strictly sterile phlebotomy is essential, since most of the germs in the donated blood are thought to enter the unit during the donation procedure. But the best disinfection methods do not prevent bacteria from entering the collection bag. A further measure for the reduction of bacterial contamination is predonation sampling. The first 10–20 mL of donated blood is let into another bag to be discarded since it contains the most bacteria.

During blood storage, the few organisms introduced into the donated blood may multiply. Keeping up the cold chain reduces such bacterial growth. However, it is difficult to store normal platelets in the cold, since they rapidly lose their viability and are thus removed from the human circulation quickly. Cold storage of platelets may still be possible, given the addition of protecting agents (DMSO, Thrombosol). Nevertheless, cold platelet storage is time-consuming and brings toxic effects to platelets and patients [21].

The last step toward reduction of transfusion of bacterially contaminated blood is to detect bacterial contamination. Changes in pH, appearance of the unit, screening with Gram's staining or fluorescent microscopy, microbiological detection methods (RNA probes), and automated culture systems have been employed in this regard. Monitoring the production of CO_2 or the reduction of oxygen in the unit—as it is caused by metabolism of growing bacteria—can be used in an automated fashion to detect bacteria in the units [30]. Many other technologies have been developed to detect bacteria in blood [21]. Ideally, detection of bacteria in blood units is performed shortly before transfusion, since detection is most sensitive at that point.

Leukocyte reduction and depletion

Another procedure performed during the storage of blood is leukocyte depletion. Controversy exists whether leukocyte depletion is better performed before or after storage. But it is generally agreed upon that a lower number of leukocytes in red cells or platelets comes with advantages. The amount of leukocytes in blood products differs. Whole blood contains 3×10^9 leukocytes per unit, buffy-coat removal reduces the leukocyte count to less than 2×10^8 and leukocyte depletion filtration to less than 5×10^6 [31]. Leukocyte depletion filtration removes not only necrotic leukocytes but also oxygen radicals, infection mediators, and pathogens (CMV, HTLV [1], and possibly prions causing variant Creutzfeldt–Jacob disease [16]). It seems to be valid that leukocyte reduction reduces CMV infection, febrile nonhemolytic transfusion reactions, and HLA (human leukocyte antigen) alloimmunization. Other immunological benefits of leukocyte reduction or depletion are suggested, but are not ac-

cepted by all. These include a reduction of the danger of graft-versus-host reactions, reperfusion damage, alloimmunization, decreased nonresponsiveness to platelet transfusions, and impairment of red cell metabolism in stored blood.

Some countries adopted a policy of universal leukocyte depletion, while others deplete leukocytes only in transfusions for patients at high risk for adverse effects [32].

Irradiation of blood products

In special situations, blood is irradiated during storage. This is done to prevent viable lymphocytes to enter the recipient and to elicit GvHD. Irradiation damages the DNA of lymphocytes. All granulocyte concentrates are irradiated since they contain many lymphocytes. Other products are irradiated to prevent GvHD in susceptible individuals, among them transplant recipients and babies who undergo intrauterine transfusions.

From whole blood to cellular components

Apart from apheresis donations, all donated blood is whole blood collected in an anticoagulant. Developing countries transfuse 37–75% of the donated blood as whole blood. In developed countries, only about 16% of all transfusions are whole blood transfusions [15]. Most whole blood donations in developed countries are therefore not used for immediate transfusion, but are simply the raw material for the production of blood products.

The basic method to separate whole blood is differential centrifugation. After centrifugation, the cells are found in layers according to their density: red cells, white cells, platelets, plasma.

The simplest way to separate whole blood is to divide it into cells and plasma (e.g., in a system with two blood bags). Plasma is frozen immediately after donation ($-30°C$) to maintain the maximum possible coagulation factor activity. The cellular part of this centrifugation is called erythrocyte concentrate. Granted, white cells and platelets are also in the cellular compartment. However, they are mostly inactivated during storage.

A more sophisticated way to separate blood is to divide it into three parts: red cells, plasma, and the buffy coat. Buffy coat is the layer that contains white cells and platelets. This is done since buffy coat causes many of the unwanted effects of transfusion. Dividing whole blood in three parts is also performed by differential centrifugation using a three-bag-system. After centrifugation, the upper layer (plasma) is transferred into the first bag and then the buffy coat (containing about 70% white cells, 90% platelets, and 10% red cells) is transferred into the second bag. The remaining red cells in the third bag constitute the red cell concentrate.

Additives

Donated blood, as well as certain blood products, contains additives. They are needed to prevent coagulation and to prolong storage time.

The obviously most important additive for blood donation is an anticoagulant. Modern anticoagulants contain not only an anticoagulating principle but also compounds that provide metabolic substrates for cell metabolism. Formerly, ACD (acidum citricum, sodium citrate, dextrose) was used. ACD red cells can be stored up to 21 days. Another anticoagulant, CPD (citrate, phosphate, and dextrose), is also available. The phosphate is added to buffer the lactate that develops during metabolism of stored red cells. It is also possible to add purine nucleotides, such as adenine, to the anticoagulant (CPD-A). They aid in the synthesis of ATP and 2,3-DPG and prolong the viability of the red cells. The standard anticoagulant for collection of whole blood, today, is CPD-A. This solution allows for whole blood storage up to 35 days.

Red cell concentrates can also be stored in special additives, such as SAG-M (sodium, adenine, glucose, mannitol), PAGGS-sorbit (phosphate, adenine, guanosine, glucose, sorbit), Adsol or AS-3. These solutions may allow storage of red cells for up to 49 days. The solutions contain sodium chloride, glucose derivatives, adenine, mannitol, and other ingredients. Red cell concentrates in additive solutions contain less isoagglutinins than red cell concentrates resuspended in plasma.

There are also additives for platelets. These include different so-called platelet additive solutions and Composol. While the solutions are perceived to have some advantages (e.g., making washing and prolonged storage of platelets possible), they seem to impair the functionality of stored platelets [33, 34].

Red cell concentrates

There are different kinds of red cell concentrates. They are sourced either from whole blood donations or are gained by an apheresis procedure. Red cell concentrates made by apheresis come with relatively stable red cell content, with interunit variation of only 6%. In contrast, red cell concentrates made from whole blood donations vary widely in their content of red cells, with up to twofold variations [35]. The crudest red cell concentrates are made from whole blood donations and simply contain the cellular portion of centrifuged blood including white cells and platelets. Other red cell concentrates from whole blood donations are buffy-coat-free, that is, with reduced amounts of white cells and platelets. Leukocyte depletion filtration of red cell concentrates further reduces the amount of leukocytes in the unit. Efforts are under way to standardize red cell concentrates and to reduce the variability of the contents. It was proposed that a single unit of red cells should be delivered with 50 g hemoglobin and in additive solutions that may be able to reduce storage lesions [36].

Red cell concentrates contain residues of plasma and plasma proteins, including antibodies. Sometimes, the amount of plasma in red cell concentrates is reduced by diluting the red cells in additive solution rather than in plasma. When patients react allergically to foreign proteins or when the presence of plasma proteins (antibodies) may be detrimental, red cell concentrates can also be washed with saline to remove almost all plasma. Last but not least, red cells can also be treated so that their antigens are disguised, presumably making red cell concentrate transfusions blood group independent.

Red cell concentrates are usually stored at low temperature, namely, normal refrigerator temperature (4°C). This temperature reduces the metabolic rate of the red cells and possible bacterial growth. On the other hand, freezing must be prevented which would lead to hemolysis of the red cells. Nevertheless, despite improved storage conditions, red cells suffer storage lesions [37]. After some days of storage, the oxygen dissociation curve is shifted to the left and red cells cannot easily release oxygen. Depending on the storage time, red cells tend to aggregate and to form stacks, called "rouleau" formation [38]. Changes of the red cell membrane occur during storage as well. The membrane loses lipids and finally the cell becomes stiff and spherocytic. Besides, new antigens may be expressed on the membrane during storage [39]. So, compatibility testing performed before storage may no longer be valid after storage.

Platelet concentrates

Platelet concentrates come in two different forms: random donor platelets, which are pooled from four to eight whole blood donations, and single donor apheresis platelets.

Random donor platelet concentrates contain a minimum of 5.5×10^{10} platelets per unit in the pool and have a volume of about 150–450 mL. The random donor platelet concentrate can be made either from platelet-rich plasma (PRP-platelets) or by centrifugation of the buffy coat (BC-platelets). For the BC-platelets, the buffy coat gained through standard centrifugation of blood is resuspended in plasma. This is stored for some hours while it is rocked, increasing the amount of platelets gained. Afterward, the mix is centrifuged ("soft spin") and the platelet and plasma are used, while the leukocytes are discarded. As an alternative, buffy coats can also be pooled, mixed with plasma or an additive, and then centrifuged. For PRP-platelets, whole blood is first centrifuged slowly so that platelet-rich plasma separates from the red cells. After transfer of this platelet-rich plasma, it is spun again to separate plasma from platelets.

Single donor platelet units are made by apheresis. The minimum of platelets is 3×10^{11} platelets [40] in a volume of 150–300 mL. The yield of apheresis depends on the donor and on the method used. One to three units of donor platelets can be obtained from one donor, depending on his/her initial platelet count.

Pooled platelet concentrates and apheresis platelets may be therapeutically equivalent and may have a similar pattern of side effects [41]. However, this is not universally agreed upon [42]. It was claimed that apheresis platelets are better preserved than platelet concentrates made from whole blood. A significant difference between apheresis and random donor platelets is that transfusion of a unit of pooled platelets leads to a higher donor exposure than single-donor platelets.

Storage of platelet concentrates occurs at room temperature (about 22°C) under gentle agitation. The length of platelet storage depends on the container and the method of collection and processing. A closed system can store platelets for up to 5 days, whereas an open system (e.g., for washing and resuspension of platelets in platelet suspension medium) typically can store platelets for 24 hours only [41]. During storage, some platelet concentrates undergo special treatment. Some units are split or hyperconcentrated for intrauterine or neonatal use. Some units are irradiated or leukocyte-depleted.

After collection and during storage, several steps of quality control of platelet concentrates are indicated. Which these are and how they are performed depend on the legislation and the money available. Platelets should be tested for microbial contamination (serological tests, NAT) and red cell serological tests are performed (blood group, etc). Visual inspection for any abnormalities (turbidity, color changes, damaged container, excessive air, etc.) prior to issue of the platelet unit is usually standard. The pH of the platelet concentrates must be between 6.4 and 7.4 [41]. During storage, platelets gain their energy in metabolic processes that produce CO_2 and H_2CO_3. This leads to a decrease of the pH. To counteract this, bags with increased gas permeability are used and the bag design is changed to a better concentrate–surface ratio.

Additive solutions for platelets may come with benefits and may even allow for cold storage. To reduce pathogens in the platelet concentrate, agents may be added. Photoinactivation of viruses and bacteria may be possible when methylene blue is added (MB-platelets). Also, solvent–detergent methods were described as a means to inactivate pathogens in the platelet concentrate (SD-platelets). However, there are not yet enough experiences with pathogen-inactivated platelets.

Granulocytes

Collection of granulocytes is difficult. The normal amount of circulating granulocytes is 30×10^7/kg. For therapy, a daily dose of more than 15×10^7/kg is recommended. Therefore, special measures must be taken to obtain a significant amount of granulocytes. Either the buffy coats of several donations are pooled or a single donor is prepared specifically to donate granulocytes by apheresis. The blood of patients with chronic lymphatic leukemia circles enough granulocytes to provide for the donation. Such patients are sometimes asked to donate. More often, though, donors are asked to take prednisone or they are administered granulocyte colony-stimulating factor. In order for a donor to donate sufficient amounts, daily donations or alternate day donations are requested. This reduces the risk of multiple donor exposure for the patient, but puts the donor at risk [43].

This shows that granulocyte donations are problematic. They are rarely prescribed. When they are given, they are given ABO and RhD compatible, since they contain many red cells [43].

Granulocyte concentrates cannot be stored and are therefore prepared for immediate transfusion. They should be transfused within 6 (–24) hours after donation.

Fresh frozen plasma

Fresh frozen plasma (FFP) is plasma that is derived from one unit of donated blood by centrifugation. It is frozen to at least −18°C within 8 hours after donation. When thawed, it can be kept refrigerated for up to 24 hours [40] before use. Storage in the frozen state is needed to prevent rapid loss of the coagulation factor activity which would occur within hours after storage at room temperature. In some countries, standard FFPs are held in quarantine for 4 months, since they are allowed to be infused only after the next donation when the donor presents healthy.

Some countries also provide plasma units derived from pooled plasma and are treated with solvent–detergent (SD-FFP) or methylene blue (MB-FFP) to reduce viral transmission. It is not necessary to keep such plasma under quarantine.

Plasma fractionation

Plasma is a mix of thousands of compounds, is unique for every individual, and differs in the individual over time, sometimes even changing within minutes. Plasma is thus a most heterogenous and volatile liquid. Whole plasma used for therapeutic reasons consists mostly of compounds not really needed for therapeutic use. Transfusing whole plasma comes, therefore, with avoidable dangers and is often a waste of resources. Therefore, dividing plasma into different compounds (fractionation) makes sense. Fractionation saves resources, reduces risks for the recipient, and increases the financial gain for the manufacturer of the blood product.

Commercially available plasma fractions are produced by fractionation of pools of source plasma, consisting of thousands of plasma portions from different donors. Plasma for fractionation is collected either by centrifugation of whole blood donations or by plasma apheresis. Apheresis plasma is often preferred. It is collected commercially and several blood tests are not required for apheresis plasma (e.g., tests for intracellular pathogens).

Methods to fractionate plasma

Fractionation makes use of different properties of plasma constituents. Differences in hydrophilia, size, sedimentation behavior, affinity to specific media, and movement in electrophoresis are starting points for fractionation.

PRECIPITATION

When certain salts (sodium chlorate, sodium sulfate), organic solvents (alcohol), metal ions (calcium, magnesium), polymers (polyethylene glycol), fatty acids (caprylat), or other acids are added to plasma, some plasma protein monomers aggregate. The aggregates are heavier than the rest of the plasma and sink to the bottom of the vessel. The aggregates can be removed from the plasma pool. Care must be taken that the proteins are not denatured during precipitation and that the precipitating agents are easily

removable after the precipitation process is finished. The prototype of the use of precipitation is the famous Cohn's fractionation see below [6, 7].

Precipitation is used by industry to divide plasma into different crude parts or to concentrate a certain protein or a group of proteins in a solution. A combination of different precipitating compounds is used to receive a product that has a relatively high concentration of the needed protein. It is not possible, however, to purify a protein through precipitation only.

Crystallization is a special form of precipitation. It leads to very pure proteins, since not much of the mother liquid is included in the protein crystals. However, the time needed to crystallize plasma proteins does not make this method suitable for industrial mass production of plasma fractions.

CHROMATOGRAPHY

The term chromatography refers to a variety of physical methods to separate complex mixtures such as plasma. The components to be separated are distributed between two phases: a stationary phase and a mobile phase, which percolates through the stationary phase.

One important kind of chromatography is ion exchange chromatography. Anions or cations bound to a matrix (stationary phase) bind proteins that are either cations or anions, respectively. When plasma is brought into contact with the matrix, proteins with certain acidic or basic groups (e.g., gamma-carboxyl groups of prothrombin complex proteins) are bound to the ions on the matrix, while other proteins are not. After flushing plasma that is not bound to the matrix, the proteins on the matrix are released and used. It is even possible to release the proteins on the matrix in a fractionated fashion, so that the proteins are further purified. With ion exchange chromatography, proteins are handled very gently.

Gel chromatography can be used to separate proteins according to their size. Porous molecules with different pore sizes are used to retain small molecules in the pores and to have bigger molecules travel through. Gel chromatography is often used to remove small contaminating molecules from a blood product.

Affinity chromatography is a relatively new, yet very often used, method to fractionate plasma. It uses specific interactions of proteins with a ligand bound to a matrix. Such interactions can be determined by natural transport properties (e.g., vitamin B_{12} is used as ligand and binds vitamin B_{12}-binding globulin), enzyme–substrate- or enzyme–inhibitor relations, or antigen–antibody interactions. Affinity chromatography is especially used to

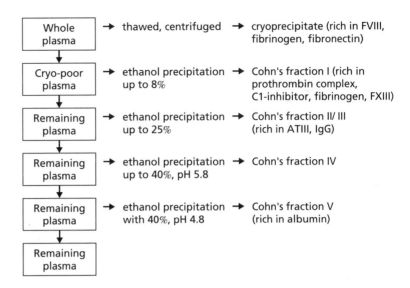

Fig 17.1 Cohn's fractionation.

gain proteins out of the plasma that are present in very low concentrations only.

Production of blood fractions

Plasma can be fractionated in many different ways. Since source plasma is expensive, industrial fractionation tries to use as many plasma proteins of the source plasma as possible. The methods by which this is done differ and depend on the proteins needed and the manufacturer's preference.

Today's fractionation still resembles the fractionation proposed by Cohn in 1940. In a stepwise approach, plasma is first divided into crude fractions. Later, the crude fractions may be used therapeutically (e.g., cryoprecipitate) or serve as the basis for the production of even purer plasma proteins.

An example of Cohn's fractionation is shown in Fig. 17.1.

Based on this classical fractionation model of Cohn, many different plasma products can be produced. Consider the following example shown in Fig. 17.2 [44].

Interaction between blood banks and clinicians

Blood banks provide the clinicians with valuable information for transfusion therapy [45]. The most often requested information is that about blood groups and blood compatibility, as determined by the type and screen (T&S) as well as by the type and cross-match (T&C).

A T&S determines the ABO and rhesus blood groups of the patient's red cells (typing), and the patient's serum

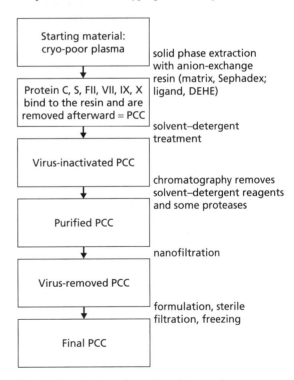

Fig 17.2 Fractionation of a prothrombin complex concentrate (PCC).

is screened for the presence of unexpected antibodies (screening) by incubating it with selected reagent red cells (screen cells). Screen cells have a known antigenic makeup and are selected in a way so that all common red cell antigens capable of inducing clinically significant red cell antibody reactions are present. If the antibody screen is positive, the unexpected antibody must be identified before antigen-negative compatible red cells can be located. This usually takes several hours.

A T&C includes not only typing of the cells but also cross-matching the patient's blood with a specific unit of blood. In a cross-match, the patient's serum is incubated with red cells from a specific donor unit to verify in vitro compatibility. A cross-match is performed either as a short (immediate spin) incubation intended solely to verify ABO compatibility or as a long incubation to verify compatibility with other red cell antigens. The immediate spin cross-match takes 5–10 minutes, while the long incubation takes at least 45 minutes.

Blood banks play an important role not only in determining the blood group of patients and test compatibility of patient blood and transfused blood but also in the detection of autoantibodies and alloantibodies. For a blood manager, this is important to treat hemolytic anemia and difficult pregnancies. Such information is vital to avoid hemolytic diseases in the newborn.

Maximum blood order schedule

A maximum blood order schedule is a table of elective procedures that lists whether a T&S is called for or how many units of blood are typically ordered. This schedule helps to limit needless cross-matching and to manage the stock of blood more effectively. A maximum blood order schedule is developed by retrospectively analyzing how much blood is typically transfused (T) in patients undergoing a certain procedure and how much blood is typically cross-matched for the procedures (C). The C/T ratio tells how effectively blood is ordered. The ideal ratio is 1.0; a realistic one is 2–3. The higher the value, the more blood is cross-matched unnecessarily. When more than two units are cross-matched on average for one unit actually transfused, the schedule needs to be revised [46].

A T&C is acceptable if there is at least 10% chance for the patient to get a transfusion. The number of units cross-matched should be chosen so that 90% of patients have sufficient units available. In locations where regularly sufficient blood is available, a T&C may only be ordered when transfusion is actually administered. A T&S is usually ordered when there is only a small chance of transfusion. The procedures for which it is ordered depend on the anxiety level of the surgeon and his/her confidence in the blood bank to supply what he/she calls for in case of extreme emergency.

Hospital transfusion committee

A place where blood banks and clinicians meet is the hospital transfusion committee. This committee is the extension of the national hemovigilance system and corroborates policies and guidelines advocated by national and hospital standards. In detail, the hospital-based transfusion committees review the transfusion practice in the hospital, develop and implement quality assessment procedures, and try to improve patient care through specific in-service education. It also investigates transfusion reactions and, when indicated, files reports. Besides, the committee helps to conserve blood components and reduce costs.

Key points

• Layers of blood safety include (1) donor education, (2) selection and deferral, (3) postdonation product quarantine, (4) a national vigilance system, and (5) blood-related procedures, namely, screening and pathogen reduction or inactivation.
• The layers of blood transfusion safety are endangered by missing donor honesty, insufficient screening for transfusion-transmittable infections, and unsatisfactory pathogen reduction and elimination.
• Blood storage introduces further problems into the blood pool. Bacterial contamination and storage lesions seem to be the most important.
• Blood is rarely transfused as whole blood. Rather, it is divided into its cellular components and plasma. Plasma is further divided into plasma fractions. This allows for a targeted therapy.
• Blood bank personnel are a valuable source of information for a blood manager.

Questions for review

• What are the safety layers of blood safety? What flaws do they have?

• What is the difference between pathogen reduction and pathogen inactivation? What agents and methods are used for these processes and what are their limitations?
• What is a blood fraction?
• What is Cohn's fractionation and how is it performed?
• Explain the following terms: type and screen, type and cross-match, hemovigilance, maximum blood order schedule, postdonation product quarantine.

Suggestions for further research

How are blood banks networking internationally? What are the politics about this business? Read more about the blood business. A good starting point is Gilbert M. Gaul's series on the blood business, which was published in 1989 in the *Philadelphia Inquirer*. Many more articles can be found on the Web.

Homework

Visit a place where platelet concentrates are made and have somebody explain how it works.
Go to the hospital blood bank and find out what steps are required in releasing a unit of blood for a patient.
Check the status of the national blood transfusion system, including the following:
• Who is the highest responsible person or organization for transfusion safety?
• Who is there to do the actual work of blood transfusion service?
• What measures are taken to control the facilities that provide blood?
• What is the percentage of donors who are voluntary, nonremunerated?
• What tests are regularly performed on all blood products?
• What monitoring systems are there for adverse effects of transfusions and for the appearance of pathogens in blood?

Exercises and practice cases

You are presented with the following numbers. What does your maximum blood-ordering schedule look like?

Type of surgery (number of times performed during the last 12 mo)	Cross-matches preformed during the last 12 mo	Number of patients transfused during the last 12 mo
Appendectomy (126)	16	1
Cholecystectomy (54)	36	3
Gastrectomy (14)	14	5
Hip replacement (22)	21	8
Coronary artery bypass graft (54)	54	16
Meningeoma resection (8)	7	1
Prostatectomy (abdominal) (30)	30	10

References

1 Pomper, G.J., Y. Wu, and E.L. Snyder. Risks of transfusion-transmitted infections: 2003. *Curr Opin Hematol*, 2003. **10**(6): p. 412–418.
2 European Parliament and the Council. Directive 2002/98/EC 27 January 2003. *OJEU*, 2003. p. L 33/30.
3 Huestis, D.W. Russia's National Research Center for Hematology: its role in the development of blood banking. *Transfusion*, 2002. **42**(4): p. 490–494.
4 Fantus, B. Therapy of the Cook County Hospital (blood preservation). *JAMA*, 1937. **109**: p. 128–132.
5 Starr, D. Medicine, money, and myth: an epic history of blood. *Transfus Med*, 2001. **11**(2): p. 119–121.
6 Cohn, E.J., *et al.* Preparation and properties of serum and plasma proteins. III Size and charge of proteins separating upon equilibration across membranes with ethanol-water mixtures of controlled pH, ionic strength and temperature. *J Am Chem Soc*, 1940. **62**: p. 3396–3400.
7 Cohn, E.J., *et al.* Preparation and properties of serum and plasma proteins. IV. A system for the separation into fractions of the protein and lipoprotein components of biological tissues and fluids. *J Am Chem Soc*, 1946. **68**: p. 459–475.
8 Walter, C.W. and W.p. Murphy, Jr. A closed gravity technique for the preservation of whole blood in ACD solution utilizing plastic equipment. *Surg Gynecol Obstet*, 1952. **94**(6): p. 687–692.
9 Strauss, R.G. Controversies in the management of the anemia of prematurity using single-donor red blood cell transfusions and/or recombinant human erythropoietin. *Transfus Med Rev*, 2006. **20**(1): p. 34–44.
10 Ludlam, C.A. and M.L. Turner. Managing the risk of transmission of variant Creutzfeldt Jakob disease by blood products. *Br J Haematol*, 2006. **132**(1): p. 13–24.

11 Rock, G., *et al.* Automated collection of blood components: their storage and transfusion. *Transfus Med*, 2003. **13**(4): p. 219–225.

12 Klein, H.G. Will blood transfusion ever be safe enough? *Transfus Med*, 2001. **11**(2): p. 122–124.

13 Busch, M., *et al.* Oversight and monitoring of blood safety in the United States. *Vox Sang*, 1999. **77**(2): p. 67–76.

14 Linden, J.V. and G.B. Schmidt. An overview of state efforts to improve transfusion medicine. The New York state model. *Arch Pathol Lab Med*, 1999. **123**(6): p. 482–485.

15 WHO Blood transfusion safety and clinical technology, S., Blood Transfusion Safety: Information Sheet for National Blood Programmes. Available at www.who.int.

16 Uhl, L. Infectious risks of blood transfusion. *Curr Hematol Rep*, 2002. **1**(2): p. 156–162.

17 Pelletier, J.P., S. Transue, and E.L. Snyder. Pathogen inactivation techniques. *Best Pract Res Clin Haematol*, 2006. **19**(1): p. 205–242.

18 Fischer, G., W.K. Hoots, and C. Abrams. Viral reduction techniques: types and purpose. *Transfus Med Rev*, 2001. **15**(2, Suppl 1): p. 27–39.

19 Pamphilon, D. Viral inactivation of fresh frozen plasma. *Br J Haematol*, 2000. **109**(4): p. 680–693.

20 Roback, J.D., *et al.* The Role of photochemical treatment with amotosalen and UV-A light in the prevention of transfusion-transmitted cytomegalovirus infections. *Transfus Med Rev*, 2006. **20**(1): p. 45–56.

21 Palavecino, E. and R. Yomtovian. Risk and prevention of transfusion-related sepsis. *Curr Opin Hematol*, 2003. **10**(6): p. 434–439.

22 Caspari, G., *et al.* Pathogen inactivtion of cellular blood products – more security for the patients or less? *Transfus Med Hemother*, 2003. **30**: p. 261–263.

23 Fielding, R., T.H. Lam, and A. Hedley. Risk-behavior reporting by blood donors with an automated telephone system. *Transfusion*, 2006. **46**(2): p. 289–297.

24 Leiby, D.A. Babesiosis and blood transfusion: flying under the radar. *Vox Sang*, 2006. **90**(3): p. 157–165.

25 Becker, J.L. Vector-borne illnesses and the safety of the blood supply. *Curr Hematol Rep*, 2003. **2**(6): p. 511–517.

26 Imarengiaye, C.O., *et al.* Risk of transfusion-transmitted hepatitis C virus in a tertiary hospital in Nigeria. *Public Health*, 2006. **120**(3): p. 274–278.

27 Mueller-Eckhardt, C. and V. Kiefel. *Transfusionsmedizin*, 3rd edn. Springer-Verlag, Heidelberg, 2004.

28 Goodnough, L.T. Risks of blood transfusion. *Crit Care Med*, 2003. **31**(12, Suppl): p. S678–S686.

29 Walther-Wenke, G., *et al.* Bacterial contamination of platelet concentrates prepared by different methods: results of standardized sterility testing in Germany. *Vox Sang*, 2006. **90**(3): p. 177–182.

30 Fournier-Wirth, C., *et al.* Evaluation of the enhanced bacterial detection system for screening of contaminated platelets. *Transfusion*, 2006. **46**(2): p. 220–224.

31 Innerhofer, p. and G. Kühbacher. Immunomodulation mechanisms following transfusion of allogeneic and autologous erythrocyte concentrates. *Infus Ther Transfus Med*, 2002. **29**: p. 118–121.

32 Heddle, N.M. Evidence-based clinical reporting: a need for improvement. *Transfusion*, 2002. **42**(9): p. 1106–1110.

33 Keuren, J.F., *et al.* Platelet ADP response deteriorates in synthetic storage media. *Transfusion*, 2006. **46**(2): p. 204–212.

34 Ringwald, J., *et al.* Washing platelets with new additive solutions: aspects on the in vitro quality after 48 hours of storage. *Transfusion*, 2006. **46**(2): p. 236–243.

35 Sweeney, J.D. Standardization of the red cell product. *Transfus Apher Sci*, 2006. **34**(2): p. 213–218.

36 Hogman, C.F. and H.T. Meryman. Red blood cells intended for transfusion: quality criteria revisited. *Transfusion*, 2006. **46**(1): p. 137–142.

37 Ho, J., W.J. Sibbald, and I.H. Chin-Yee. Effects of storage on efficacy of red cell transfusion: when is it not safe? *Crit Care Med*, 2003. **31**(12, Suppl): p. S687–S697.

38 Hessel, E. and D. Lerche. Cell surface alterations during blood-storage characterized by artificial aggregation of washed red blood cells. *Vox Sang*, 1985. **49**(2): p. 86–91.

39 Krugluger, W., M. Koller, and p. Hopmeier. Development of a carbohydrate antigen during storage of red cells. *Transfusion*, 1994. **34**(6): p. 496–500.

40 Fritsma, M.G. Use of blood products and factor concentrates for coagulation therapy. *Clin Lab Sci*, 2003. **16**(2): p. 115–119.

41 British Committee for Standards in Haematology. Guidelines for the use of platelet transfusions. *Br J Haematol*, 2003. **122**: p. 10–23.

42 Arnold, D.M., *et al.* In vivo recovery and survival of apheresis and whole blood-derived platelets: a paired comparison in healthy volunteers. *Transfusion*, 2006. **46**(2): p. 257–264.

43 Yeghen, T. and S. Devereux. Granulocyte transfusion: a review. *Vox Sang*, 2001. **81**(2): p. 87–92.

44 Josic, D., L. Hoffer, and A. Buchacher. Preparation of vitamin K-dependent proteins, such as clotting factors II, VII, IX and X and clotting inhibitor protein C. *J Chromatogr B Analyt Technol Biomed Life Sci*, 2003. **790**(1–2): p. 183–197.

45 Yazer, M.H. The blood bank "black box" debunked: pretransfusion testing explained. *CMAJ*, 2006. **174**(1): p. 29–32.

46 Napier, J.A.F., *et al.* Guidelines for implementation of a maximum surgical blood order schedule. *Clin Lab Haematol*, 1990. **12**: p. 321–327.

18 Transfusions. Part I: cellular components and plasma

Medical use of blood has always been controversial. Formerly, blood letting was considered to be the cure for all ailments. Nowadays it seems quite the contrary is believed, namely, that transfusion of blood is a panacea. Despite rapidly increasing theoretical knowledge about human blood and its medical use, the practice of blood use seems little changed. In fact, today's medical use of blood can be compared with an "early 1900 ironclad ship operating in the rough seas of the 21st century" [1]. Comparison of the facts gleaned from current literature on blood with current medical practice reveals a huge gap between knowledge and practice. Hopefully, this chapter will close any gap in the clinician's knowledge and practice and it will not be necessary to wait further decades until the general medical community has realized that changes are urgently needed. A further purpose of this chapter is to help clinicians see why adjustment of current practice toward a more outcome-oriented approach to the medical use of blood, that is, blood management, is needed.

Objectives of this chapter

1 Describe what is known about the benefits of allogeneic transfusions.
2 List different methods used to define a "transfusion trigger" and state the limitations of such.
3 Explain the risks and side effects of allogeneic transfusions.
4 Examine current guidelines for the use of red cells, platelets, white cells, and plasma, and the basis for the guidelines.
5 Define the risk–benefit ratio of blood transfusions.

Definitions

Transfusion: Infusion of blood or blood components into a living being. Blood can be derived from various sources.

- Autologous transfusion: Blood taken and stored from the same individual, the patient, is infused. The patient receives his own blood.
- Allogeneic (= isogenic, homologous) transfusion: Blood from another genetically distinct individual of the same species, a blood donor, is infused.
- Heterologous transfusion: Blood from an organism of a different species, e.g., a cow, is infused into a human.

A brief look at history

Blood has always been viewed as something special. It has been credited with magic qualities and healing properties. People believed blood determined the qualities of an individual, and that such qualities could be transferred in the blood. Therefore, blood from wounded heroes was collected and drunk [2]. Blood has also been drunk in attempts to cure anemia and epilepsy. Royalty from various dynasties have bathed in blood in attempts to cure their ailments. The principle "like cures like" underlies attempts to use blood for wound care. Because blood runs out of a wound, it was thought a cure could be obtained by returning blood to the wound. Some cultures used human blood mixed with oil. In Asian cultures, children who had been kidnapped were hung head-down over a pot with hot oil and their blood was let and flowed into the oil. This "human oil" was used to cure wounds [2]. Most ancient cultures used such cruel methods to obtain and use blood for medicinal purposes. Only the ancient Hebrews were forbidden to use blood for medical purposes [3].

Aside from peroral and external use of blood, its injection of it has kindled the interest of poets and scientists alike. In Greek mythology there are descriptions of attempts to open a blood vessel and to instill some fluids in exchange, including, on occasions, blood. A first, yet questionable attempt to infuse blood was made to rejuvenate Pope Innocent VIII in 1492. Nevertheless, he died, as did the boys who "donated" their blood. Later, in the seventeenth century, attempts were made to transfuse blood, first animal to animal, later animal to human. The indications for transfusion were psychological disorders. Blood of a sheep, a tame animal, was thought to calm a madman. Well, it did, and he died. The first blood transfusions were unsuccessful and were therefore soon banned by the authorities, among them the Pope [3].

New attempts to transfuse were made in the nineteenth century. At the beginning of the 1800s, James Blundell transfused a man who suffered from vomiting [4]. He died, but this did not keep Blundell from trying again. He finally succeeded in transfusing blood in 50% of his cases—a miracle indeed, considering he had no idea about blood groups. Blundell's success encouraged other physicians. In time, hundreds of patients were transfused. Problems arising during the development of blood transfusions, e.g., with blood banking, were to some extent overcome.

Apart from the challenges in the blood bank sector, other challenges had to be faced concerning the indications for transfusions. The historical work of Adams and Lundi, who claimed that oxygen transport is impaired if hemoglobin falls below 10 g/dL or if the hematocrit is below 30%, has been used in the form of the 10/30 rule as a transfusion trigger. Recent findings have shown that Adam and Lundi's work is a valuable physiological study, but cannot be used to define a transfusion trigger. However, use of the 10/30 rule continues—no matter how deleterious the effects. John Maynard Keynes seemed to be right when he claimed: "The difficulty lies, not in the new ideas, but in escaping the old ones." History has shown that—in response to the AIDS pandemic—no ill effects were observed when the transfusion trigger was lowered and substantially less blood transfused.

Guidelines were formulated to guide the decision to transfuse. Transfusion guidelines have changed considerably in developed countries within the last 20 years. Before the AIDS era, guidelines often included a special transfusion trigger in the form of a hemoglobin level warranting transfusions in all patients. After the dangers of transfusion were recognized, the focus of guidelines has shifted more toward a patient-oriented approach to transfusion medicine that takes into account the clinical condition of the individual patient. This has been mirrored in the development of guidelines and in some subsequent changes in behavior [5]. Decreased reliance on an arbitrary transfusion trigger has been observed in parallel to increased interest in autologous transfusions.

Why do physicians transfuse?

According to one editor "Physicians have the best of intentions in applying the therapy, but the decision to transfuse is driven by fear (i.e., of not acting, lawsuit, or adverse outcome) and emotion. The transfusion trigger, a particular hemoglobin level of discomfort in the prescribing physician, is not defined by clear physiologic parameters. To date, we do not have a real time monitor of oxygen supply and demand to the microcirculation of the whole body or individual organs. Therefore, physicians make transfusion decisions based upon their past teaching and enculturation. We are encultured to believe that giving blood saves lives, yet there is little data published to support such conclusion" [6]. Reading this, clinicians may wonder what really is behind allogeneic transfusions—science or emotions? To better understand transfusion behavior, examine some facts and follow the lines of thought behind transfusion therapy.

How could today's transfusion practice be described? In one word: Variable. For a certain kind of heart surgery, for instance, there are institutions able to treat patients while giving transfusions to only 3% of patients while others transfuse 83% of patients with comparable illnesses [6]. Similar differences in transfusion practice are observed in many other procedures. So, why is there such immense variation? Undoubtedly, transfusion practice is influenced by industry and advertisement [7] as well as by hierarchy and peer pressure. Variations in transfusion practice mirror the lack of clear indications for blood transfusion. Besides, there is still a strong emotional component to transfusions. It simply feels good to say: "I have even given him blood." However, the physician's well-being is hardly a valid indication for transfusions. A more "official" indication for transfusions is that the "transfusion trigger" has been reached. Automatically blood is ordered once a certain laboratory value appears on the patient's sheet. This seems a more scientific approach, since the physician just follows the guidelines. But treating a laboratory value is as beneficial to the patient as is the emotional well-being of the physician.

What is an appropriate approach to taking a decision on which therapeutic option is the best in a given situation? It is clearly the patient-centered approach. As in any medical intervention, the outcome in the context of patient preference, cost-effectiveness, and legislation or policy is what determines the benefit of a given procedure. This also applies to transfusions.

In this chapter, the intention is to follow a systematic line of reasoning to evaluate the use of transfusions as opposed to other therapeutic options in the light of patient-centered blood management. Rational rather than emotional consideration of treatment potentially involving the use of allogeneic blood products may help to change the clinician's way of thinking. Thinking in a structured manner requires the use of appropriate strategies or tools. Many different tools are available for medical decision-making, however, the tools are only as good as the knowledge and expertise used to feed information into them, therefore, initially some of the basics about blood products are reviewed. Thinking will follow the lines of the BRAND mnemonic (Benefits, Risks, Alternatives, Nothing done, Decision), commonly used for medical decision-making. Afterwards, two decision-making tools (PMI, Grid Analysis) are introduced to think through and digest the information presented in order to come up with a useful decision.

What do you get when ordering a blood product?

When clinicians order a vial of penicillin, they just have to look at the vial's label to obtain a complete list of contents. Such a label is not available for most blood products, though, and no label could ever list all the ingredients in the blood bag. However, better knowledge of what actually is transfused to a patient, apart from the contents on the blood bag label, will hopefully influence the clinician's therapeutic decision. While considering such an "extended list of contents" the clinician can visualize what effects a blood component may have in the transfused patient.

Red cells

Red cell concentrates come at varying volumes, typically between 200 and 450 mL per bag. In a red cell concentrate, the hematocrit should be between 50 and 70% and certainly less than 80%. Obviously, in practice, the hemoglobin content of a red cell unit varies widely [8]. The viability of the red cells in the concentrate also varies considerably. In theory, less than 0.8% of the red cells should be hemolyzed after the median storage time. After the maximum storage time, 24-hour red cell survival after transfusion is about 70% (recovery rate), the remaining

up to 30% of red cells being destroyed during the first 24 hours after transfusion.

The red cells found in a banked red cell concentrate are not of the same quality they were when still in the blood vessels. Storage does not leave red cells unaltered. Depending on the time and manner of storage, red cells develop various types of storage lesions. During storage, red cells lose ATP and at the same time their shape. First, they develop spiculae and become echinocytes. Then, they swell and become more spherocytic. Finally, they shed their spiculae as lipid vesicles and become completely spherocytic [9]. They lose their deformability and their osmotic resistance [10]. Red cell surface receptors, among others those making red cells stick to the vessel wall, are also activated during storage.

During storage, red cells also lose compounds from inside the cell. Lost antioxidants result in oxidative damage to the red cell cytoskeleton and membrane. Hemoglobin is reduced to methemoglobin, which cannot bind oxygen. Additionally, blood stored more than 7 days is deplete of 2,3-DPG, a compound needed to release oxygen to the tissues [10].

White cells simultaneously stored within blood packs also impair the red cell function. White cells, present even in leukocyte-depleted products, increase hemolysis and potassium level due to leakage from the red cells. Cytokines released from leukocytes accumulate in the stored blood product. Soluble lipids, being similar to platelet activating factor, are also present in the red cell units. These lipids do not seem to come from white cells and can therefore not be reduced by leukoreduction [10].

During storage, red cells and residual white cells and platelets undergo proteolysis resulting in the release of the lysed cell's contents into the supernatant of red cell concentrate. The amount of proteins found in the red cell concentrate supernatant increases gradually over the time of storage. Most likely the proteins originate from decaying cells. Residual plasma contributes further to components found in supernatant.

Theoretically, all compounds of the red cell, the proteome [11] (see Table Appendix A.4), lipids, minerals, carbohydrates, and nucleic acids, can be found in the supernatant of red cell concentrates. Proteomics has shed new light on the proteins found in red cells and subsequently, in the supernatant of red cell concentrates. Initial proteomic analyses have so far revealed about 200 proteins in the red cell, of which about 25% are unknown [11]. The extreme complexity of the red cell proteome and the predominance of hemoglobin makes it difficult to detect all the proteins in the red cell. However, looking at what

Table 18.1 Examples of ingredients found in the supernatant of stored red cell concentrates.

Ingredient	Biologic activity
Adenine	Nutrient
Albumin, haptoglobin, transferrin, apolipoprotein, actin, hemoglobin (as fragments or isoforms)	Common proteins found abundantly with known functions
Alpha-1B glycoprotein	Function unknown, possibly immunoglobulin-related
Anticoagulant (e.g., citrate)	Anticoagulation
Bacteria	Sepsis
Carbonic anhydrase I	Catalyzes hydration of carbon dioxide and dehydration of bicarbonate, removal of carbon dioxide by red cells, regulation of functions in the gastrointestinal tract and kidneys (stomach acidity, acid–base and fluid balance)
cDNA clone (hypothetical protein)	Not known
Complement C4 A	Inflammation
CTAP	Promoter of neutrophil adhesion
Fibrinogen	Coagulation protein
Free iron	Promotes bacterial growth, modulates endogenous iron metabolism
Glucose	Added nutrient
Immunoglobulins and their fragments	Immunomodulation
Phosphate	Added nutrient
Plasticizers	Toxic (released from blood bags)
S100 calcium-binding protein	Modulates activity of leukocytes, inflammation, cell proliferation, and differentiation including neoplastic transformation, phosphorylation, regulates enzyme activities, function of cytoskeleton and membranes, intracellular calcium homeostasis, trophic or toxic depending on present concentration
Serum amyloid P (SAP)	Acute phase scavenger
Thioredoxin peroxidase B	Antioxidant, regulation of intracellular H_2O_2, may regulate gene expression
Transthyretin	Transport, binding

is already known about the red cell proteome gives new insight into blood transfusions and into the reasons why transfusions come with so many side effects. Table 18.1 lists some of the ingredients found in the supernatant of red cell concentrates [12]. It can easily be seen that the infused material is—to a varying degree—a proinflammatory, procoagulatory cocktail.

Platelets

There are two basic forms of platelet concentrates. Random donor platelets, pooled from whole blood donations, contain platelets from multiple donors with at least $5.5–6 \times 10^{10}$ platelets per unit. The platelet concentrate volume depends on the number of pooled units. In contrast, single donor platelets are gained by apheresis of one donor. The units have a volume of about 200 mL and contain at least $2–3 \times 10^{11}$ platelets.

In the additive solution, platelet concentrates contain not only platelets, but also a considerable amount of plasma and red cells as well as leukocytes, the amount depending on whether the platelets are leukocyte depleted or not.

Similar to red cells and white cells, platelets undergo lesions due to procurement and storage. Storage lesions lead to changes in the shape of the platelets so that they lose their natural discoid form. The granule content is released and adhesive glycoproteins are expressed, severely impairing function. Stored platelets do not aggregate normally in response to aggregating agents (e.g., epinephrine). Recovery and survival are impaired, especially if the pH is below 6.0. The pH in stored platelets is lowered due to platelet metabolism. In time, stored platelets undergo proteolysis, disintegrating and shedding proteins into platelet concentrate supernatant. Membrane proteins also change, presenting a changing pattern of antigens; therefore, antigenicity seems to increase with storage [13].

Storage also increases the incidence of transfusion reactions. The longer cells are stored, the more side effects. It has been suggested that reactions to platelet transfusions result from pyrogenic and vasoactive substances accumulated during storage [14]. Since proteolysis is a common feature of platelet storage lesions, it would be interesting to know what proteins are released that may affect the patient. Exactly which proteins are released is difficult to say. In fact, this may change depending on the donor and storage time. Potentially, all contents of a platelet can be released once the platelet is damaged. However, as is also the case with red cells, since the proteome (all proteins in the platelet), transcriptome (all mRNA transcripts in the platelet), and all other contents of normal human platelets have not yet been described, it cannot be said with certainty what the supernatant of platelet concentrates contains. Using advanced techniques such as proteomics and transcriptomics, hundreds, if not thousands of proteins have been found in the platelet, yet the significance of these proteins is poorly understood [15–17]. As far as is understood, platelet-derived proteins have many different functions and releasing such proteins may influence functions in the entire body. It remains to be seen whether platelet-derived clusterin influences transfusion recipients' apoptosis, whether frataxin derived from the transfusion changes iron homeostasis of the patient or whether the progesterone receptor associated protein P48 found in platelets influences progesterone receptor signaling in transfused patients [16]. Many hypothetical proteins and identified proteins with such names as WUGSC:H_DJ0777O23 and KIAA0193 with unknown function may or may not influence the transfused organism. All the components that finally influence the transfused body are simply not yet known and may perhaps never be known.

Fresh-frozen plasma

Fresh-frozen plasma (FFP) contains all the components usually found in the blood; however, the number of cellu-

lar components is starkly reduced. Despite this reduction in cellular components, some red cells, white cells, and platelets remain. FFP contains at least 60 g protein per liter. This proteome is a mixture of known and unknown proteins (compare list and footnote to Table Appendix A.3) [18]. About 120 proteins have been identified, many others have not. The main proteins in FFP are albumin, immunoglobulins, fibrinogen, and transferrin. In addition to proteins, it contains metabolites, cellular components, tumor markers, (pregnancy) hormones, etc.

To produce FFP, freshly donated plasma must be frozen within 6–8 hours, otherwise it would deteriorate rapidly. The influence of therapeutically significant proteins in FFP varies and is not only dependent on the donor, but also on the duration and conditions of storage. After 8 hours storage at room temperature, 13% of factor VIII activity is lost; after 24 hours about 30% of the factor activity is lost. The overall loss of plasmatic factors participating in coagulation, anticoagulation, and clot lysis is nonproportional, some proteins deteriorating faster than others. Therefore, stored plasma turns into a procoagulatory infusion, because anticoagulatory proteins (protein S, protein C) deteriorate faster than procoagulatory components.

What is the problem?

Before a medical decision is made, the problem to be remedied needs to be defined. There are basically two types of problems related to patients' blood management: *artificial* problems and *real* problems.

Artificial problems are those that only exist on paper. For example, when an arbitrary "laboratory-based transfusion trigger" is reached this is considered a problem. What is a transfusion trigger? Well, it is a value thought to indicate whether patients need a transfusion. Generally, a certain hemoglobin or platelet level or a certain coagulation parameter (e.g., the INR) is advocated guiding the use of red cells, platelets, or plasma, respectively. However, such predetermined values do not reflect what they should, namely, indicate that a patient now benefits from transfusion therapy.

Real problems are those that actually endanger the patient. Such include moderate to severe anemia, possibly resulting in impaired tissue oxygenation, cardiovascular instability, heart failure [19] with or without left ventricular hypertrophy, progressive kidney failure [20], respiratory failure with or without ventilator dependence and difficulties weaning from the ventilator [21], and increased mortality [22]. Coagulopathy, possibly resulting in bleeding,

bleeding-associated complications and death, is also a real problem. The more severe the anemia and coagulopathy, the greater the risk of adverse events. Further, the sicker the patient, that is, the more he suffers from cardiovascular or other diseases, the less he can tolerate anemia and coagulopathy. Such real problems have recently been used to define a "physiologic transfusion trigger," one that also takes the patient's clinical condition into consideration. However, there is also no single real problem that reliably indicates that a patient now benefits from transfusion.

A closer look at transfusion triggers used for red cell transfusion will illustrate the futility of trying to define a valid transfusion trigger. The classical trigger for red cells is the hemoglobin level. A hemoglobin level as a transfusion trigger is preferred because of ease of measurement. But there is little clinical evidence facilitating prediction of the critical hemoglobin level at which ischemia develops in any given patient [23]. To illustrate: Imagine a patient has been infused with 2 L of hydroxyethyl starch. Due to the effect of dilution, the hemoglobin level decreases substantially. Does the patient now need a red cell transfusion? Hardly. Many factors influence the hemoglobin level by simply changing the ratio of red cell mass to blood volume, among such are catecholamines, diuretics, stress or bed rest, and many more. Therefore, hemoglobin levels do not work as transfusion triggers.

Since the paramount reason for giving red cell transfusions is to restore tissue oxygenation, values reflecting the actual oxygen transport and utilization process have been tried as a transfusion trigger. A mixed venous gas analysis deriving the oxygen extraction ratio has also been suggested. An oxygen extraction ratio of <50% in combination with a low hemoglobin level has been under discussion [24]. This, however, also does not indicate that the patient will benefit from transfusion. Global ischemia is assumed when acidosis or hyperlactatemia are present. Other markers try to identify regional ischemia, which, in combination with a low hemoglobin level, may suggest a "need" for red cell transfusions. Organs with a critical oxygen demand, e.g., brain, heart, kidney, and the gut have been studied. The electroencephalogram can diagnose brain dysfunction, but it is also altered by drugs and other influences. The continuous electrocardiogram can demonstrate ST segment changes as a measurement for myocardial ischemia. Kidney function markers can demonstrate organ dysfunction and tonometry has been used to diagnose ischemia of the gastrointestinal tract. However, many other factors can influence such indicators of ischemia. Oxygen transport variables and ischemia markers are therefore not suitable for indicating whether a red cell transfusion will improve the patient's condition [25]. They simply indicate that the patient may have a real problem.

No transfusion trigger can replace good clinical judgment as the basis for deciding whether a patient is in a state of partial or global ischemia or whether the patient has a relevant clotting abnormality. Each patient must be evaluated and therapeutic options must be justified to meet the unique needs of every patient. The reaction to a decrease in hemoglobin level is what determines how well a patient copes with anemia. The decision for any prophylactic or therapeutic measure in blood management is a clinical one, based on physical examination and history taking. Before a therapy is prescribed, the following questions need to be asked to look for real problems: "Has hypovolemia been corrected? Is the patient hemodynamically stable? Is there evidence of organ ischemia? Is there potential for continuing or sudden blood loss? Is arterial blood normally saturated with oxygen? Can the patient be expected to appropriately increase cardiac output?" [25]. These questions show that the duration of anemia, intravascular volume, extent of a pending surgical procedure, likelihood of massive blood loss, and the presence of coexisting diseases all need to be considered, since they may be the real problems of the patient. Other values, e.g., laboratory values and oxygen measurement, may be added to supplement the diagnosis. However, a pathologic laboratory value is at best an indicator that the patient has a real problem, but it is not the problem in itself. The patient's vital signs, the results of the physical examination, urine output, and the mental status are the most important variables. "A patient who is conscious, comfortable and rational, with warm fingers and toes and who has a stable pulse rate and blood pressure and a urine output of at least 0.5 ml/kg/h is perfusing his heart, brain, kidneys and periphery" [25]. The patient is therefore unlikely to be in acute distress.

Having read the above, it is not difficult to understand that there is no transfusion trigger in the sense that a certain value or patient condition predicts that the patient will now benefit from a transfusion.

BRAND: benefits of transfusions

When it has been established that the patient has a real problem, such as moderate to severe anemia or a coagulopathy, or if the patient already suffers from such symptoms (impaired tissue oxygenation or bleeding, respectively), then a medical decision is warranted.

Table 18.2 List of therapeutic goals for which blood products are transfused.

Therapeutic goal	Do stored allogeneic blood products reach this goal?
Improve survival	Transfusions are a risk factor for death and are not associated with improved survival. Transfusions increase mortality
Increase red cell mass	Yes
Improve tissue oxygenation	No, on the contrary
Prevent or treat impaired tissue oxygenation, e.g., stroke, myocardial infarction	No, on the contrary
Reduce length of hospital stay	No, on the contrary
Reduce time of ICU stay	Possibly not, transfused patients are often longer in the ICU than nontransfused patients
Reduce ventilator dependency	No, but controversial; transfusion associated with prolonged mechanical ventilation
Prevent renal failure in anemic patients	No, on the contrary
Improve/restore microcirculation	Red cells: no, on the contrary
Reverse coagulopathy (e.g., due to liver failure, coumadin overdose)	Fresh frozen plasma: coagulopathy frequently insufficiently treated
Prevent bleeding in thrombocytopenic patients	Platelet concentrates likely not necessary

The first step in medical decision-making is to ascertain the benefits of the envisioned therapy. This also holds true for the decision to transfuse or not to transfuse. Therefore, what benefits are expected from the transfusion of allogeneic blood? It would be beneficial if the transfusion would achieve at least one, better several, therapeutic goals. What are the formulated therapeutic goals for patients considered candidates for allogeneic transfusions? Simply changing a laboratory value should not be the therapeutic goal. Blood management being patient-centered does not treat laboratory values, but rather the patient and the real problems.

Therapeutic interventions are expected to benefit the patient with the ultimate goal of improving patient outcome. There are two hypotheses underlying the reasoning used for a treatment decision involving blood transfusion. The one used most often in favor of red cell transfusion is that the body needs oxygen and therefore the stated goal of the transfusion is to improve tissue oxygenation. Platelets and plasma are given to ensure coagulation to stop or prevent bleeding, granulocytes are expected to fight infections. All this is believed to translate into a better outcome for the patient. The other hypothesis is that optimal outcome is associated with giving maximum support to the body's own mechanisms for protecting tissue from oxidative and other damage until homeostasis is restored. Adding transfused blood to the equation may interfere

with defensive measures already initiated by the body and may contribute to worsening the outcome. However, the latter theory has not as yet been extensively studied.

Allogeneic transfusions are given to achieve therapeutic goals. Some of them are listed in Table 18.2. Look at this table and check whether the goals can be achieved by transfusions [20, 21, 26–36]

After looking at the table, the question as to what the benefits of transfusions are is certainly justified. Interestingly, although the risks associated with transfusion are well described, far less is known about the benefits. In 1996, an article entitled "Benefits and risks of blood transfusion in surgical patients" [37] observed that "little direct evidence in support of the benefits of transfusion is apparent" and "in many ways the benefits of RBC transfusion have been assumed." The author did not mention one single benefit of transfusions in the article, yet more than 10 transfusion-associated risks were discussed. It seems "the belief that RBC *and other allogeneic* (italics by the authors) transfusions are efficacious ... is not supported by the bulk of emerging clinical evidence" [31]. Now, 10 years later, no further proof has been furnished in support of the beneficial effects of allogeneic blood transfusion. It is therefore highly questionable whether the transfusion of allogeneic blood products benefits patients.

If the stringent tenets of evidence-based medicine, the precautionary principle or simply common sense were used to decide whether or not to transfuse, this intervention would be abandoned after just examining the evidence for the benefit of transfusion—if it were not for many other factors causing physicians and other healthcare providers to hold to the attitude that "blood transfusions saves lives," to continue letting "firm belief" and cultural conditioning dictate their behavior so that they "trust that blood transfusion is a 'life-giving' force" [38].

BRAND: risks of transfusions

Effects of allogeneic transfusions in the human body

Transfusing stored blood into living human beings causes many changes in the recipient's organism. The most striking changes appear to be induced in the microcirculation. While fresh, deformable autologous red cells squeeze through the narrow vessels of the microcirculation to deliver oxygen, stored red cells lack this ability. The hardened red cells impair the microcirculation and tissue oxygenation. Stored red cells decrease capillary perfusion, increase sticking and transmigration of leukocytes, induce edema formation in the endothelium, and deformed red cells slow the blood flow and block vessels [33]. Red cell surface receptors are also activated during storage and the cells therefore tend to adhere more to the vessel wall, contributing to a microvascular traffic jam. Besides, the stored red cells that have lost 2,3-DPG cannot unload oxygen to the tissue. So, transfused red cells can load oxygen, but are no longer able to unload it. Apart from the oxygen delivery of fresh red blood cells, stored red cell units obviously do not deliver sufficient oxygen but cause severe microvascular damage. Although loss of 2,3-DPG, deformability as well as the increased aggregatability are partly reversible after transfusion, stored red cells do not function as expected. Oxygen uptake is not increased after transfusion, neither globally nor regionally [39]. Mixed venous oxygen saturation does not increase and lactate levels do not decrease after transfusion of stored red cells [29]. What is even worse, stored red cells not only fail to function as hoped for, they impair tissue oxygenation. Indeed, after 7–14 days storage, red cells appear to cause so many changes in the microvascular system that measurable tissue "deoxygenation" occurs after transfusion [28].

Transfusion of stored blood also changes coagulation. Stored blood contains procoagulant factors and factors promoting vasoconstriction. Exocytotic microvescicles, e.g., from red cells formed during storage, seem to be only one of the reasons why transfusions are believed to be thrombogenic [9]. In addition, different blood components are primed during storage to initiate coagulation once infused.

Allogeneic transfusions also undoubtedly exert a profound effect on the transfusion recipient's immune system [40]. Such effects have been collectively called TRIM (transfusion-related immunomodulation) (see below). TRIM is a multifactoral process caused by, among many other factors, priming of neutrophils during storage, release of cytokines accumulated in the stored blood product, and the surplus of decayed blood cells flooding the reticuloendothelial system for clearance.

Outcome variables

The profoundly negative effects of allogeneic transfusions on the human microcirculation, coagulation, and immune systems result in deterioration of many outcome variables. Allogeneic transfusions have therefore been termed a risk factor for negative clinical outcomes. On the other hand, transfusions have never been shown to be associated with improved outcome.

The risk of postoperative bacterial infection (wound, urinary tract, pneumonia, sepsis, abscess formation) is increased after allogeneic transfusions, a phenomenon shown for standard and leukodepleted red cell concentrates as well as for stored autologous red cells [41–45]. A meta-analysis demonstrated that transfusions increase the risk for infection after simple surgery by the factor 3.45. Trauma surgery patients receiving transfusions are 5.3 times more likely to develop an infection than nontransfused patients [46]. Patients who are transfused are more susceptible to developing dose-dependent multiorgan failure [47], are longer ventilator-dependent, need more vasopressors and remain longer in the ICU, and have longer stays in hospital [48].

Transfusions also worsen the outcome of patients undergoing surgery for malignancy. This has been shown in a variety of cancers (such as cancer of the lung [49], stomach [50], and female genitals [51]). Cancer patients' survival rates decrease when patients are transfused [50] and disease-free survival time is shortened [49]. The risk of developing metastases increases.

Transfusions diminish the strength of gastrointestinal anastomoses leading to increased anastomotic leakage [52, 53]. Animal experiments suggest the breaking strength of such anastomoses is reduced [54]. Transfusions after gastrointestinal bleeding increase the likelihood for rebleeding and increase mortality. This is due to the transfusion reversing the hypercoagulable state that naturally develops after hemorrhage [27].

Some particular effects of allogeneic transfusions have been described in neonates. The development of chronic lung disease and retinopathy of prematurity is associated with transfusion exposure [55]. The manifold increase in levels of growth-promoting substances (insulin-like growth factor) in adult blood as compared with baby blood may, when transfused, accelerate angiogenesis and may damage babies' eyes via retinal neovascularization [56]. Oxidative damage [57] of lipids caused by transfusions may damage the lungs of the premature. Necrotizing enterocolitis is also likely more frequent in babies that have received allogeneic transfusions [58].

A history of transfusion is a risk factor for many diseases, such as stroke and myocardial infarction [59], as well as for intracranial hemorrhage [60]. Interestingly, even infertility is associated with transfusions [61]. The reasons suggested for these associations were long-term immunomodulation and patient infection with various infectious agents causing chronic inflammation. Platelet transfusion has also been implicated as a cause of perioperative stroke [48]. Thromboembolism, deep vein thrombosis, and pulmonary embolism have been associated with many blood products [62].

Patients who suffer from ischemic heart disease are more likely to suffer deleterious effects when anemia is present [63]. This has led to the assumption that such patients therefore benefit from generous red cell transfusion. However, quite the contrary may be the case. Evidence is accumulating which shows that the sicker the patient, the less allogeneic transfusions are tolerated. A liberal transfusion strategy is more often associated with reduced exercise tolerance and increased myocardial ischemia than a restrictive one [64, 65]. Patients who are transfused while suffering from an acute coronary syndrome are more likely to die than nontransfused patients with the same syndrome, even after correcting statistics to take account of comorbidities [26]. It has even been suggested that patients transfused to keep the hematocrit above 25% are four times more likely to die than those not transfused [66]. An author summarizes current findings as follows: "Previous randomised studies support the conclusion that blood transfusion may, at best, be neutral with respect to survival or, at worst, be associated with either decreased survival or worsening cardiac function" [66].

Kidney function is also dependent on oxygen transport and deteriorates as patients become more anemic. However, as in the case of ischemic heart disease, transfusing anemic patients in an attempt to prevent renal damage is futile. Allogeneic transfusions even increase kidney damage. The reasons for this phenomenon are multifactorial; among those postulated are impaired oxygen unloading capacity of stored red cells, impaired microvascular perfusion with hardened red cells and other factors, leading to tissue deoxygenation rather than oxygenation [67]. Free iron from lysed transfused red cells may contribute to the kidney damage [20].

Overall, transfusions are negatively correlated with short- and long-term survival. Of course, transfused patients are usually in a more severe condition than nontransfused patients. However, when accounting for disease severity, transfusions are still associated with increased perioperative death [48]. It has been shown that patients who underwent heart surgery are twice as likely to die within 5 years compared to patients who underwent the same procedures without receiving a transfusion. Patients receiving transfusions were more severely ill, yet, when statistics were corrected to take account of comorbidities, transfusions still caused 70% more mortality [68]. Transfused trauma victims are almost three times as likely to die than other patients with the same hemoglobin level and shock severity [69].

Risks and side effects of transfusions

Risks and side effects of transfusions are a major concern and have attracted even more attention than drug-associated risks. Since blood is a precious and delicate substance, strenuous efforts have been made to avoid the dangers associated with it. Governments have instituted mechanisms to control transfusions and associated transfusion risks. A very good example is transfusion surveillance in the United Kingdom. An initiative termed Serious Hazards of Transfusions (SHOT) was launched in 1996 and since then information has been collected about transfusion-related hazards in the following categories: incorrect blood component transfused, acute transfusion reaction, delayed transfusion reaction, post-transfusion purpura, transfusion associated graft-versus-host disease, transfusion-related acute lung injury and transfusion-transmitted infection. Although participation by hospitals is voluntary, SHOT has collected interesting data [70], some of which is reviewed below.

Transfusion-transmittable infections (TTIs) are considered by the public to be the greatest problem related to transfusions. This may be true in developing countries but is not the case in developed countries. Only about 1% of events reported to the SHOT initiative were TTIs [70]. The blood bank is responsible for donor selection and test procedures, both important to reduce the risk of TTIs (see the chapter on blood banking). A clinician must rely on the blood bank for appropriately tested blood and cannot do much to reduce the incidence of TTIs per given unit. However, the clinician is in the unique position of being able to reduce the incidence of TTIs calculated per patient. Skilful blood management can considerably reduce the amount of blood transfused and the number of patients receiving transfusions, thereby reducing TTIs.

Bacterial contamination

Bacterial contamination of blood products is possible at each stage of processing, from blood collection to storage and transfusion. Bacteria may multiply in the blood bag and develop toxins. Platelets are especially prone to toxin development, because they are stored at 20–24°C, a temperature ideal for bacterial growth. Methods used by blood banks to reduce the risk of bacterial contamination are discussed in Chapter 18. However, there are some things that can be done on the part of the physician to reduce the incidence of bacterially contaminated transfusions. The simplest way to reduce bacteria transfusion is to avoid transfusions. If this is not desired, pretransfusion inspection of the blood component for signs indicative of bacterial contamination, adherence to preset storage times and re-warming periods and sterile handling of blood aid in reducing the incidence of bacterial infusion.

Clerical error

Clerical error occurs when blood is transfused to a patient other than the one intended. Statistics from developed countries show that this occurs in about 1:14,000–19,000 (United States) or 18,000 (United Kingdom) units of transfused allogeneic blood. The error rate in autologous units is similar (Canada 1:17,000) [71]. Impressive proof of the magnitude of clerical error in the scope of transfusion complications is provided in the SHOT study. In the reporting year 2001–2002, 71.8% of all reported transfusion-associated hazards were clerical errors [70].

Clerical errors result from human mistakes and mainly occur at the patient's bed side [72]. Methods to better identify patients and blood have been proposed to reduce clerical errors.

Immunological reactions

ALLOIMMUNIZATION

Alloimmunization occurs when antibodies develop against blood antigens other than those of the ABO and Rhesus system. Antibodies against such antigens are found in 1–2% of all cross-matched hospital patients. Incidence of alloantibodies increases with increased exposure to donor blood. After 10–20 transfusions, more than 10% of patients have alloantibodies and more than 30% after 100 transfusions [73]. Formation of alloantibodies is especially problematic in multiple-transfused patients, such as patients with hemoglobinopathies.

Alloimmunization leads to red cell destruction by delayed extravascular hemolysis. It is best prevented by avoiding exposure to donor blood, especially in patients with chronic blood disorders.

FEBRILE NONHEMOLYTIC TRANSFUSION REACTION

Febrile nonhemolytic transfusion reaction (FNHTR) is a diagnosis of exclusion. It is defined as an increase of body temperature of more than 1°C above pretransfusion values, sometimes accompanied by shaking chills. Such febrile reactions occur especially after platelet and granulocyte transfusions. They are attributed to donor white cells and proinflammatory cytokines.

ANAPHYLACTIC TRANSFUSION REACTIONS

All blood components can elicit allergic reactions ranging from minor urticaria to fatal anaphylaxis. Allergic reactions to blood products occur as often as reactions to penicillin. The estimated incidence varies from 1:1598 to 1:170,000 transfused blood products, depending on the kind of blood product transfused. More allergic reactions occur during platelet transfusion than during red cell or plasma transfusion.

Allergic reactions manifest rapidly, within minutes, often after only a few milliliters have been transfused. They are rapid, sometimes dramatic and potentially fatal reactions to foreign substances in sensitized patients. Allergic reactions to blood components present with the same symptoms as other allergic reactions: hypotension, bronchospasm, edema, gastrointestinal symptoms, rash, etc. Fever does not occur. The latter helps in the differential diagnosis of transfusion reactions and differentiates allergic reactions from hemolytic or septic reactions.

The exact reason for allergic reactions to blood components is not known. Since leukoreduction does not reduce the risk of allergic reactions, they may therefore not be leukocyte-related. Some patients have anti-haptoglobin antibodies or anti-IgA antibodies, both of which can cause allergic reactions. Negatively charged activated platelets and platelet microparticles have also been suspected as a cause, since they are thought to activate complement cascade.

TRANSFUSION-RELATED ACUTE LUNG INJURY

Transfusion-related acute lung injury (TRALI) is a clinical condition that develops within 6–24 hours after transfusion of blood products and results in a condition clinically indistinguishable from acute respiratory distress syndrome. Leukocytes infiltrate the lung, pulmonary edema develops and hyaline membranes form, thus damaging lung tissue.

The incidence of TRALI is not known, particularly because there is no consensus definition for the condition. It has been estimated that TRALI occurs in between 1:1323 and 1.3:1,000,000 transfusions [74] and is most probably a severely underreported condition. The exact mortality rate from TRALI is unknown, but has been estimated to range from 5 to 25% of all patients developing TRALI [74].

All blood products can cause TRALI, including autologous products. Plasma-containing products are most commonly implicated. The reasons why blood products cause TRALI have not been fully elucidated. Pathogenesis seems to be multifactoral. Different pathophysiological models have been described. One model claims that antibodies directed against leukocytes cause pulmonary damage. The antibodies are either present in the transfused blood and react with recipient leukocytes, or donor leukocytes react with antibodies present in the recipient. Another hypothesis claims that the development of TRALI is a two-event process. The first event is patient-related and causes activation of the patient's pulmonary endothelium. There, leukocytes sequestrate and attach to the pulmonary vasculature. This priming occurs as a result of hypoxia, infection, inflammation, surgery, massive transfusion, or administration of cytokines. The second event leading finally to TRALI is the transfusion. This transfusion activates the leukocytes adhering in the lung and results in endothelial damage with capillary leakage and finally, TRALI.

HEMOLYTIC TRANSFUSION REACTIONS

Hemolytic transfusion reactions occur due to accelerated immune-mediated red cell destruction. Two different entities with distinct clinical features are differentiated—acute and chronic (or delayed) hemolysis.

Acute hemolysis occurs within 24 hours of transfusion and is usually an intravascular hemolysis. The reason is most frequently ABO incompatibility. The presence of red cell alloantibodies [75] or an interdonor incompatibility (that is, a patient receives blood from different donors and the donor blood types do not match among themselves) may lead to acute hemolysis. Acute hemolysis is usually caused by red cell transfusions, but also by incompatible plasma or platelets, especially those with high titers of anti-A or anti-B. The symptoms develop acutely with fever, chills, abdominal and chest pain, nausea, vomiting, hypotension, tachycardia, hemoglobinemia, hemoglobinuria, flushing, and the feeling of impending doom. Renal failure, disseminated intravascular coagulation with uncontrolled bleeding, shock, and death may result.

Chronic (= delayed) hemolysis results in extravascular hemolysis with a gradual decline in hemoglobin. Antibodies are present that are usually directed against the Rhesus, Kell, Kidd, or Duffy group antigens [75]. Delayed hemolysis develops within days or weeks after transfusion and presents with fever, chills, dyspnea, jaundice, and failure to maintain an appropriate post-transfusion hematocrit. Patients with sickle-cell disease are especially vulnerable to delayed hemolysis and occasionally react with suppressed erythropoiesis and hemolysis that also includes autologous red cells (bystander hemolysis).

TRANSFUSION-ASSOCIATED GRAFT-VERSUS-HOST DISEASE

A rare, but particularly lethal complication of allogeneic transfusions is transfusion-associated graft-versus-host disease(TA-GvHD). Symptoms develop 3–30 days after the transfusion and include fever, watery diarrhea, erythematous maculopapular skin rash progressing to generalized erythroderma, and desquamation. Hemorrhage, infection, and pancytopenia follow. More than 90% of patients die within 1–3 weeks.

TA-GvHD is caused by proliferating transfused donor T-lymphocytes. The donor lymphocytes recognize the recipient's cells as foreign and attack them, while the recipient's system does not identify the donor cells as foreign and such are tolerated. Those affected are mainly immunocompromised patients or patients receiving a blood product from a genetically similar donor (one-way HLA), e.g., from a relative or in a closed population. Many different immunosuppressive therapies have been tried to treat TA-GvHD, but success has been limited [75]. Irradiation of blood components can prevent the development of TA-GvHD.

MICROCHIMERISM

Transfusions with components containing white cells should be considered a "mononuclear cell transplantation" [76]. In analogy to TA-GvHD, microchimerism means that "transplanted" donor cells proliferate and survive in the transfusion recipient's bone marrow for months or even many years after the transfusion of blood products containing white cells, including leukoreduced blood components [77–80]. There they compete with the recipient's leukocytes. It has been shown that after receiving blood from a male, females carry Y chromosomes in their blood. The long-term effects of microchimerism are unknown. It may predispose to autoimmune diseases, chronic graft-versus-host disease, and recurrent abortion [75].

POST-TRANSFUSION PURPURA
Post-transfusion purpura is a rare transfusion complication. About 1–2 weeks after the transfusion, thrombocytopenia develops accompanied by the typical symptoms of a bleeding diathesis. The cause for this complication is thought to be platelet-specific alloantibodies resulting in destruction of the patient's platelets.

The condition is usually self-limited, but has a mortality rate of about 13% [75]. If an intervention is warranted, the therapy of choice is intravenous immunoglobulin. Steroids and plasmapheresis have also been used occasionally. Platelet transfusions are generally ineffective.

Circulatory effects

Infusions usually come with circulatory effects. This is also true of infusions of blood. The effects caused are those common to fluid therapy in addition to those caused uniquely by blood.

Transfusion-associated circulatory overload (TACO) occurs when too much fluid is transfused or when transfusion is too rapid. Patients with renal failure or cardiopulmonary disease are prone to volume overload. The same is true for patients with chronic anemia (because they are already hypervolemic) who are not currently bleeding. Overload results in acute respiratory failure with dyspnea, tachycardia, hypertension, and cyanosis.

Cellular blood products come with a higher viscosity than acellular fluids. The increase in blood viscosity resulting from transfusion decreases cardiac output [81] and blunts the patient's own compensatory response to anemia.

Iron overload

Long-term transfusion therapy regularly results in iron storage. Iron stored in the tissues leads to transfusion-associated hemosiderosis with oxidative tissue damage. The heart and endocrine organs, such as the pancreas, are especially prone to damage.

Therapy is recommended well ahead of the development of clinically relevant hemosiderosis. Chelation therapy, usually with desferrioxamine, is begun once the serum ferritin level reaches a certain mark.

Immunomodulatory effects

An effective immune response requires the fine-tuned interaction of all parts of the immune system. Among them are CD4+ T-helper cells, which recognize antigens in combination with major histocompatibility complex molecules (MHC) type 2, the latter being expressed only on few cells, such as B-lymphocytes and macrophages. The CD8+ cytotoxic T-cells recognize antigens with MHC type 1, the latter being present on all cells with a nucleolus, and on platelets. As a result of interaction, different responses occur all with the aim of ridding the system of intruders. Depending on the mechanisms leading to activation of the immune system, different responses occur. A Th1 response results in CD4+ cell proliferation, release of IL-2, γ-interferon, macrophage activity, delayed-type hypersensitivity, and cytotoxicity. A Th2 response results in increased interleukin 4, 5, 6, and 10, B-cell activation, and antibody formation.

Immunosuppression results when the normal responses to an antigen are downregulated or modulated. Transfusions cause such changes, a condition called transfusion-related immunomodulation (TRIM). Overall, allogeneic transfusions elicit a persistent, but ineffective, immune response.

Each cellular blood component contains at the least some residual platelets and leukocytes that carry MHC molecules, and so does plasma. These allow the body to identify them as foreign. Since transfusions are usually not MHC-matched, they elicit immunological reactions. These may result either in alloimmunization, tolerance, or immunosuppression.

Transfusion antigens confuse the immune system. On the one hand, transfused cells are considered self, that is, from the same species. On the other, they are considered foreign since they have another MHC. This kind of situation does not happen in response to other foreign material, such as bacteria. And since blood is given intravenously, the immune system lacks costimulation from signals originating from infected tissues and dendritic cells. This lack of costimulation results in anergy and apoptosis of T cells.

Leukocytes from the donor also influence the blood recipient. The necrotic remains of stored white cells preferentially stimulate Th2 response. This results in increased levels of IL-4, 5, 6, and 10, B-cell activation, and antibody formation. In addition to this, the patient's Th1 response is downregulated, resulting in diminished CD4+ cell proliferation, release of IL-2, γ-interferon, macrophage activity, delayed-type hypersensitivity, and cytotoxicity.

In summary, allogeneic transfusions impair T-cell proliferation, change the CD4+/CD8+ ratio, reduce delayed hypersensitivity reactions, release Th2 cytokines while reducing Th1 cytokines to a lesser degree. Macrophage function, natural killer-cell activity, and cellular cytolysis are also affected. The more leukocytes are present in donated blood, the more extensive is the immunomodulation response to transfusion. Reducing the amount of donor leukocytes in blood products is therefore helpful in reducing immunologic side effects of transfusions. However, leukocyte-depleted red cells also affect the immune system, for example, by suppression of T-cell proliferation [82].

Immune response to autologous transfusions [82, 83]

In contrast to the immune response to allogeneic transfusions, the response to an autologous transfusion is short term. Autologous red cells increase the proliferation of T-cells, cytokine secretion, and B-cell activation.

Stored autologous blood seems, in part, to have the same effects on the immune system as stored allogeneic blood. Patients who receive their own preoperatively stored blood experience an impaired natural killer cell function similar in extent to that for allogeneic blood. However, when patients receive fresh autologous blood procured by intraoperative hemodilution, natural killer cell function is increased. This may explain why the postoperative infection rate is reduced in patients who only receive their own fresh blood.

BRAND: "alternatives"—other therapeutic options

There are many therapeutic and prophylactic options for anemia, coagulopathy, and immunodeficiency. Most of these options do not involve the use of allogeneic blood products. As shown in previous chapters, these options are safe and effective and therefore indispensable for improving the patient outcome. When decisions are made about a patient's blood management, asanguinous therapeutic options are certainly the first line of treatment, and not an alternative to transfusions. Therefore, such treatment deserves its due place in the decision-making process.

BRAND: no transfusion or no therapy at all

When the use of transfusions is being contemplated, the consequences of "no transfusion" should also be considered. However, the consequences of "no transfusion" should not be confused with the consequences of "no therapy." While it may indeed be better not to transfuse the patient, appropriate blood management may still be required. Many, if not all, conditions that typically have resulted in allogeneic transfusions being given require therapy, but not the transfusion of blood.

Anemia, for example, although only a symptom, most often needs therapy, either by remedying the underlying condition or by directly treating the anemia. If anemia is not treated, problems can ensue. Untreated anemia seems to worsen the patient outcome. Depending on the severity of the anemia, the time over which it has developed and the comorbidities of the patient, symptoms such as fatigue, palpitations and tachycardia, left ventricular hypertrophy, deterioration of kidney function, changes in mental status, dyspnea, etc. result. What is more, anemia also potentiates the ill effects of other medical conditions [19]. To date it has not yet been clarified whether all kinds of anemia benefit from therapy. Since anemia may be protective to a certain degree, the value of anemia therapy, in addition to therapy for the underlying disease, is not fully understood. However, proof is accumulating, showing that some therapies of anemia are beneficial. The benefit depends on the kind of therapy. While patients with cardiovascular and renal dysfunction and anemia benefit from erythropoietin therapy and the resulting correction of anemia (preventing remodeling of the myocardium, improving kidney function, reducing fatigue, etc.), patients transfused as a therapeutic strategy to correct anemia do not [19, 31].

Also, coagulopathy and immunodeficiency require therapy to prevent or treat the ill effects of these conditions. Simply not to transfuse is not the answer to the finding that allogeneic blood products do not improve the outcome of the patient. Therefore, like anemia, coagulopathy and immunodeficiency require intervention.

Table 18.3 PMI: to transfuse or not to transfuse.

Plus: positive results of transfusing allogeneic red cells	Minus: negative results of transfusing allogeneic red cells	Implications: outcomes (positive or negative)
Laboratory results are normalized	Impaired microcirculation	Oxygen delivery may be impaired (-3)
Treatment may be in accordance with guidelines	Exposure to infectious risks	Patient may acquire a TTI (-2)
	Immunosuppression	Expectations of peers are met ($+2$)
	A therapy with no proven benefit is applied	Increased risk of infection, cancer recurrence, etc. (-2)
	Costs are incurred	The patient may be worried about receiving a transfusion, causing long-term stress (-1)
	Immunologic reactions to blood elicited	The long-term effects of transfusions will affect the patient (stroke, heart attack, microchimerism, etc.) (-2)
		Mortality is increased (-3)
		The threat of possible law suits is increased because of a transfusion (-1)

BRAND: decision-making

The therapeutic options: to transfuse or not to transfuse?

Now that several facts about allogeneic transfusions have been considered, the focus will now be on structured decision-making, as mentioned at the outset. Decision-making is a cognitive process to select a course of action from available options. It begins with the recognition that something needs to be changed and it ends with a decision about what is to be done. Such decisions may be rational or irrational and have an influence on future success, in this case, the patient outcome. All the information available is required to make a sound decision.

Aids for decision-making, known as decision-making tools, have been devised. Two of such tools will now be used and applied in a treatment decision that typically would result in the prescription of allogeneic transfusions.

PMI: plus, minus, implications

The first decision-making tool is PMI, standing for plus, minus, implications. This tool is used when only two alternatives exist or to make a "yes or no" decision. In the example, the decision is whether or not to transfuse a patient with red cells. The positive effects of transfusing the patient are listed as are the negative effects and the implications of these options (Table 18.3).

Consider Table 18.3. Most likely a decision can be made at a glance. If not, here is a further aid to reaching a sound decision. Score each implication and then add the scores. A positive score means the effect is highly desirable, a negative score means the effect is undesirable. Granted, scores may be subjective. However, they may nevertheless help indicate in which direction the balance of the decision is tending to go.

Grid analysis

Another decision-making tool is grid analysis. It is best used if it is believed that a number of good options are available. List all therapeutic options and add the factors that are important to decision-making (Table 18.4). Assign each factor a relative importance, from poor (0) to excellent (3). Then score all options in the list according to the factors. If one factor does not hold for the option, score 0.

The example of a severely anemic patient is used to illustrate the use of grid analysis; the patient is anemic but shows no sign of impaired oxygen delivery and no bleeding is anticipated in the near future.

The following therapeutic options are available for this patient:

Allogeneic transfusions

rHuEPO therapy and wait

Table 18.4 Grid analysis: to what degree are the factors achieved by each of the options (score 0–3)?

Factors	Oxygen	Speed	Safety	Costs	Guidelines	Superiors	Patient wishes	Total
Transfusion	0	3	0	1	3	3	1	
EPO + wait	2	2	3	2	1	2	2	
Iron	1	1	2	2	1	2	2	
Do nothing	0	0	1	3	0	0	0	

Iron, multivitamins and wait

Do nothing

The following factors need to be considered to analyze the decision:

Oxygen delivery improved

Speed of onset of therapeutic results

Create a safety margin

Save costs

Adhere to guidelines

Avoid trouble with superiors

Give treatment corresponding to the patient's wishes

How important is each factor (weighting)? When assigning the relative importance (weight) to each factor, multiply the weight with the above scores. Then, add up (Table 18.5).

Using this decision-making tool, it is concluded that the best option for this patient is to treat with rHuEPO and then wait until the patient has recovered from anemia.

Using decision-making tools, such as the two described above, may help clinicians avoid overly emotional decisions and finally result in a conclusion contrary to that dictated by emotion. However, it may represent the most beneficial option for the patient, because it takes into account what is known to be beneficial and what is known to be detrimental. Decision-making tools also help clinicians internalize new thinking patterns and aid in transferring recent scientific evidence into routine patient care. There-

fore, by all means use such decision-making tools and incorporate new information pertinent to blood management as soon as it becomes available.

Biases in medical decision-making and influence on the transfusion decision

Decision-making styles differ from person to person and depend on each individual's cognitive style, that is, the extent to which thoughts and feelings, judgment, and perception, etc. are incorporated in the thinking process. Apart from these differences, human decision-making processes are always biased. Some of the known biases are also typically found in the transfusion decision. Recognizing such biases may serve as encouragement to make a conscious effort to avoid falling prey to them.

• Conservatism: "Undoubtedly, transfusions save lives." Often such and similar statements are used to introduce articles dealing with blood transfusions. Even if the article provides support for the notion that blood does not save lives this sentence is added almost apologetically because what follows does not confirm the general belief. Such statements result from the conservatism typically found in transfusion medicine. It demonstrates an unwillingness to change thought patterns.

• Wishful thinking or optimism: Since blood is often believed to be the last resort, the hope is that it will perform

Table 18.5 Grid analysis: assigning the relative importance to each factor.

Factors Weight	Oxygen 3	Speed 1	Safety 2	Costs 2	Guidelines 1	Superiors 1	Patient wishes 3	Total
Transfusion	0	3	0	2	3	3	3	14
EPO + wait	6	2	6	4	1	2	6	27
Iron	3	1	4	4	1	2	6	21
Do nothing	0	0	2	6	0	0	0	8

a miracle. Therefore, often even patients who have already suffered cardiac arrest are transfused (personal observation). People simply want to see transfusions in a positive light.

• Willingness to believe what has been repeated most often and by the greatest number of different of sources: When "Donate blood and save lives" is declared on posters and in advertisements finally, people believe it. The main thing is to say it time and again. The more such information is spread, the more difficult it is to come to the realization that there is no reason to believe that transfusions save lives.

• Initial information shapes the view of subsequent information: If medical students are taught in school that transfusions are beneficial, they tend to hold to this belief for the rest of their career.

• Peer pressure: Individuals who question the necessity of a transfusion are often subjected to immense pressure if peers think differently.

• Source credibility: An idea is rejected if bias exists against the person, organization, or group to which the person belongs. For instance, if a layman claims transfusions are detrimental, this idea is easily rejected. However, if a professor makes the same statement, the idea is more likely to be accepted.

• Reluctance to apply the same decision-making criteria in similar situations: Safety and efficacy of intravenous drugs are often rigorously tested and controlled. However, the same standards simply do not apply for blood products. Although transfusions have never been tested for efficacy and do not fulfill the stringent criteria of drug testing they are used nevertheless. If transfusions were subject to regulatory controls and approval, they would not be approved for use. When it comes to transfusions, there is reluctance to apply the same decision-making criteria and the same precautionary principles used for approving drugs.

• Conforming to decision-making expectations of others in the medical profession: For a medical professional to state that he does not believe transfusions save lives is considered unusual. The medical professional is expected to believe that transfusions save lives.

Transfusion guidelines

Medical practice has long been determined by guidelines. Originally, these represented a consensus of expert opinion that defined the standard of practice. During recent years, a change has been made toward a more scientific approach to guideline formulation. The approach has a defined methodology and is evidence-based. However, at present, only a few guidelines actually abide by established scientific methods [84].

Guidelines are formulated by individuals as well as by medical societies, boards, or consensus conferences (e.g., American Association of Blood Banks, Canadian Red Cross Society, British Committee for Standards in Haematology). Many of the guidelines are published and are made easily accessible to encourage dissemination and use. Some guidelines have been formulated to guide the use of special blood products in a variety of settings (see Appendix B), while others have been created to guide treatment of a specific disease involving transfusion therapy (see Appendix B).

A brief glance at an example of a modern guideline reveals the level of evidence on which single recommendations are based. For example, in 2003, 60 recommendations were issued in the "Guidelines for the use of platelet transfusions" drawn up by the British Committee for Standards in Haematology. Only three were supported by level 1 or 2 evidence, that is, by appropriate scientific data. A further seven recommendations were based on weak scientific proof (level 3, grade B). The remaining 50 recommendations were based only on expert opinion (level 3, grade C, and level 4 evidence). Interestingly, all three recommendations supported by level 1 and 2 evidence advocate reduced use of transfusions.

The following paragraphs describe the content of current transfusion guidelines. Most guidelines mirror the opinion of a select group of people and not the opinion of the authors. Although such are not necessarily based on sound scientific evidence, transfusion guidelines define indications for blood products. They might also include approaches for minimizing the use of allogeneic transfusions and relate circumstances in which transfusions are not recommended. This information is important, but constitutes an aid at best. Sound clinical judgment is still necessary.

Guidelines for red cell transfusions

Presumably, the most significant hazard of severe anemia is diminished oxygen carrying capacity. Severe anemia needs to be corrected. This being so, intuitively many physicians order stored red cells. This is mirrored in current guidelines, which state that the main indication for red cell transfusions is to increase the oxygen carrying capacity in patients with anemia.

Since the benefits of red cell transfusions are questionable, guidelines state that transfusions should not be considered when a patient is able to tolerate anemia. Although the literature demonstrates that healthy patients can tolerate normovolemic anemia down to surprisingly low hemoglobin levels (5 g/dL or even lower to 3.5 g/dL)) [10], guidelines often recommend maintaining hemoglobin levels between 7 g/dL and 9 g/dL. The guidelines state that transfusions are rarely recommended if hemoglobin level is above 10 g/dL.

Guidelines also relate the previously accepted contraindications for red cell transfusions, namely, stable, acute, and chronic anemia. These include autoimmune anemia, megaloblastic anemia, iron deficiency and anemia in patients with renal failure, all of which can be corrected by nonblood management [85].

Guidelines for platelet transfusions

Platelets are given for the treatment of hemorrhage in certain types of thrombocytopenia or platelet function defects. Although controversial, platelets are also given prophylactically. Before the decision to transfuse is reached, the cause of thrombocytopenia needs to be established, because there are thrombocytopenias for which platelet transfusions are contraindicated or ineffective.

What do current guidelines say about platelet transfusions? According to current guidelines, platelet transfusions may be considered under the following conditions.
• Bone marrow failure (because of disease, cytotoxic therapy, or irradiation): Without risk factors, a threshold of 5×10^9/L for platelet transfusions is considered safe [86]. Patients with chronic stable thrombocytopenia (e.g., myelodysplasia or aplastic anemia) should be transfused very restrictively, so that alloimmunization is best avoided. For this group of patients, no threshold for prophylactic platelet transfusions is indicated. The transfusion indication depends on the degree of clinical hemorrhage. When risk factors such as fever >38°C, fresh minor hemorrhage, sepsis, antibiotics, and other hemostatic impairment exist, the transfusion threshold may be lowered.
• Thrombocytopenic patients are believed to need a certain number of platelets to undergo procedures safely: Sound scientific evidence is lacking for the indications for prophylactic platelet transfusions prior to surgical interventions [86]. In the search for guidelines, refuge was therefore taken in expert opinion. This resulted in the following recommendations: Bone marrow aspirations can be performed without platelet support given that adequate surface pressure is maintained after puncture. A platelet count between 40 and 50×10^9/L is considered desirable for lumbar puncture, epidural catheter inser-

tion, endoscopy, intravascular catheters, liver biopsy, and laparotomy [87]. For surgery in areas where even minor bleeding could be detrimental, brain or eye surgery for example, guidelines recommend a platelet count of at least 100×10^9/L. The fact that some physicians perform procedures safely in patients with much lower platelet counts than those stated demonstrates there is no unequivocal agreement to these thresholds. Lumbar punctures, for example, have been performed safely with a patient platelet count of only about 20×10^9/L.
• In neonatal alloimmune thrombocytopenia it was recommended that special platelet products be given as soon as possible.

There are conditions where platelets are not recommended unless there is a life-threatening bleeding. If at all possible, other approaches should be sought to avoid alloimmunization.
• Platelet transfusions are rarely recommended in platelet function disorders [86]. If such occur, antiplatelet drugs should be stopped and the underlying condition corrected. In renal failure patients, the hematocrit should be corrected to >0.30 (EPO). Desmopressin (DDAVP) will usually work in the presence of platelet function disorders. Patients with congenital Glanzmann's thrombasthenia are good candidates for recombinant factor VIIa. This avoids alloimmunization and subsequent platelet refractoriness.
• Several immunosuppressive therapies are available for autoimmune thrombocytopenias. Platelet transfusions are recommended only where there is life-threatening bleeding and should be given together with intravenous methylprednisolone and immunoglobulin.
• Post-transfusion purpura usually responds to high-dose intravenous immunoglobulins (2 g/kg over 2–5 days). Platelet transfusions are usually ineffective and should only be used if attempting to control severe bleeding.

There are some clear contraindications for platelet transfusions. Platelets can cause life-threatening thrombosis in conditions with thrombotic consumption of platelets. This may occur in thrombotic thrombocytopenic purpura, heparin-induced thrombocytopenia, and active disseminated intravascular coagulation.

Guidelines for granulocyte transfusions

There are no evidence-based indications for granulocyte transfusions [88]. Some conditions considered indications are infections in patients with granulocyte function deficiency, septic granulomatosis, and severe neutropenia with less than 500 neutrophils per microliter blood (despite colony-stimulating factor therapy), given that anti-infective therapy has been unsuccessful. Granulocyte transfusions were recommended by some scientists when neonates with severe sepsis and neutropenia deteriorate despite at least 24 hours of antibiosis. However, such neonates also respond to granulocyte colony stimulating factors [89].

Guidelines for FFP

FFP has been used extensively earlier. However, the benefits of FFP have been shown to be questionable, or more suitable products are now available. Consequently, current guidelines list only few indications for FFP.

The 2004 guideline of the British Committee for Standards in Haematology [90] makes the following recommendations: FFP is indicated for

- Single inherited clotting factor deficiency, if there is no virus-safe fractionated product available. In developed countries, this refers to factor V.
- Severe bleeding in the presence of multiple coagulation factor deficiency or disseminated intravascular coagulation.
- Microvascular bleeding during surgery without other obvious reasons, given the need for factor replacement is confirmed in laboratory tests.
- Plasma exchange for thrombotic thrombocytopenic purpura.

FFP is considered second-line treatment to reverse vitamin K antagonists in the presence of severe bleeding and for the treatment of hemorrhagic disease of newborn. Vitamin K always has to be administered concomitantly. First-line treatment for the conditions mentioned is prothrombin complex concentrate. In developing countries without access to factor concentrates, FFP has also been recommended as the ultima ratio for life-threatening bleeding in hemophiliacs [91].

According to the guidelines FFP is often used inadequately. Knowing when it is not indicated [90] helps prevent unnecessary patient exposure to donor blood products. FFP is not indicated

- when prothrombin time (PT) or activated partial thromboplastin time (aPTT) is <1.5 times normal
- for volume expansion in adults or children
- for nutrition
- in disseminated intravascular coagulation without bleeding

- for the reversal of vitamin-K antagonist (warfarin) anticoagulation or prolonged INR (international normalized ratio) without severe bleeding
- to treat vitamin K deficiency in critically ill
- to prevent periventricular hemorrhage in preterm infants
- for plasma exchange (except for thrombotic thrombocytopenic purpura)
- when administered according to formulas in case of massive transfusions

---

A word about leukoreduction

Several countries have made leukoreduction of all suitable blood products mandatory. In other countries, both leukoreduced and nonleukoreduced products are available. In its guidelines, the British Committee for Standards in Haematology [92] gave the following summary recommendations regarding the use of leukoreduced blood:

Indications
- Prevention of febrile nonhemolytic transfusion reactions
- Reduction of graft rejection after hematopoetic cell transplantation (e.g., in aplastic anemia). Transfusions for patients who are potentially candidates for hematopoetic cell transplantation should always consist of leukodepleted blood.
- Prevention of transmission of viral infections by transfusion (CMV, effective alternative to CMV negative blood)
- Fetal and neonatal transfusions (below age 1)

Probably indicated (insufficient evidence)
- Platelet refractoriness
- Kidney transplants
- Immunomodulation
- Progression of HIV

Not indicated
- Prevention of TA-GvHD
- In noncellular blood components such as FFP, cryoprecipitate and blood products prepared from pooled blood

---

Key points

- Stored allogeneic blood products are unpredictable in use and most of the ingredients are unknown.
- Medical decision-making is often made using the mnemonic BRAND
  ○ Benefits of transfusions: Decades of research in the field has not shown any major benefit for patients.

◦ Risks of transfusions: Allogeneic blood transfusions substantially alter the recipient's organism. They also cause many diseases (TRIM, infections, etc.).

◦ Alternative therapies: There are many therapeutic options available that do not resort to use of allogeneic blood.

◦ No therapy: At times, doing nothing rather than transfusing is a sound medical option. However, under certain circumstances, patients greatly benefit from therapy with drugs or methods not involving blood transfusions. No Therapy is not the alternative to allogeneic transfusion. Blood management options are.

◦ Decision: Blood management is the path to be taken, because blood saves lives, while transfusions do not.

Questions for review

• Why do physicians transfuse?
• What are the benefits of allogeneic transfusions?
• What effects do stored blood products have on the microcirculation?
• How do allogeneic transfusions affect patient outcome?
• What results if anemia and coagulopathy are left untreated?
• What do the following abbreviations stand for and how do the conditions present clinically? FNHTR, TACO, TRIM, TRALI, TA-GvHD, TTI.

Suggestions for further research

Look into current guidelines for blood transfusions. Choose those that state the level of evidence (Tables Appendix A.8 and Appendix A.9) on which recommendations are based. Sort the recommendations by level and compare which recommendations are based on scientific evidence and which are merely the opinion of the authors of the guidelines.

Exercises and practice cases

Use grid analysis to decide on the most suitable therapeutic option for the following patient:

Mr B requests bilateral hip replacement. He agrees that you to choose from the following therapy options and any combinations you may find beneficial:

Use a cell saver (intra- and postoperatively)

Operate one hip at a time, allowing for restoration of red cell mass

Preoperative autologous donation

Do nothing to prevent blood loss and transfuse allogeneically if the blood count drops

Use acute normovolemic hemodilution

You consider the following factors to be important:

Prevention of infection in the hip is of utmost importance

The hazards of allogeneic transfusions should be avoided

The patient wants to invest as little time as possible in the treatment

The overall cost of treatment, including length of stay, should be minimized

What conclusion do you come to?

Homework

• Find out who is in charge of blood transfusion risk management and quality assurance at your hospital and ask for an opinion on blood management.

• Explain the risks and benefits of blood transfusion and appropriate blood management procedures to a patient.

• Find a reliable source from which to figure out the risks of infection with blood-borne diseases in your country.

References

1 Hathaway, E.O. Changing educational paradigms in transfusion medicine and cellular therapies: development of a profession. *Transfusion*, 2005. **45**(Suppl 4): p. 172S–188S.

2 Mahdihassan, S. Blood as the earliest drug, its substitutes, preparations and latest position. *Am J Chin Med*, 1986. **14**(3–4): p. 104–109.

3 Barsoum, N. and C. Kleeman. Now and then, the history of parenteral fluid administration. *Am J Nephrol*, 2002. **22**(2–3): p. 284–289.

4 Blundell, J. Some account of a case of obstinate vomiting in which an attempt was made to prolong life, by the injection of blood into the veins. Lecturer, in conjunction with Dr. Haighton, on physiology and midwifery, at Guy's Hospital, 1818. p. 296–301.

5 Nuttall, G.A., *et al.* Current transfusion practices of members of the American society of anesthesiologists: a survey. *Anesthesiology*, 2003. **99**(6): p. 1433–1443.

6 Speiss, B.D. Transfusion and outcome in heart surgery. *Ann Thorac Surg*, 2002. **74**(4): p. 986–987.

7 Yamey, G. Albumin industry launches global promotion. *BMJ*, 2000. **320**: p. 533.

8 Hogman, C.F. and H.T. Meryman. Red blood cells intended for transfusion: quality criteria revisited. *Transfusion*, 2006. **46**(1): p. 137–142.

9 Greenwalt, T.J. The how and why of exocytic vesicles. *Transfusion*, 2006. **46**(1): p. 143–152.

10 Ho, J., W.J. Sibbald, and I.H. Chin-Yee. Effects of storage on efficacy of red cell transfusion: when is it not safe? *Crit Care Med*, 2003. **31**(12, Suppl): p. S687–S697.

11 Kakhniashvili, D.G., L.A. Bulla, Jr., and S.R. Goodman. The human erythrocyte proteome: analysis by ion trap mass spectrometry. *Mol Cell Proteomics*, 2004. **3**(5): p. 501–509.

12 Anniss, A.M., *et al.* Proteomic analysis of supernatants of stored red blood cell products. *Transfusion*, 2005. **45**(9): p. 1426–1433.

13 Snyder, E.L., *et al.* Protein changes occurring during storage of platelet concentrates. A two-dimensional gel electrophoretic analysis. *Transfusion*, 1987. **27**(4): p. 335–341.

14 Muylle, L., *et al.* Reactions to platelet transfusion: the effect of the storage time of the concentrate. *Transfus Med*, 1992. **2**(4): p. 289–293.

15 Garcia, A., *et al.* Extensive analysis of the human platelet proteome by two-dimensional gel electrophoresis and mass spectrometry. *Proteomics*, 2004. **4**(3): p. 656–668.

16 O'Neill, E.E., *et al.* Towards complete analysis of the platelet proteome. *Proteomics*, 2002. **2**(3): p. 288–305.

17 Gnatenko, D.V. and W.F. Bahou. Recent advances in platelet transcriptomics. *Transfus Med Hemother*, 2006. p. 33.

18 Anderson, N.L., *et al.* The human plasma proteome: a nonredundant list developed by combination of four separate sources. *Mol Cell Proteomics*, 2004. **3**(4): p. 311–326.

19 McCullough, P.A. and N.E. Lepor. The deadly triangle of anemia, renal insufficiency, and cardiovascular disease: implications for prognosis and treatment. *Rev Cardiovasc Med*, 2005. **6**(1): p. 1–10.

20 Habib, R.H., *et al.* Role of hemodilutional anemia and transfusion during cardiopulmonary bypass in renal injury after coronary revascularization: implications on operative outcome. *Crit Care Med*, 2005. **33**(8): p. 1749–1756.

21 Ouellette, D.R. The impact of anemia in patients with respiratory failure. *Chest*, 2005. **128**(5, Suppl 2): p. 576S–582S.

22 Carson, J.L., *et al.* Severity of anaemia and operative mortality and morbidity. *Lancet*, 1988. **1**(8588): p. 727–729.

23 Wahr, J.A. Myocardial ischaemia in anaemic patients. *Br J Anaesth*, 1998. **81**(Suppl 1): p. 10–15.

24 Sehgal, L.R., *et al.* Evaluation of oxygen extraction ratio as a physiologic transfusion trigger in coronary artery bypass graft surgery patients. *Transfusion*, 2001. **41**(5): p. 591–595.

25 Engelfriet, C.P., *et al.* Perioperative triggers for red cell transfusions. *Vox Sang*, 2002. **82**(4): p. 215–226.

26 Yang, X., *et al.* The implications of blood transfusions for patients with non-ST-segment elevation acute coronary syndromes: results from the CRUSADE National Quality Improvement Initiative. *J Am Coll Cardiol*, 2005. **46**(8): p. 1490–1495.

27 Blair, S.D., *et al.* Effect of early blood transfusion on gastrointestinal haemorrhage. *Br J Surg*, 1986. **73**(10): p. 783–785.

28 Marik, P.E. and W.J. Sibbald. Effect of stored-blood transfusion on oxygen delivery in patients with sepsis. *JAMA*, 1993. **269**(23): p. 3024–3029.

29 Mazza, B.F., *et al.* Evaluation of blood transfusion effects on mixed venous oxygen saturation and lactate levels in patients with SIRS/sepsis. *Clinics*, 2005. **60**(4): p. 311–316.

30 Vamvakas, E.C. and J.H. Carven. Allogeneic blood transfusion, hospital charges, and length of hospitalization: a study of 487 consecutive patients undergoing colorectal cancer resection. *Arch Pathol Lab Med*, 1998. **122**(2): p. 145–151.

31 Silver, M.R. Anemia in the long-term ventilator-dependent patient with respiratory failure. *Chest*, 2005. **128**(5, Suppl 2): p. 568S–575S.

32 Schonhofer, B., H. Bohrer, and D. Kohler. Blood transfusion facilitating difficult weaning from the ventilator. *Anaesthesia*, 1998. **53**(2): p. 181–184.

33 Arslan, E., *et al.* Microcirculatory hemodynamics after acute blood loss followed by fresh and banked blood transfusion. *Am J Surg*, 2005. **190**(3): p. 456–462.

34 Dara, S.I., *et al.* Fresh frozen plasma transfusion in critically ill medical patients with coagulopathy. *Crit Care Med*, 2005. **33**(11): p. 2667–2671.

35 Slichter, S.J. Relationship between platelet count and bleeding risk in thrombocytopenic patients. *Transfus Med Rev*, 2004. **18**(3): p. 153–167.

36 Wandt, H., *et al.* A therapeutic platelet transfusion strategy is safe and feasible in patients after autologous peripheral blood stem cell transplantation. *Bone Marrow Transplant*, 2006. **37**(4): p. 387–392.

37 Greenburg, A.G. Benefits and risks of blood transfusion in surgical patients. *World J Surg*, 1996. **20**(9): p. 1189–1193.

38 Spiess, B.D. Blood transfusion: the silent epidemic. *Ann Thorac Surg*, 2001. **72**(5): p. S1832–S1837.

39 Fernandes, C.J., Jr., *et al.* Red blood cell transfusion does not increase oxygen consumption in critically ill septic patients. *Crit Care*, 2001. **5**(6): p. 362–367.

40 Blumberg, N. Deleterious clinical effects of transfusion immunomodulation: proven beyond a reasonable doubt. *Transfusion*, 2005. **45**(2, Suppl): p. 33S–39S; discussion 39S–40S.

41 Morris, C.D., *et al.* Prospective identification of risk factors for wound infection after lower extremity oncologic surgery. *Ann Surg Oncol*, 2003. **10**(7): p. 778–782.

42 Innerhofer, P., *et al.* Risk for postoperative infection after transfusion of white blood cell-filtered allogeneic or autologous blood components in orthopedic patients undergoing primary arthroplasty. *Transfusion*, 2005. **45**(1): p. 103–110.

43 Sauaia, A., *et al.* Autologous blood transfusion does not reduce postoperative infection rates in elective surgery. *Am J Surg*, 1999. **178**(6): p. 549–555.

44 Ikuta, S., *et al.* Allogeneic blood transfusion is an independent risk factor for infective complications after less invasive gastrointestinal surgery. *Am J Surg*, 2003. **185**(3): p. 188–193.

45 Banbury, M.K., *et al.* Transfusion increases the risk of postoperative infection after cardiovascular surgery. *J Am Coll Surg*, 2006. **202**(1): p. 131–138.

46 Hill, G.E., *et al.* Allogeneeic blood transfusion increases the risk of postoperative bacterial infection: a meta-analysis. *J Trauma*, 2003. **54**(5): p. 908–914.

47 Moore, F.A., E.E. Moore, and A. Sauaia. Blood transfusion. An independent risk factor for postinjury multiple organ failure. *Arch Surg*, 1997. **132**(6): p. 620–624; discussion 624–625.

48 Spiess, B.D., *et al.* Platelet transfusions during coronary artery bypass graft surgery are associated with serious adverse outcomes. *Transfusion*, 2004. **44**(8): p. 1143–1148.

49 Nosotti, M., *et al.* Correlation between perioperative blood transfusion and prognosis of patients subjected to surgery for stage I lung cancer. *Chest*, 2003. **124**(1): p. 102–107.

50 Murata, N., *et al.* Influence of perioperative blood transfusion on the prognosis of patients with gastric cancer receiving anticancer chemotherapy. *Gastric Cancer*, 2000. **3**(1): p. 24–27.

51 Santin, A.D., *et al.* Influence of allogeneic blood transfusion on clinical outcome during radiotherapy for cancer of the uterine cervix. *Gynecol Obstet Invest*, 2003. **56**(1): p. 28–34.

52 Yeh, C.Y., *et al.* Pelvic drainage and other risk factors for leakage after elective anterior resection in rectal cancer patients: a prospective study of 978 patients. *Ann Surg*, 2005. **241**(1): p. 9–13.

53 Okano, T., *et al.* Blood transfusions impair anastomotic wound healing, reduce luminol-dependent chemiluminescence, and increase interleukin-8. *Hepatogastroenterology*, 2001. **48**(42): p. 1669–1674.

54 Apostolidis, S.A., *et al.* Effect of ranitidine on healing of normal and transfusion-suppressed experimental anastomoses. *Tech Coloproctol*, 2004. **8**(Suppl 1): p. s104–s107.

55 Collard, K.J. Is there a causal relationship between the receipt of blood transfusions and the development of chronic lung disease of prematurity? *Med Hypotheses*, 2006. **66**(2): p. 355–364.

56 Hubler, A., *et al.* Does insulin-like growth factor 1 contribute in red blood cell transfusions to the pathogenesis of retinopathy of prematurity during retinal neovascularization? *Biol Neonate*, 2005. **89**(2): p. 92–98.

57 Collard, K.J., S. Godeck, and J.E. Holley. Blood transfusion and pulmonary lipid peroxidation in ventilated premature babies. *Pediatr Pulmonol*, 2005. **39**(3): p. 257–261.

58 Dempsey, E.M. and K.J. Barrington. Short and longterm outcomes following partial exchange transfusion in the polycythemic newborn: a systematic review. *Arch Dis Child Fetal Neonatal Ed*, September 20, 2005.

59 Yamada, S., *et al.* History of blood transfusion before 1990 is a risk factor for stroke and cardiovascular diseases: the Japan Collaborative Cohort Study (JACC Study). *Cerebrovasc Dis*, 2005. **20**(3): p. 164–171.

60 Yamada, S., *et al.* Risk factors for fatal subarachnoid hemorrhage: the Japan Collaborative Cohort Study. *Stroke*, 2003. **34**(12): p. 2781–2787.

61 Gorgun, E., *et al.* Fertility is reduced after restorative proctocolectomy with ileal pouch anal anastomosis: a study of 300 patients. *Surgery*, 2004. **136**(4): p. 795–803.

62 Abu-Rustum, N.R., *et al.* Transfusion utilization during adnexal or peritoneal cancer surgery: effects on symptomatic venous thromboembolism and survival. *Gynecol Oncol*, July 29, 2005.

63 Sabatine, M.S., *et al.* Association of hemoglobin levels with clinical outcomes in acute coronary syndromes. *Circulation*, 2005. **111**(16): p. 2042–2049.

64 Hebert, P.C., *et al.* A multicenter, randomized, controlled clinical trial of transfusion requirements in critical care. Transfusion requirements in critical care investigators, Canadian critical care trials group. *N Engl J Med*, 1999. **340**(6): p. 409–417.

65 Johnson, R.G., *et al.* Comparison of two transfusion strategies after elective operations for myocardial revascularization. *J Thorac Cardiovasc Surg*, 1992. **104**(2): p. 307–314.

66 Rao, S.V., *et al.* Relationship of blood transfusion and clinical outcomes in patients with acute coronary syndromes. *JAMA*, 2004. **292**(13): p. 1555–1562.

67 Tsai, A.G., p. Cabrales, and M. Intaglietta. Microvascular perfusion upon exchange transfusion with stored red blood cells in normovolemic anemic conditions. *Transfusion*, 2004. **44**(11): p. 1626–1634.

68 Engoren, M.C., *et al.* Effect of blood transfusion on longterm survival after cardiac operation. *Ann Thorac Surg*, 2002. **74**(4): p. 1180–1186.

69 Malone, D.L., *et al.* Blood transfusion, independent of shock severity, is associated with worse outcome in trauma. *J Trauma*, 2003. **54**(5): p. 898–905; discussion 905–907.

70 Stainsby D., *et al.* Summary of annual report: key observations and recommendations. 2001–2002. www.shotuk.org, 2003. Published 17th July.

71 Goodnough, L.T. Risks of blood transfusion. *Crit Care Med*, 2003. **31**(12, Suppl): p. S678–S686.

72 Sazama, K. Transfusion errors: scope of the problem, consequences, and solutions. *Curr Hematol Rep*, 2003. **2**(6): p. 518–521.

73 Brand, A. Immunological aspects of blood transfusions. *Transpl Immunol*, 2002. **10**(2–3): p. 183–190.

74 Silliman, C.C., D.R. Ambruso, and L.K. Boshkov. Transfusion-related acute lung injury. *Blood*, 2005. **105**(6): p. 2266–2273.

75 Janatpour, K. and P.V. Holland. Noninfectious serious hazards of transfusion. *Curr Hematol Rep*, 2002. **1**(2): p. 149–155.

76 Nusbacher, J. Blood transfusion is mononuclear cell transplantation. *Transfusion*, 1994. **34**(11): p. 1002–1006.

77 Vietor, H.E., *et al.* Survival of donor cells 25 years after intrauterine transfusion. *Blood*, 2000. **95**(8): p. 2709–2714.

78 Dzik, W.H. Microchimerism after transfusion: the spectrum from GVHD to alloimmunization. *Transfus Sci*, 1995. **16**(2): p. 107–108.

79 Lee, T.H., *et al.* Survival of donor leukocyte subpopulations in immunocompetent transfusion recipients: frequent long-term microchimerism in severe trauma patients. *Blood*, 1999. **93**(9): p. 3127–3139.

80 Lee, T.H., *et al.* High-level long-term white blood cell microchimerism after transfusion of leukoreduced blood components to patients resuscitated after severe traumatic injury. *Transfusion*, 2005. **45**(8): p. 1280–1290.

81 Langenfeld, J.E., *et al.* Correlation between red blood cell deformability and changes in hemodynamic function. *Surgery*, 1994. **116**(5): p. 859–867.

82 Innerhofer P, *et al.* Immunomodulation mechanisms following transfusion of allogeneic and autologous erythrocyte concentrates. *Infus Ther Transfus Med*, 2002. **29**: p. 118–121.

83 Nielsen, H.J., Influence on the immune system of homologous blood transfusion and autologous blood donation: impact on the routine clinical practice/differences in oncological and non-tumour surgery? *Anasthesiol Intensivmed Notfallmed Schmerzther*, 2000. **35**(10): p. 642–645.

84 Calder L, *et al.* Review of published recommendations and guidelines for the transfusion of allogeneic red blood cells and plasma. *CMAJ*, 1997. **156**(11, Suppl 1): p. S1–S8.

85 National Kidney Foundation. K/DOQI clinical practice guidelines for anemia of chronic kidney disease. *Am J Kidney Dis*, 2001. **37**: p. S182–S238.

86 British Committee for Standards in Haematology, Blood Transfusion Task Force, Murphy, M.F., *et al.* Guidelines for the use of platelet transfusions. *Br J Haematol*, 2003. **122**: p. 10–23.

87 Schiffer, C.A., *et al.* Platelet transfusion for patients with cancer: clinical practice guidelines of the American Society of Clinical Oncology. *J Clin Oncol*, 2001. **19**(5): p. 1519–1538.

88 Bishton, M. and R. Chopra. The role of granulocyte transfusions in neutropenic patients. *Br J Haematol*, 2004. **127**(5): p. 501–508.

89 Gibson, B.E., *et al.* Transfusion guidelines for neonates and older children. *Br J Haematol*, 2004. **124**(4): p. 433–453.

90 British Committee for Standards in Haematology, Duguid, .J. *et al. Guidelines for the Use of Fresh Frozen Plasma, Cryoprecipitate and Cryosupernatant.* British Committee for Standards in Haematology, 2004.

91 Chuansumrit, A. Treatment of haemophilia in the developing countries. *Haemophilia*, 2003. **9**(4): p. 387–390.

92 British Committee for Standards in Haematology, B.T.T.F. Guideline on the clinical use of leucocyte-depleted blood components. *Transfus Med*, 1998. **8**: p. 59–71.

19 Transfusions. Part II: plasma fractions

If a patient presents with a certain lack of a plasmatic factor, all that is needed is to replenish the missing factor, if even that. The preferred therapy is to take care of the isolated deficiency, either by nonblood therapies or by the use of plasma fractions.

This chapter will introduce you to available plasma fractions and will explain how to use them.

Objectives of this chapter

1 List medical therapeutics fractionated from plasma.
2 Describe the indications for commonly used plasma fractions.
3 Explain basic rules why some plasma fractions are used for a certain indication and others not.
4 Learn about asanguinous therapeutic options for the indications that typically call for therapy with plasma fractions.

Definitions

Plasma fraction: A more or less pure extract of human or animal blood plasma, rich in a certain plasma component. The term fractionation refers to the process of separating plasma into its components.

Orphan drug: Is a term coined by the legislation to describe a product that treats a rare disease (e.g., affecting <200,000 Americans). In the United States, an Orphan Drug Act was signed into law in 1983 in order to support drugs that otherwise would not receive the necessary attention by industry. Grants and other monetary incentives support companies devoting themselves to work with orphan drugs, aiming at stimulating research, development, and approval of such products. Some plasma fractions are orphan drugs.

A brief look at history

Whole blood has been used in the transfusion therapy of early times. Blood divided into its main components was later used as a means to expand scarce resource blood. Dividing blood into cells and plasma was rather easy, since even simple blood sedimentation could be used to produce concentrates of cellular blood components and plasma. Fractionation, a process used to further divide human plasma into its components, started its way into blood banking in the late 1940s with the advent of Cohn's fractionation [1]. In the first decades, albumin was the main protein produced by Cohn's fractionation. Later, byproducts of plasma fractionation were increasingly used. Using certain fractions rather than whole blood helped to target transfusion therapy to medical problems secondary to a specific factor deficiency.

A vivid example of a clinical problem the therapy of which benefited from the ever more sophisticated fractionation is hemophilia A. Once treated with whole blood and later with plasma, hemophilia A can now be treated with a plasma fraction containing mainly the missing factor VIII. Already in the 1950s, a crude plasma fraction containing factor VIII as well as fibrinogen and many other compounds was used. However, the large volume needed to be transfused caused volume overload. Another plasma fraction, now known as cryoprecipitate, was used thereafter. During the 1970s, the process of plasma fractionation was further refined, so that fractions with improved potency of factor VIII were available. The first commercially available factor concentrate was introduced in the United States and marketed in 1968 under the trade name Hemofil. This was a derivative made from cryoprecipitate and was rich in factor VIII. Although bringing positive clinical results, pathogens were shown to be transmitted to the patients. Virtually every hemophiliac treated with such antihemophiliac preparations was infected with various kinds of hepatitis [2]. However, in comparison to the effects of untreated hemophilia, hepatitis was considered a minor problem [3]. The situation changed as in the early 1980s HIV was found in antihemophiliac preparations. Half of all hemophiliacs treated with plasma-derived products contracted the human immunodeficiency virus. Therefore, methods to virus-inactivate or eliminate plasmatic fractions were developed. Among them was chromatography. This method enabled the blood industry to purify crude plasma fractions into more specific components. Using this method, high- and ultrahigh-purity factor concentrates of factor VIII were brought on the market. Nowadays, recombinant factor concentrates developed in parallel to the plasma-derived products are often favored over blood products [2, 3].

Apart from the fractionation of factor VIII, many other fractions have been produced. In addition to the initially produced albumin, cryoprecipitate became available in the 1970s. Later, prothrombin complex concentrates were also produced. By the end of the 1970s and the beginning of the 1980s, intravenous immunoglobulin was fractioned, which was used primarily for the treatment of congenital immunodeficiencies. However, over time, additional indications of intravenous immunoglobulins were explored [4]. Some of the factor concentrates produced became en vogue for a time and were abandoned thereafter. Either their side effects were considered too severe, or better products became available. For example, in some countries, cryoprecipitate has been abandoned in favor of fibrinogen and other factor concentrates. Other countries still use cryoprecipitate and this may be the only low-volume factor concentrate available for therapy. The trend is to use a concentrate of only the missing factor, being produced either in recombinant fashion or sourced from plasma, rather than crude products like fresh frozen plasma (FFP) or cryoprecipitate.

The anatomy of plasma

About 120 different proteins have so far been detected in plasma and described. Many more have been found in proteomic and other analyses and await their identification. The major portion of plasma proteins totaling 60 g/L, is made up of albumin (30–40 g), immunoglobulins (8–17 g), fibrinogen (2.5–3.5 g), transferrin (2–3 g), α1-proteinase inhibitor (1.5–2 g), and α2-macroglobulin (1.3–2 g). Most other plasma constituents are found only in trace amounts in the plasma (compare

Table Appendix A.3). But plasma is not a fluid with a limited number of distinct compounds. Rather, plasma is a unique fluid with a changing mix of ingredients. Its constitution differs from individual to individual. There are virtually hundreds of compounds that are regularly found in plasma (coagulation factors, albumin, coeruloplasmin, etc.). Additionally, there are

- compounds that are only found during certain periods in life (such as during pregnancy),
- compounds that differ with the individual (such as blood group antibodies),
- compounds that are found in plasma depending on the life-style of the individual (parts of his diet, drugs he took),
- compounds that are just transported by the plasma (hormones, etc.),
- compounds that show past diseases (such as antibodies to whatever came the way of the individual),
- compounds that are produced as the result of a current disease (cancer cells, acute phase proteins, etc.),
- compounds that are on their way to be excreted (debris, cellular remains, bilirubin, etc.),
- infectious agents (such as viruses, bacteria, prions, fungi, and other parasites),
- many other compounds not yet identified.

It is obvious how difficult it is to fractionate this mix of thousands of compounds that are only partially identified, not known at all, and that differ with every single donor. It is (nearly) impossible to do so. Therefore, keep in mind that whatever plasma fraction is used for therapy, the product is only vaguely defined. Apart from the proteins declared on the label of the product, the product consists of other, undeclared plasmatic components. Once in a while, new ingredients are found in the concentrates, with no exact knowledge as to their clinical significance [5].

Plasma fractions

Plasma fractions that are therapeutically used are usually proteins with enzymatic or transport activity. For those fractions with enzymatic activity, a series of terms have been used to describe their properties. Before starting to consider the different fractions, we would like to review important concepts needed to understand the fractions.

The need for factor replacement is determined by the lack of at least one essential plasmatic factor. Diagnosis of factor deficiency is made by measuring the activity level of a (coagulation) factor in the plasma. It is given as the

Table 19.1 Characteristics of coagulation factors needed to calculate dose regimen.

Factor	Molecular weight	Recovery (%)	Through level (below which abnormal surgical bleeding may occur)	$t \frac{1}{2}$ (h)
vWF	240–270,000	80–100	40	72
I (Fibrinogen)	340–320,000	80–100	25–30	75
II	70–72,000	50–60	40	60
V	330–350,000	80–100	15–20	12
VII	50,000	30–50	10	6
VIII	285–300,000	70–100	25–30	8–19
IX	52–55,000	30–50	25–30	11–27
X	55–59,000	30–50	15–20	50
XI	143–160,000	80–100	30	50–60
XIII	320,000	80–100	5	250

amount of clotting factor in the plasma of the patient when compared with normal plasma. The clotting factor levels in the plasma (= specific activity, potency) or in a concentrate are measured in international units (IU). One unit activity is the amount of factor present in 1 mL of normal plasma.

An important property of plasma fractions is their *purity*. The purity of a plasmatic fraction describes how much protein is present in addition to the factor needed for the therapeutic action. It relates the total number of units of the desired protein per milligram of total protein. Purity has nothing to do with the degree of contamination. A low purity concentrate is only a crude part of plasma that contains the needed factor or group of factors in a higher concentration than plasma. The purity is usually below 1 U/mg total protein. Intermediate purity concentrates have a purity of about 1–10 U/mg and a high-purity concentrate about 50–150 U/mg. An ultra-high (= very high) purity concentrate is intended to be virtually free of proteins other than the desired factor and has a purity of more than 2000 U/mg. Such concentrates are produced by affinity chromatography or monoclonal antibody techniques. They contain 2000–4000 U/mg of protein. However, ultra-high purity concentrates are not stabile and require stabilizers such as albumin. Adding albumin lowers the concentration of protein per milligram of the final concentrate and thereby their purity.

When factor concentrates are infused, not all infused factor protein is found in the plasma immediately after transfusion. How much actually is found is called *intravascular or biologic recovery*. The recovery means the percentage of a plasmatic factor found in the vessels immediately after infusion. Recovery is determined by the

distribution space of the body. The more plasma volume per body weight, the less is the recovery of a factor. Small plasmatic factors distribute not only in the intravascular space, but also extravascular. Therefore, they have a lower recovery than factors that remain mostly in the vessels. The recovery is also determined by the presence or absence of antibodies against the infused factor. When such are present, the recovery is lowered. Table 19.1 displays the average recoveries of coagulation factor products.

The recovery of a plasmatic factor differs with the individual, but is relatively stable over time. However, individual recoveries can also change, depending on the development of antibodies to the factor or an increased use. The latter is true, for instance, when a clotting factor is constantly used in the presence of activated coagulation. To determine the individual recovery, a *survival study* is performed. A determined dose of a factor is administered and serial phlebotomies over about 24 hours determine the changing factor levels. Survival studies are often performed prior to an elective surgical procedure or as the initial work-up of a patient scheduled for prophylactic factor therapy. Based on the results of a survival study, an appropriate dose regimen for the patient can be developed.

The dose of the plasmatic factor is determined by the residual activity of the patient, the clinical condition of the patient (symptoms present, not present, or likely to develop due to given circumstances), the factor's half-life, and the mode of administration (Table 19.1). Most therapy regimen set a minimum level of factor activity that must not be fallen short of. This minimum level is called through (level).

When a need for a plasmatic factor is established, a therapy regimen must be chosen. Sometimes it is possible to provide the factor continuously, sometimes as bolus injections. Plasmatic factors have been injected intravenously, subcutaneously, or intramuscularly. Not every route of administration works for all kinds of factors and for all situations.

Depending on the factor needed, prophylactic as well as therapeutic regimens may be indicated. In the case of coagulation factors, primary prophylaxis starts at an early age, as soon as it is seen that a patient bleeds recurrently, but before joint bleeding occurs. Secondary prophylaxis starts when a patient already had recurrent bleeding in a joint.

Coagulation factors

Coagulation, the act of blood clotting at the site of injury, is a vital mechanism to prevent fatal hemorrhage. Hemostasis is achieved when a group of plasmatic coagulation factors, cells, and cellular components interact in a preset way. When important players in this interaction are missing, coagulation may be impaired and spontaneous or exaggerated traumatic bleeding may occur. The therapy of missing coagulation factors includes supplementation by infusion of factor concentrates, either produced in a recombinant fashion or made from donor blood. A variety of different coagulation factor concentrates have been developed.

Factor mixes

CRYOPRECIPITATE

Cryoprecipitate consists of a mix of proteins, collectively called cryoglobulins. It is a compound that precipitates when FFP is thawed at 4°C. Factor VIII, factor XIII, von Willebrand's factor (vWF), fibrinogen, and fibronectin are the main constituents of cryoprecipitate [6].

Cryoprecipitate is very similar to FFP. In contrast to most other factor concentrates, it is not virus-attenuated. The risk of transmitting a virus to the patient is therefore higher in cryoprecipitate than in other factor concentrates.

The use of cryoprecipitate was recommended in 1996 by the Task force of the American Society of Anesthesiologists [7] for patients with von Willebrand's disease (vWD), unresponsive to desmopressin or bleeding, and for bleeding patients with fibrinogen levels below 80–100 mg/dL. Today, cryoprecipitate is used to substitute fibrinogen, either as therapy for congenital deficiency, dysfibrinogenemia, or for acquired hypofibrinogenemia such as develops in disseminated intravascular coagulation or thrombolysis. Cryoprecipitate is also used to treat some rare factor deficiencies, e.g., factor XIII. Deficiencies of factor VIII or vWF are not usually treated with cryoprecipitate any more, since, although theoretically effective, better, and safer alternatives exist [6]. Cryoprecipitate may not be available any more in countries where purer and safer factor concentrates for treatment of the above-mentioned factor deficiencies exist.

PROTHROMBIN COMPLEX CONCENTRATE

There are two types of prothrombin complex concentrates (PCC): one with "four" factors and other with "three." The "four" factor PCC contains mainly vitamin K-dependent coagulation factors (II, VII, IX, X, proteins S and C). Factor VII is missing in the "three" factor PCC. PPSB, another name for PCC, can serve as a mnemonic standing for the main ingredients of PCC, namely, prothrombin (FII), proconvertin (FVII), Stewart Prower Factor (FX), and antihemophiliac B factor (FIX). Ideally, the factors II, VII, IX, and X should be evenly distributed in a ratio of 1:1:1:1, and the proteins S and C should be present in about 1 U per 1 unit factor IX. Apart from the mentioned compounds, there are many other proteins in PCC, some of them as yet undefined. Among them are ceruloplasmin, inter-α-trypsin inhibitor (ITI), kininogen, vitronectin, and protein Z [8].

A major problem of PCCs is their thrombogenicity and their ability to trigger allergic reactions. PCC therapy has been associated with myocardial infarction and disseminated intravasal coagulation. Activated coagulation factors have been attributed such effects.

A "three-factor PCC," also called a low-purity factor IX product, was once the favored therapy for hemophilia B. Its use has been abandoned in favor of highly purified FIX concentrates. The thromboembolic complications of PCC can so be avoided.

The "four-factor" PCC is still in use. Since it contains all vitamin K-dependent factors it can be used for indications that call for replacement of those proteins: vitamin K antagonist overdose [9], severe coagulopathy in liver disease [10], and replacement of proteins C and S. Also, rare deficiencies of factors II, VII, or X [11] can be treated with PCC, as well as patients with hemophilia A or B who developed inhibitors.

The coagulation factors in PCCs can also be activated, so that the concentrate is called activated prothrombin complex concentrates (aPCC). It is thought that hemophiliacs who have an inhibitor against the missing factor can be treated with aPCC. The defect in the coagulation process is thought to be thereby circumvented [10]. A concentrate called FEIBA (Factor Eight Inhibitor Bypassing Activity) also belongs to the aPCCs.

"Single" factor concentrates

Technically, it is possible to fractionate most clotting factors from plasma. Additional production steps reduce a certain amount of other compounds found in the fraction. However, it is not possible to provide a plasma-derived product containing solely the needed factor. Therefore, the term "single" factor concentrate is misleading.

FACTOR VIII CONCENTRATE

The plasmatic coagulation factor VIII is a small molecule. It consists of A-, B-, and C-domains. When activated, it loses most of the B-domain. The small factor FVIII:C circulates in blood bound non-covalently to the big vWF molecule. The vWF carries and protects the FVIII:C molecule and targets it to the site of injury. When the protecting influence of vWF is missing, the half-life of FVIII is reduced from 8 hours to about 8 minutes. Factor VIII is synthesized in the liver and the endothelium, while vWF is synthesized in megakaryocytes and the endothelium as well. The activated factor VIII activates factor IX and together with factor IX, activates factor X.

FVIII concentrates come in different purity levels. Intermediate purity FVIII concentrates are prepared by precipitation. Their specific activity ranges from 2 to 5 U/mg protein. Such concentrates contain not only FVIII but also vWF and can therefore be used as treatment for hemophilia A and vWD. Other purification steps of FVIII yield a product with a specific activity of 15–150 U/mg protein. Such concentrates do not contain relevant amounts of vWF. High and ultra-high purity FVIII concentrates made by chromatographic methods do not contain vWF at all. Such factor concentrates contain 2000–3000 U/mg protein. However, albumin is added and the specific activity is so reduced to 10 U/mg protein.

Factor VIII concentrates can also be made from animal plasma, usually of porcine or bovine origin (made from pigs or cows, respectively). However, the products can cause slight to severe thrombocytopenia and the production of such factor concentrates was discontinued in some countries [12].

VON WILLEBRAND FACTOR CONCENTRATES

vWF is a mix of multimeric plasma glycoproteins with molecular weights ranging from 40,000 to 20,000,000. It facilitates the platelet adhesion to the vessel wall by anchoring the platelet to the subendothelium. Besides, vWF is a cofactor of FVIII. When vWF is lacking or defective, patients develop vWD.

Patients with severe vWD not responding to desmopressin or other pharmacological therapies are usually treated with factor VIII concentrates containing relevant amounts of vWF. Attempts have been made to produce concentrates that contain mainly vWF with only small amounts of factor VIII [13]. Such concentrates are available in some countries.

FACTOR IX CONCENTRATES

Factor IX is a naturally occurring vitamin K-dependent coagulation factor and acts as a serine protease. Factor IX can be activated either by factor XI or by a complex of tissue factor and factor VIIa. In the activated form, factor IX activates factor X.

Factor IX concentrates for the therapy of hemophilia B are available in different purities, ranging from low (= PCC) to very high purity. Modern chromatographic purification methods have led to a product that does not have the thrombogenicity of early days. But prolonged infusion of FIX has been associated with thromboembolic complications.

FIBRINOGEN

Fibrinogen is a protein which is synthesized in the liver. When thrombin proteolytically cleaves fibrinogen, fibrin develops. Fibrinogen is therefore the precursor of fibrin. When it is lacking or defective, thrombi can not be formed properly and coagulation is impaired.

Human fibrinogen concentrates are available in some countries [14]. It may also contain residues of fibronectin and other proteins.

Formerly, the therapy of hypo-, dys-, or afibrinogenemia was cryoprecipitate or FFP. It is still used in some countries. Where fibrinogen concentrates are available, they are preferred. Therefore, afibrinogenemia or dysfibrinogenemia [15] as well as other conditions leading to low fibrinogen levels, e.g., DIC, are indications for fibrinogen concentrates. Fibrinogen concentrates may also be effective to overcome the coagulopathy developing after infusion of certain starch solutions [16].

FACTOR XIII

Factor XIII is a plasma transglutaminase. In its form as a proenzyme, it is activated by thrombin. Factor XIII enhances hemostasis, wound healing, and plays an important role in pregnancy by preventing decidual bleeding.

Formerly, factor XIII concentrates have been produced from human placentas. Today, commercially available concentrates are fractionated from human plasma. Factor XIII is used to substitute a congenital deficiency of this factor. Furthermore, it has been used to treat badly healing wounds, problems with collagen synthesis, and vessel leakage. Factor XIII concentrates are also used to prevent miscarriages and perinatal bleeding in pregnant women with factor XIII deficiencies. The recommended level for pregnant women is 3–10% during pregnancy and during labor, 20–30% of factor activity are recommended to prevent perinatal bleeding [17].

FACTOR XI, PROTHROMBIN, THROMBIN, FACTOR X, FACTOR VII

Factor XI is a vitamin K-dependent serine protease whose activated form activates factor IX (along with FVIII). A congenital deficiency has been described with increased prevalence in Ashkenazic Jews (∼4%). Even if severe, the deficiency may be clinically asymptomatic until the patient is challenged by surgical trauma. In this event, a factor concentrate may be beneficial. In some countries, virally inactivated factor XI concentrates are available for treatment [18].

Apart from thrombin which is used for surgical glues, other coagulation factors are usually not purified on an industrial scale. However, it is possible, and can be performed on the basis of the Orphan Drug Act in the United States [8]. In some European countries, coagulation factor concentrates of factors X and VII are readily available.

Anticoagulation factors and other therapeutically used plasma fractions

ANTITHROMBIN III

Antithrombin III is probably the most important antithrombin of the four originally found antithrombins. It is synthesized in the liver. Antithrombin III is a serine proteinase inhibitor and acts as an anticoagulant by directly binding and inactivating the serine proteases, above all thrombin, but also factors XIa, Ixa, and Xa. In the absence of heparin, the serine proteinase activity proceeds slowly. When heparin is present, the activity of Antithrombin III is increased 10–10,000 times. Antithrombin III possesses not only anticoagulative, but also anti-inflammatory effects.

Antithrombin III deficiency is either congenital or acquired. Patients with hereditary antithrombin III deficiency have an increased risk of thrombosis. This risk is especially high when other risk factors for thromboembolism occur, such as pregnancy and surgery. Acquired deficiency of antithrombin III develops when its production is impaired (protein catabolism is reduced, liver disease), when antithrombin III is lost (in nephrotic syndrome), or when antithrombin III is consumed (DIC, thrombosis). Septic or otherwise critically ill patients may also have low antithrombin III levels.

Antithrombin III is available as plasma-derived concentrate. They have a reported incidence of side effects of about 3%. The effects include chest tightness, dizziness, abdominal cramps, fever, and shortness of breath. All side effects were regarded as mild.

Antithrombin III concentrates are used for patients with the hereditary antithrombin deficiency or with abnormal antithrombin. However, oral anticoagulation therapy is the first-line treatment and should be used whenever possible. In situations with additional thrombotic risk factors, antithrombin III concentrates are the recommended therapy in addition to heparin. Sometimes, antithrombin III is also given without concurrent thromboembolic risk factors [19].

In acquired antithrombin III deficiency, a low antithrombin III level is associated with worse outcome in critically ill patients. Whether or not the correction of subnormal antithrombin concentrates to normal or supranormal levels in critically ill patients actually improves the outcome remains to be seen. To date, the literature shows contradictory results [20–22]. Nevertheless, in some regions of the world, AT III is still widely used [23] for indications not proven.

PROTEIN C

Protein C is a vitamin K-dependent factor structurally similar to other coagulation factors. It prevents the formation of blood clots by inactivating factors Va and VIIIa. Protein C needs calcium, a phospholipid surface, and protein S to cleave its target factors.

When protein C is lacking, different causes may have led to it. Protein C deficiency may be inherited or acquired [24]. A homozygous deficiency with factor levels below 1% is lethal, unless appropriate therapy is administered. Already in the neonatal period, the deficiency of protein C presents with purpura fulminans, DIC, and thrombosis [25]. Heterozygous forms of protein C deficiency often do not lead to thrombosis. The clinical relevance of the heterozygous form is therefore still a subject of debate. Apart from the inherited form of protein C deficiency, there are acquired forms of the deficiency. Low levels of protein C have been observed in DIC, after surgery, in tumor patients, in sepsis, and when protein C cannot be synthesized properly (vitamin K deficiency, liver disease).

Protein C is available as a plasma-derived concentrate. It has a recovery of about 44% and a half-life of 4–8 hours. Protein C is also available as recombinant product.

Inherited protein C deficiency can be treated with heparin, oral anticoagulants, or factor substitutes [26]. For many years, homozygous protein C deficient patients have been treated with FFP or prothrombin complex concentrates to replace protein C. Today, they are treated with protein C concentrates. It may also be possible to treat them with coumadin, low-molecular-weight heparin, steroids, or liver transplantation [24]. Patients with heterozygous deficiency are preferably treated with anticoagulation. Probably, factor substitution may be beneficial for these patients as well, especially in the presence of additional thrombotic risk factors. However, since there are only a few patients with protein C deficiency, large-scale clinical trials are not possible. The therapy of protein C deficiency is therefore not scientifically proven and rather based on case reports and small case series.

Patients with acquired protein C deficiency are sometimes also treated with activated protein C. It shows some promise in the therapy of severe sepsis [27].

PROTEIN S

Protein S is a cofactor of protein C and inactivates factors Va and VIIIa. In blood, protein S circulates either free or bound to the complementary system protein C4. Protein S may be lacking, either secondary to an inherited disorder or as an acquired disorder (after starting vitamin K antagonist therapy, in liver disease, in pregnancy, when consumed in cases of DIC or thrombosis). When protein S is lacking, phlebothrombosis and pulmonary embolisms may develop. In a neonate with homozygous protein S deficiency, purpura fulminans has been described. The therapy is a vitamin K antagonist or heparin to prevent clotting.

C1-ESTERASE INHIBITOR

The C1-esterase inhibitor is the most important factor regulating the classical pathway of complementary system activation. Patients lacking C1-esterase inhibitor have an increased activation of the complementary system. This results in a condition called hereditary angioneurotic edema (Quincke's disease). Sometimes triggered by trauma or infection, the patients develop symptoms such as abdominal pain and attacks of swollen tissues with swelling of the larynx compromising breathing. The treatment and prophylaxis options include antihistamines, androgens, tranexamic acid, and some newer agents (kallikrein inhibitor, bradykinin B2 receptor antagonist). Formerly, FFP or solvent-/detergent-treated plasma have been administered in acute attacks of angioneurotic edema. Nowadays, a recombinant product and a plasmatic concentrate rich in C1-esterase inhibitor are the treatment options of choice in severe angioneurotic edema [28]. The choice of treatment depends on the severity of the condition, the site of swelling, and the response to treatment [29, 30].

α1-PROTEINASE INHIBITOR ($=$ α1-ANTITRYPSINE)

Alfa1-antitrypsine is a glycoprotein. It inhibits serin proteinases such as trypsin, thrombin, and renin. Clinically important is its inhibition of the elastase of neutrophils. When a congenital defect of α1-antitrypsine expression is present, tissue, especially in the lung, liver, and skin, are damaged by the uninhibited action of neutrophils and emphysema occurs. Plasma-derived α1-antitrypsine concentrates are available. Experiments with them will demonstrate whether the therapy benefits patients with a deficiency of α1-antitrypsine.

HUMAN ALBUMIN

Albumin is the blood protein with the greatest mass in plasma. About 2/3 of all plasma protein is albumin. Albumin is produced in the liver. It transports many compounds, e.g., products of hemoglobin degradation, metal ions, NO, and drugs. It renders toxins harmless while transporting them to their point of detoxification or excretion. It has a strong antioxidant activity in the serum [31]. Besides, albumin maintains the colloid-osmotic pressure of the plasma.

Concentrates of human albumin are available for therapy. More than 95% of the protein in the albumin concentrate is albumin. The remaining 5% consists of aggregates of prekallikrein activator, heme, aluminium, potassium, sodium, and other compounds. For therapeutic use, albumin is available in 4 or 5% solutions and in 20–25% solutions.

Albumin has anticoagulative properties. It may support the development of edema when albumin leaves the vessels due to capillary leakage. Hypervolemia with pulmonary edema may result secondary to albumin therapy. Besides, sodium and water excretion may be reduced after albumin infusion. Other side effects of albumin infusions include viral transmission, allergic reactions, and fever. Occasionally, hypotension occurs. This was attributed to bradykinin and other compounds present in the concentrate. Although the levels of bradykinin have been reduced in recent years, patients who are on ACE inhibitors and who therefore have an altered bradykinin metabolism may still react with hypotension to albumin infusions. Another argument against human albumin therapy is the costs. Albumin is very expensive in comparison to other volume expanders.

Albumin has been advocated as the ideal volume replacement. But the use of albumin is highly debated. Opponents of albumin therapy mention a condition called analbuminemia. It is characterized by the complete absence of albumin right from birth. Such patients are able to live with almost no ill effects, but have a low blood pressure and tend to have edema. Obviously, life without albumin is possible. Besides, the use of albumin is not only expensive, but also carries risks that do not outweigh the benefits of the albumin substitution. Human albumin seems to promote invasive fungal infections in critically ill patients [32] and may therefore be detrimental to the patient's condition.

Formerly, human albumin was used for parenteral nutrition. This indication for albumin therapy is now obsolete, along with many other indications that were proposed over time. However, albumin is still widely used, although there is often no sound reason to do so. Hypovolemia is probably the most frequently cited indication for albumin. Nevertheless, there is no proof that human albumin is superior to synthetic crystalloids or colloids for this indication. Human albumin can also be used for therapeutic plasma exchange [33], although synthetic colloids may be at least equally effective. Burn centers often use albumin for the first 24 hours after burn injury. They claim that edema can be mobilized more rapidly with albumin. Also, hypalbuminemia in patients who have more than 30–50% of their body surface burned is often treated with albumin. However, multiple organ dysfunction cannot be prevented by using albumin instead of crystalloid solutions to resuscitate burn patients [34]. Hypalbuminemia due to other causes, such as kidney and liver diseases, does not warrant albumin therapy. Under most circumstances, diuretics are sufficient to treat the complications of hypalbuminemia. When ascites needs to be drained, patients may react with hypovolemia. This can be treated with synthetic colloids and does not need albumin therapy. Neurologists sometimes also find albumin helpful. Vasospasms after subarachnoid hemorrhage and cerebral edema or ischemia are treated with hemodilution. Such hemodilution does not need albumin to be performed. Other suitable, nonblood-derived fluids do as well. In the pediatric setting, albumin is sometimes recommended. But also in this setting, albumin is not indicated. Albumin has been used as an adjunct to the therapy of Morbus hemolyticus neonatorum or other causes of hyperbilirubinemia. It binds bilirubin and thus reduces the likelihood of kernicterus. Other therapies of neonatal hyperbilirubinemia are available and albumin in this setting should be obsolete.

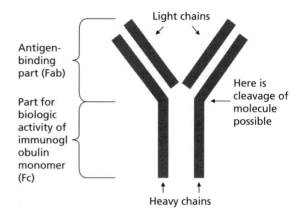

Fig 19.1 Immunoglobulin monomer.

All in all, although there is still a widespread use of human albumin solutions, there is hardly a proven indication for its use. In fact, there seems to be no advantage of albumin over synthetic colloids or crystalloids.

IMMUNOGLOBULINS

Immunoglobulins are a group of heterogenous molecules made up of a various number of immunoglobulin monomers. The latter look like a Y with its arms being the Fab parts and the leg being the Fc part (Fig. 19.1). In the blood, different classes of immunoglobulins are present, namely G, M, and A (IgG, IgM, IgA). IgG is the main immunoglobulin in human serum. It binds bacterial and viral antigens and antibodies and induces their phagocytosis. IgG increases the synthesis of leukocytes and regulates mediators of inflammation. IgM increases the phagocytosis of bacteria and viruses, neutralizes toxins, inactivates autoantibodies, and regulates the complementary system. Since IgM is a pentamer or hexamer (consisting of 5–6 immunoglobulin monomers), it makes up big agglutinates that are easily recognized by phagocytes (opsonization). Compared to IgG, IgM is much stronger as regards its ability to immobilize bacteria. IgA binds toxins, activates the complementary system, and modulates the inflammatory response as well.

In vivo, immunoglobulins have a variety of functions as part of the immune system. They are able to scavenge bacteria, viruses, and other infectious agents, as well as their toxins. They mediate cellular responses that lead to the destruction and elimination of the invaders. Besides, immunoglobulins play an important role in balancing the immune system. They can activate players in the immune system, such as macrophages and granulocytes. They can also inactivate parts of it, affecting the activation and effector functions of T and B cells, inhibit the release of proinflammatory factors and scavenge cytokines. Autoantibodies can be regulated as well. With this knowledge, it seemed prudent to use immunoglobulins when the patient's own immunoglobulin synthesis is insufficient (neonates, primary immune deficiency), or when a patient suffers an infection or an autoimmune diseases.

A vast variety of human plasma-derived immunoglobulin concentrates are on the market. They can be divided into two main groups: normal immunoglobulins and hyperimmunoglobulins. Normal immunoglobulins are a concentrate of one or more classes of immunoglobulins collected from a pool of the general donor population. They are made from at least 1000 donor plasmas and contain the whole spectrum of antibodies developed in this population, those against infectious agents and their toxins, as well as those directed against self (autoantibodies). Hyperimmunoglobulins are made from plasmas of selected donors who have been immunized against a certain antigen. However, it is not mandatory that hyperimmunoglobulins actually have a higher than normal titer of the required antibody.

A major problem of the preparation of plasma-derived immunoglobulin concentrates is that they have to remain in a form enabling them to react with their antigen. The purification process activates them, and aggregates form. The aggregates are mainly irreversible, leave the immunoglobulins without the ability to bind their antigen, and can activate the complementary system. This may contribute to the side effects of immunoglobulin therapy. The standardization of immunoglobulins is difficult. It has been ruled that at least 95% of the protein in an immunoglobulin concentrate must be immunoglobulins (unless albumin is added). There exist major differences between the products of the manufacturers and between batches. It is desirable that the manufacturers of immunoglobulin solutions provide information about the actual content of the immunoglobulin concentrate. Information about their IgA content, the titer of certain clinically relevant antibodies, etc. may be beneficial to decide which immunoglobulin product is suitable for the specific patient under consideration [4]. Besides, information about the production process (the form of fractionation and purification, and addition of stabilizers) would be beneficial since all these processes change the immunoglobulin concentrate [35].

Immunoglobulin concentrates can be administered subcutaneously, intravenously, intrathecally, or intramuscularly. Formulations for "intramuscular only" use are crude, not purified, contain many aggregates, and cannot be given intravenously, since the contaminants may elicit unwanted responses. The half-life of intravenously administered immunoglobulins is 3–5 weeks.

Immunoglobulin solutions are generally safe. But there is a residual risk of transmission of a disease, with newly emerging viruses contributing to this risk [36]. The literature abounds with reports of hepatitis B transmission through immunoglobulin therapy, and some reports were made about hepatitis C. The risk of hepatitis transmission has been reduced by newer methods of production and virus inactivation. Nowadays, acute side effects of intravenous immunoglobulins are more common than viral transmission. About 5% of patients treated with immunoglobulins experience relevant side effects. Stabilizers, such as sucrose, have been accused of partially causing those side effects [37]. Minor side effects such as malaise, rash, fever, flu-like pains, and minor allergic reactions usually resolve after several days [38]. Major side effects, although rare, can end fatally and include anaphylactic reactions, arthritis, aseptic meningitis, irreversible renal failure, stroke, myocardial infarction and other thrombotic events [39], hemolysis, and leukopenia.

IgA deficiency is considered a contraindication to intravenous immunoglobulin. Patients lacking IgA may develop antibodies to the immunoglobulin and have an allergic reaction. If IgA deficiency is present, a concentrate with a low IgA content should be used when immunoglobulin therapy seems indicated.

Normal intravenous immunoglobulins of human origin (IVIG) Immunoglobulin concentrates made from pooled blood, collected from normal donors, are given either to prevent or battle a disease caused by an infectious agent or a toxin, or to modify the immune system. The exact mode of action of intravenous immunoglobulins is not well understood and is certainly complex. The injected immunoglobulins modulate Fc receptor expression and function, the complementary system, cytokines and the activation, differentiation and function of T- and B-cells. They also influence cell growth and cellular adhesion molecules [40].

Intravenous immunoglobulins have been used in the antibacterial and antiviral therapy and prophylaxis of patients with primary [41] or secondary immunodeficiency (such as in malignant diseases) [42]. In preterm or low-birth-weight infants, it is used to boost the immune system. Also, bacterial infections of the newborn or sepsis are considered indications for immunoglobulins. However, a review concluded that there is no reason to believe that it can prevent any infection or improve the outcome for the infants [43]. IVIGs can also be used as a treatment for immunocompetent patients with specific infections for which no other therapy works, e.g., as it happens when antibiotics are having no effect [44] or a new infectious agent infected someone [45].

Immunoglobulins given for immunomodulation have been recommended in a variety of settings. These include autoimmune thrombocytopenia, immune thrombocytopenic purpura [46], Brucella melitensis-induced thrombocytopenic purpura [47], granulocytopenia, certain types of anemia [48], acquired inhibitors for coagulation factors, Kawasaki syndrome [49], Guillain-Barre-syndrome [50], myasthenia gravis [51], multiple sclerosis [52], polymyositis, dermatomyositis [53], lupus erythematosus, rheumatoid arthritis, Morbus Crohn, AIDS and infectious complications associated with organ transplantation [54] and transplant rejection [55], autoimmune mucocutaneous blistering diseases (pemphigus vulgaris, etc.) [56], antineutrophil cytoplasmic antibody-associated vasculitis (Wegener's granulomatosis, microscopic polyangiitis), polyarteritis nodosa, Henoch–Schonlein purpura, toxic epidermal necrolysis [57], Stevens–Johnson syndrome [58], Clostridium difficile diarrhea [59], hyperbilirubinemia caused by a hemolytic disease of the newborn and many more. However, for most of the indications, the proof of benefit to the patient is lacking [49, 58]. For many of these diseases, other treatment approaches are available in addition to immunoglobulins. These include other immunomodulatory regimen based on corticoids, cyclophosphamide, etc.

Hyperimmune immunoglobulins of human origin Hyperimmune products usually have a very high titer for a specific antibody (5–8 times higher than in normal IVIG). It can be used either for i.v. or i.m. application. Hyperimmune immunoglobulins are routinely available e.g., for cytomegalic virus (CMV), varicella zoster (VZV), and hepatitis B virus (HBV). It can also be produced in response to a newly emerging pathogen using reconvalescent serum, as was the case with Severe Acute Respiratory Syndrome (SARS) [60]. Hepatitis B immunoglobulin is used to prevent the recurrence of hepatitis B [61]. In hematopoietic stem cell transplantation, chemotherapy, and in patients with otherwise impaired immune function, CMV hyperimmunoglobulins are given for prophylaxis and treatment of cytomegalic virus infection [37].

Antisera Rather purified immunoglobulins given to combat or prevent a disease caused by a distinct antigen are also called antisera. Antisera are used prophylactically as passive immunization (e.g., for hepatitis A, B, tetanus, Rabies) [62] or to treat a specific disease (tetanus; botulism [63], etc.). The subgroup of antisera used to treat envenomation with animal venoms are also called antivenoms or antivenins.

Antisera against infectious agents or toxins are rather purified hyperimmune sera produced from human or animal sources (e.g., horses, sheep, chicken). Animals (or sometimes humans) are vaccinated with or against the infectious agents or toxins. The antigens injected are either derived from infectious agents (diphtheria or tetanus toxine), from animal toxines (snakes, spiders, scorpions, fish, jelly fish, insects) or from iatrogenously or suicidally administerable toxins (digoxine) [64]. Vaccinated animals (or humans) synthesize antibodies and these are used to produce antisera. Antisera are often processed to remove proteins that may cause allergies and to concentrate the desired type of antibodies. Inactive proteins may be precipitated or removed by chromatography. Immunoglobulin molecules can be cleaved further into antibody fragments [65]. Target-specific immunoglobulins (IgG) and their fragments (Fab2, Fab) as well as the choice of the source animals determine the differences in pharmacokinetic and pharmacodynamic properties of the antisera [66]. Fab molecules have a shorter half-life than IgG molecules. However, Fab preparations seem to produce fewer allergic side effects. Lyophilized antisera consisting of Fab fragments can easily be dissolved for injection and are very stable, even in the heat [67]. This is very advantageous for use in tropical regions.

The rates of allergic, anaphylactic, and pyrogenic reactions to antisera depend on the animal species used for antiserum production, the method of production, and the presence of molecular aggregates and total protein in the final drug. The reactions usually occur when Fc receptors activate the complementary system [68]. The quality of antisera thus greatly influences the rate of reactions to it. The incidence of adverse reactions to snake bite antivenom, for instance, varies, being about 10% in Australia and over 80% in India [68]. Some authorities therefore recommend pretreatment with subcutaneous adrenaline [65] or intravenous antihistaminics or corticoids [68, 69]. Other authorities recommend only having emergency medications available. Serum sickness is a common occurrence after the administration of antisera. Its development depends on the amount of antiserum administered [70]. Serum sickness presents with fever, arthralgia, and pruritus. Although usually self-limiting, antihistaminics and corticoids are used to alleviate the symptoms [70].

Poisonous snake or spider bites pose major problems to the inhabitants of certain areas. It has been estimated that about 2.5 million people are bitten by snakes annually worldwide, causing an excess of 100,000 deaths [71]. In an attempt to provide treatment for persons bitten by poisonous animals, monospecific and polyspecific antivenoms have been made available. Monospecific antivenoms contain antibodies to only one antigen, polyspecific antivenoms contain the antibodies against several antigens. Polyspecific antivenoms are of practical value when resources are scarce or when it is not exactly known what toxin is present. Polyspecific antivenoms for snake bites sometimes contain a mix of antibodies against the toxins of snakes commonly present in a certain area, e.g., Southern Africa or Southern Europe [72].

Antivenoms against animal stings or bites can be given intravenously or intramuscularly [73]. It was recommended to apply the antivenom to the muscle that has been injected with the toxin (that is, the area of the snake bite). Otherwise, intravenous injection is recommended unless the antivenom preparation is so crude that intravenous injection is dangerous [74]. Antivenom injected intravenously may act longer than that being injected intramuscularly [73].

The dosing of antivenom is important. As other drugs, toxins, and antitoxins have a pharmacokinetic profile that needs to be known in order to dose the antivenom correctly. A pharmacokinetic or pharmacodynamic mismatch between the antivenom and the toxin may cause recurrence of the symptoms. These occur when the toxin has a longer half-life than the antivenom. To prevent late local tissue damage or coagulopathy with bleeding after snake bites, recurrence phenomena need to be prevented and treated. Repeated dosing and close observation of the patient in the hours after the envenomation are recommended. The duration of the therapy depends on individual risk factors and on the clinical response to the therapy [66, 67].

Anti-D-immunoglobulin When fetal red blood cells with the Rhesus (Rh) antigen (blood group antigen D) cross the placenta, an immunological response may be induced in an Rh-negative mother with the production of IgM and IgG. The IgG molecule crosses the placenta and can act against fetal red cells. The fetus may then suffer from hemolysis, anemia, and hydrops fetalis.

Maternal sensitization occurs when the mother is first exposed to fetal blood. In an uncomplicated pregnancy, this happens during delivery. In this case, the first child is not affected by the antibody developing after birth, but the next baby is. When the mother is exposed to fetal blood prior to delivery, usually due to testing or obstetric complications, the current fetus is at risk for an antibody attack.

To prevent the production of antibodies, anti-D-immunoglobulin is administered to non-sensitized Rh-negative women. The anti-D-immunoglobulin will destroy any fetal red blood cells that have entered the maternal bloodstream, preventing the formation of maternal antibodies to the Rh factor.

Anti-D-immunoglobulin was recommended to be given to non-sensitized Rh-negative women who have an Rh-positive child or when the fetal blood type is unknown. The injection should be given soon after birth. Non-sensitized D-negative women should receive the immunoglobulin after miscarriage, threatened or induced abortion, molar pregnancy, and ectopic pregnancy, at amniocentesis and after chorionic villous sampling, and following cordocentesis. Additional anti-D immunoglobulins may be required for events leading to severe feto-maternal hemorrhage (>15 mL of fetal red blood cells) [75].

Anti-D-immunoglobulin is also used in the therapy of diseases other than feto-maternal Rh incompatibility. Patients with immune thrombocytopenic purpura may also be treated with such anti-D-immunoglobulins [76].

Plasma fractions in blood management

Blood banks and pharmaceutical companies all over the world offer hundreds of different concentrates of plasma factors. However, only very few diseases seem to benefit from them. Most functions in blood are performed by different proteins, so that when one is lacking, others kick in to take over the job. Others can be substituted by nonblood therapy. Actually, for most, if not all, plasmatic factor deficiencies there are nonblood alternatives.

Since only a limited number of plasma proteins have a unique, life-conserving function, only few plasma proteins are produced commercially in considerable quantities. Although it is often technically possible to produce concentrates of other plasma proteins, it is usually not done. The reason for this is that there is either no clinical benefit from the infusion of a certain plasma protein, or there is not a market big enough to warrant the mass production of a concentrate. In the latter case, the United States mandated the so-called Orphan Drug Act. It will help provide patients with rare blood protein deficiencies with a corresponding factor concentrate.

Hemophilia A and B

While pharmaceutical [77] and physical therapies are the first-line treatment for most hemophiliacs, factor substitution plays an important additional role in the therapy of severe hemophilia. There are many products that contain factor VIII and would theoretically work in the therapy of hemophilia A. Among them are FFP, cryoprecipitate, factor VIII concentrates with intermediate, high or ultra-high purity, porcine FVIII concentrates, and recombinant FVIII. For the therapy of hemophilia B, FFP, prothrombin complex concentrates, activated prothrombin complex concentrates, and factor FIX concentrates, either human plasma-derived or recombinant, are available. FFP is no real choice for the patients since, unless exchange transfusion is performed, not enough FFP can be given to raise the FIX levels sufficiently in severe hemophilia.

The choice of therapy for hemophiliac patients depends on availability, costs, and patient characteristics. Whenever possible, recombinant products should be preferred. If not all patients can be treated with recombinant factors and a selection must be made, recombinant factors should be used for all patients who have never before been treated with a plasma-derived product and patients who are seronegative for HCV and HIV. When plasma-derived products are chosen for the therapy of hemophilia, the product with the highest possible purity is indicated, especially in situations when thrombosis risks exist (e.g., surgery) and when long-term therapy is anticipated (immune tolerance regimen, prophylaxis). High and very-high purity products are preferred to reduce unnecessary risks to the patient. High purity factor concentrates are expensive. It is not clearly determined whether the intermediate purity concentrates come with disadvantages for rather healthy hemophiliacs when compared with high-purity concentrates. Intermediate purity concentrates have immunosuppressive effects [78]. These can be of clinical significance in already immunocompromised patients (HIV) [79]. HIV-positive patients benefit from a high purity, since this may preserve their CD4 lymphocyte count.

Details of the therapy of hemophiliacs have been made available in the form of treatment recommendations [80]. The following recommendations for hemophilia therapy have been made [81]:
• In life-threatening bleeding, without exact knowledge of the factor lacking, recombinant factor VIIa is the first

choice treatment (90–120 mcg/kg). When the needed factor is known, 50–70 IU/kg of a factor concentrate are infused.
• In intracerebral bleeding, a high-dose regimen of the factor needs to be started and continued until the resorption of the bleeding is seen. Afterward, low-dose substitution is warranted to prevent re-bleeding.
• Patients with polytrauma should have a level of 100% factor activity until the wounds have healed.
• For surgery, the individual level should be determined before the operation and substitution is begun right before surgery.
• When bones are fractured or bones are operated on, levels of 80–100% of factor VIII or IX are recommended. For the time the bone heals, a minimum of 10–20% of factor should be maintained.
• For dental work, a minimum of 30% factor activity VII is recommended, together with antifibrinolytic therapy to counteract the fibrinolytic activity of the saliva.
• For gastrointestinal bleeding and bleeding into the psoas or retroperitoneum, 50% factor activity is recommended.

Recommendations like these may be not feasible in developing countries. This is so because of a limited availability of factor concentrates calling for rationing available resources. In such settings, reduced infusion doses of factor concentrates have been found adequate [82].

Hemophiliacs A and B with low levels of clotting factors (<1%) are sometimes recommended to use clotting factor concentrates prophylactically. It has been claimed that this reduces severe bleedings in joints and soft tissues. However, proof that prophylactic use of clotting factor concentrates is superior to placebo in reducing bleeding is still missing [83].

Inhibitor treatment of hemophiliac patients

The treatment of hemophilia with injection of the missing coagulation factor comes with one great disadvantage. The body may recognize the injected material as foreign and develop antibodies (IgG alloantibodies). Such antibodies are able to inactivate the injected factor and are therefore called inhibitor. Besides, also patients who are not hemophiliacs can develop an inhibitor. They form alloantibodies against the endogenous factor VIII. The latter may happen idiopathically (in elderly patients), in autoimmune diseases (systemic lupus erythematosus, rheumatoid arthritis), in malignancies, as a drug reaction (penicillin, chloramphenicol, phenytoin), and during or after pregnancy.

About 10–30% of patients with severe hemophilia A and 2–5% with severe hemophilia B or mild to moderate hemophilia A develop inhibitors [84]. Inhibitors are detected with the Bethesda assay and the level of the inhibitor is expressed in Bethesda Units (BUs). One BU is the amount of antibody that neutralizes 50% of FVIII in a 1:1 mixture of the patient's plasma and normal plasma (after 2 hour incubation at 37°C). According to the Bethesda assay, patients are sorted into two groups: low responders with low titers of inhibitors (<10 BU), who do not increase the titer after a challenge with FVIII, and high responders who develop a high titer of inhibitor when challenged with FVIII.

To overcome the problems in patients with inhibitors, products other than the factor concentrates can be infused. Factor VIII and factor IX normally catalyze the activation of factor X. Since factor VIII or IX inhibitors block this action, bypassing their action by directly activating factor X seems to be a way to provide hemostasis without active hemophiliac factors. Some products are able to do this. Activated PCCs directly activate factor X and prothrombin [2]. However, despite the availability of aPCC for more than 20 years, the reported experience with this agent is limited [84]. The products are effective in only about half of uncomplicated bleeding events.

Recently, recombinant factor VII was put on the market with its indication for inhibitor treatment of hemophiliacs and is now the therapy of choice for such patients [85]. With the appropriate does of rHuFVIIa, even major surgery is safely possible in hemophiliacs with inhibitors [84].

Also, immunosuppressive agents to control the antibody production against clotting factors (corticosteroids, cyclophosphamide, and azathioprine) have been recommended for the therapy of patients with inhibitors. They are given in order to reduce the offending (auto)antibody [86]. Intravenous immunoglobulin solutions have also been used in such, since the concentrate may contain antibodies against the inhibitor to inactivate it.

If these approaches fail and the patients is bleeding profusely, high-dose porcine factor FVIII or human FIX may be effective, given the inhibitor is low enough (<5 BU) or lowered by plasmapheresis or protein A immunoabsorption.

Another way to overcome the inhibitor is to induce immune tolerance. To this end, patients receive frequent infusions of the offending factor (e.g., daily or weekly). After months or years, the inhibitor is eliminated. However, the induction of immune tolerance fails in 20% of cases is costly and comes with multiple adverse effects.

von Willebrand disease

Congenital vWD develops when vWF is lacking or defective. Three main types of congenital vWD are known. The most common form is Type I vWD. Patients have only a moderate decrease in vWF in plasma and experience only minor bleeding. However, a surgical challenge or trauma can lead to major bleeding. Type II vWD is rare. The level of vWF is normal, but the molecule does not work properly. In the subgroup IIa vWD, vWF molecules are either not secreted or are rapidly destroyed in the circulation. The subgroup IIb vWD vWF molecules bind increasingly to platelets and aggregate them. Patients with Type III vWD synthesize no vWF at all. The platelet aggregation is diminished with a bleeding pattern similar to thrombocytopenia. Additionally, factor VIII is impaired as well, leading to a hemophilia-like symptom pattern. There is also an acquired form of vWD which occurs when antibodies inhibit vWF or when tumors (such as lymphoid tumors) adsorb vWF on to their surface.

DDAVP is the agent of choice for the prophylaxis and therapy of most forms of vWD. A test dose of DDAVP and determination of the stimulated factor levels is recommended before surgery is performed under DDAVP protection. Therapeutic options other than DDAVP include antifibrinolytics and hormones. As regards plasma fractions, vWF concentrates [87], cryoprecipitate and factor VIII concentrates containing high vWF levels [88] may be considered as a therapeutic option. Recently, it has been recommended to combine the therapy with factor concentrates with infusions of intravenous immunoglobulins [89]. When DDAVP does not work and vWD has to be substituted, a virus-inactivated factor concentrate with sufficient levels of vWF is to be preferred over cryoprecipitate. Probably, the best choice is a vWF concentrate with very low levels of factor VIII in order to reduce thrombotic complications [88]. Patients with a high risk of bleeding complications due to vWD may also be eligible for prophylactic measures, including infusions of factor concentrates in order to reduce the incidence of severe bleeds [90]. In developing countries, cryoprecipitate may be the only available blood fraction for the therapy [91]. It is costly and may not be sufficiently tested for transfusion-transmittable diseases. In such settings it is especially important to explore all available nonblood-based therapeutic options before a plasma fraction is considered for therapy.

Other single (congenital) clotting factor deficiencies

Other, much less frequently occurring single factor deficiencies can be treated with either a plasma-derived factor concentrate or another, cruder plasma fraction. Most of the single factor deficiencies can be treated with recombinant factor VIIa. This is probably the safest, yet most expensive, option. Appendix A contains Table Appendix A.2, which delineates therapeutic options for the therapy of rare clotting factor deficiencies.

Therapy of vitamin K deficiency

The synthesis of many plasmatic factors depends on the presence of vitamin K. Mainly, these are factors II, VII, IX, and X as well as proteins S and C. Vitamin K deficiency can be caused either by insufficient intake or by iatrogenic influences, such as therapy with vitamin K antagonists (cumadin anticoagulants) or antibiotics [92].

The treatment of vitamin K deficiency is the correction of the underlying cause and vitamin K application. Usually, this is all it takes. Within hours, the factors are replenished. But when the therapy does not bring the desired results or the delay in response would endanger the patient, clotting factor concentrates, either recombinant or serum-derived ones, are prescribed.

Formerly, for emergency oral anticoagulation reversal, FFP was often prescribed. However, it was shown that FFP often does not correct the underlying deficiency. To achieve therapeutic factor levels in over-anticoagulated patients, several liters of FFP would have to be infused in order to develop the desired factor levels. If the half-life of a missing factor is short and repeated infusions are necessary, fluid overload would develop. When FFP is used, diuretics and a partial plasma exchange have been necessary to treat the developing volume overload.

What is the therapy of vitamin K deficiency or oral anticoagulation reversal in emergency situations? In cases of emergency, vitamin K application is the treatment of choice. If not enough time is available to allow for the endogenous correction of the factor deficiency, PCCs are recommended [93]. They correct the factor deficiency without causing volume overload [94]. Several dosing regimen were proposed. A standardized infusion of PCC of 500 IU factor IX equivalent has been recommended [93]. However, an individualized regimen based on the initial INR, the target INR, and the patient's body weight may be more effective in reaching the target INR than the use of a standard dose of PCC [95].

As an alternative to PCCs, recombinant factor VIIa can be given. This is probably safer than PCCs. Trials are under way to show that the recombinant factor is to be preferred, especially in cases where very fast reversal of vitamin K-dependent factor deficiency is needed, such as in intracranial bleeding.

Bleeding in liver-related coagulopathies

All coagulation factors (apart from vWF) are synthesized in the liver. When the liver fails, the plasmatic coagulation is impaired as well. Besides, severe liver insufficiency is accompanied by hyperfibrinolysis, since inactivation of pro- and anticoagulant factors in the liver is impaired. The condition is occasionally also accompanied by thrombocytopenia secondary to increased use of platelets and toxically impaired platelet production.

Patients with liver-disease-related coagulopathies can be treated without blood products, using such options as antifibrinolytics, DDAVP, vitamin K, or hormones. When blood products are considered, plasma fractions such as antithrombin III, PCC, and fibrinogen are recommended (and sometimes even platelets). However, since a liver insufficiency also affects anticoagulative factors (protein C, protein S), the risk for thromboembolism is increased when coagulative factors are given.

Disseminated intravascular coagulation

A disseminated intravascular coagulation (DIC) usually develops in connection with a life-threatening disorder, such as severe sepsis or polytrauma. It presents with spontaneous bleeding and deterioration of the function of organs, leading to multiorgan failure.

A DIC is initiated by a systemic activation of the coagulation process. Endotoxin or thromboplastin-containing amniotic fluid may initiate this, resulting in increased thrombin formation in blood. The thrombin induces the formation of fibrin and further activates other plasmatic coagulation factors. Fibrin will impair the microcirculation and a multiorgan failure results. As a reaction to so much fibrin in the circulation, fibrinolysis increases tremendously, and bleeding results. The massive use of platelets and coagulation factors depletes the blood of them, thereby accelerating bleeding. These processes continue until the offending agent is cleared from the circulation.

When a DIC is diagnosed, the underlying condition has to be treated immediately to stop the continuous activation of coagulation. In parallel, hematologic support needs to be initiated. However, the therapy of DIC is difficult, since bleeding and coagulation occur simultaneously. To stop the coagulation, anticoagulation has been advocated, yet, it accelerates bleeding. There is a paucity of data supporting the therapy of DIC. Therapeutic algorithms recommend FFP and antithrombin, followed by heparin and possibly activated protein C when no bleeding is present. When the patient bleeds, aprotinin, platelets, fibrinogen, and PCC were proposed. However, such recommendations are not supported by hard data. There is no proof that FFP, ATIII, or aPC really improve the outcome of patients with a DIC [81].

Plasmatic fractions used to reduce the use of other blood products

Sometimes, there are different blood-derived products available for the therapy of one condition. When this is the case, the factor with the lowest risk of adverse effects should be preferred. Since most plasmatic fractions are virus-inactivated, they seem to be somewhat safer than blood products that are not. Using the saver, plasmatic fractions can reduce the use of other blood products. Besides, some plasmatic fractions may be acceptable to a patient, while cellular blood components are not. It makes sense, to know about possible variations in the use of blood products. Here are some examples:

• It was shown that factor VIII concentrates with vWF are as effective as cryoprecipitate for the therapy of patients with vWD unresponsive to DDAVP [96]. The use of cryoprecipitate can therefore be safely reduced when therapy is provided with factor VIII concentrates.

• Plasmatic factor concentrates may also reduce the use of cellular blood components. Intermediate-purity factor VIII concentrates reduce bleeding in patients with vWD and reduce their exposure to red cell transfusions [97]. Factor IX concentrates containing other activated factors can improve hemostasis when used in mild to moderate thrombocytopenia [98].

• Therapeutic apheresis procedures can be performed with a variety of agents for plasma exchange. Synthetic colloids are suitable for plasma exchange. In case someone does not want to resort to asanguinous therapies, albumin may be an alternative to FFP [33]. As an alternative approach to exchange transfusion, intravenous immunoglobulin therapy has been proposed in newborns suffering from hyperbilirubinemia secondary to hemolysis [99].

• For acute attacks of hereditary angioedema, FFP and solvent-/detergent-treated plasma may be effective treatment, but the potentially safer C1 esterase inhibitor concentrate should be used [30].

All these examples show that plasmatic fractions can reduce the use of potentially more hazardous blood products.

Approaches to reduce the use of plasmatic fractions

Plasmatic fractions mostly undergo one or a series of purification steps that reduce the risk of transmitting a disease. By this, they seem to be safer than untreated cellular components for transfusion. However, there is still a residual risk of transmitting diseases. Besides, also plasmatic fractions can impair the immune system and elicit severe side effects. They have to be prescribed with the greatest care and only in settings when the therapy promises success. If possible, plasmatic fractions should be avoided just as all other blood products.

Although the reduction of the use of plasma fractions does not receive the same attention as the reduction of cellular component use, there are many methods devised to reduce the use of these blood products. The strategies used to avoid the transfusion of plasmatic fractions are very similar to the ones used to avoid cellular component transfusion. It takes a skilled MANAGER to reduce the use of such components. Try to remember the strategies below, using the mnemonic MANAGER, standing for

M: Monitoring and evaluation
A: Avoid blood loss
N: Need established
A: Administration
G: Generating endogenous resources
E: Existence of pharmaceutical alternatives
R: Recombinant products

M: monitoring

Monitoring and a thorough evaluation of the patient often reduces or avoids his exposure to plasmatic fractions. Three examples may illustrate this.

• Pregnant women who are Rh-negative usually receive anti-D-immunoglobulin. However, not all women need it. If it is possible to establish whether the patient in question falls among the group of patients where anti-D-immunoglobulin administration is not recommended, the patient does not need to receive this blood product.

Among the women who should not receive anti-D-immunoglobulin are those with a "weak D" (Du-positive), a complete mole, or when the father of the child is also Rh-negative. Such diagnosis can eliminate unnecessary blood product administration [75].

• Patients who have been bitten by a poisonous animal can sometimes be treated with antiserum. But it is often difficult to find out whether the animal actually injected its toxin into the patient. To "treat the patient, not the poison," a thorough evaluation of the patient is needed to establish whether he really has toxin in his blood [100]. When the need for antivenom is established, monitoring of the residual amount of toxin in the blood can guide the use of antivenom. This typically reduces the amount of antivenom given [101]. In certain areas of the world where snake bites are not typically deadly, it is prudent simply to monitor the patient closely instead of treating him prophylactically after snake bites. Only severely envenomated patients may be candidates for therapy [102].

• Patients with clotting abnormalities may be given plasma-derived clotting factors. Using an algorithm to monitor their clotting abnormalities with tests such as thrombelastography may reduce unnecessary clotting factor therapy [103].

A: avoid blood loss and circumstances that may lead to exposure to blood products

As it is the case with cellular blood products, the use of plasmatic fractions can be reduced when overall blood loss is minimized. Expertise in surgical technique or the use of minimally invasive procedures can reduce blood loss and with it, the loss of plasmatic factors. Surgery can even be performed in patients who are coagulopathic, if the surgical technique is meticulous. When blood loss occurs, it is sometimes possible to recover the lost blood, including plasmatic fractions. Concentrating and returning residual blood in a cardiopulmonary bypass by means of certain techniques allows for recovery of autologous plasma proteins, among them also clotting factors, for the patient [104]. Also, ascites can be concentrated and autologous plasma proteins returned [105].

Forethought may also reduce a person's exposure to blood products. Ask yourself: Is my patient endangered of developing a condition that may result in a therapy with plasmatic fractions? If so, can this condition be avoided? Two examples illustrate this.

• Certain patients may be likely to contract an infectious disease. Active vaccination against this disease, well before the patient is exposed to the infectious agent, may prevent a disease that typically would be treated with plasmatic

fractions. When a patient is vaccinated against tetanus, for instance, passive vaccination is not needed and exposure to blood products is avoided.

• Patients with severe hemophilia often develop bleeding into their joints. Hemophiliac arthropathies result. Patients with such a condition may benefit from early knee arthroplasty. This procedure may reduce their future use of clotting factor concentrates [106].

N: need established (indication given?)

When a plasmatic fraction is considered for treatment, ask yourself: Is there a real need to expose my patient to blood products? A thorough knowledge of the real benefits and detriments drastically reduces the use of blood fractions.

Very often, plasmatic fractions are given although there is no need. Clinical practice guidelines help to reduce unnecessary exposure of patients to blood products. Albumin use has been reduced by way of such guidelines [107]. Female patients suffering from severe factor XI deficiency are often given factor XI concentrates prior to giving birth. Prophylactic use of the concentrates may not be necessary, however [108]. Knowing when plasmatic fractions are not indicated is vital to reducing their unnecessary use.

Another example illustrates how vital a thorough knowledge about plasma products is. It helps to resist the temptation to follow mere intuition when using such products. The use of antivenom for snake bites, although tempting, is often not indicated, especially when only local symptoms are experienced by the patient [109]. Close monitoring and supportive nonblood care alone may result in an acceptable outcome, even in the presence of severe coagulopathy [110, 111]. Although clotting factor concentrates and FFP intuitively appeal as therapeutic options in coagulopathic patients, they may be ineffective or even dangerous since they seem to increase mortality [71, 112, 113].

A: administration

Timing, dosing, and the route of administration have a bearing on the total amount of plasmatic fractions given. Here are some examples:

• Patients who undergo surgery with a cardiopulmonary bypass need to be anticoagulated. This is often done by heparin. When such patients require plasmatic factor replacements, the infusion should be withheld until after the neutralization of heparin. This reduces the amount of concentrate needed.

• The administration of coagulation factor concentrates to maintain the blood level of a patient above the through

level is inversely related to the time between the boli given, which means that more frequent smaller bolus injections reduce the total amount of coagulation factor when compared to less frequent, but high-dose injections [114]. A continuous infusion of factors has totally eliminated time intervals between bolus injections and therefore reduces the requirements of factor concentrates maximally [115].
• Dosing of snake antivenom may be varied. It has been shown that a low single-dose administration of an antivenom for neurotoxic symptoms of snake bites is as effective as high multiple-dose regimen [116].

G: generate endogenous resources

When plasmatic proteins are lacking in patients, it may still be possible to increase the production of the lacking protein pharmacologically. Desmopressin may raise the level of FVIII and the vWF. Vitamin K may raise the level of vitamin K-dependent plasmatic factors. Liver transplant patients who typically receive antiviral agents and immunoglobulins for protection against hepatitis B infection can undergo an enhanced program of vaccination and often develop sufficient autologous hepatitis B antibodies so that immunoglobulin therapy can be finished [117]. Therefore, before you think about giving a plasma-derived product, check whether there is a way to animate the patient's body to help itself.

E: existence of pharmaceutical alternatives

There are quite a few pharmaceuticals that can reduce the use of plasma fractions. Tranexamic acid may reduce the use of cryoprecipitate in patients undergoing liver transplantation [118]. The same is true for aprotinin [119]. Antiviral drugs may be as effective or even superior to immunoglobulin therapy against cytomegaly virus infection in transplant recipients [120]. Immunoglobulins extracted from human milk may be a good source of immunoglobulin A for babies with immunodeficiencies or with mucosal infections [121]. This may be superior to intravenous immunoglobulin therapy. Always make sure that you do not miss a suitable pharmacological approach to the therapy of your patient that may be able to reduce your patient's exposure to blood products.

R: recombinant products

When you are sure that the patient cannot be treated with the above measures, try to find him a recombinant product that can replenish the missing factor. Almost every plasma factor can be produced in a recombinant fashion. Granted, they are expensive or may not be registered in your country. But if you can make a recombinant product available, you may have spared your patient contact with the blood of another person or animal.

Key points

• Each plasma sample is unique in its composition.
• Using fractionation methods, a variety of plasma fractions can be made available for therapy. Most of the therapy with plasmatic fractions is empirical. Attempts to demonstrate an improved outcome in patients receiving therapy with such products have failed for most indications.
• Optimization of the use of plasmatic fractions follows the same line of thought as the attempts to reduce the use of cellular blood components. As a mnemonic, use MANAGER:
M: Monitoring. Is it beneficial to obtain more information about the patient (e.g., a laboratory parameter) that could guide my therapy more exactly? Would it be beneficial just to monitor the patient rather than rushing him into therapy?
A: Avoid blood loss and circumstances that may require exposure to blood products. Is there any way to reduce the overall blood loss of the patient?
N: Need established. Is the plasma product really indicated? Is there a proven benefit to the patient if I give him the product? Am I sure the product is not contraindicated?
A: Administration. What timing, dosing, and route of administration is the one that brings maximum benefit without exposing the patient to unnecessary plasma products?
G: Generate endogenous resources. Is there any way to treat the patient so that the missing blood component is produced in an autologous fashion?
E: Existence of pharmaceutical alternatives. Is there any drug available that may reduce the use of the plasma product? Is there anything that may replace the function of the missing protein?
R: Recombinant products. Is there any recombinant plasma product available that may fit the needs of my patient?

Questions for review

• What do the following terms mean: Bethesda unit, international unit, intravascular recovery, potency, purity, specific activity, survival study, through level.

• What is the difference between (a) FFP and cryoprecipitate, (b) intravenous immunoglobulins and hyperimmune globulins, (c) "three" factor PCC and "four" factor PCC?

• What indications have been proposed for the following plasma fractions: factor XIII, C1-esterase inhibitor, high-purity factor VIII, albumin, fibrinogen, intravenous immunoglobulins?

• What therapeutic options exist for the following conditions (What options are based on blood and which ones are not?): hemophilia A without inhibitors, patients with coumadin overdose, vWD, and hereditary angioneurotic edema.

Suggestions for further research

Find out what the term "gammaglobulins" means. Where does this term stem from?

How do platelets and fibrinogen interact to form a clot? How can this be used clinically in cases of thrombopenia?

Below Table Appendix A.3, you find a list of proteins found in human plasma. Try to determine the function of some of them. Which ones might benefit or harm the patient receiving human plasma containing these proteins?

Exercises and practice cases

Refer to Table 19.1. Compare the recoveries and the molecular weight of the factor. Can you see a relationship?

Refer to Table Appendix A.2 which lists the treatment options for factor deficiencies. What nonblood-based therapeutic options are available? What factor deficiency cannot be treated adequately without taking resort to donor blood products?

Use the MANAGER strategy to evaluate the therapy of the following patients. What could be done to prevent or reduce the following patient's exposure to the blood products? List all the points that you find during a thorough literature search, using the mnemonic MANAGER.

• A small preschool child suffering from hemophilia B is scheduled for dental surgery. The surgeon claims the child needs to have general anesthesia with nasal intubation. (Compare Ref. [122])

• A baby girl presents with ecchymosis and hemorrhagic bullae 15 hours after birth. She subsequently develops gangrene in her buttock and inguinal region. The original case report continues: "Disseminated intravascular coagulation was diagnosed and treated with human antithrombin III, gabexate mesilate, FFP, and platelet concentrates. Although the infant's condition improved at first, a new purpuric lesion developed on the right arm at seven days of age. Further tests revealed that the protein C activity of the infant was 3% (normal range 80–130%) ... The diagnosis of purpura fulminans syndrome due to homozygous protein C deficiency was made on the patient's ninth day of life. In addition to treatment with FFP and warfarin potassium, administration of activated protein C concentrate, affinity-purified from human plasma, ... was initiated on the 11th day of life." (Compare Ref. [123])

• A male patient with a history of unexplained thrombocytopenia is transfused with platelet concentrates for severe postoperative hemorrhage after hernia repair. However, his coagulopathy is not corrected. Years later, he eventually is diagnosed with vWD Type 2B. What management options would have prevented his being exposed to the platelet concentrates? What future therapy and prophylaxis would you recommend to optimize his blood management when this patient would present for dental extraction? (Compare Ref. [124])

Homework

List all available pharmacologic and blood-based therapeutic options available in your hospital to treat patients with a deficiency of plasmatic proteins.

References

1 Farrugia, A. and P. Robert. Plasma protein therapies: current and future perspectives. *Best Pract Res Clin Haematol*, 2006. **19**(1): p. 243–258.

2 Kingdon, H.S. and R.L. Lundblad. An adventure in biotechnology: the development of haemophilia A therapeutics—from whole-blood transfusion to recombinant DNA to gene therapy. *Biotechnol Appl Biochem*, 2002. **35**(Pt 2): p. 141–148.

3 Mannucci, P.M. and E.G. Tuddenham. The hemophilias—from royal genes to gene therapy. *N Engl J Med*, 2001. **344**(23): p. 1773–1779.

4 Siegel, J. The product: all intravenous immunoglobulins are not equivalent. *Pharmacotherapy*, 2005. **25**(11, Pt 2): p. 78S–84S.

5 Romisch, J., *et al.* A protease isolated from human plasma activating factor VII independent of tissue factor. *Blood Coagul Fibrinolysis*, 1999. **10**(8): p. 471–479.

6 Fritsma, M.G. Use of blood products and factor concentrates for coagulation therapy. *Clin Lab Sci*, 2003. **16**(2): p. 115–119.

7 Practice Guidelines for blood component therapy: a report by the American Society of Anesthesiologists Task Force on Blood Component Therapy. *Anesthesiology*, 1996. **84**(3): p. 732–747.

8 Josic, D., L. Hoffer, and A. Buchacher. Preparation of vitamin K-dependent proteins, such as clotting factors II, VII, IX and X and clotting inhibitor protein C. *J Chromatogr B Analyt Technol Biomed Life Sci*, 2003. **790**(1–2): p. 183–197.

9 Lubetsky, A., *et al.* Efficacy and safety of a prothrombin complex concentrate (Octaplex) for rapid reversal of oral anticoagulation. *Thromb Res*, 2004. **113**(6): p. 371–378.

10 Tjonnfjord, G.E. Activated prothrombin complex concentrate (FEIBA) treatment during surgery in patients with inhibitors to FVIII/IX: the updated Norwegian experience. *Haemophilia*, 2004. **10**(Suppl 2): p. 41–45.

11 Kouides, P.A. and L. Kulzer. Prophylactic treatment of severe factor X deficiency with prothrombin complex concentrate. *Haemophilia*, 2001. **7**(2): p. 220–223.

12 Hay, C.R. Porcine factor VIII: current status and future developments. *Haemophilia*, 2002. **8**(Suppl 1): p. 24–27; discussion 28–32.

13 Goudemand, J., *et al.* Clinical management of patients with von Willebrand's disease with a VHP vWF concentrate: the French experience. *Haemophilia*, 1998. **4**(Suppl 3): p. 48–52.

14 Kreuz, W., *et al.* Efficacy and tolerability of a pasteurised human fibrinogen concentrate in patients with congenital fibrinogen deficiency. *Transfus Apher Sci*, 2005. **32**(3): p. 247–253.

15 Parameswaran, R., *et al.* Spontaneous intracranial bleeding in two patients with congenital afibrinogenaemia and the role of replacement therapy. *Haemophilia*, 2000. **6**(6): p. 705–708.

16 Fenger-Eriksen, C., *et al.* Thrombelastographic whole blood clot formation after ex vivo addition of plasma substitutes: improvements of the induced coagulopathy with fibrinogen concentrate. *Br J Anaesth*, 2005. **94**(3): p. 324–329.

17 Ichinose, A., T. Asahina, and T. Kobayashi. Congenital blood coagulation factor XIII deficiency and perinatal management. *Curr Drug Targets*, 2005. **6**(5): p. 541–549.

18 Aledort, L.M. and J. Goudemand. United States' factor XI-deficiency patients need a safer treatment. *Am J Hematol*, 2005. **80**(4): p. 301–302.

19 Lechner, K. and P.A. Kyrle. Antithrombin III concentrates—are they clinically useful? *Thromb Haemost*, 1995. **73**(3): p. 340–348.

20 Wiedermann, C.J., *et al.* High-dose antithrombin III in the treatment of severe sepsis in patients with a high risk of death: efficacy and safety. *Crit Care Med*, 2006. **34**(2): p. 285–292.

21 Kulka, P.J., M. Tryba, and S. Lange. Are there certified indications for the use of antithrombin III in intensive care. *AINS*, 2001. **36**(3): p. 143–153.

22 Levi, M. Antithrombin in sepsis revisited. *Crit Care*, 2005. **9**(6): p. 624–625.

23 Messori, A., *et al.* Antithrombin III in patients admitted to intensive care units: a multicenter observational study. *Crit Care*, 2002. **6**(5): p. 447–451.

24 Pescatore, S.L. Clinical management of protein C deficiency. *Expert Opin Pharmacother*, 2001. **2**(3): p. 431–439.

25 Foster, P.R., *et al.* Activated protein C concentrate reverses purpura fulminans in severe genetic protein C deficiency. *J Pediatr Hematol Oncol*, 2004. **26**(1): p. 25–27.

26 Radosevich, M., *et al.* Chromatographic purification and properties of a therapeutic human protein C concentrate. *J Chromatogr B Analyt Technol Biomed Life Sci*, 2003. **790**(1–2): p. 199–207.

27 Bernard, G.R., *et al.* Efficacy and safety of recombinant human activated protein C for severe sepsis. *N Engl J Med*, 2001. **344**(10): p. 699–709.

28 Bork, K., *et al.* Treatment with C1 inhibitor concentrate in abdominal pain attacks of patients with hereditary angioedema. *Transfusion*, 2005. **45**(11): p. 1774–1784.

29 Gompels, M.M., *et al.* C1 inhibitor deficiency: consensus document. *Clin Exp Immunol*, 2005. **139**(3): p. 379–394.

30 Longhurst, H.J. Emergency treatment of acute attacks in hereditary angioedema due to C1 inhibitor deficiency: what is the evidence? *Int J Clin Pract*, 2005. **59**(5): p. 594–599.

31 Fasano, M., *et al.* The extraordinary ligand binding properties of human serum albumin. *IUBMB Life*, 2005. **57**(12): p. 787–796.

32 Rodrigues, A.G., R. Araujo, and C. Pina-Vaz. Human albumin promotes germination, hyphal growth and antifungal resistance by Aspergillus fumigatus. *Med Mycol*, 2005. **43**(8): p. 711–717.

33 McLeod, B.C. Therapeutic apheresis: use of human serum albumin, fresh frozen plasma and cryosupernatant plasma in therapeutic plasma exchange. *Best Pract Res Clin Haematol*, 2006. **19**(1): p. 157–167.

34 Cooper, A.B., *et al.* Five percent albumin for adult burn shock resuscitation: lack of effect on daily multiple organ dysfunction score. *Transfusion*, 2006. **46**(1): p. 80–89.

35 Boros, P., G. Gondolesi, and J.S. Bromberg. High dose intravenous immunoglobulin treatment: mechanisms of action. *Liver Transpl*, 2005. **11**(12): p. 1469–1480.

36 Boschetti, N., *et al.* Virus safety of intravenous immunoglobulin: future challenges. *Clin Rev Allergy Immunol*, 2005. **29**(3): p. 333–344.

37 Sokos, D.R., M. Berger, and H.M. Lazarus. Intravenous immunoglobulin: appropriate indications and uses in hematopoietic stem cell transplantation. *Biol Blood Marrow Transplant*, 2002. **8**(3): p. 117–130.

38 Hamrock, D.J. Adverse events associated with intravenous immunoglobulin therapy. *Int Immunopharmacol*, 2006. **6**(4): p. 535–542.

39 Katz, U. and Y. Shoenfeld. Review: intravenous immunoglobulin therapy and thromboembolic complications. *Lupus*, 2005. **14**(10): p. 802–808.

40 Bayary, J., *et al.* Intravenous immunoglobulin in autoimmune disorders: an insight into the immunoregulatory mechanisms. *Int Immunopharmacol*, 2006. **6**(4): p. 528–534.

41 Bayrakci, B., *et al.* The efficacy of immunoglobulin replacement therapy in the long-term follow-up of the B-cell deficiencies (XLA, HIM, CVID). *Turk J Pediatr*, 2005. **47**(3): p. 239–246.

42 Berger, M. Subcutaneous immunoglobulin replacement in primary immunodeficiencies. *Clin Immunol*, 2004. **112**(1): p. 1–7.

43 Ohlsson, A. and J.B. Lacy. Intravenous immunoglobulin for preventing infection in preterm and/or low-birth-weight infants. *Cochrane Database Syst Rev*, 2004. (1): p. CD000361.

44 Bayry, J., *et al.* Intravenous immunoglobulin for infectious diseases: back to the pre-antibiotic and passive prophylaxis era? *Trends Pharmacol Sci*, 2004. **25**(6): p. 306–310.

45 Roos, K.L. West Nile encephalitis and myelitis. *Curr Opin Neurol*, 2004. **17**(3): p. 343–346.

46 Beck, C.E., *et al.* Corticosteroids versus intravenous immune globulin for the treatment of acute immune thrombocytopenic purpura in children: a systematic review and meta-analysis of randomized controlled trials. *J Pediatr*, 2005. **147**(4): p. 521–527.

47 Altuntas, F., *et al.* Intravenous gamma globulin is effective as an urgent treatment in Brucella-induced severe thrombocytopenic purpura. *Am J Hematol*, 2005. **80**(3): p. 204–206.

48 Arzouk, N., *et al.* Parvovirus B19-induced anemia in renal transplantation: a role for rHuEPO in resistance to classical treatment. *Transpl Int*, 2006. **19**(2): p. 166–169.

49 Aries, P.M., B. Hellmich, and W.L. Gross. Intravenous immunoglobulin therapy in vasculitis: speculation or evidence? *Clin Rev Allergy Immunol*, 2005. **29**(3): p. 237–245.

50 Shahar, E. Current therapeutic options in severe guillain-barre syndrome. *Clin Neuropharmacol*, 2006. **29**(1): p. 45–51.

51 Gajdos, P., *et al.* Treatment of myasthenia gravis exacerbation with intravenous immunoglobulin: a randomized double-blind clinical trial. *Arch Neurol*, 2005. **62**(11): p. 1689–1693.

52 Haas, J., M. Maas-Enriquez, and H.P. Hartung. Intravenous immunoglobulins in the treatment of relapsing remitting multiple sclerosis—results of a retrospective multicenter observational study over five years. *Mult Scler*, 2005. **11**(5): p. 562–567.

53 Mydlarski, P.R., N. Mittmann, and N.H. Shear. Intravenous immunoglobulin: use in dermatology. *Skin Therapy Lett*, 2004. **9**(5): p. 1–6.

54 Sarmiento, E., *et al.* Hypogammaglobulinemia after heart transplantation: use of intravenous immunoglobulin replacement therapy in relapsing CMV disease. *Int Immunopharmacol*, 2005. **5**(1): p. 97–101.

55 Ibernon, M., *et al.* Therapy with plasmapheresis and intravenous immunoglobulin for acute humoral rejection in kidney transplantation. *Transplant Proc*, 2005. **37**(9): p. 3743–3745.

56 Ahmed, A.R. Use of intravenous immunoglobulin therapy in autoimmune blistering diseases. *Int Immunopharmacol*, 2006. **6**(4): p. 557–578.

57 French, L.E., J.T. Trent, and F.A. Kerdel. Use of intravenous immunoglobulin in toxic epidermal necrolysis and Stevens–Johnson syndrome: our current understanding. *Int Immunopharmacol*, 2006. **6**(4): p. 543–549.

58 Faye, O. and J.C. Roujeau. Treatment of epidermal necrolysis with high-dose intravenous immunoglobulins (IV Ig): clinical experience to date. *Drugs*, 2005. **65**(15): p. 2085–2090.

59 McPherson, S., *et al.* Intravenous immunoglobulin for the treatment of severe, refractory, and recurrent clostridium difficile diarrhea. *Dis Colon Rectum*, March 15, 2006.

60 Zhang, Z., *et al.* Purification of severe acute respiratory syndrome hyperimmune globulins for intravenous injection from convalescent plasma. *Transfusion*, 2005. **45**(7): p. 1160–1164.

61 Kruger, M. European hepatitis B immunoglobulin trials: prevention of recurrent hepatitis B after liver transplantation. *Clin Transplant*, 2000. **14**(Suppl 2): p. 14–19.

62 Hankins, D.G. and J.A. Rosekrans. Overview, prevention, and treatment of rabies. *Mayo Clin Proc*, 2004. **79**(5): p. 671–676.

63 Arnon, S.S., *et al.* Human botulism immune globulin for the treatment of infant botulism. *N Engl J Med*, 2006. **354**(5): p. 462–471.

64 Gonzalez Andres, V.L. Systematic review of the effectiveness and indications of antidigoxin antibodies in the treatment of digitalis intoxication. *Rev Esp Cardiol*, 2000. **53**(1): p. 49–58.

65 Nuchpraryoon, I. and P. Garner. Interventions for preventing reactions to snake antivenom. *Cochrane Database Syst Rev*, 2000. (2): p. CD002153.

66 Boyer, L.V., S.A. Seifert, and J.S. Cain. Recurrence phenomena after immunoglobulin therapy for snake envenomations: Part 2. Guidelines for clinical management with crotaline Fab antivenom. *Ann Emerg Med*, 2001. **37**(2): p. 196–201.

67 Dart, R.C. and J. McNally. Efficacy, safety, and use of snake antivenoms in the United States. *Ann Emerg Med*, 2001. **37**(2): p. 181–188.

68 Cheng, A.C. and K.D. Winkel. Antivenom efficacy, safety and availability: measuring smoke. *Med J Aust*, 2004. **180**(1): p. 5–6.

69 Gawarammana, I.B., *et al.* Parallel infusion of hydrocortisone ± chlorpheniramine bolus injection to prevent acute adverse reactions to antivenom for snakebites. *Med J Aust*, 2004. **180**(1): p. 20–23.

70 LoVecchio, F., *et al.* Serum sickness following administration of Antivenin (Crotalidae) Polyvalent in 181 cases of presumed rattlesnake envenomation. *Wilderness Environ Med*, 2003. **14**(4): p. 220–221.

71 White, J. Snake venoms and coagulopathy. *Toxicon*, 2005. **45**(8): p. 951–967.

72 Laing, G.D., *et al*. A new Pan African polyspecific antivenom developed in response to the antivenom crisis in Africa. *Toxicon*, 2003. **42**(1): p. 35–41.

73 Ellis, R.M., *et al*. A double-blind, randomized trial of intravenous versus intramuscular antivenom for red-back spider envenoming. *Emerg Med Australas*, 2005. **17**(2): p. 152–156.

74 Chaves, F., *et al*. Intramuscular administration of antivenoms in experimental envenomation by Bothrops asper: comparison between Fab and IgG. *Toxicon*, 2003. **41**(2): p. 237–244.

75 Fung Kee Fung, K. Prevention of Rh alloimmunization: are we there yet? *J Obstet Gynaecol Can*, 2003. **25**(9): p. 716–719.

76 Shad, A.T., C.E. Gonzalez, and S.G. Sandler. Treatment of immune thrombocytopenic purpura in children: current concepts. *Paediatr Drugs*, 2005. **7**(5): p. 325–336.

77 Frachon, X., *et al*. Management options for dental extraction in hemophiliacs: a study of 55 extractions (2000–2002). *Oral Surg Oral Med Oral Pathol Oral Radiol Endod*, 2005. **99**(3): p. 270–275.

78 Berntrop, E. Die Auswirkungen einer Substitutionstherapie auf das Immunsystem von Blutern. *Hämostaseology*, 1994. p. 74–80.

79 Sultan, Y. High purity factor VIII concentrates for the treatment of HIV-positive patients with haemophilia. *Blood Coagul Fibrinolysis*, 1995. **6**(Suppl 2): p. S80–S81.

80 United Kingdom Haemophilia Centre Doctors Organisation (UKHCDO). Guidelines on the selection and use of therapeutic products to treat haemophilia and other hereditary bleeding disorders. *Haemophilia*, 2003. **9**: (1–23).

81 Mueller-Eckhardt, C. and V. Kiefel. *Transfusionsmedizin*, 3rd edn. Springer-Verlag, Heidelberg, 2004.

82 Mathews, V., *et al*. Surgery for hemophilia in developing countries. *Semin Thromb Hemost*, 2005. **31**(5): p. 538–543.

83 Stobart, K., A. Iorio, and J.K. Wu. Clotting factor concentrates given to prevent bleeding and bleeding-related complications in people with hemophilia A or B. *Cochrane Database Syst Rev*, 2005. (2): p. CD003429.

84 Rodriguez-Merchan, E.C., *et al*. Elective orthopaedic surgery for inhibitor patients. *Haemophilia*, 2003. **9**(5): p. 625–631.

85 Shapiro, A. Inhibitor treatment: state of the art. *Dis Mon*, 2003. **49**(1): p. 22–38.

86 Holme, P.A., F. Brosstad, and G.E. Tjonnfjord. Acquired haemophilia: management of bleeds and immune therapy to eradicate autoantibodies. *Haemophilia*, 2005. **11**(5): p. 510–515.

87 Goudemand, J., *et al*. Pharmacokinetic studies on Wilfactin, a von Willebrand factor concentrate with a low factor VIII content treated with three virus-inactivation/removal methods. *J Thromb Haemost*, 2005. **3**(10): p. 2219–2227.

88 Federici, A.B. Management of von Willebrand disease with factor VIII/von Willebrand factor concentrates: results from current studies and surveys. *Blood Coagul Fibrinolysis*, 2005. **16**(Suppl 1): p. S17–S21.

89 Lipkind, H.S., *et al*. Acquired von Willebrand disease: management of labor and delivery with intravenous dexamethasone, continuous factor concentrate, and immunoglobulin infusion. *Am J Obstet Gynecol*, 2005. **192**(6): p. 2067–2070.

90 Berntorp, E. and P. Petrini. Long-term prophylaxis in von Willebrand disease. *Blood Coagul Fibrinolysis*, 2005. **16**(Suppl 1): p. S23–S26.

91 Mannucci, P.M. Management of von Willebrand disease in developing countries. *Semin Thromb Hemost*, 2005. **31**(5): p. 602–609.

92 Alperin, J.B. Coagulopathy caused by vitamin K deficiency in critically ill, hospitalized patients. *JAMA*, 1987. **258**(14): p. 1916–1919.

93 Yasaka, M., *et al*. Optimal dose of prothrombin complex concentrate for acute reversal of oral anticoagulation. *Thromb Res*, 2005. **115**(6): p. 455–459.

94 Makris, M., *et al*. Emergency oral anticoagulant reversal: the relative efficacy of infusions of fresh frozen plasma and clotting factor concentrate on correction of the coagulopathy. *Thromb Haemost*, 1997. **77**(3): p. 477–480.

95 van Aart, L., *et al*. Individualized dosing regimen for prothrombin complex concentrate more effective than standard treatment in the reversal of oral anticoagulant therapy: an open, prospective randomized controlled trial. *Thromb Res*, September 20, 2005.

96 Foster, P.A. A perspective on the use of FVIII concentrates and cryoprecipitate prophylactically in surgery or therapeutically in severe bleeds in patients with von Willebrand disease unresponsive to DDAVP: results of an international survey. On behalf of the Subcommittee on von Willebrand Factor of the Scientific and Standardization Committee of the ISTH. *Thromb Haemost*, 1995. **74**(5): p. 1370–1378.

97 Coppola, A., *et al*. Long-term prophylaxis with intermediate-purity factor VIII concentrate (Haemate P) in a patient with type 3 von Willebrand disease and recurrent gastrointestinal bleeding. *Haemophilia*, 2006. **12**(1): p. 90–94.

98 Galan, A.M., *et al*. Concentrates containing factor IX could improve haemostasis under conditions of thrombocytopenia: studies in an in vitro model. *Vox Sang*, 2002. **82**(3): p. 113–118.

99 Mundy, C.A. Intravenous immunoglobulin in the management of hemolytic disease of the newborn. *Neonatal Netw*, 2005. **24**(6): p. 17–24.

100 Bowden, C.A. and E.P. Krenzelok. Clinical applications of commonly used contemporary antidotes. A US perspective. *Drug Saf*, 1997. **16**(1): p. 9–47.

101 Theakston, R.D. An objective approach to antivenom therapy and assessment of first-aid measures in snake bite. *Ann Trop Med Parasitol*, 1997. **91**(7): p. 857–865.

102 Petite, J. Viper bites: treat or ignore? Review of a series of 99 patients bitten by Vipera aspis in an alpine Swiss area. *Swiss Med Wkly*, 2005. **135**(41–42): p. 618–625.

103 Sorensen, B. and J. Ingerslev. Tailoring haemostatic treatment to patient requirements—an update on monitoring haemostatic response using thrombelastography. *Haemophilia*, 2005. **11**(Suppl 1): p. 1–6.

104 Samolyk, K.A., S.R. Beckmann, and R.C. Bissinger. A new practical technique to reduce allogeneic blood exposure and hospital costs while preserving clotting factors after cardiopulmonary bypass: the Hemobag. *Perfusion*, 2005. **20**(6): p. 343–349.

105 Borzio, M., *et al*. A simple method for ascites concentration and reinfusion. *Dig Dis Sci*, 1995. **40**(5): p. 1054–1059.

106 Bae, D.K., *et al*. Total knee arthroplasty in hemophilic arthropathy of the knee. *J Arthroplasty*, 2005. **20**(5): p. 664–668.

107 Debrix, I., *et al*. Clinical practice guidelines for the use of albumin: results of a drug use evaluation in a Paris hospital. Tenon Hospital Paris. *Pharm World Sci*, 1999. **21**(1): p. 11–16.

108 Salomon, O., *et al*. Plasma replacement therapy during labor is not mandatory for women with severe factor XI deficiency. *Blood Coagul Fibrinolysis*, 2005. **16**(1): p. 37–41.

109 Rojnuckarin, P., *et al*. A randomized, double-blind, placebo-controlled trial of antivenom for local effects of green pit viper bites. *Trans R Soc Trop Med Hyg*, 2006.

110 Heard, K., G.F. O'Malley, and R.C. Dart. Antivenom therapy in the Americas. *Drugs*, 1999. **58**(1): p. 5–15.

111 Camilleri, C., *et al*. Conservative management of delayed, multicomponent coagulopathy following rattlesnake envenomation. *Clin Toxicol (Phila)*, 2005. **43**(3): p. 201–206.

112 Jelinek, G.A., *et al*. FFP after brown snake envenoming: think twice. *Anaesth Intensive Care*, 2005. **33**(4): p. 542–543.

113 Jelinek, G.A., *et al*. The effect of adjunctive fresh frozen plasma administration on coagulation parameters and survival in a canine model of antivenom-treated brown snake envenoming. *Anaesth Intensive Care*, 2005. **33**(1): p. 36–40.

114 Morfini, M., A. Messori, and G. Longo. Factor VIII pharmacokinetics: intermittent infusion versus continuous infusion. *Blood Coagul Fibrinolysis*, 1996. **7**(Suppl 1): p. S11–S14.

115 Batorova, A. and U. Martinowitz. Continuous infusion of coagulation factors. *Haemophilia*, 2002. **8**(3): p. 170–177.

116 Agarwal, R., *et al*. Low dose of snake antivenom is as effective as high dose in patients with severe neurotoxic snake envenoming. *Emerg Med J*, 2005. **22**(6): p. 397–399.

117 Starkel, P., *et al*. Response to an experimental HBV vaccine permits withdrawal of HBIg prophylaxis in fulminant and selected chronic HBV-infected liver graft recipients. *Liver Transpl*, 2005. **11**(10): p. 1228–1234.

118 Boylan, J.F., *et al*. Tranexamic acid reduces blood loss, transfusion requirements, and coagulation factor use in primary orthotopic liver transplantation. *Anesthesiology*, 1996. **85**(5): p. 1043–1048; discussion 30A–31A.

119 Marcel, R.J., *et al*. Continuous small-dose aprotinin controls fibrinolysis during orthotopic liver transplantation. *Anesth Analg*, 1996. **82**(6): p. 1122–1125.

120 Varga, M., *et al*. Comparing cytomegalovirus prophylaxis in renal transplantation: single center experience. *Transpl Infect Dis*, 2005. **7**(2): p. 63–67.

121 Carbonare, C.B., S.B. Carbonare, and M.M. Carneiro-Sampaio. Secretory immunoglobulin A obtained from pooled human colostrum and milk for oral passive immunization. *Pediatr Allergy Immunol*, 2005. **16**(7): p. 574–581.

122 Delgado, A.V. and J.C. Sanders. A simple technique to reduce epistaxis and nasopharyngeal trauma during nasotracheal intubation in a child with factor IX deficiency having dental restoration. *Anesth Analg*, 2004. **99**(4): p. 1056–1057, table of contents.

123 Kumagai, K., *et al*. Perioperative management of a patient with purpura fulminans syndrome due to protein C deficiency. *Can J Anaesth*, 2001. **48**(11): p. 1070–1074.

124 Mauz-Korholz, C., *et al*. Management of severe chronic thrombocytopenia in von Willebrand's disease type 2B. *Arch Dis Child*, 1998. **78**(3): p. 257–260.

20 Law, ethics, religion, and blood management

Decision making is, at times, difficult, all the more so when human lives are at stake. Having principles and laws aids in decision making. This chapter deals with principles and laws needed to make sound decisions in blood management. It will consider blood management from three different angles: the ethical, the legal, and the religious angle. All three aspects are interwoven and must be taken into account before decisions are made.

Objectives of this chapter

1 Relate basic principles of ethics and law pertaining to blood management.
2 Be able to list points that need to be kept in mind caring for a Jehovah's Witness patient.
3 Tell how a compassionate use protocol is instituted.

Definitions

Ethics: is the practice of making principled choices between right and wrong, or, as Webster's dictionary put it in 1913, the "science of human duty" or "the body of rules or duty drawn from this science."

Medical ethics determines the principles of proper professional conduct concerning the rights and duties of the physicians, patients, and fellow practitioners, as well as the physician's actions in the care of patients and interaction with their families.

Patients' rights: Patients' rights are fundamental claims of patients, as expressed in statutes and declarations, or generally accepted moral principles.

Compassionate use: Compassionate use (= single patient IND, single patient access) means providing an investigational new drug (IND) to a patient on humanitarian grounds before the drug has received official approval, when the patient would otherwise not qualify or cannot enter the clinical trial.

Principles as a basis for decision making in blood management

A body of principles and regulations governs everyday decision making in medicine, and quite a few of them relate also to blood management. Picturing these as a pyramid (Fig. 20.1), we see that one set of principles and regulations builds on another one. The very basis for these regulations is found in the Holy Scriptures, as I. Taylor wrote: "The completeness and consistency of its morality is the peculiar praise of the ethics which the Bible has taught." Building on the Bible's teachings and the in-built human conscience, ethics developed which—as a science—describes human duties. As a subset of such ethics, human rights were determined and eventually formulated in writing. Human rights obviously apply also in humans who are sick. Their rights, namely, patients' rights, are based on human rights and specify these to apply in the situation sick persons find themselves in. Charters and bills dealing with patients' rights go another step further and give detailed guidance. As such, they are a help for governmental and nongovernmental institutions to integrate patients' rights into their legislation or codes by adjusting them to the unique situation in the country or their field of work, respectively.

The pyramid can also be considered from top to bottom. Quite a few principles may not be adequately incorporated in the law of a country, yet deserve consideration. A look into charters or bills of patients' rights may help, and, if not available or applicable, basic human rights or principles of ethics and religion may apply.

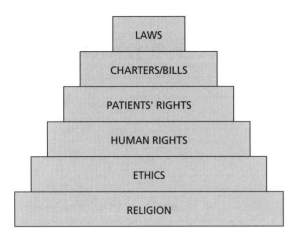

Fig 20.1 Pyramid of principles.

Principles of bioethics

Many ethical principles apply to the medical field. Among them are autonomy, veracity, fidelity, right to know, beneficence, and justice. The *Belmont Report* [1], formulated in 1979, summarized them as the three "basic ethical principles," being respect for person, beneficence, and justice.

Principle of respect for persons

Respect for persons is expressed in two distinct ways: accepting the autonomy of humans and protecting those who cannot act fully autonomously.

"Autonomy, the moral right to choose and follow one's own plan of life and action, is a deeply embedded and dominant element in western culture, law, ethics, and medicine" [2]. Respecting this autonomy in medicine means that patients are allowed to voice their opinions and choices and to accept them unless they are outrightly detrimental to others. This includes that the patients are given the chance to articulate their decisions intentionally, without controlling influences and with the needed knowledge. Before a medical intervention is started, an informed consent must be obtained whenever possible. When an informed consent is not available, it must be ruled what to do now to uphold the respect for person. There are three different ways to determine what the patient wants. The most common is to accept what the patient said before he/she became unconscious (subjective standard). If this is not known, persons who know the patient well can tell about the patient's values and what he/she

had said in the past. Judgment can be rendered according to this information (substituted judgment standard). If all this is not available, it is assumed what the patient would have wanted if he/she had the chance to decide.

Accepting the autonomy of a patient is based on the assumption that a patient is capable to self-determine. When this capability is wholly or in part lacking, the patients are still entitled to full respect. They must be protected from harming themselves or others, but apart from this, they must be allowed to follow their plan of life to the extent possible in their limited capability. Respect for persons also requires asking permission of other parties who are legitimate substitute decision makers for the patient.

Principle of beneficence

The principle of beneficence is the obligation of a physician to benefit the patient. In addition, the Hippocratic maxim "primum nihil nocere" (first, do no harm; nonmaleficence) is also expression of the principle of beneficence. Nonmaleficence means that no needless harm is administered intentionally.

Unless in an emergency, the physician usually has the right to decide whom he/she has a duty to and whom not; that is, whom he/she takes as a patient and whom not. Sometimes, a physician has the legal duty to take all patients and can refuse to do so only if his/her conscience is violated. The latter may be the case when a physician has a contract with governmental agencies that provide health care for the public. However, no matter how the physician entered a patient–physician relationship, it is always his/her duty to adhere to the principle of beneficence.

To act in an ethical manner, procedures performed in blood management must benefit the patient and must avoid any undue harm. How does this look in reality? Well, studies are urgently needed to evaluate the benefits of transfusions. There is a solid body of evidence that methods like cell salvage and acute normovolemic hemodilution as well as many drugs are able to reduce patients' exposure to donor blood, something regarded to be of benefit to the patient. When such methods and drugs are used with skill, their side effects are usually mild. The benefit of avoiding exposure to donor blood seems to exceed the harm possibly caused. To use such methods and drugs therefore seems to be ethical.

What about the benefits of allogeneic transfusions? Despite decades of medical transfusions and the well-entrenched belief that allogeneic transfusions are beneficial, most contemporary transfusion practices are not based on solid evidence. It is known that untreated, severe anemia increases mortality. However, it is unclear whether the correction of anemia by transfusion lowers mortality rates. There is an obvious lack of evidence that allogeneic transfusions benefit the patient. In contrast, there is overwhelming evidence that such transfusions cause harm to the recipient. With currently available evidence, it is questionable whether donor blood transfusions meet the criteria for an ethical intervention.

Principle of justice

The principle of justice describes the fair distribution of the goods in a society as the allocation of scarce resources. It also means that nothing good is withheld from a person who has a right to receive it or to impose undue burden to patients.

Sometimes, it has been called unjust when patients request therapy other than allogeneic transfusion. It was proposed that such patients should pay for any expenses incurred by the choice of other therapeutic options. However, this view was abandoned. Personal choices affect and sometimes increase the risks persons take. As an example, smoking increases the risk of certain diseases. Nevertheless, the expense of the treatment of smoking-related diseases are usually covered by governmental health care. Besides, nobody would ask a patient to pay for the transfusion only because it may, in the long run, be more expensive than nonblood management. The consensus is therefore as follows: Patients who refuse allogeneic transfusions on personal reasons or who want to use alternative treatment are not held liable for any costs that incur for the choice made [3]. Blood management, whether it includes the use of allogeneic blood products or not, must be made available to all patients. It is perfectly just to offer several therapeutic options to patients and to let the patients have the final say on what they want to use.

Human rights and patients' rights

Based on basic ethical principles, human rights were formulated. In 1945, when the members of the United Nations signed the Charter of the United Nations, they declared their faith in such human rights. The official UN Declaration of Human Rights was finally signed in 1948. It includes the right for health care. Patients' rights as a subset of human rights were declared parallel to the declaration of human rights.

The human rights movement gave impetus to the development of patients' rights. Another driving factor for

this was the fact that medicine turned into a business, with patients as its customers. Thus, consumer rights also played a role in the definition of patients' rights. In 1962, US president Kennedy identified consumer rights when he voiced a proclamation before the US Congress and identified the rights of safety, information, choice, and voice. Over the years, consumer rights were expanded to include other rights such as patients' rights.

Derived from basic human as well as consumer rights, patients' rights were formulated by organizations such as the WHO and Consumers International. Patients' rights include

- the right to health care
- access to information
- choice
- participation
- dignity and human care
- confidentiality
- complaints and redress

Such expressions of patients' rights are general and are considered basic. They are thought to be valid for all humans on earth. So, no matter where you live or under which legislation you practice medicine, you are always obliged to keep up the universal patients' rights.

Charters, bills, and laws

With an increased recognition of patients' rights, many governments and nongovernment organizations included such in their body of regulations. Various international organizations drafted bills and charters to aid in decision making in specific countries. The European Charter of Patients Rights (the Nice Charter of Fundamental Rights) [4], the Declaration on the Promotion of Patients' Rights in Europe, (Amsterdam, 1994), the Ljubljana Charter on Reforming Health Care (1996), the Jakarta Declaration on Health Promotion into the 21st Century (1997) are examples. These help to develop laws that suit the countries needs. Charters, policy-related documents recommending minimum standards for patient care, are the basis for nongovernmental organizations to develop patients' rights documents. In contrast, bills are considered to be for governments and are the basis for drafting laws.

On the basis of charters and bills, governments enacted laws focusing on patients' rights. In 1992, Finland became the first country to enact such law. The Netherlands followed in 1995. By November 2003, only Denmark, Finland, France, Greece, Ireland, Israel, Italy, Lithuania,

Malaysia, Portugal, San Marino, South Africa, Spain, Sweden, Switzerland, Vietnam, the United Kingdom, and Uruguay have enacted patients' laws [5].

Taking The Nice Charter of Fundamental Rights as an example, it can be seen that there are accepted principles that also pertain to blood management. The Charter "affirms a series of inalienable, universal rights (...). These rights transcend citizenship, attaching to a person as such. They exist even when national laws do not provide for their protection." Fourteen rights of patients were formulated. The 3rd right (right to information) supports the ethical principle of informed consent. "Health care services, providers and professionals have to provide patient-tailored information, particularly taking into account the religious, ethnic or linguistic specificities of the patient" [4]. The 4th right (right to consent) states: "Every individual has the right of access to all information that might enable him or her to actively participate in the decisions regarding his or her health." After being informed, the patient can either consent (4th right) or refuse (5th right; right of free choice). Especially interesting is the 10th right (right to innovation): "Each individual has the right of access to innovative procedures, including diagnostic procedures, according to international standards." The 12th right is the right to personalized treatment: "Each individual has the right to diagnostic or therapeutic programs tailored as much as possible to his or her personal needs. The health services must guarantee, to this end, flexible programs, oriented as much as possible to the individual." In the following, we will go into detail regarding the application of these principles into blood management.

Charters, bills, and laws concerning blood management

For a decision in blood management to be ethical, humane, and legal, certain criteria need to be met. In the following, we define and explain important legal and ethical concepts pertaining to blood management. Understanding these concepts aids in making the required principled decisions.

Informed consent

An informed consent is an expression of patient autonomy, and adhering to it is paramount for upholding this autonomy.

A valid informed consent [6] comprises four elements: (1) Consent must be given voluntarily, (2) the patient must have capacity (adults are assumed to be competent until proven otherwise), (3) consent must be specific (to the treatment and provider of the treatment), and (4) consent must be informed.

The duty of a physician is to inform his/her patient. The extent of information about a medical procedure should be proportional to its risks and its degree of invasiveness. It is commonly held that prescribing an aspirin requires an informed consent, too, but it is not as extensive as the informed consent for liver transplantation. Blood is not a drug as is aspirin. The transfusion of blood is more akin to the transplantation of an organ. Furthermore, the informed public is concerned about the risks of transfusions. Informed consent for a blood transfusion is therefore required to be fairly extensive. To this end, many hospitals provide printed consent forms, not for aspirin, but for blood transfusions and other invasive measures [7].

Recommendations were given about the contents of the information given to a patient prior to surgery. The information should include the following:

- To describe the recommended therapy, be it a transfusion or a measure to reduce the transfusion likelihood and anemia tolerance or tolerance of a coagulopathy.
- The risks and benefits, especially those that lead to death or serious impairment.
- Possible alternatives to the proposed procedure with their risks and benefits. In our case, this means measures to reduce the likelihood of receiving allogeneic blood.
- What would happen if no treatment is administered at all?
- The probability of success of the intervention.
- The length of recuperation.
- Other important information.

Some countries enacted laws that describe the content of the information the patients should receive before they can decide about transfusions in their health-care plan. For instance, §13(1) of the German Transfusion Act forces physicians to inform patients about the possibility of autologous transfusions. Similar legislation exists in other countries, such as in some states of the Unites States. With regard to an informed consent, a physician can be held liable if he/she does not inform the patient properly, if he/she does not obtain consent, or if he/she acts contrary to what the patient consented to or refused.

It was established that a patient must be informed as early as possible about the chance of receiving a transfusion. At least 24 h must be allowed in between the information about the transfusion and the actual transfusion whenever possible. This would give the chance to decide without time pressure. In case of an emergency, the 24-h time cannot be allotted and the patient has to decide within a short period.

The goal of informed consent is not just to have someone make a decision about his/her medical care. It is not a "legal bulwark to be contested over and used to mark the boundaries of liability and choice" [8]. Adherence to the principle of informed consent is more than a formalistic approach to patient authority. An informed consent is to honor the patients' wishes. It includes the right to "say no without censure or sanction" [8]. On the part of the physician, it requires not to consciously or unconsciously manipulate and coerce patients to achieve a desired medical end [8]. If it is done, it would betray the trust and dignity of the patient.

If an informed consent cannot be obtained, as in the case of an emergency, a physician has the privilege to treat the patient without consent. Such a situation arises when the patient's life or health is endangered, the patient cannot give consent, and there is no substitute decision maker (such as a person who is permitted to give legal substitute consent or an advance directive).

The competent adult has the right to refuse treatment. When the patient has lost consciousness or is otherwise unable to decide for him-/herself, a guardian or a court order is often obtained. In a life-endangering emergency, the physician has to assume what the patient's will is. An emergency does not allow for extensive evaluation of the patient's wishes. In such situations physicians are required to do what is in the best interest of the patient. It is assumed that it is in the patient's best interest to keep him/her alive. Physicians are allowed to do the best they can to avert danger for life or health. Since transfusions are considered lifesaving, they are administered without hesitation unless there is reason to assume that the patient would decide differently (as he may have outlined in an advance directive).

Advance directive

An advance directive or a living will is the legal expression of a patient's wishes regarding health care. It is written to guarantee that the patient's wishes in regard to medical care, medication, and resuscitation are carried out when the patient is unable to communicate his/her desires. Sometimes the advance directive entails a power of attorney that gives someone decision-making powers upon the person's incompetence. Among others, decisions pertaining to blood transfusions are recorded in an advance directive. Countries differ with regard to the form of a valid advance directive. For practical reasons, the written form is preferred, sometimes signed by two witnesses or a solicitor.

Writing an advance directive is one thing, adhering to it is another. Paternalism has widely been replaced by an emphasis on patient participation, respect for autonomy, and quality of life and death [9]. However, difficulties arise when a patient is cognitively impaired. Health-care professionals often do not consult with the advance directive or tend to engage in "soft" paternalism by making decisions that they think are in the best interest of the patient. Nevertheless, advance directives are binding, no matter whether the physician agrees with its content or not. Many legislations have laws that guide the draft of advance directives, but few laws exist to enforce adherence to it. To avoid variations in the interpretation of advance directives caused by the ambiguity of terminology, physicians should encourage patients to clarify their wishes, whenever possible. This is especially important when an intervention is planned for.

Pregnancy and motherhood

A patient's right to refuse treatment was sometimes challenged when the person refusing blood was pregnant or had dependent children. The reason for the challenge was that children need care. It was assumed that the mother would die if she does not accept blood transfusions and would therefore abandon her children. Forcing the mother to accept blood was justified with the will to keep the mother alive for her to take care of the children. However, if there is someone willing to take care of the children (the father or another relative, a friend), the mother may be allowed by the court to exercise her right of autonomy to decide freely [10]. In many jurisdictions, maternal-fetal duties and rights are not well defined. However, the principle of autonomy is upheld in general and applies to pregnant women as well. Physicians are not obliged to seek a court order to force a pregnant woman to take a blood transfusion. The ethical tenets of the American Medical Association and the American College of Obstetricians and Gynecologists even discourage such action [11].

Minors

Patients' rights are also applicable to minors. However, parental care and decision substitutes for the informed consent of the patient. Parents are responsible for their children. They are morally and legally obliged to take good care of them, providing them with the necessities of life as best as they can. To do this, they are endowed with the right to make decisions for their children. Many of the decisions parents make affect the well-being of their children. The bond between parents and children, ideally, is so tight that outsiders should refrain from intervening. In the great majority of cases, laws do not call for intervention even if the children's well-being is obviously endangered. This is the case where children have to live with smoking parents or when parents verbally abuse or divorce each other. However, when parental decisions outrightly violate the well-being of their children, the principle of *parens patriae* kicks in. This means that the state has the duty to assume a father-role for the child and protect it from harm.

The principle of *parens patriae* also applies in situations where physicians participate in blood management [12]. It was at times claimed that refusing a transfusion for their child constitutes an abuse of parental rights or neglect. Nonetheless, when parents demonstrate that they are willing to accept treatment and look for the best possible care without blood, they take considerable pains to help their child in accordance with their values. "Refusal of one form of treatment in preference for a viable alternative is exercising the parental right of informed choice, not neglect" [13]. In the United States, the legal view that parents have the right to decide for their child was upheld in many cases. For instance, the Banks case (Supreme Court, 1994) confirmed that unless there is an emergency that calls for the immediate transfusion of blood, a physician is not allowed to overrule parental refusal of a blood transfusion.

To speak in practical terms, what should be done to avoid morally, ethically, and legally questionable treatment of minors when parents refuse transfusions? A series of steps were proposed. In most cases, conflicts can be settled with adherence to these suggestions [13]:

1 Ask yourself: "Does a truly life-threatening emergency actually exist?"
2 Review nonblood medical alternatives and treat the patient without using allogeneic blood.
3 If needed, consult with other doctors experienced in nonblood alternative management and treat without using allogeneic blood.
4 If necessary, transfer the patient to a cooperative doctor or facility before the patient's condition deteriorates.
5 Have the outcome uncertainties, the medical risks, and the emotional trauma of a forced blood transfusion been fully considered? Has proper respect been shown for the parents' choice of treatment?

In case of a serious conflict, physicians and families should seek consultative assistance. Only in rare circumstances should judicial determination be sought.

Young minors are not capable to give an informed consent. An exemption is made with minors that are mature enough to give consent. Some legislation recognizes the term mature minor or an equivalent of it. Persons may be minors under law since they did not pass the age threshold set by the government to be considered an adult. However, also adolescents and even children are able to decide on their health. If they are mature enough to decide, their wish should be taken into consideration and respected.

The mature minor rule was created as a result of a 1967 court case, "Smith v. Selby." It allows health-care providers to treat youth as adults, based upon an assessment and documentation of the young person's maturity. The mature minor rule enables the provider to ask the young person questions in order to determine whether or not the minor has the maturity to provide his/her own consent for treatment. Guidelines for an individual to be considered a mature minor include: age, living apart from parents or guardian, maturity, intelligence, economic independence, experience (general conduct of an adult?), and marital status. The age guideline does not provide a certain lower limit. Treating both 13- and 14-year-olds as mature minors when they demonstrate key qualities of the mature minor is reasonable. Treating youths who are of age 12 and younger is up to the provider's best judgment.

Excursus: the physician and his/her conscience

When patients make use of their right for autonomy, they may at times decide differently than a health-care provider would. In the setting of blood management, such situations arise, for instance, when Jehovah's Witnesses opt against an allogeneic transfusion. Feelings such as guilt, frustration, and anger may arise on the part of their health-care providers. "A patient's refusal of care alters routine understandings of beneficence and non-maleficence and complicates caregiver roles. Suddenly, giving a blood transfusion, a routine act of beneficence, has become an act of maleficence for the patient in question" [3]. How can physicians and other health-care providers continue when they feel they have difficulties accepting a patient's decision?

Here are some proposals how to handle one's conscience when there seems to be a clash of belief systems:
• From a legal point of view, physicians are allowed to refuse treatment (unless in an emergency). Said a journal: "The frustration and guilt that caregivers experience in such situations are justified and understandable, and there is always the alternative of requesting that the patient see

another caregiver who feels comfortable about providing care despite the patient's refusal of certain treatments" [3]. The early transfer of a patient to someone who can take the case is morally and ethically justified and often prevents further sequelae for the physician as well as for the patient.

• Understand that there is something worse than death. A nurse, caring for a patient refusing transfusion, commented: "I felt that she and the rest of the people in the church didn't view death as the worst thing... " [3].

• Try to understand why you feel the way you feel. Accepting death is often difficult. Said Martin McKneally: "Surgery is a warrior culture, whose practitioners are committed to battle heroically and physically against death and disease" [2]. If a physician defines his/her value by the extent he/she succeeds in fighting death, he/she often must be disappointed and frustrated, as one physician explains: "Even with full therapy, it wasn't very clear that this patient was going to be cured despite the best that we had to offer, but there was an opportunity for us to focus our frustration on an external factor" [3]. Make sure you do not project your own frustration about death upon your patient's.

• Change your perspective: "Were... (the patients) caregivers harming her by respecting her wishes? If one considers only her physical body, the answer is yes. However, if one considers the person that... (the patient) saw and understood herself to be, the answer is no" [3].

• Expand the compassion for your patient as a whole person. A nurse caring for a patient, who decided differently from how she would have decided, explained: "Understanding why she made her decisions and what they really meant helped us" [3].

• Learn about transfusions: Transfusions are not the panacea the media claim. A comparison of the risks and benefits of transfusions helps you to understand that you do not deprive/withhold something especially precious if you do not transfuse. On the contrary, you might even come to the conclusion that you do something good for the patient if you provide other therapeutic options.

• Learn about alternative treatments. There are many treatments you can offer your patient instead of transfusing him/her.

Jehovah's Witnesses

Medical and ethical issues arise when patients ask for a therapy that is different from the current standard of care. In the field of blood management, Jehovah's Witnesses are a vivid example of such issues. Considering how they think, what they believe, and what special care they require will help to broaden the mind. It serves as a model of how patient care can be individualized.

Jehovah's witnesses and their attitude toward medical care

Jehovah's Witnesses love and cherish life. They consider it holy, a gift from their God, which needs to be handled with care. Unhealthy practices such as the use of tobacco, recreational drugs, and excessive alcohol are prohibited by Biblical principles. Overeating, risky hobbies, and a sedentary lifestyle are discouraged, while a healthy, balanced diet, moderate physical exercise, and personal hygiene are encouraged. When it comes to health care, Jehovah's Witnesses are encouraged to make a conscientious decision. Most matters of health care are subject to personal choice, among them organ donation, organ transplant including bone marrow transplant, and contraception.

However, when blood is concerned, Jehovah's Witnesses adhere to the Biblical command to "keep abstaining from blood." They consider blood being as holy as life itself. For a Jehovah's Witness patient, it is more important to adhere to the Biblical command—not to take blood—than having the chance of temporary prolongation of life. Besides, Jehovah's Witnesses consider a friendship with God a precious good and a violation of this relationship by disobedience to Biblical laws a great loss. To better understand the strong feelings involved in transfusions, one may consider the context of one of the Biblical commands to keep abstaining from blood. The same paragraph also outlines that Christians are to keep abstaining from adultery. Forced adultery, namely rape, is a severe insult to a person and leaves scars that may last for the rest of the life. The person may even not be able to continue as she did before. In the same manner, forced blood transfusion is a severe insult on the integrity of a Jehovah's Witness and leaves scars similar to that in severity of rape.

Jehovah's Witnesses do not take in blood, neither by mouth nor parenterally. This, however, does not mean that they refuse all medical treatment. As a group, they simply refrain from the use of blood and do not accept blood transfusions. When Jehovah's Witnesses refuse transfusions, they do not claim the "right to die" but ask to be treated with other therapeutic options.

What the physician has to do

Open-minded physicians hold that treatment is successful only if a patient is holistically treated with his/her unique physical, social, and spiritual requirements. Taking the religion of a patient into consideration is one aspect of successful treatment. Jehovah's Witnesses are entitled to have this principle applied in their health care as well. When Jehovah's Witness patients refuse conventional treatment with donor blood, physicians are called upon to tailor an individual treatment concept for the patient. This starts with an understanding of the patient's wishes.

Jehovah's Witnesses use a certain terminology that helps them to express their wishes regarding the use of blood in their treatment. The word "blood" in the Biblical command to "keep abstaining from blood" is interpreted as being whole blood or one of the four main components of blood, namely, plasma, red cells, white cells, and platelets. These are refused by all Jehovah's Witnesses who adhere to Bible teachings. All products made of these four main components of human blood are called fractions. Among them are proteins taken from plasma (such as coagulation factors, albumin, immunoglobulins), red cells (such as hemoglobin solutions), and platelets (such as products for wound healing). Whether a Jehovah's Witness considers such fractions to be blood or to be no blood is a matter of his/her conscience: "When it comes to fractions of any of the primary components, each Christian, after careful and prayerful meditation, must conscientiously decide for himself" [14].

Another term frequently used in connection with the care of Jehovah's Witness patients is that of a "closed circuit." According to the Biblical rule that blood that has left the body is to be discarded (Leviticus 17:13)—neither donor blood nor patient's own blood is to be transfused if it has left the body and has been stored (as in the case of preoperative autologous donation). Some patients allow physicians to use autologous blood in the course of surgery or another treatment. So it may be possible to salvage blood from a wound, irradiate it, and give it back immediately. Often, though, patients require that blood may only be retransfused if it did not leave their body entirely. It is then possible to use the patient's blood if certain conditions are met, namely, that the patient's blood is always in contact with the body via tubing. Again, it is the patient's own conscience which decides whether blood has left the body, once it has been taken through tubes or not. One Jehovah's Witness may decide it has left the body and will not allow the physician to give it back. Others have decided the blood has not left the body and consider the tubing being an extension of the circulation. A prerequisite of the latter group of patients is that the blood is in constant contact with the body (via tubing), a setup which is called a closed circuit (Fig. 20.2). If the tubing is disconnected from the patient, the blood cannot be given back. Some details of the definition of a closed circuit are

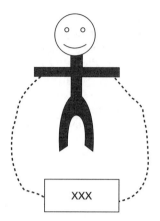

Fig 20.2 Model of a closed circuit: As an extension of the vasculature, tubing is connected to the patient. A device (the with "XXX" marked box) is included in the circuit. This device may be equipment for dialysis, cell salvage, oxygenation (heart–lung machine), or apheresis.

again a matter of conscience. For one Jehovah's Witness a dialysis is a closed circuit since the blood virtually goes through a circuit and does not stop; that is, it is not stored outside the body. Others accept also a cell saver, although the blood is not in continuous flow. They argue that the continuous flow is not required since a cardiac arrest also does not make blood unacceptable although the blood flow stopped temporarily. This sounds a bit confusing. However, simple communication between physicians and the patients often is enough to understand the issues that are important to a patient. Being asked about the use of a patient's own blood, the governing body of Jehovah's Witnesses summarized the issue as follows: "The details may vary, and new procedures, treatments, and tests will certainly be developed. It is not our place to analyze each variation and render a decision. A Christian must decide for himself how his own blood will be handled in the course of a surgical procedure, medical test, or current therapy. Ahead of time, he should obtain from the doctor or technician the facts about what might be done with his blood during the procedure. Then he must decide according to what his conscience permits" [15].

The above-mentioned points need to be taken into consideration when one cares for a Jehovah's Witness patient (compare Table 20.1). To obtain an informed consent, the patient needs to be informed about the different possible uses of blood products. It is prudent to explain to the patient all fractions and all ways to use the patient's own blood. Although being extraordinarily well informed about the use of blood in medicine, most Jehovah's

Table 20.1 Jehovah's Witnesses and their attitude toward blood.

What is never accepted
  Whole blood
  Red cells
  White cells
  Platelets
  Plasma
  Blood that has been stored outside the body (e.g.,
      for preoperative autologous donation)
What is accepted by some and not by others (so-called matters
      of conscience)
  Fractions
  Albumin (as volume substitute or as part of drugs)
  Sera, e.g., for vaccination, rhesus incompatibility
  Immunoglobulins
  Hemoglobin-based solutions
  Coagulation factor concentrates, e.g., factor VIII,
      factor IX, AT III, cryoprecipitate
  Plasma protein solutions
  Fibrin
  Glues containing blood derivatives
  Bone marrow, stem cells
  Methods, with or without a closed circuit
  Heart–lung machine
  Extracorporeal oxygenation
  Dialysis (e.g., CVVH), hemofiltration
  Cell salvage, with or without irradiation
  Perioperative platelet and plasma apheresis
  Acute normovolemic hemodilution
What is accepted
  Crystalloids, colloids
  Erythropoietin
  Recombinant clotting factors
  Perfluorocarbons
  Surgical devices to achieve hemostasis
  And many more

CVVH, continuous veno-venous hemofiltration.

Witnesses are medical laymen. The physician should explain clearly what products derived from blood are available and how the patient's blood is used. It is wise to have all patients fill in a form as to what is acceptable to them and what not. A patient presenting for the treatment of pneumonia, for instance, should be informed about such issues in the same manner as a patient who presents for a coronary artery bypass graft. Knowing the patient's opinion is extremely helpful if an emergency arises that allows no time for an in-depth evaluation of the patient's wishes.

Knowing the patient's opinion regarding the use of his/her own blood often enables a physician to adapt procedures to make them acceptable to the patient. One example is a cell-saving device. Usually, blood is sucked from the surgical field and collected in a container. If there is enough blood to be recycled, the cell saver is set up, the blood is processed, and given back to the patient. Some Jehovah's Witness patients may object to this procedure since it includes what they consider storage of blood outside the body. However, if the cell saver is set up right before the operation starts and its tubing is connected to the patient prior to use, it may be acceptable to the patient. In like manner, other procedures can be adapted to the wishes of Jehovah's Witnesses (such as acute normovolemic hemodilution). Doing this is ethical, preserves patients rights, and widens the array of methods that the patient allows the physician to use.

Patient and physician support organized by Jehovah's Witnesses

Jehovah's Witnesses are interested in the best possible medical care. Their refusal of allogeneic transfusions, however, challenges physicians to look for the best possible care without the use of donor blood. Jehovah's Witnesses support physicians in their endeavor to do that. The Watchtower Society, the legal entity of Jehovah's Witnesses, has instituted several services that are actively involved in issues pertaining to transfusions. First and foremost, they support the patient and his/her family to receive appropriate medical care and psychological support while they heed their Bible-trained conscience, forbidding donor blood transfusions. Secondly, they support health-care providers with valuable information regarding medical care without blood and facilitate communication between the patient, the physician, nurses, etc. To achieve these goals, several organizations were launched.

Jehovah's Witnesses initiative in the field of blood management is spearheaded by the Hospital Information Services (HIS). Its center is in Brooklyn, New York, the world headquarter of the Watchtower Society. Many branch offices of Jehovah's Witnesses throughout the world host an HIS as well. HIS collects and provides information on transfusion-free management. They have a huge collection of articles form the medical literature and keep it updated and filed. On mouse-click, they are able to come up with information about how to treat a specific disease or how to perform a certain procedure without donor blood. The information can be retrieved within minutes and mailed or faxed to physicians who are looking for the appropriate treatment of a Jehovah's Witness.

The HIS is also versed in legal and ethical issues pertaining to the refusal of transfusions. Under certain circumstances, lawyers can be asked to help in case a legal dispute arises.

Besides, the HIS keeps a record of physicians who are willing to treat Jehovah's Witness patients without blood transfusions. Throughout the world there exist specialists who can take care of the Jehovah's Witnesses. Upon request, Jehovah's Witness patients are provided with addresses of such cooperative physicians. This helps in preventing problems that may arise when Jehovah's Witnesses are treated by physicians who are not able or willing to treat without donor blood.

Another responsibility of the HIS is to coordinate the so-called Hospital Liaison Committees (HLC). These operate on a regional level. Members of Jehovah's Witnesses are especially trained to perform the tasks assigned to the HLC. The HLC keeps direct contact with the physicians in the region where the HLC operates. During regular visits they search for physicians who are able and willing to treat Jehovah's Witness patients. Current information on transfusion-free management is provided. It is their aim to inform physicians and help them understand the Jehovah's Witnesses' position. HLCs are the link between patients, physicians, and the HIS. They take good care of Jehovah's Witnesses who are sick, visit them, and support them in their way through the health-care system.

Another group of Jehovah's Witnesses belong to the so-called patient-visiting group (PVG). Whether transfusions are involved or not, the PVG visits patients who are hospitalized in the facility the PVG is assigned to. Typically, a congregation of Jehovah's Witnesses close to the hospital provides the members of the PVG responsible for that very hospital. Among the PVGs goals is to visit the patients, bear them company, comfort and encourage them, do pastoral work, and help them with things needed, such as providing literature to read. It is their aim to make the patients comfortable and ensure them that they are members of a loving brotherhood.

Compassionate use

As learned before, according to the Nice Charter of Fundamental Rights, patients have the right to innovation. This includes the use of new drugs if they promise to be beneficial. At times it may even seem useful to provide a patient with a drug that is not approved yet. The terms compassionate use, single patient IND, or single patient access

Table 20.2 FDA protocol: physician request for a single patient IND for compassionate or emergency use.

Send a facsimile with a letter to follow. Include the following:
1 A formal written request for a single patient IND for compassionate or emergency use should be made.
2 Provide the clinical history of the patient, his treatment and response to treatment, as well as the reason for requesting the proposed treatment.
3 Outline a treatment plan with dosage, duration, and route of administration of the drug, etc. Provide literature which supports your intent.
4 Add a Drug Supply Reference Statement, naming the supplier or manufacturer of the drug and a statement that a letter of authorization to cross-reference an appropriate IND of the supplier or Drug Master File of the manufacturer is included.
5 Informed Consent Statement (state that an informed consent and the approval of an ethics committee will be obtained before initiating the therapy).
6 Curriculum vitae of the treating physician (to demonstrate his/her qualification).
7 FDA Form 1571 (treating physician listed as sponsor).
8 Contact phone and fax.

were coined to describe the process of getting permission to use a drug that is not approved yet.

In the United States, the Food and Drug Administration (FDA) is responsible for compassionate use protocols. When a physician would like to use an unapproved drug for a single patient, he/she has to follow the protocol set up by the FDA. First, the physician must ask the manufacturer for permission to use the drug and to provide the product. Then, the official protocol of the FDA has to be followed (compare Table 20.2).

If the request is approved, an IND number will be issued by the FDA, and the treating physician will be contacted by phone or fax, with a letter to follow. The IND is considered active upon issuance of the number. The IND sponsor, that is, the treating physician, will then contact the drug supplier and provide the IND number. The supplier may then ship the drug directly to the treating physician.

For further information, compare the FDA home page (www.fda.gov).

Key points

• Upholding the ethical principle of autonomy by adherence to informed consent and advance directives is the sine qua non of medical ethics.

- To balance the ethical principles of beneficence and non-maleficence, a comprehensive evaluation of the benefits and risks of transfusions and means to reduce patient's exposure to donor blood is required.
- The care of Jehovah's Witness patients poses medical and ethical challenges to the team of health-care providers. Meeting these challenges enhances the performance of the team and spurs on the development of new methods in blood management.
- The compassionate use of a nonapproved drug is ethically justified under specific circumstances. In the United States, the FDA is the board to be contacted for the initiation of a compassionate use protocol.

Questions for review

- Which ethical principles govern medical decision making?
- How are patients' rights defined?
- What is a mature minor and how can he/she contribute to decisions regarding his/her therapy?
- What special considerations are needed when treating patients who are Jehovah's Witnesses?

Suggestions for further research

Who is responsible for patients' rights? Is there a patients' right movement in your country? Do they do anything pertaining to blood management?

Homework

Learn about the legal situation of transfusions and transfusion avoidance in your country. Is there a law or a guideline on how to formulate an advance directive, a power of attorney, or a living will that is related to blood management? What is the required form of such? Are there any aids available, such as brochures, checklists? If so, get them and file them.

Is there any legal rule how a patient needs to be informed about blood management options? What information needs to be included? Is there a minimum time required after information of the patient before he/she should receive a transfusion?

Is there a law in your country that upholds patients' rights? Have there been a series of court cases that ruled

about matters of blood management? If so, get some information on it. If there is a law, try to get the original paragraphs, read them, and file them.

Contact the nearest HLC of Jehovah's Witnesses and record their contact information in the address book in the Appendix E. Ask them to explain their work and service. Also ask for the name, address, and contact phone of the PVG.

Find out how to prescribe a drug that is still in experimental status/not approved. Pay particular attention to the way a compassionate use protocol is set up in your institution.

Ask the following questions:

Who is entitled to institute such a compassionate use protocol? Record the address of the agency in your address book.

Whom do you have to contact? (Address?)

How long does it take to get permission in an emergency?

What formalities do you have to fulfill?

References

1 National Commission for the Protection of Human Subjects of Biomedical and Behavioral Research. *The Belmont Report: Ethical Principles and Guidelines for the Protection of Human Subjects of Research.* Department of Health, Education, and Welfare, 1979.
2 McKneally, M.F. Witnessing death as lifesaving treatment is withheld. *Ann Thorac Surg,* 2002. **74**(5): p. 1430–1431; discussion 1432–1433.
3 Knuti, K.A., *et al.* Faith, identity, and leukemia: when blood products are not an option. *Oncologist,* 2002. **7**(4): p. 371–380.
4 Cittadinanzattiva-Active Citizenship Network Group, Cotturi, G., *et al. European Charter of Patients Rights. Basis Document.* Rome, 2002.
5 Rider, M.E. and C.J. Makela. A comparative analysis of patients' rights: an international perspective. *Int J Consumer Studies,* 2003. **27**(4): p. 302–315.
6 Grainger, B., E. Margolese, and E. Partington. Legal and ethical considerations in blood transfusion. *Can Med Assoc J,* 1997. **156**(Suppl 11): p. S50–S54.
7 Goldman, E.B. Legal considerations for allogeneic blood transfusion. *Am J Surg,* 1995. **170**(6, A Suppl): p. 27S–31S.
8 Guinn, D.E. Honor the patient's wishes. *Ann Thorac Surg,* 2002. **74**(5): p. 1431–1432; discussion 1432–1433.
9 Thompson, T., R. Barbour, and L. Schwartz. Adherence to advance directives in critical care decision making: vignette study. *BMJ,* 2003. **327**(7422): p. 1011.
10 Gyamfi, C., M.M. Gyamfi, and R.L. Berkowitz. Ethical and medicolegal considerations in the obstetric care of a

Jehovah's Witness. *Obstet Gynecol*, 2003. **102**(1): p. 173–180.

11 Levy, J.K. Jehovah's Witnesses, pregnancy, and blood transfusions: a paradigm for the autonomy rights of all pregnant women. *J Law Med Ethics*, 1999. **27**(2): p. 171–189.

12 Jones, J.W., L.B. McCullough, and B.W. Richman. A surgeon's obligation to a Jehovah's Witness child. *Internal Med J*, 2003. **33**: p. 362–364.

13 Ariga, T. and S. Hayasaki. Medical, legal and ethical considerations concerning the choice of bloodless medicine by Jehovah's Witnesses. *Leg Med (Tokyo)*, 2003. **5**(Suppl 1): p. S72–S75.

14 Watch Tower Bible and Tract Society of New York. The Watchtower, 2004. **125**(12): p. 29–31.

15 Watch Tower Bible and Tract Society of New York. *The Watchtower*, 2000. (October 15): p. 30.

21 Step by step to an organized blood management program

Blood management is a multimodal, multidisciplinary team approach whose aim to improve patient outcome. It is driven by the philosophy that the patient is the center of attention. Blood management is best implemented within the framework of an organized and recognized program. In this chapter, help is given to assemble all the different elements of blood management into an organized program. The needed background information is provided as are the management tools.

Objectives of this chapter

1 List ten steps that will lead to implementation of a blood management program.
2 Identify ways to educate and train different groups in blood management.
3 Acquire management skills essential for running a blood management program.

Definitions

Program: A system of services created to meet a public need, involving a series of steps that have to be carried out or goals to be achieved.
Marketing: Communicating information, an idea, product, or service in order to encourage sharing, purchase, or use of it by others. It consists of a group of activities designed to find out what customers want (market research), to increase customer awareness, and to attract them to the object being marketed; planning and executing a concept in order to meet customers' needs.
Education: It includes all activities revolving around teaching or instructing, aimed at imparting knowledge or skills.

Why take the trouble to organize a blood management program?

Arranging for and keeping order requires energy. Since this is true also for the order needed to organize blood management, you might ask why you should invest your energy in such an endeavor. Well, an organized blood management program is well worth the effort. Successfully implemented, a program will result in the establishment of a competence center for blood management, offering a holistic care program for patients. It will provide the ideal skill mix of well-educated and trained up-to-date health-care providers, needed to manage patients' blood effectively. In such a center, the experience gained over time will translate into improved patient outcomes [1]. A blood management program will win new patients for the hospital, reduce overall treatment costs, and help eliminate the adverse effects associated with transfusions. Patient and health-care provider satisfaction will increase. Surely, these are more than enough reasons to start an organized blood management program.

Who can take the initiative to start an organized blood management program?

Once the idea that a blood management program would be a valuable asset to a hospital has been hatched, who should initiate the program? The best approach is to start from within the institution [2], meaning that someone already working with the hospital—usually an influential physician—should spearhead the program. It is certainly true that a successful program is driven by internal forces. However, history shows that many programs have not been initially started in this manner. Often, nurses, nursing coordinators, individual Jehovah's Witnesses, or others initiated development of the program. In recent times, consultants or companies in the consulting field have offered to initiate a program. These support the hospital from outside and contribute their expertise. Hospitals can hire consultants to support the hospital's own efforts to launch a program. Among the advantages of hiring a company is that external consultants can address "hot" issues with much more ease than physicians who have to be careful about internal hospital politics. This may mean that the program can progress faster than otherwise. Further, external consultants devote their whole day to program development and are not distracted by daily clinical activities. In addition, they may bring the needed expertise required to tailor the program to the needs of the hospital. They are usually acquainted with time-proven concepts, can easily implement them, and have access to forms, computer programs, agendas, statistics, and methods that may be difficult for the hospital to obtain.

Finally, *who* starts the program is not so important, as long as a program *is* started. If there are no physicians willing to adopt the program, then most probably not even the hospital administration or the head of the most influential department can bring about the needed philosophical changes. However, if resourceful department heads or others are available who see the potential of the program, implementation is possible even if proposed by a less influential person.

Step 1: information and education of the initiator

You as the initiator of a blood management program need to acquire the necessary knowledge and compile information about general and specific blood-management-related issues. The right motivation is also required to start a blood management program because it must be sufficient to overcome the initial hurdles that have to be cleared.

Several ways of gathering the needed information are feasible. If available, consulting a dedicated program of education on blood management would be the easiest source. Such a program has been developed in Canada as part of a provincial program for blood conservation (The Ontario Transfusion Coordinators) [3]. If such education is unavailable, self-education is warranted. There is more than enough educational material available. Pertinent journals and blood-management-related books and brochures are good sources of information. More informal, yet very practical education can be gained at blood management conferences, before and after dedicated lectures and during visits to existing blood management programs. There are several Web sites that provide information about blood-management-related issues and several societies that provide information and serve as a conduit for information exchange (see Appendix B for detailed information).

Another field in which you as the initiator of the program need to acquire knowledge is the specific situation of the hospital. This is best done by performing a structured initial analysis (as shown in Appendix C). In the initial analysis, hospital-specific information is gathered about the patient population, established blood management measures, the current use of blood, the financial implications of these issues, and about the personnel and their willingness and ability to adopt blood management. Information about the hospital also includes the area it serves, its market share, other blood management programs in the vicinity, and a comparison with local competitors. Information about funding opportunities is also beneficial. In addition, forces and interests outside the hospital that may help or hamper establishment of a blood management program should be known. Such an initial analysis performed in the early stages of a blood management program forms the basis for future activities. If the initial analysis identifies aspects that seem to indicate that the program cannot be implemented successfully, it may still be possible to choose another hospital to implement the program.

After educating yourselves about blood management, you are equipped to work toward instituting an organized blood management program. A continuous source of motivation is required so that you do not tire out in your efforts. Early on, join others who are engaged in the same kind of project. This can be done by joining blood management forums on the Internet, any of the many societies, or by regularly communicating with colleagues who share the same commitment.

Step 1: How to proceed:

• Learn as much about blood management in general as possible.
• Perform an initial analysis of the hospital you want to work with.
• Arrange for occasions that provide ongoing motivation for you.

Step 2: your business plan

Now that the information has been gathered and sufficient motivation is available to start a blood management program, make specific plans. Put them down in a form that can be presented orally as well as in writing; the latter will be the business plan [4].

An informal business proposal

When attempting to convince others to help found a blood management program, the informal format will most likely be chosen. Present your ideas orally and arrange your arguments well in order to win support. An oral presentation is best made before key individuals in the hospital where the program is to be initiated. It must be in a position to help further the program and may include high administrative staff (chief executive officer (CEO), marketing director, head of the financial department, etc.). Also, key clinical staff (heads of the various medical and surgical departments, head of nursing, chief of staff, quality assurance officer, etc.) should be invited. Persons with a keen interest in blood management may also be invited. Since it may be important for the administration to see how many key hospital staff are already willing to adopt a new approach, inviting both representatives of the administration and clinicians to a discussion may be beneficial. This may help identify the support (and resistance) the hospital administration (and you) will encounter in initiating the program. The presentation will probably have to be made several times to reach all those of importance in the hospital.

The purpose of such initial informal presentations is to establish your position as an authority in the field and to make the plan to establish a blood management program known to those invited. It is also the occasion to establish some important facts such as that blood management is better care and is beneficial to both, the patients and the hospital. Current hospital data (especially the cost and transfusion-use issues) and recent key publications should be available and presented to support the argument that proceeding with blood management is the course to be taken. After Step 1, pertinent information will be available from the fundamental analysis.

Use some visual aids to support the initial presentation. An overhead projector, slides, or handouts may be used to appeal to the audience. A sample outline for this initial presentation is to be found in Table 21.1. Further sample presentations can be downloaded from the Internet (e.g.,

Table 21.1 Sample outline for the first presentation.

Definition (and history) of blood management
Risks of transfusion
Benefits of a blood management program (for this very
    hospital, for the patients, physicians, etc.)
Cost issues of transfusion and blood management (general and
    hospital-specific)
Recommendation to go ahead with a blood management
    program—cite the next few steps and a time
    frame for them

from the home page of PNBC—Physicians and Nurses for Blood Conservation).

A formal business proposal

In addition to the informal presentation, it may be useful to prepare a formal written business plan. This plan serves several purposes. Initially, the most important purpose is to provide the hospital administration with answers to key questions. This information may well be the basis for their decision to support or to reject your proposal. The business plan is also a guide for you or others who want to start the blood management program. It may stake the claims, as it were, building the framework in which the blood management program will develop. A formal business proposal usually addresses those individuals who are empowered to make decisions. After receiving the proposal, they should be able to decide whether to permit you to start, and they should also be able to cooperate toward the funding of the project and afford the needed network access (business relations, introduction to the right people, introduce the program to further key persons). The written proposal, therefore, mainly addresses the hospital's administration.

A formal written business proposal can be designed in various formats. If the hospital makes a form available to employees for business proposals, this form could be used. If not, select your own format. Whatever format is chosen, keep the business proposal simple and concise and tailor its contents to the specific business context the hospital operates in.

The contents of the business proposal may vary, depending on the format. Refer to Appendix C that outlines different model structures for the written business plan. More model business plans can be found on the PNBC Web site (Appendix B) or can be obtained by simply asking colleagues at conferences or via Internet discussion platforms.

Table 21.2 Why do we need the program?

Efficacy of allogeneic transfusions not proven
Blood shortages
Current and future costs rising
Patient preference
Public concern
Liability
Need to improve clinical outcomes

No matter what format is chosen for the business proposal, some of the key features discussed below could be included.

Why do we need a blood management program?

The full scope of problems arising from unwarranted medical use of blood may not be realized by all in the hospital. They may also be unaware of the specific issues of the current and emerging transfusion-related situation the hospital finds itself in. In the introduction to the business plan, briefly explain the reasons why a move toward blood management is needed. After explaining the problems (see Table 21.2) [5], a statement could be made to the effect that the envisioned blood management program is the solution to the multiple problems surrounding use and misuse of blood.

**What can be anticipated if the blood
management program is implemented?**

General as well as hospital-specific data are required to illustrate the results expected from the program. The more hospital-specific data are included, the more trustworthy the projections. General information may include statistics on patient safety, liability issues, improved outcome, and patient satisfaction. Hospital-specific projections may include an increased market share, the number of patients expected to choose the hospital because of the blood management program, and the reduction of allogeneic transfusions. What may be even more impressive are data on how transfusion-related problems can be reduced, e.g., reduction of posttransfusion infection rates and a reduced length of stay.

Who will be served by the program?

It is prudent to answer the question of who initially will be served by the program directly in the formal business proposal. Although blood management is preferably mainstream medicine, for practical reasons, starting the program for a restricted population only may be better. This creates an environment in which the hospital staff can become comfortable with the new philosophies and techniques involved [6]. Later, further patient groups can be added. This makes the start easier and prevents the hospital being overwhelmed by a flood of patients presenting for blood management. Many hospitals have chosen to start with a program for Jehovah's Witnesses and have gradually added other patient groups until universal blood management is adopted finally for all patients. To begin with, other patient populations may be those treated in a single department or even just those undergoing a specific procedure (e.g., hip replacement) or suffering from a specific disease (e.g., sickle-cell patients). Refer to Step 9 for more information on how to choose where to start.

Can the success of the program be monitored?

Progress can be monitored by setting goals for the program. This may help not only the program to check progress and to adapt to challenges but also ensure the continuing support of the hospital administration. By mentioning what monitoring tools (Table 21.3) have been chosen, control of program success may be placed in the hands of the administration, making managers even more willing to start the program in the first place.

**What is the time frame in which the proposed
changes will be realized?**

It may take 3–5 years until the full benefit of a program is realized. The hospital administration should be aware of this. This will prevent coordinators from being pressured unduly when the expected goals are not met within several months.

Will the program be financially taxing?

Cost projections are often of interest to the hospital administration. Try to answer questions such as: How much do we have to invest? Is such investment worthwhile? What is the return on investment?

To answer the hospital administration's financial questions, prepare a rough estimate of the budgeted investment. It may be better to estimate the budget on the high side. Identify essential line-item expenses for operation of the program (compare Table 21.4). Typically, only costs directly related to the program are included in the budget. Other incidental costs are not included. The latter include costs for medical treatment, e.g., for

Table 21.3 Simple ways to monitor program progress.

Goal	Monitoring	Source of statistics
Reduce allogeneic transfusions	Units of blood used, procedures performed	Blood bank, transfusion meeting reports, hospital or departmental statistics of performed procedures, billing department
Increase patient share	Number of patients enrolled in program	Admission services, patient questionnaire regarding motivation to use the program
Increased patient satisfaction	Patient satisfaction score increases	Questionnaire
Reduced transfusion-associated infections	Number of infections, relation to transfusion, historical numbers of infections	Infection-tracking sheet, billing department, transfusion meeting reports
Reduced length of stay	Length of stay, in comparison with historical population or with population not in the blood management program	Admission services, billing department

blood-management-related drugs and autotransfusion. Such costs will arise, but are usually offset either by savings realized by reduced allogeneic blood use or are already included in the respective departmental budgets. Worth mentioning is that implementation of the program will shift savings and expenses within hospital budgets. For instance, blood bank costs will be reduced, but pharmacy costs may increase. Such shifts need not be calculated, but the administration should be informed as necessary.

In addition to making a budget, make a realistic estimate of the time frame involved and the financial goals to be reached. For instance, based on the initial analysis it may be estimated that costs can be saved by reducing the current transfusion rate by 20% within the next 3 years. Another way to project costs and revenue is to multiply the number

Table 21.4 Line-item budgeting.

Line item	Comment
Salaries of (full-time) program coordinators	When budgeting for several years, include increases in salaries.
Equipment	Includes office equipment only, since the medical-surgical equipment is usually covered by the budgets of the respective departments.
Staff education	Include costs for educating and training physicians, nurses, and ancillary staff; the coordinator's participation in national and international conferences, use of libraries, purchase of books and journals.
Management fees	To compensate medical directors or committee members for the hours they spend for the program.
Patient tracking and identification	The costs incurred depend on how patients are tracked and identified. Costs for computer specialists, printing of stickers, wristbands for patients, forms, and the like.
Marketing	It will be easier to budget marketing costs if the avenues to be used to market the program have been determined; include also costs for community education, clubs, etc.
Office costs	All the miscellaneous things needed to run the program, i.e., telephone, fax, mail, pagers, stationery, postage, printing of brochures, office rent, cleaning, etc.
Miscellaneous	Depending on the scope of the program, costs for research, data analysis, grants for patients (travel costs, accommodation of families, etc.) may have to be included.

of new patients by the average income per patient gained by the hospital. To do so, average the income over the last 3 or 6 months and divide this figure by the average number of patients treated during this period.

The method chosen to demonstrate the financial benefits of the program depends on the type of health system in which the hospital operates. Government runs hospitals with a fixed budget, and a mandate to care for the general public may not be interested in increasing patient load. Cost reductions and a reduction in the length of stay in the hospital might be more welcome. Other hospitals that are dependent on patients for income may be more concerned about increasing numbers of patient. Yet others receive income from various sources and may be interested in prestige rather than financial gain or another motive may be of more interest. Some background information about payment modes and sources of income may help in the choice of argument to convince the hospital administration that the program is lucrative. However, no matter how revenue is estimated, budget on the low side. This will make it easier to either meet or exceed the administration's expectations.

Who will put the program into practice?

The business proposal also has to address the issue of who will share the responsibilities within the program. Outlining the structure of the program as described in Step 5 will help the reader of the business plan to understand how the program will finally operate.

Step 2: How to proceed:

- Prepare an informal presentation using visual aids.
- Prepare a realistic budget and project hospital revenue.
- Write a formal business plan.

Step 3: get help: your champions

Professionals who have been successful in implementing a blood management program emphasize the necessity of having at least one champion to implement the program [7]. Champions are those health-care providers who work together with the initiator to achieve the goals. They are the locomotives of the venture. Champions are motivated to implement blood management or are at least make sure that reducing allogeneic transfusions is essential and per-

forming blood conservation is beneficial. Such champions are indispensable to change the behavior of health-care providers [8, 9] and to spread the philosophy of the program [6]. Champions are opinion leaders and serve as credible messengers to establish the program. They play a vital role in setting realistic goals, participating in the development, distribution and implementation of blood management guidelines, and in staff education.

Since champions are thus essential to the program, seek out such individuals. While working through this book and doing the homework, you have already contacted a variety of professionals who may be potential champions. Ideally, persons will be found who already practice blood management. There may be others who are convinced that changes are needed, but who are waiting for a little encouragement and support to translate their resolve for change into action by founding a blood management program. Champions are often found among anesthesiologists [3]; however, blood bank professionals, surgeons, or other professionals have given substantial support to blood management programs. Ask such professionals and offer to help them. They may be more than willing to provide support and do their share.

However, what if a suitable champion cannot be found? Then the initiator will have to create the champions. List those who may be suitable, preferably individuals in the top league, as it were—heads of departments, the CEO, or another person in a similar position. Others may also be recruited. A short guide on how to identify such individuals can be found in an article by Hiss published in 1978 [10].

Having identified potential champions, think about what may motivate them to change their opinion and practice methods. Usually, physicians are satisfied with the treatment they give; they claim to transfuse only if it is unavoidable and in any case they are the authorities when it comes to reducing transfusions. This is the common belief. Change it by benchmarking. Gather convincing data. The hardest data available are those associated with death or major morbidity. Maybe a comparison can be made between transfusion rates in the hospital and with rates in other hospitals. If possible, begin a small-scale study. The format given in Table B.1 could be used as the basis. After collecting the data, come up with some simple statistics. For instance, show how many red cell transfusions were given because of accepted transfusion guidelines, how many were given to patients initially presenting with anemia, or how many received transfusions mainly because of high intraoperative blood loss. Such transfusions can easily be avoided. Such simple mathematics may convince the potential champion or at least move him/her to give the program a try.

If all else fails, be your own champion. In time, you may be successful in recruiting further champions. For the time being continue by yourself. Remember that no effort, however small, goes unnoticed; so, even if a ful-fledged program cannot be implemented, do not give up. Everything takes time, even recruiting champions. Once physicians have had the chance to come to terms with blood management, then they will volunteer to be champions.

Step 3: How to proceed:

- If possible, find at least one champion, either by recruiting one or by creating one.
- If none is available initially, be your own champion.

Step 4: get more support—convince the hospital administration

No blood management program has ever been established and continued without the ongoing support of the hospital administration. It is usually the hospital administration that initiates the profound change needed in the hospital's philosophy regarding blood use. The hospital administration must fully advocate the intended changes, otherwise needed support is missing and the program will finally vanish. Therefore, a very important step in implementing a blood management program is to sell the program to the hospital administration [6].

In many cases, the hospital administration is represented by the CEO. The CEO is most likely confronted with new proposals every day, which, to the presenter, are very important. The CEO has now to be convinced of the importance of your program [2]. Putting yourselves into the CEO's shoes for a moment will help understand what it may take to convince him. The CEO is responsible not only for monetary issues such as allocating limited resources, but also for patient safety, patient relations, litigation, public relations, ethical and political issues, distinguishing the hospital from competitors, etc. His/her ultimate goal is to keep the hospital running effectively. To convince the CEO, his/her concerns must be addressed in terms he/she can understand. The main aim should be to convince him/her that the program will contribute to keeping the hospital viable, now and in the future. Convey to the CEO what clear advantages result from adopting a blood management program. Be very specific using data pertinent to

the hospital. For a CEO to be convinced to invest money and time in the program, he/she has to see what the return on investment will be. Show how many patients it would take to recover the invested costs. Try to model some calculations that demonstrate the extent of savings achievable. Apart from cost issues, it may also be important to reassure the CEO that the program will not interfere with hospital politics. It may be beneficial to demonstrate to the CEO that there is already interest and support in the hospital, e.g., the heads of anesthesiology, hematology, blood bank, surgery, or other surgical specialties. It is therefore prudent to come up with some champions before approaching the CEO. However, where this is not possible, suggest to the CEO to address the issue as soon as possible to find out whether there is support among the physicians.

When you have convinced the hospital administration to implement the blood management program, ask for approval in writing. The administration may officially endorse your formal business plan or may want to create its own contract. Whatever the case, make sure that your responsibilities and authority are clearly delineated. Nothing is more frustrating than a lack of authority. If permission needs to be asked for every little detail, progress will be hampered and may even make the program futile. After receiving the hospital administration's approval, they could be asked to inform others about the program's implementation and to introduce you and your plan, stating what your responsibilities are and what authority you now have (e.g., by e-mail, hospital newsletter, by inviting staff to dinner, or by walking through the hospital with you and introducing you to the heads of departments). This will pave the way for further contact with hospital staff and win their cooperation.

Step 4: How to proceed:

- Identify those who represent the hospital administration.
- List points that may convince them to implement your blood management program.
- Sign a contract with the hospital for the implementation of the program.

Step 5: structure is essential: directors, coordinators, committees

Once the hospital administration finally approves the business proposal, the way is paved to begin the actual work of organizing the program. The first thing to be done is to structure the program. If a thoroughly planned business proposal is already available, this will serve as a guide through the next few months' work. Both a medical and an administrative structure need to be established and effective communication facilitated.

Medical structure

As shown by experience, the greatest benefit is drawn from a formal blood management program if it is physician-driven [4]. Therefore, there should be at least one physician—still better is a group of physicians taking the lead in medical matters (the champions). If just one physician is available, he/she can be appointed medical director. If more than one physician are available, a group of medical directors, a committee or working group, could be organized. Ideally, this group represents a variety of specialties. The physicians taking the lead will develop and implement the medical part of the program and will be instrumental in providing ongoing staff education and training. They will act as role models for other health-care providers in the program. The main task of the medical directors is clinical work, and only a small proportion of their time will be spent with administrative issues. They are the liaison between the program administration and the clinicians.

Another important task for the physicians taking the lead is to recruit a core team. All members of this core team must share a commitment to patient-centered blood management [11]. They must not only be willing but also capable of performing blood management, while treating patients. The members of this core team should include the champions, the physicians taking the lead in the program, and other physicians who are already trained or are prepared to be trained in blood management. This core team should present a suitable skill mix to offer multidisciplinary blood management. Typically, surgeons, anesthesiologists, internists, pediatricians, nursing staff, etc., are included. The names of members of the core team should be known to the administration of the blood management program so that patients wishing to use the services of the program can be referred to them. The core team members should also be well informed about the program's policies and procedures. It is advisable to have them sign a written agreement with the program, stating the rights and responsibilities of members of the core team. This may be necessary to ensure that patients wishing to benefit from a blood management service are treated according to the policies and procedures of the program. Such a written

agreement serves as the durable basis for the relationship between the program and physicians, and vice versa.

Administrative structure

The administrative part of the blood management program is essential to keep the program going. Probably the most important factor is the presence of at least one dedicated coordinator [3], because experience shows no program can develop without one. The coordinator is typically not a physician but is a member of senior nursing or technical staff or an otherwise dedicated individual with a background knowledge in blood management. He/she is essential to the daily affairs of the program [7]. His/her many responsibilities include development, organization, and supervision of program progress. The coordinator develops policies and procedures for the program, renders patient-specific decisions, gives support, assesses patients for blood management, serves as liaison between patients, physicians, the administration, and the public, organizes education and training, and collects data for quality management and research. The model job description for the coordinator can be found in Appendix C or in the literature [3]; this gives deeper insight into the many responsibilities of a blood management coordinator.

Facilitating communication

Since blood management is a team approach, communication among the members of the team is essential. Therefore, structuring a blood management program also includes paving the way for communication among all parties. These are the coordinator(s), the physicians who are the program leaders, core team members, other hospital staff who only indirectly contribute to the success of the program, and also the patients, their families, as well as the public. The lines of communication should always be open. To be practical, the blood management program should be located in an office within the hospital and the coordinator should be present. The regular business hours should be known to patients and staff alike. It should be possible to contact members of the blood management program in an emergency, e.g., during the night or at weekends. All these provisions facilitate communication.

Those taking the lead in the program must communicate regularly. It is wise to schedule regular meetings. This is especially important in the initial phases of program development. During such programmed meetings, the responsibilities of each single member of the steering group should be established. Regular meetings involving the committee of medical directors and the program's administrative personnel (the coordinator(s)) keep the lines of communication open. In addition, communication may be scheduled with other established committees, e.g., with the hospital transfusion committee, administration, public relations, nursing committees, and patient relation groups.

Step 5: How to proceed:

- Recruit medical directors for the program and get them to form a committee.
- Appoint at least one dedicated blood management coordinator.
- Identify a medical-surgical and nursing core team.
- Organize an in-hospital office for the coordinator.

Step 6: policies and procedures

Now that personnel have been recruited and the organizational background for the program has been set up, it is necessary to establish how these will work to fulfill the purposes of the program. This is determined in the policies and procedures that should now be developed. Since blood management is a multimodal approach [12] spanning the field of patient care—from first contact with the institution until completion of care—policies and procedures should mirror every modality of care [7]. The policies and procedures define acceptable and unacceptable care. They answer the question of how the program will benefit patients and how universal blood management will be established in the clinical routine. Policies and procedures are designed to finally shape the behavior of all parties participating in blood management [13].

Which policies and procedures are needed depends on the scope of the blood management program. If the program serves only the patients attending one department, only a limited set of policies and procedures is needed initially. For example, if at the beginning the program only applies to orthopedics, then the use of a cardiopulmonary bypass does not need to be addressed. If the program initially serves only one specific group of patients, then policies and procedures that are unacceptable may not be required (e.g., if the program is only for Jehovah's Witnesses, policies and procedures for preoperative autologous donation for storage are not needed).

Listing surgical and medical continua helps in getting an idea as to which policies and procedures need to be developed. Continua include all methods and approaches to patient blood management offered by the program, organized according to sequence of occurrence in medical care (e.g., preoperatively, intraoperatively, postoperatively). An example of a surgical continuum is found in Appendix C. Continua can be developed for elective procedures (e.g., in gynecology, orthopedics, urology), for emergencies, for polytraumatized patients, for intensive care of adults, for radiation and chemotherapy in cancer patients, for obstetrics, and for the premature, neonates, and other pediatric patients. To begin with and as an aid to the development of continua, some review articles list methods available for blood management [14–17].

Developing policies and procedures is no easy task; however, many sample policies and procedures are already available. Therefore, do not reinvent the wheel. First, use policies and procedures developed for your hospital. The initial analysis may show what policies and procedures are already available and need to be adapted or are still missing and need to be developed. Appendix B contains a list of published algorithms and guidelines. Refer to them to establish your own set of policies and procedures. A list of administrative, clinical, legal, and ethical guidelines that have been established by other blood management programs can be found in Appendix C.

Typically, administrative policies and procedures are developed by the coordinator in cooperation with the medical directors and the hospital administration. Medical policies and procedures are best developed by the coordinator, the group of champions, and steering physicians with an interest in blood management and with the pertinent nursing staff and technicians in cooperation. The legal department should assist with legal policies and procedures. Staff will be more than happy to ensure that pitfalls are avoided and will probably be able to give valuable advice. They may be concerned about the impact of the program on hospital litigation. If necessary, contact experienced lawyers or hospital administrations to convince the hospital's legal department that the blood management program is no threat to the hospital.

In time, policies and procedures will change, because they need to be adapted to program development and growth as well as to changing needs. During the initial development of policies and procedures select a format that is simple to modify, allowing for adding and deleting policies and procedures as needed. If the hospital has International Standards Organization (ISO) certification, contact a professional to help you to bring the program's policies and procedures in line with ISO requirements (this may be mandatory to receive funding). Lists of policies and procedures may not be all that is required; lists of those responsible and of the tools may be needed. Refer to Appendix C for a model format for a policy or procedure.

After the policies and procedures have been finalized, it is important to implement them. Initially, circulate them among those involved in the policy or procedure. Then the champions need to take the lead in putting them into practice. This requires hard work, frequent educational interventions, and encouragement.

Step 6: How to proceed:

- Develop medical and surgical continua pertinent to the program.
- Identify medical, administrative, and legal/ethical issues to be regulated by policies and procedures.
- Collect available policies and procedures, tapping either those currently applicable in the hospital or published in the literature.
- Develop a unique set of policies and procedures.

Step 7: education—preparation for life

Health-care practitioners' general knowledge about blood-management-related issues is surprisingly scant. Medical and nursing school curricula often omit blood-management- and transfusion-related issues. Even professionals who train in a dedicated fellowship-training program do not often learn much about the fundamentals of patient-centered blood management [18]. Further, use of autologous blood is infrequently taught, and in-depth knowledge must therefore not be assumed. Residents and young physicians in particular, those who typically carry the major clinical workload, do not know much about blood management. Therefore, when beginning a blood management program, most staff members need to enhance their knowledge and skills in blood management.

Specific educational interventions can be planned whose goal is to build a highly motivated, well-trained team of health-care practitioners sharing a commitment to blood management. Behavioral changes are initiated through education and encouragement, and in the end all participants in the blood management program practice according to their assigned role. This ideally results in improved patient outcomes. As research has demonstrated, improvement of blood-management-related behavior is

achievable by education [19, 20]. There is a strong association between knowledge of transfusion indications and their use in situations where they are considered appropriate [13]. Thorough education and training can substantially reduce the use of allogeneic blood components and encourage multifactoral use of blood conservation measures [21, 22]. Willingness to listen to counsel and actively seeking advice are also associated with a reduction in transfusions [13]. Therefore, educational interventions, encouragement, and fostering a spirit of mutual consultation are essential to establish and improve a blood management program.

Since education is an integral part of a blood management program, it is essential to know how to educate. Merely introducing guidelines or presenting a lecture about blood management will not change practice [23]. Forcing physicians to adhere to guidelines seldom wins their favor. How, then, can behaviors be changed? There is extensive research on this subject. Six general methods have been studied: education, feedback, participation of physicians in the effort to change, administrative interventions, financial incentives, and penalties [9]. Success in terms of changing the health-care provider's behavior or better patient outcome varies. Mere lectures or supplies of written material do not change physicians' behavior, unless the curriculum has been specially designed to effect change. Clinical guidelines do not automatically change behaviors. The reasons may be that guidelines are impractical, physicians may not trust guidelines or they ignore them, giving in to other influences such as financial constraints or incentives or fear of litigation. Guidelines only effect changes when they are distributed and endorsed by opinion leaders. Feedback may or may not be effective, depending on the circumstances. When physicians themselves recognize that their methods need improvement and prospective feedback is given at a time when physicians can change their behavior immediately (and not retrospectively), then feedback may be effective. In contrast, surprisingly effective in changing behavior is so-called academic detailing, an educational method involving an opinion leader talking to one person at a time. Including physicians in the change process is also very important to change. While in some instances outside pressure may change physicians' behavior (e.g., a law requiring quality assurance measures for autologous blood products), changes in practice are best started from within. Hence, educational interventions should place control in the hands of health-care personnel. Including health-care providers in the process of education would not undermine their authority or call their judgment into question, thus they do not feel threatened. Administrative efforts to enforce change are effective, but most should be used as a last resort. Financial incentives (e.g., payment by case) or penalties (being financially personally responsible for treatment) are very effective in changing physicians' behavior. Having said all this, no single method is inherently successful in changing behavior. A combination of methods seems to be better than a single method.

Who should receive education?

Since the success of a blood management program depends on each player, all participants in the program need to be educated. First of all, this would mean the blood management coordinator. This individual should be well informed initially and should keep up-to-date with current developments so as to remain an expert in blood management. The coordinator should be capable of speaking to physicians and other health-care providers as well as the hospital administration.

In addition to the coordinator, all champions, directors, and members of the core team should be educated and trained in blood management in relation to their specialty. If possible, they should have a better knowledge of blood management than the average health-care provider. Ideally, they should also know what other specialties contribute to the success of blood management. This will enable them to coordinate patient care across specialties.

Minimum levels of education and training should be defined for all other participants in the program (Table 21.5). However, these levels should not be unreasonably high so as not to deter potential participants, but rather they should be sufficiently demanding to ensure a good blood management service to patients. Education given to other persons in the program should focus on their role, specialty, and field of expertise.

Table 21.5 Whom to include in educational interventions.

- Physicians
- Nurses (including intensive care, anesthesia, and ward nurses)
- Students (medical and nursing)
- Laboratory personnel
- Blood bank professionals
- Visiting professionals
- Administration
- Ancillary staff, e.g., admission personnel
- Patients and family
- The public

Structured educational interventions

Maintaining the philosophy of universal blood management requires continuous education over years, and so planning is essential. Three steps are involved: (1) assessment of educational needs and wants, (2) defining the content of educational interventions, and (3) evaluation (that is, assessment of what the blood management team learnt and put into practice as a result).

Needs assessment

The goal of the needs assessment is to determine what the blood management team wants and needs to learn. A variety of methods can be used. The formal ones are surveys in written or oral form [24], questionnaires [25], and a literature search of pertinent information [26]. The informal ones include discussions in the hospital lounge, cafeteria, or at medical meetings, or simply, intuition. "Keeping one's ear to the ground or one's hand on the pulse of medical practice" [19] is essential. Another important way to identify educational content is by making a baseline review of current blood management practice. Using treatment policies and procedures which are to be implemented as the basis, an audit may help to identify how well current treatment conforms to such policies and procedures. For example, suppose it was planned that a cell salvage device be used in a certain type of procedure and hemodilution in another and that an antifibrinolytic would also be introduced. An audit may reveal that the cell salvage device and hemodilution are already being used where possible for the majority of eligible patients, but only a few patients receive the antifibrinolytic. Education on the use of the antifibrinolytic agent should, therefore, be given the highest priority. Such an audit needs to be done regularly and continuously throughout the lifetime of the blood management program to identify current educational needs.

To change behavior, it is also wise to ask why members of the blood management team behave in a manner perceived to be unacceptable. For example, a liberal transfusion practice often results from a lack of knowledge of the pathophysiology of anemia [19]. Nonimplementation of a cell-salvage device may be based on the belief that returning blood to the patient can often be detrimental. Avoidance of acute normovolemic hemodilution could be based on the understanding that it does not reduce allogeneic transfusions. Other reasons are fear of litigation or criticism for allowing a patient to continue with a low hemoglobin level. Further, some may understand that there are benefits inherent to allogeneic transfusions experienced by all patients and that transfusion risks are so small that they do not outweigh the benefits. Such misconceptions need to be removed.

Another obstacle to change of practice is anxiety. Seymour Handler, in his article "Does continuing medical education affect medical care: a study of improved transfusion practices" [19] summarized the situation experienced in blood management as follows: "Reduced hemoglobin values cause more symptoms in the attending physician than in the patient. . . . The surgeon's anxiety is translated into an order for blood transfusions. . . . Indeed, the major problem of postoperative anemia may be the surgeon's anxiety. . . . Studying massive surgical hemorrhage without blood replacement apparently requires more courage than most surgeons can muster." Apparently, there is a strong emotional component to blood management. To implement changes in the behavior of the blood management team, consideration should be given to the anxiety and timidity exhibited when changes in policy are proposed. Knowing about such misconceptions and anxieties can help those who are responsible to design appropriate educational interventions and motivation campaigns.

Content of education

The content of the education and training offered in the blood management program depends on the result of the needs assessment and on the target students. Make a list of the envisioned educational contents, prioritize them, and add a note about the target audience to help plan such interventions. Content is also best tailored to the current situation of the program. Initially, more basic education is needed; later, updates may be sufficient. Additional ad hoc interventions in response to challenges encountered or to highlight exemplary patient care may reinforce lessons learned in more formal, programmed training. Such patient-based discussions are the spice of the educational program.

In addition to medical issues, organizational issues may be the content of education, as well as team building concepts and communication.

Evaluation of education

The effects of the educational intervention should be evaluated to monitor progress, to spot weak points, and to adapt to developing needs. Several methods can be used to do so: (a) comparison of behavior before and after training, (b) comparison of performance and behavior in the hospital's program with that in other hospitals or programs, (c) comparison of professional behavior after training with that of those in the hospital who did not receive special training. Professionals who did not change their behavior in response to the educational intervention may thus be identified. There may be a problem that has not received due attention. When the situation is taken care of, the professional may be more than willing to comply with the contents of the training.

"Crucial prerequisites for success in postgraduate education include the voluntary participation and active learner involvement of resident and staff physicians, as well as the education program coordinator's respect for the resident's autonomy, familiarity with their already crowded educational agenda, and accommodation of their time-consuming professional commitments" [27]. Taking these points into consideration, put the educational plan down in writing. It could be included in the schedule that every new employee receives as part of the orientation; a brief introduction to blood management and an invitation to participate could also be included. At least one annual mandatory lecture on blood management could be scheduled for nursing staff, and invitations for blood management conferences could be posted on nurses' bulletin boards. Fixed dates for scheduled education and training should be set to ensure the highest possible participation of all involved in the blood management program and that no one is overlooked.

Educational methods and tools

There is a wide variety of educational methods to choose from [28] and they can all be used to teach blood management. The best results seem to be achieved by a combination of methods, depending on local circumstances, target audience, and manpower available.

Formal one-to-one education

Formal one-to-one education is a very effective means of changing the behavior of medical professionals. It is used by pharmaceutical companies in that they regularly send representatives to physicians who are potentially in a position to effect a change in practice. This type of intervention is time consuming, although a session rarely exceeds 90 minutes. It has been shown that even short 30-minute visits to surgeons increases the likelihood of their increasing the rate of autologous donations.

Formal one-to-one education may be scheduled as a brief visit of 30–90-minutes duration [29] for which preparation is needed. Defining the goal of the visit and the take-home messages (not too many) helps in arranging visits such that the goals are reached. Material needs to be gathered which supports the credibility of the source information presented. The pros and cons of the information presented need to be discussed, as do the benefits of the proposed change of behavior. Those visited should be encouraged to interact and to continue working with others in the blood management team. At the end of the session, the take-home messages should be repeated and the individual visited should be aware of the behavioral changes expected. Ideally, visual aids should be used and a short summary of the content discussed should be left with the visited person. Questions should be allowed and contact information for the visiting professional should be available after the visit.

An example of an outline for a formal one-to-one educational intervention can be found in Appendix C.

Informal one-to-one education

Situations for informal discussion of blood-management-related issues arise spontaneously. They arise at the bedside, in the canteen or lounge, in the hallways, after formal meetings, etc. It is up to those concerned to take advantage of such situations. The impact of such informal one-to-one education is difficult to study, but it seems to substantially influence the person contacted. In fact, informal one-to-one education is thought to be the most effective type of educational intervention [19].

Lectures and grand rounds

Most hospitals in the world arrange for regular lectures and grand rounds for professionals. Such educational interventions are either scheduled for the whole hospital or part of the in-service education of the various departments. Lectures have the advantage that many can be taught at one time, making them a relatively inexpensive type of education. However, the knowledge conveyed is limited and behavioral changes often do not occur. When lectures are used, they are best combined with other methods of education.

Conferences on blood management

Educational conferences dedicated to blood management are often of high quality. Most of the topics presented relate to blood management, making such conferences a very condensed form of education. They offer multiple opportunities to network with colleagues and discuss current topics of blood management as well as opportunities to ask questions, formally or informally. However, such conferences are often used only by individuals who are already interested in blood management. The high cost of participation and travel may preclude most of the staff from attending. A solution to this problem is to send one or two members of the team who on return present selected issues to all members of the team.

Daily clinical rounds

Patients who are candidates for a certain procedure (cell salvage, minimization of iatrogenic blood loss) or who are at high risk for transfusions can be visited daily by a trained member of the blood management team. Typically, a chart review is performed and the past day's therapy is discussed as well as the next steps in blood management. When deviations from established policies and procedures are observed, personnel attending to the patient can be instructed as needed [30]. However, this approach is time consuming, especially in the initial phase of establishing a program. However, it is very likely to be effective, and in time, staff will be alert to the treatment needed for blood management and only a few patient cases will need to be discussed.

Retrospective peer review and audit

In transfusion medicine, peer review processes and audits have proven valuable in reducing transfusions. In some hospitals, medical records personnel check transfusion forms retrospectively for compliance with transfusion guidelines [31]. Other hospitals describe an approach where blood bank pathologists review the indications for blood transfusions and provide a written or oral review to the physician who ordered the transfusion [20]. Regular chart review can provide valuable clues about blood management practice. Using and circulating the results of such reviews, educational interventions can be tailored explicitly to address the weak points identified.

Algorithms

No matter how well designed they are, policies and procedures are of no use if they are not implemented. A great deal of time needs to be invested in implementation. Algorithms can be an aid in doing this. Implementing them may include providing technical and organizational support (e.g., immediate availability of drugs and equipment, bedside monitoring), training, and initial guidance until the algorithm has been internalized by staff.

Prospective review of blood management practice

Reviewing transfusion decisions prospectively has been shown to reduce inappropriate transfusion behavior. Blood bank personnel required to check the indication before blood is issued can review every transfusion order prospectively. They may be able to withhold blood products or provide instant information on a more appropriate therapy. A mandatory pathology consultation has been established elsewhere before clotting factor concentrates were issued [32]. Using well-trained decision makers for the transfusion decision has reduced the use of the blood products.

Computer systems can also be used to double-check the transfusion order [33]. They can list accepted indications and alert the physician regarding any deviations from such. The computer system can utilize laboratory results, e.g., the latest hemoglobin value or the coagulation profile, to provide further support. Similarly, computers can be used to double-check the hematologic status of patients before booking of the operating room for elective procedures is permitted. A computer system can be used to double-check whether a patient gave informed consent for the scheduled procedure.

Self-educating documentation and order slips

Existing guidelines are often not translated into practice. Typically, published guidelines are buried in files or disappear in physicians' drawers. A convenient way to turn blood-related guidelines into practice is to design order sheets for blood management procedures, containing a short and simple form of procedure-related guidelines. Such a self-educating blood- or procedure request form is a simple administrative intervention that can reduce allogeneic transfusions [34] or can encourage adherence to policies and procedures.

Simply printing transfusion guidelines with information on acceptable and unacceptable transfusion practice on the blood request form forces the transfusing physician to read the guidelines. The front page of such a form might consist of fields to be filled in, depending on what blood product the physician plans to administer. If red cells are ordered, the fields may be the latest hemoglobin level, heart rate, blood pressure, and the presence of symptoms of anemia. The reason for the transfusion and the clinical situation (e.g., type of surgery) should be stated for all blood products. The institution's transfusion guidelines can be printed on the reverse side of the form. Mandatory completion of forms before blood is released has been instrumental in enforcing adherence to transfusion policies [20]. The beauty of this self-educating request form lies in its simplicity. No manpower is needed to instruct users, and it is well accepted, especially by junior medical staff. By reading the form, staff members instantly educate themselves. They may realize that their request does not comply with current guidelines, so they may refrain from asking for blood. Thus, they do not lose face, and therefore, this educational instrument may be well accepted.

In a similar manner to blood product request forms, request and documentation forms for blood-management-related procedures may be designed to support adherence to established guidelines. Documentation forms for autologous blood use may include inclusion and exclusion criteria, a checklist of the steps involved in performing the procedure, and mandatory fields to be filled in. Other forms may include the content of the informed consent process, the algorithm used to optimize a patient's hemoglobin level prior to surgery, the procedures to draw blood samples in patients at high risk for iatrogenic blood loss, and the schedule for preoperative assessment and optimization before elective surgery is performed (e.g., booking the operating room is possible only when the patient has reached at least minimum hemoglobin level).

Combining the form with an audit process further enhances the value of the educational intervention. Requests that do not comply with guidelines may have to be first cross-checked by a blood management specialist. The compiled request and documentation forms for each month may be audited by the blood management or transfusion committee.

Reading assignments and journal clubs

While reading assignments may be feasible only in the formal education setting, a journal club may make reading assignments acceptable for professionals. During a 1-hour session, one or a number of selected articles dealing with blood management can be discussed. Typically, journal club participants know in advance which articles are to be discussed and they are asked to read them before the meeting. A short presentation of the content is given to summarize the article and a discussion follows. A good communicator should be chosen to steer the discussion and to provide constructive feedback. Explicit learning objectives for each meeting together with a structured review and meeting process may contribute to the educational success of the journal club [35, 36]. When all participants are asked to contribute, they change from being passive listeners to active learners. This will help them to retain the content of the articles. Combining reading with a meal at each club meeting will make the journal club an even more pleasant experience and the opportunity to socialize may be a further incentive for participation.

Dedicated teaching programs

A very successful type of education is a specifically developed rotation, exclusively dedicated to blood management. This is a time- and resource-intensive endeavor, but seems to bring rich reward. Such a dedicated program typically includes seminars, attendance at transfusion meetings, research projects, reading assignments, dedicated lectures, hands-on experience in blood management techniques (in the laboratory and in the clinical setting), and acting as consultants for physicians and patients in the blood management program and it could conclude with formal graduation tests. Implementing such a dedicated teaching program needs much planning. The goals and objectives need to be outlined and staff need to be assigned to this program. A time period should be fixed for the participants of the program. For example, anesthesiology residents interested in transfusion issues were offered a 2-month rotation dedicated to transfusion medicine [37]. Similar programs have been designed in the field of bloodless health care and in blood management in general.

While such programs may, at first, seem hard to install, the benefits outweigh the disadvantages. Staff trained in such intensive programs are most likely dedicated and well trained in effective blood management. The program trainees are apt candidates for research projects. These projects can be designed to audit and substantially improve the hospital's blood management.

Use of educational tools

There are many educational tools. Per se, they do not educate but they provide help to teach. Educational tools can be distributed to persons who are motivated enough to use them themselves or the tools can be used in education and training by blood management teachers. In the latter case, they are only useful in combination with other educational interventions. Otherwise, they are ineffective in changing health-care provider practices.

CURRENT LITERATURE ARTICLES

Literature articles are valuable teaching tools. Therefore, the coordinator of the blood management program will want to stay up-to-date with the literature on blood management. Useful articles could be collected and distributed to others who want the information or need to have it. However, discretion is required and the choice should be selective. Flooding others with literature does not help. On the contrary, it may even make them reluctant to read articles that are especially important for them. Therefore, if the coordinator finds an interesting article about heart surgery, it should not be sent to the urologists and dermatologists in the program but rather should be reserved for the cardiac surgeons. Interesting literature may also be sent for reading in response to a recent case. If a team is confronted with a difficult case and there is something in the literature that might help design the patient's care plan, it should be sent to all team members. The team members may be more inclined to read the article despite their tight schedule because it appears to be beneficial.

VIDEOTAPES

In situations where many persons are to be taught, videotapes may be very useful [38]. A slide show running in parallel with a recorded tape explanation could be used as an alternative.

Often videos are commercially available. Companies selling medical equipment for blood management provide videos for free. If there is no video available to fit current educational needs, a video could even be produced by program staff. In teaching environments such as universities, there are often media centers that can aid in producing the video. If a practical topic is to be taught, e.g., cell salvage or patient identification, the one performing the procedure can be followed with a video camera and comments can be added. Photographs and computerized graphics may be used to supplement the educational content. If self-production of educational videos is not possible, commercial videos may be an adequate substitute.

Videos provide a uniform method of teaching. Since the video can be used on multiple occasions, persons working in different shifts, in different departments, and even in different hospitals can be taught using the same educational content. This may compensate for the efforts required to produce a video.

Although it might seem a good idea simply to send copies of the video to health-care providers and ask them to view it, it may be more practical to invite practitioners to prearranged video sessions. Health-care providers may be more inclined to watch the video—discussion of the educational contents will be promoted among the audience, and the number of persons who actually watched the video can be monitored.

SAMPLES OF EQUIPMENT OR DRUGS

Samples of equipment or drugs may be useful educational tools. They may be used to provide hands-on experience or it may be possible to simply ask a sales representative to bring in some drug samples and printed information. The drugs can be issued to health-care providers who are then asked to use them in practice. What may have greater educational value may be to arrange not only for samples but also for the assistance of a professional to demonstrate how the samples are used. For example, to introduce a tissue adhesive into practice, a sales representative might be willing to demonstrate how best to assemble the syringes, prepare the area where the adhesive is to be applied, apply the adhesive, and check its effectiveness. The representative may be able to provide some insider tips, making it easier for staff to use the product. Such an approach would help avoid suboptimal results with the adhesive; this in turn might lead to health-care providers becoming frustrated and abandoning a method which would have been beneficial had it been used properly.

If equipment is bought, health-care providers who are expected to use it will have to be trained in its use. If there are multiple options available and no decision has been made as to which brand is to be bought, why not borrow each model and ask those health-care providers concerned to try them out. Sales representatives, technicians, or health-care providers experienced in the use of the equipment should be available in the initial stages when new equipment is introduced. There are already educational guidelines available for some blood management techniques, e.g., for autotransfusion [39]. Coordinators may want to use such guidelines. These usually show concisely how to teach the essential details of the method. Often companies that produce equipment can provide educational material; using these along with the equipment in a hospital setting may be the most effective way of training staff to use new technology.

BROCHURES AND PICTURES

Brochures, pictures, charts, tables, and similar printed material may be efficient tools for educating patients, nursing staff, medical staff, and the public. They may be used to convey basic ideas and to explain various methods used in blood management. They can also be used as marketing tools. Such printed material may be made available through the marketing department of the hospital; it may be designed by the coordinator, or previously published material can be used, if permitted.

The coordinator should ensure that he/she has all the printed material available, fitting the needs of the program. This would include pictures of a cell-saving device and a heart–lung machine for patient education. Charts showing how to perform acute normovolemic hemodilution may be used to educate health-care providers. Program brochures may be available as a giveaway for patients who are treated in the blood management program and for media representatives. Written material including current treatment algorithms may be handed out to health-care providers receiving their initial orientation. As the blood management program develops, printed material can be designed to be used as an effective tool in all types of educational interventions.

Role-plays

Selected educational topics can best be taught in role-play settings. One example is improving the process of informed consent for blood management. Role-plays may be welcome to practice this essential part of blood management. As demonstrated in a study, a 1-hour didactic lesson coupled with a 90-minute workshop with role-plays tremendously improved health-care providers' ability to inform the patients about the options in blood management and to obtain a valid informed consent for the planned treatment [40].

Combinations of educational interventions

As the literature demonstrates, combinations of some of the above-mentioned educational interventions are effective in reducing blood use [41]. For instance, the combination of audit, review of published guidelines, case presentations, and an in-service program has proven successful in substantially reducing fresh frozen plasma transfusions [42]. In another campaign to improve the awareness of physicians about transfusions guidelines, a small leaflet with the guidelines was distributed, the topic was discussed within the departments, a continuing medical education program for all staff members was set up, and questions were answered on a one-to-one basis. This combination of educational interventions reduced unjustified transfusions [43]. When planning educational interventions, a variety of methods in combination is most effective.

> ### Step 7: How to proceed:
>
> - Identify educational needs.
> - List groups of persons participating in the blood management program who should be trained.
> - List educational methods within the reach of the program.
> - Outline a schedule ensuring initial and continuing education of all those who should be trained.

Step 8: marketing

Marketing, in other words "going to the market," can mean that something is obtained or something is sold. On going to the market, it is helpful to know what exactly is to be marketed. Realistic goals should also be defined before going to the market.

Posing a series of questions will help identify the product or service to be marketed—in this case, blood management. The answers to such questions as "What service do I want to market?" "How is this product identified (name, logo)?" "What is unique and important about this service?" "Why would people be willing to use this service?" and "What is especially attractive to customers?" will clarify how the product is identified in the market. Even if the answers are obvious, it is wise to take the time to put the answers in writing. This is the starting point for the marketing concept.

Next, set the marketing goals. The goals may include making money, increasing the hospital's market share, retaining patients, winning new patients, or enhancing the hospital's image. Improving patient care can also be a marketing goal. Since blood management is good clinical practice that improves patient outcome, successfully marketing blood management, in turn, also improves the outcome by convincing the patients to use this superior mode of treatment.

The next step is to define the target group. Who would look for blood management services of his/her own initiative or who can be convinced to do so? These individuals are the marketing target and include referring physicians, potential patients, the media, the public, your colleagues, or others (compare Appendix C).

At this point, marketing tools need to be chosen and there are many. However, since not all marketing methods fit all target groups, a method applicable to the group has to be selected. The program's budget as well as the time and manpower available may limit the choice of marketing

methods. Marketing media are chosen taking these factors into account; they might include print media, electronic media, person-to-person communication, distribution of giveaways and gimmicks, and word of mouth (compare Appendix C). Presentations can be scheduled at staff orientations. The public or health-care providers can be invited to blood management seminars. Customers of companies providing equipment for blood management can be contacted.

Another very interesting marketing tool is a club. Clubs can be founded for the chronically ill, e.g., for sickle-cell-disease patients. Organizing regular club meetings for the patients and their families not only wins "customers" for the hospital but also serves to educate those concerned about disease management and enhances adherence to a chronic drug regimen. In turn, such clubs attached to a blood management program reduce transfusions and improve the patient outcome, potentially resulting in a reduction in mortality [1].

Most probably help will be needed to successfully market a blood management program. If available, the hospital's public relations manager can be asked for help. Also, a commercial consultant can be instrumental in designing and marketing the program. Those who are experienced in running a blood management program can share their experiences when asked for advice.

> ### Step 8: How to proceed:
>
> - Define the marketing goals.
> - List the target groups for the marketing initiative.
> - Select marketing methods to address the target groups identified.
> - Recruit help for marketing initiatives.

Step 9: running the program

Once the initial hurdles have been cleared, many daily challenges encountered while running the program will have to be faced. In the following, some suggestions are given to as to how such challenges can be met.

Setting priorities

At the beginning of the program there is so much to do that it cannot possibly be done at once, therefore it is imperative to set priorities. The burden of organization and prioritizing will fall mainly on the coordinator. Prioritizing means to limit the initial tasks to items that are really important. The contract on which the blood management program is based may already limit the field of work, thus setting the priorities. If the hospital administration has agreed to launch blood conservation in the cardiac surgery department only, then this limit should be respected, even if other departments urgently need blood conservation. If the program is limited to a special patient population, then this should be the priority. In time, the opportunity to expand the program may arise, but for practical reasons, the tasks assigned to the program must have priority.

But what if the purpose of the blood management program is described as "perioperative blood management" or even as "hospital-wide" blood management? Then suddenly the program coordinator will most probably be confronted with an enormous workload. This can be compiled in a desk journal to help organize the work at hand. Whenever a new task arises, it should be noted in the journal. Once in a while, upcoming tasks need to be prioritized. If there is so much work that the coordinator is unable to do it, it needs to be limited. How can this be done?

If the first task is to demonstrate that the program can reduce transfusions, then it is best to start where most transfusions can be reduced and this place needs to be identified. Sometimes, this will be self-evident from the available hospital statistics. If, for instance, orthopedic surgeons transfuse much more than ear, nose, and throat surgeons, then the orthopedic department may deserve initial attention. If the workload needs further limiting, blood product use can be classified by disease. The hospital's information department may be able to print a list of transfusions, sorted according to diagnosis-related groups [44]. These can be ranked, starting with the diseases for which most transfusions are administered, and priorities can be listed top down. Another starting point could be where the most variations in transfusion use occur. To this end, transfusions can be classified according to surgeon. Some surgeons may transfuse more than others for the same procedure. This may be the point where transfusion use varies most and where a start can be made to lower transfusion rates. For instance, a surgeon who transfuses small amounts could be asked to describe the technique used to help those who transfuse more to adapt their technique.

Another approach in Belgium, which began small and systemically expanded, has been described [17]. Using this approach, blood management is divided into three stages. A basic analysis of the situation in the hospital will reveal the stage at which the hospital operates. As the program progresses, the first stage will give way to the second and the third.

Stage 1: Most or all patients receiving a type of surgery are transfused.
  • *Strategy:* Use of systematic blood management measures that benefit all patients. A reduction of blood use is expected in all patients.

Stage 2: A new class of patients who are not transfused emerges.
  • *Strategy:* Try to identify prospectively which patient population is transfused and which is not. Rethink the transfusion decision and the decision on which blood management measures are used. Do they increase risks and costs for nontransfused patients? Focus blood management measures on patients who typically receive transfusions.

Stage 3: Most patients receive no allogeneic transfusions. However, a small group of patients still receives major amounts of blood.
  • *Strategy:* Analysis of critical incidents. Are there indicators for the critical incidents? Are there procedural changes that may reduce such critical incidents? Can blood management be improved in such situations? At what cost? Is there a safety net that can be established for the patients?

After these three stages are over, further progress can still be made. Every drop of blood should be considered precious. A database established in the initial phase of program development will help identify emerging problems early, as well as interteam variability and other challenges that need to be addressed. Continually adapting blood management is vital for continued progress.

Data collection propels the program

Data should be gathered from the beginning of the blood management program and stored in a database [11]. A well-designed database will provide valuable information about the progress of the program and about potential challenges. It will be a research tool, will permit comparison of the effectiveness of newly modified blood management measures, and will assist in quality control.

Designing such a database may take more time than initially anticipated, but it is well worth the effort. Permission from the hospital's ethical review board will have to be obtained initially. When this is granted, the content of the database will need to be defined. An interdisciplinary working group including the computer department may be required for this task. Listing the questions the database is to answer will help determine what data need to be

Table 21.6 Contents of the database.

Demographic data of patients
Patient risk factors (preexisting diseases, drugs)
Surgery or procedures performed
Details of blood management measures (e.g., acute
    normovolemic hemodilution with volumes, volume
    replacement, etc.)
Drugs used for blood management
Outcome data (length of stay, morbidity, mortality)
Use of blood products

collected. Working definitions for each data entry need to be defined (e.g., What is considered a deep vein thrombosis? What is considered preoperative aspirin ingestion?). Table 21.6 lists potential contents of a blood management database.

Data to be entered into the database should be collected for every patient over the lifetime of the program. The information sets collected should be as complete as possible. In addition to the fixed content, flexible space may be left in the database. This will allow for temporary collection of additional data, e.g., for a short-term research project. Keep the database simple. Data sheets attached to patient files or hand-held computers used to enter data collected on chart review may facilitate data collection.

It should be simple to retrieve data from the database. The computer department may be able to design the database so that important data can be regularly summarized and tables, charts, and reports can be printed for the hospital administration or for research projects.

Building routine

Running a blood management program involves many routine tasks. These include patient tracking, referrals, patient transfers, patient education, obtaining informed consent, patient assessment, staff education, bookkeeping, and many more. To ensure these tasks do not become a heavy burden, the coordinator needs to establish a routine and to design appropriate forms and checklists to perform tasks properly.

It is also practical to establish and publicize office hours, a phone number, e-mail address, and emergency contacts. This will give patients and health-care providers alike the chance to contact program staff. It will also help the coordinator find time when he/she can work without disturbance.

Every morning on coming to the hospital the coordinator should know which patients are participating in the blood management program. This is where patient tracking comes in. Which patients need to be tracked daily depends on the scope of the program. Thus, selection criteria have to be established for patients that should be in the program. If the program is for orthopedic patients only, then the coordinator should be informed about all current and upcoming orthopedic patients. If the coordinator takes care of Jehovah's Witness patients, then he/she has to track them. If the coordinator wants to track all patients whose blood management needs close monitoring, he/she may want to know about all patients with low hemoglobin levels or with a coagulopathy. Whatever the case, the coordinator needs to find all the patients that fit the selection criteria. Patients may come to the blood management office to contact the program coordinator. Physicians and nurses may be instructed to inform the coordinator whenever a patient happens to fit the selection criteria. It may also be possible to retrieve the names of patients who fit the selection criteria from the hospital medical or admission computer system. The hospital's computer department may be able to connect the laboratory computer to a blood management program e-mail account to notify the coordinator about patients whose laboratory values indicate severe anemia or coagulopathy, and a visit can be scheduled. It may even be possible to adjust the admission routine to screen patients eligible for blood management. The admission clerk may ask patients if they are willing to participate in the blood management program. If they agree, the admission clerk may note this in the computer and an e-mail is automatically sent to the blood management program.

Identifying patients in the blood management program is also important. Again, which patients need to be identified depends on the scope of the program. If all eligible patients are treated according to the tenets of blood management, some hospitals differentiate between level 1 and level 2 patients, based on whether individual patients refuse transfusion under all circumstances or not. Other hospitals have decided to identify intensive care patients who receive special treatment to reduce iatrogenic blood loss. In other places, patients with at least a 10% risk of receiving a transfusion are identified. In practice, patient identification can involve marking the patient's chart, attaching a wristband, attaching a warning sign to the patient's bed, or entering a special note into the computer.

Some blood management programs have greatly benefited from the use of a dedicated computer program (Table 21.7) to organize the daily routine. The program supports daily tasks and contains information and tools needed daily. Tasks such as letter writing and filling in

Table 21.7 Contents of an office program.

Data file with patient contact information
Data file with information about health-care providers willing
    to do blood management
Forms (linked to the patient and physician database) for
    transfer, referrals, informed consent, information materials,
    marketing, etc.
Tools to schedule appointments (e.g., for preoperative rHuEPO
    or iron therapy)
Filing of pertinent literature

rHuEPO, recombinant human erythropoietin.

forms, keeping track of patients and physicians participating in the program, transfers, referrals, literature organization, and research can all be supported with software.
It can either be designed by the hospital's computer department or by a commercial provider. Programs tested
in practice are commercially available.

Forms, questionnaires, and checklists need to be designed in order to transfer established administrative policies and procedures from the paper into practice. Many of
the forms used elsewhere have been published in the literature [45] or on the Internet (e.g., on the PNBC Web site).
They can simply be adjusted to the needs of the program.
As an example, Appendix C contains a transfer form with
a checklist for reference.

Step 9: How to proceed:

- If overwhelmed by the amount of work, set priorities
and tackle one point at a time.
- Obtain a computer program that fills the program's
needs.
- Design forms and checklists that facilitate routine tasks.

Step 10: evaluation and safety

Evaluation and benchmarking

In all likelihood the goals for the blood management program were established at the business proposal stage. After some time has elapsed, it will be worthwhile to check
whether these goals have been reached. Data have to be
collected to do this. The database mentioned earlier can
be designed to evaluate the blood management program.
Which data are collected for evaluation depends on what
needs to be measured. If increasing the patient load was

the goal, patient numbers need to be tracked. It may also
be useful to check new patients' area codes to see where
they come from. Or if the goal of the program is to reduce transfusions, transfusion statistics, the procedures
performed, and the patients who were treated need to be
registered.

Evaluation of the program, however, does not only consist of checking to see whether the program has reached
its business goals. It would be interesting to know how the
program performed medically and how it is performing
in comparison with other blood management programs.
The purpose of this is to improve patient care and to provide information to policymakers, patients, and the public and may lead to available resources being used more
efficiently. To benefit from such an evaluation, benchmarking is needed. Benchmarking simply means setting
a point of reference or comparison to define excellent patient service. What constitutes best service currently can
be determined by consulting the program's benchmarking partners. Benchmarking implies that performance is
improved by adopting the best practice of benchmarking partners. Procedures that benchmarking partners use
to outperform the program being evaluated are identified
and adopted. In turn, benchmarking partners use features
of other programs to improve where necessary.

Safety systems

Preventing hazards in the blood management program
improves patient safety. Safety provisions contribute to
the performance of a blood management program. By
definition, blood management includes a commitment to
safe patient care. Safety assurance must be a central part
of the blood management program.

Organized measures to systematically prevent hazards
and improve patient safety are relatively new to medicine
in general and to blood management in particular. However, safety programs per se are not new. Aviation and
many other businesses with the potential for causing serious accidents have systems in place to prevent serious
hazards and have established a convincing safety record.
What can be learned from aviation and other industrial
safety systems? The overall goal is to prevent major fatal
accidents. As these occur infrequently, there is no way to
analyze them statistically for triggers. However, major accidents are often preceded by major and minor incidents,
termed near misses. In comparison to major, fatal accidents, such incidents occur much more frequently and
are amenable to systematic analysis when reported. Modern safety systems analyze incidents, and a safety culture is

developed. In such a safety culture the awareness of participants is raised so that notice is taken even of minor errors and near misses as well as reporting is encouraged. Of course, the individual reporting the incident should not have to fear any adverse consequences. An analysis is made and the reason for the near miss sought. Any intrinsic problem is identified to prevent further near misses. This is how major fatal accidents are reduced. There needs to be a clear line between acceptable and unacceptable practice, and all participants should be aware of it. Further elements of safety systems include continuing monitoring of service performance, a report system for near misses and fatalities, an initiative to analyze reported events in order to draw the necessary conclusions, and making changes to policies mirroring the commitment to avoid a recurrence of the reported event as well as adopting appropriate measures to implement these policies.

The safety concept used in aviation is also applicable in blood management. An error log can be kept to record all errors. These errors can be grouped as actual errors, potential major errors, and potential minor errors [46]. Errors can be grouped according to the processes they occur in and are typically defined as deviations from established policies. Table 21.8 provides an example of errors in a process relevant to blood management.

Once a patient hazard has been identified, policy changes need to be implemented. Three key points are essential to implement policy changes that result in increased patient safety: simplify, avoid duplication, and implement changes in a multidisciplinary fashion [26]. Keeping processes simple and guidelines concise reduces

errors. Duplication of paperwork leads to errors; therefore, each set of data should be collected only once. And a multidisciplinary approach is essential when it comes to working on and modifying guidelines.

Step 10: How to proceed:

• Review the business goals regularly and document whether they have been met.
• Participate in benchmarking to improve the service offered by the blood management program.
• Put a safety system in place to keep a record of all errors. Correct policies and procedures after analysis of recorded safety failures.

Suggestions for further research

What are effective methods to motivate health-care providers? What role does motivation play in implementing a blood management program? How can others be motivated to become blood managers?

Homework

Find out what is required to obtain permission from the ethics committee to establish a blood management database.

Are there any legal restrictions on advertising by medical facilities in your country? If so, what are they?

Table 21.8 Example of errors in the process of informed consent.

Actual error
  The patient is treated contrary to his/her stated wishes.
Potential errors—major
  Patient did not receive information about blood management.
  Patient was not given the opportunity to fill out the informed consent form.
  Patient underwent surgery without the surgeon knowing about the patient's preferences regarding blood management.
Potential errors—minor
  Wrong name on patient informed consent form.
  Consent form is not filed in patient chart.
  Information is missing; not all needed details of patient's wishes are recorded.
  The signature on the informed consent form is missing.

References

1 Akinyanju, O.O., A.I. Otaigbe, and M.O. Ibidapo. Outcome of holistic care in Nigerian patients with sickle cell anaemia. *Clin Lab Haematol*, 2005. **27**(3): p. 195–199.

2 Morgan, T.O. Blood conservation: the CEO perspective. *J Cardiothorac Vasc Anesth*, 2004. **18**(4, Suppl): p. 15S–17S.

3 Freedman, J., *et al.* A provincial program of blood conservation: The Ontario Transfusion Coordinators (ONTraC). *Transfus Apher Sci*, 2005. **33**(3): p. 343–349.

4 Derderian, G.P. Establishing a business plan for blood conservation. *J Cardiothorac Vasc Anesth*, 2004. **18**(4, Suppl): p. 12S–14S.

5 Spiess, B.D. Blood conservation: why bother? *J Cardiothorac Vasc Anesth*, 2004. **18**(4, Suppl): p. 1S–5S.

6 Morgan, T.O. Cost, quality, and risk: measuring and stopping the hidden costs of coronary artery bypass graft surgery. *Am J Health Syst Pharm*, 2005. **62**(18, Suppl 4): p. S2–S5.

7 Ozawa, S., A. Shander, and T.D. Ochani. A practical approach to achieving bloodless surgery. *AORN J*, 2001. **74**(1): p. 34–40, 42–47; quiz 48, 50–54.

8 Lomas, J., *et al.* Opinion leaders vs audit and feedback to implement practice guidelines. Delivery after previous cesarean section. *JAMA*, 1991. **265**(17): p. 2202–2207.

9 Greco, P.J. and J.M. Eisenberg. Changing physicians' practices. *N Engl J Med*, 1993. **329**(17): p. 1271–1273.

10 Hiss R.G., *et al.* Identification of physician educational influentials in small community hospitals. *Res Med Educ*, 1978. **17**: p. 283–288.

11 Green, J.A. Blood conservation in cardiac surgery: the Virginia Commonwealth University (VCU) experience. *J Cardiothorac Vasc Anesth*, 2004. **18**(4, Suppl): p. 18S–23S.

12 Rosengart, T.K., *et al.* Open heart operations without transfusion using a multimodality blood conservation strategy in 50 Jehovah's Witness patients: implications for a "bloodless" surgical technique. *J Am Coll Surg*, 1997. **184**(6): p. 618–629.

13 Salem-Schatz, S.R., J. Avorn, and S.B. Soumerai. Influence of knowledge and attitudes on the quality of physicians' transfusion practice. *Med Care*, 1993. **31**(10): p. 868–878.

14 Waters, J.H. Overview of blood conservation. *Transfusion*, 2004. **44**(12, Suppl): p. 1S–3S.

15 Martyn, V., *et al.* The theory and practice of bloodless surgery. *Transfus Apher Sci*, 2002. **27**(1): p. 29–43.

16 Shander, A. Surgery without blood. *Crit Care Med*, 2003. **31**(12, Suppl): p. S708–S714.

17 Baele, P. and P. Van der Linden. Developing a blood conservation strategy in the surgical setting. *Acta Anaesthesiol Belg*, 2002. **53**(2): p. 129–136.

18 Domen, R.E., *et al.* Fellowship training programs in blood banking and transfusion medicine: results of a national survey. *Am J Clin Pathol*, 1996. **106**(5): p. 584–587.

19 Handler, S. Does continuing medical education affect medical care. A study of improved transfusion practices. *Minn Med*, 1983. **66**(3): p. 167–180.

20 Rehm, J.P., *et al.* Hospital-wide educational program decreases red blood cell transfusions. *J Surg Res*, 1998. **75**(2): p. 183–186.

21 Ferraris, V.A. and S.P. Ferraris. Limiting excessive postoperative blood transfusion after cardiac procedures. A review. *Tex Heart Inst J*, 1995. **22**(3): p. 216–230.

22 Wilson, K., *et al.* The effectiveness of interventions to reduce physician's levels of inappropriate transfusion: what can be learned from a systematic review of the literature. *Transfusion*, 2002. **42**(9): p. 1224–1229.

23 Salamat, A., J. Seaton, and H.G. Watson. Impact of introducing guidelines on anticoagulant reversal. *Transfus Med*, 2005. **15**(2): p. 99–105.

24 Irving, G. A survey of the use of blood and blood components among South African anaesthetists working in teaching hospitals. *S Afr Med J*, 1992. **82**(5): p. 324–328.

25 Rock, G., *et al.* A pilot study to assess physician knowledge in transfusion medicine. *Transfus Med*, 2002. **12**(2): p. 125–128.

26 Mancini, M.E. Performance improvement in transfusion medicine. What do nurses need and want? *Arch Pathol Lab Med*, 1999. **123**(6): p. 496–502.

27 Barnette, R.E., D.J. Fish, and R.S. Eisenstaedt. Modification of fresh-frozen plasma transfusion practices through educational intervention. *Transfusion*, 1990. **30**(3): p. 253–257.

28 Toy, P.T. Audit and education in transfusion medicine. *Vox Sang*, 1996. **70**(1): p. 1–5.

29 Soumerai, S.B., *et al.* A controlled trial of educational outreach to improve blood transfusion practice. *JAMA*, 1993. **270**(8): p. 961–966.

30 Shanberge, J.N. Reduction of fresh-frozen plasma use through a daily survey and education program. *Transfusion*, 1987. **27**(3): p. 226–227.

31 Morrison, J.C., *et al.* The effect of provider education on blood utilization practices. *Am J Obstet Gynecol*, 1993. **169**(5): p. 1240–1245.

32 Marques, M.B., *et al.* Clinical pathology consultation improves coagulation factor utilization in hospitalized adults. *Am J Clin Pathol*, 2003. **120**(6): p. 938–943.

33 Hoeltge, G.A., *et al.* Computer-assisted audits of blood component transfusion. *Cleve Clin J Med*, 1989. **56**(3): p. 267–272.

34 Cheng, G., *et al.* The effects of a self-educating blood component request form and enforcements of transfusion guidelines on FFP and platelet usage. Queen Mary Hospital, Hong Kong. British Committee for Standards in Hematology (BCSH). *Clin Lab Haematol*, 1996. **18**(2): p. 83–87.

35 Lee, A.G., *et al.* Structured journal club as a tool to teach and assess resident competence in practice-based learning and improvement. *Ophthalmology*, 2006. **113**(3): p. 497–500.

36 Lee, A.G., *et al.* Using the Journal Club to teach and assess competence in practice-based learning and improvement: a literature review and recommendation for implementation. *Surv Ophthalmol*, 2005. **50**(6): p. 542–548.

37 Growe, G.H., L.C. Jenkins, and S.C. Naiman. Anesthesia training in transfusion medicine. *Transfus Med Rev*, 1991. **5**(2): p. 152–156.

38 Brooks, J.P. and T.G. Combest. In-service training with videotape is useful in teaching transfusion medicine principles. *Transfusion*, 1996. **36**(8): p. 739–742.

39 Training recommendations for autotransfusion unit operators. *Health Devices*, 1995. **24**(4): p. 162.

40 Goodnough, L.T., A.L. Hull, and M.E. Kleinhenz. Informed consent for blood transfusion as a transfusion medicine educational intervention. *Transfus Med*, 1994. **4**(1): p. 51–55.

41 Garrioch, M., *et al.* Reducing red cell transfusion by audit, education and a new guideline in a large teaching hospital. *Transfus Med*, 2004. **14**(1): p. 25–31.

42 Ayoub, M.M. and J.A. Clark. Reduction of fresh frozen plasma use with a simple education program. *Am Surg*, 1989. **55**(9): p. 563–565.

43 Kakkar, N., R. Kaur, and J. Dhanoa. Improvement in fresh frozen plasma transfusion practice: results of an outcome audit. *Transfus Med*, 2004. **14**(3): p. 231–235.

44 Jefferies, L.C., B.S. Sachais, and D.S. Young. Blood transfusion costs by diagnosis-related groups in 60 university hospitals in 1995. *Transfusion*, 2001. **41**(4): p. 522–529.

45 Gohel, M.S., *et al.* How to approach major surgery where patients refuse blood transfusion (including Jehovah's Witnesses). *Ann R Coll Surg Engl*, 2005. **87**(1): p. 3–14.

46 Galloway, M., *et al.* Providing feedback to users on unacceptable practice in the delivery of a hospital transfusion service—a pilot study. *Transfus Med*, 2002. **12**(2): p. 129–132.

Appendix A: detailed information

Table A.1 Transfusion-transmittable diseases.

Infectious agent	Causing	Likelihood
Anaplasma phagocytophilum (HGE) (rickettsia)	Ehrlichiosis	
Babesia microti (parasite)	Babesiosis, life-threatening hemolysis in immunocompromized and elderly	USA: <1:1,000,000
Chlamydia pneumoniae	Aortic aneurysm, ischemic heart disease (?)	Unclear whether TTI, but likely, since microbe in 9–46% of all healthy donors
Coxiella burnetti (Gram-negative coccobacillus)	Q-fever	One case reported
CTF Orbivirus (Arbovirus)	Colorado tick fever	One case reported
Cytomegalovirus (CMV) (herpes virus family)	Clinically undetectable, severe diseases with mortality in immunocompromized	Found in most donations
Epstein-Barr-virus	Various diseases	Found in most donations
Filaria (nematodes, worms)	Transfused microfilaria cannot multiply since they cannot develop into adult worm, disease self-limited	
Hepatitis A virus (HAV)	Hepatitis A	USA: 1:1,000,000
Hepatitis B virus (HBV) (lipid-enveloped)	Hepatitis B	USA: 1:205,000–250,000 Canada: 1.88:100,000
Hepatitis C virus (HCV) (lipid-enveloped)	Hepatitis C	USA: 1:250,000–1,935,000 Canada: 0.35:1,000,000, UK: 1:3,000,000
Human Herpes 8 virus		
Human Immunodeficiency virus (HIV) (lentivirus, retrovirus)	AIDS	USA: 1:100 before testing era, currently 1:1–2,100,000 Canada: 1:10,000,000; South Africa: 2.6: 100,000
Human T-lymphotropic virus Type I and II (HTLV) (retrovirus)	Neurodegenerative disorder	USA: 1:640,000 Canada: 0.95:1,000,000
Leishmania	Leishmaniasis (visceral, cutaneous, mucosal)	Occasionally
Listeria monocytogenes		Found in platelets (case report)
New coronavirus, poss. paramyxovirus as cofactor	Severe acute respiratory syndrome (SARS)	Not known whether TTI
Parvovirus B19	Hemolytic anemia, aplastic anemia in susceptible individuals	Highly variable
Plasmodium spp.	Malaria	USA: 1–3:4,000,000; Worldwide one of the more common TTIs
Protease-resistant prion protein (?)	Variant Creutzfeld-Jakob disease	
Rickettsia spp.	Rocky mountain spotted fever	One case reported
SEN virus (non-enveloped DNA virus, Circovirus)	Hepatitis?	Present in blood of 1.8–24% of healthy individuals, depending on geographic region

Table A.1 (*Continued*)

Infectious agent	Causing	Likelihood
Toxoplasma gondii	Toxoplasmosis	
Transfusion-transmitted virus (TTV)	Hepatitis?	50% of blood donated in the USA
Treponema pallidum	Syphilis	No cases in USA in last decades
Trypanosoma cruzi	Chagas disease	In endemic areas
West Nile virus	Meningoencephalitis	2.7:10,000 in endemic areas in USA

Bartonella spp. (cat scratch disease, bacillary angiomatosis), Francisella tularensis (Tularemia), Borrelia burgdorferi (Lymes disease), Japanese encephalitis virus, St Louis encephalitis virus, Western equine encephalitis virus, LaCrosse encephalitis virus, yellow fever virus, dengue virus: None of them were reported to have caused a transfusion-transmitted disease, although theoretically possible.

Table A.2 Treatment options for factor deficiencies.

Missing/defect factor	Incidence	Consequence of lack	Recommended first-line treatment	Alternatives (may not be the best therapy available)
FI (Fibrinogen)	1:1 M	Bleeding disorder	Fibrinogen concentrate	Cryo, FFP
FII Prothrombin	1:2 M	Bleeding disorder	PCC	FFP
FIII thromboplastin			—	
FIV Calcium	—		—	
FV	1:1 M	Bleeding disorder	FFP	rHuFVIIa
FVII	1:500 K	Bleeding disorder	rHuFVIIa	FVII (PCC with FVII works, but thrombosis risk), FFP
FVIII	1:5–10 K	Hemophilia A	Mild: DDAVP + TA, severe: rHuFVIII Inhibitor: rHuFVIIa	FVIII Inhibitor: FEIBA, porcine FVIII, high-dose FVIII, PCC
FIX Christmas	1:30–60 K	Hemophilia B	rHuFIX Inhibitor: rHuFVIIa	High purity FIX, Inhibitor: FEIBA, PCC, FFP
FX Stuart Prower	1:1 M	Bleeding disorder	PCC (with appropriate levels of FX)	FFP, low purity FIX
FXI	1:1 M	Bleeding disorder	If FXI:C <15 U/dL: FXI; if FXI:C 15–70 U/dL: TA, in heavy bleeding FXI	FFP
FXII Hagemann		?	Not needed for hemostasis	
FXIII	1:2 M	Bleeding disorder	FXIII concentrate	cryoppt
von Willebrand	>1:1 K	Bleeding disorder	Mild: DDAVP + TA, severe: vWF concentrate or FVIII with high level vWF	FFP, cryoppt
Protein S		May be thrombosis		PCC
Protein C	1:300–500	Purpura fulminans, thrombosis	Protein C concentrate	PCC, FFP
Antithrombin III		Thrombosis, heparin resistance	ATIII concentrate	rHuATIII

If not indicated otherwise, factor concentrates are plasma-derived.

K, thousand; M, million; TA, Tranexamic acid; cryoppt, cryoprecipitate; FFP, fresh frozen plasma; PCC, prothrombin complex concentrate; rHuATIII, recombinant human antithrombin III; vWF, von Willebrand factor.

Table A.3 Plasma constituents.

Constituent	Function	Amount in plasma
Fibrinogen	Coagulation	260 mg/dL
Prothrombin	Coagulation	80–90 mcg/mL
Factor V	Coagulation	0.4–1 mg/dL
Factor VII	Coagulation	0.47 mcg/mL
Factor VIII	Coagulation	0.01 mg/dL
Factor IX	Coagulation	4 mcg/mL
Factor X	Coagulation	6.4–10 mcg/mL
Factor XI	Coagulation	0.4–0.6 mg/dL
Factor XIII	Coagulation	2.9 mg/dL
Protein C	Anticoagulation	3.9–5.9 mcg/mL
Protein S	Anticoagulation	25–25 mcg/mL
Vitronectin	Adhesion, complement system	0.2–0.4 mg/mL
Albumin	Transport, colloid-osmotic pressure	Main protein of serum (55–62%)
Haptoglobin	Binds free hemoglobin	27–140 mg/dL
Transferrin	Carries iron in blood	150–350 mg/dL
Ceruloplasmin	Transports Cu, phenoloxidase	20–60 mg/dL
Prealbumin	Transport	16–35 mg/dL
Antithrombin III	Anticoagulation	11–16 mg/dL
α-2-Antiplasmin	Important inhibitor of plasmin and other coagulation factors	7 mg/dL
α-1-Antitrypsin	Inhibition of trypsin, elastase,	160 mg/dL
α-1-antichymotrypsin	Inhibits chymotrypsine	45 mg/dL
C-1-esterase-inhibitor	Controls activation of C1 and coagulation factors; deficiency: hereditary angioneurotic edema	24 mg/dL
α-2-macroglobulin	Inhibits thrombin, plasmin, etc. clearance of exogenous proteinases	150 mg/dL
von Willebrand factor	Coagulation	1 mg/dL
Prekallikrein	Coagulation *et al.*	3.5–5 mg/dL
Plasminogen	Coagulation	7–20 mg/dL
IgG	Immunologic function	1375 mg/dL
IgA 1 + 2	Immunologic function	250 mg/dL
IgM	Immunologic function	120 mg/dL
IgD	Immunologic function	3 mg/dL
IgE	Immunologic function	0.02 mg/dL
Complement 4	Immunologic function	30 mg/dL
Complement 3	Immunologic function	130 mg/dL

Many more plasma proteins have been characterized, among them: Actin, Afamin precursor, Angiotensinogen precursor, Apolipoprotein precursors, ATP synthase precursor, Atrial natriuretic factor precursor, Bullous pemphigoid antigen fragment, Calgranulin A, Carbonic anhydrase, Cathepsin precursor, Chaperonin, Cholinesterase precursor, Clusterin precursor, Endothelin converting enzyme, Fibulin-1 precursor, Ficolin 3 precursor, Gamma enolase, Glial fibrillary acidic protein, Gravin, Heparin cofactor II precursor, Human psoriasin, Insulin-like growth factor binding protein 3 precursor, Interleukin, Kininogen precursor, Melanoma associated antigen p97, Mismatch repair protein, Oxygen regulated protein precursor, Preoxireduxin, Platelet basic protein precursor, Plectin, PSA precursor, Putative serum amyloid A-3 precursor, Selenoprotein P precursor, Signal recognition particle receptor alfa subunit, tetranectin precursor, Vascular cell adhesion pretein 1 precursor, Vinculin.

Table A.4 The proteome of human red cells.

Actin	Glycophorin C
Adducin	Heat shock proteins
Aldehyde dehydrogenase	Hemoglobin
Aldolase	Hydroxyacyl gluthatione hydrolase
Aminolevulinate dehydratase	Lactate dehydrogenase
Ankyrin	Peroxireduxin 2
Aquaporin	Phosphoglucose isomerase chain A
Arginase	Phosphoribosyl pyrophosphate synthetase
ATP citrate lyase	Placental ribonuclease inhibitor
B-CAM protein	Poly (A) specific ribonuclease
Biliverdin reductase	Polyubiquitin
C1-tetrahydrofolate synthase	Presenilin-associated protein
Calcium transporting ATPase 4	Prostatic-binding protein (neuropolypeptide)
Calpain inhibitor (Calpastatin)	Purine nucleoside phosphorylase
Carbonic anhydrase	RAP2B (RAS oncogene)
Catalase	Rh blood D group antigen
Cofilin	Spectrin
Creatine kinase	Stomatin
D-dopachrome tautomerase	Synaptobrevin
Dematin	Thioreduxin
Duodenal cytochrome b	Transgelin
Enhancer protein	Translation initiation factor 2C
Flotilin	Tropomodulin
Glucose transporter glycoprotein	Tropomyosin
Glutaraldehyde-3-phosphate dehydrogenase	Trypsinogen
Glutathione transferase	Ubiquitin activating enzyme
Glutoredoxin	Ubiquitin isopeptidase
Glyceraldehyde-3-phosphate dehydrogenase	Zinc finger protein 180
Glycophorin	Zona pellucida binding protein

Some of the many identified proteins, together with uncounted unidentified proteins.

Table A.5 Definitions and equations of oxygen transport (Chapter 2).

Definitions

Viscosity	Measure of internal friction in a laminar flow	Depends on temperature; normal for blood: 3 to 5 relative units (water is 1 relative unit), plasma is 1.9 to 2.3 relative units; can increase with slowing of blood: up to 1000 relative units because of reversible agglomeration. Blood viscosity is affected by hematocrit, plasma viscosity, cell deformability, cell aggregation
P50	Oxygen partial pressure where oxygen saturation of hemoglobin is 50%, normal value for adult hemoglobin is 26.6 mm Hg	A high P50 means a low affinity of hemoglobin for oxygen and vice versa

Equations

Oxygen saturation (SO_2)	(Actual O_2 content of Hgb $\times$ 100)/ maximum oxygen content of Hgb	
Arterial oxygen content CaO_2	$CaO_2 = (1.34 \times Hgb \times SaO_2) + 0.003 \times PaO_2$	
Oxygen delivery (DO_2)	$DO_2 = CO \times CaO2 = CO \times (Hgb \times 1.34 \times SaO_2 + 0.003 \times PaO_2) \times 10$	
Oxygen consumption (VO_2)	$VO_2 = DO_2 \times O_2ER$ $VO_2 = CO \times 1.34 \times Hgb \times SaO_2$ to SvO_2	Normal: 110 to 160 mL/min $\times$ m^2
Oxygen extraction ratio O_2ER	$(CaO_2 - CvO_2)/CaO_2$	Normal: 0.20 to 0.30
Hagen-Poiseuille equation	$Q = \pi (P1 - P2) R^4/8nL$ where $P1$ and $P2$: inlet and outlet pressures; R: tube radius, n: viscosity, L: tube length	Describes laminar flow Q in non-collapsible tubes

Table A.6 Definitions of basic qualities of fluids (Chapter 6).

Quality	Description	Remarks
Osmotic pressure	Hydrostatic pressure required to oppose the movement of water through a semipermeable membrane in response to an osmotic gradient	The osmotic pressure is referred to as colloid osmotic pressure (= oncotic pressure) if it is exerted by colloids
Mole (mol)	The amount of a substance that contains 6.022×10^{23} molecules (Avogadro's number)	
Molality	The number of moles of a solute in 1 kg of a solvent	
Molarity	The number of moles of a solute in 1 L of a solvent	
Osmole (osm)	The amount of a substance that exerts an osmotic pressure of 22.4 atm. in 1 L of solution	
Osmolality	Number of osmoles of a solute per kg of a solvent	Number of particles in the solution; independent of size and weight of particles, independent of any membrane; normal plasma osmolality is 287–290 mOsm/kg
Osmolarity	Number of osmoles of a solute per liter of a solvent	
Tonicity (mosmol/kg)	Effective osmolality; it is the sum of the concentrations of solutes which exert an osmotic force across a membrane	Tonicity is less than osmolality; it is the property of a solution in relation to a membrane
Equivalent (Eq) = millival (mval)	One equivalent is the amount of ion required to cancel out the electrical charge of an opposite charged monovalent ion (the valence charge of the ion is the number of equivalents there are in one mole of that ion)	For monovalent ions: 1eq = 1 mol For divalent ions: 1 eq = 0.5 mol For trivalent ions: 1 eq = 0.333 mol
Dalton (Da)	A unit of mass used to express atomic and molecular weights that is equal to one twelfth of the mass of an atom of carbon-12. It is equivalent to 1.6610^{-27} kg	

Table A.7 Facts about hemophilia A and B.

Classification:
Mild: 6–30% factor activity (muscle/joint bleeding after major trauma, usually no spontaneous bleeding)
Moderate: 1–5% factor activity (muscle/joint bleeding after minor trauma, rarely spontaneous or central nervous system bleeding)
Severe: <1% factor activity (spontaneous bleeding in muscles, joints, central nervous system) (about 70% of hemophilia A patients and 50% of hemophilia B patients have severe hemophilia)

Inhibitors:

Antibodies against the coagulation factor under consideration
Develops in about 30% of previously untreated patients now treated with rFVIII, inhibitor-development more
Pronounced in Hispanic and African patients
Patients on FIX concentrates develop inhibitors less frequently (1–3%)

Therapy:

Prophylactic: increasing in vivo clotting factor levels to more than 1% activity is sufficient to prevent most spontaneous joint bleeds
FVIII: 25–40 U/kg 3 × per week
FIX: 25–40 U/kg 2 × per week
Short-term prophylactic (before surgery, physical therapy or major activity): surgical procedures can safely be performed if factor concentration is perioperatively kept at a level of 50–100%

Therapeutic:

mild hemorrhage: 20–30% factor activity required (FVIII: 10–15 U/kg, FIX: 20–30 U/kg), e.g., in severe epistaxis, persistent hematuria, dental bleeding (if unresponsive to aminocaproic acid or tranexamic acid)
major hemorrhage: 40–50% factor activity required (FVIII: 20–25 U/kg, FIX: 40–50 U/kg), e.g., in advanced muscle/joint bleeding, hematoma of neck, tongue, pharynx, dental extraction*
life-threatening hemorrhage: 70–100% factor activity required (FVIII: 35–50 U/kg, FIX: 70–100 U/kg; maintenance treatment with half-initial dose for 5 days to several weeks), e.g., in intracranial or GI bleed, surgery, major traumatic bleeding

*For dental extraction, 10% activity plus oral and local antifibrinolytic agents for 7–10 days may be sufficient.
100% clotting factor activity is 1 U/mL of average normal plasma.

Table A.8 Levels of evidence.

Ia Evidence obtained from meta-analysis of randomized controlled trials
Ib Evidence obtained from at least one randomized controlled trial
IIa Evidence obtained from at least one well-designed controlled study without randomization
IIb Evidence obtained from at least one other type of well-designed quasi-experimental study
III Evidence obtained from well-designed nonexperimental descriptive studies, such as comparative studies, correlation studies, and case studies
IV Evidence obtained from expert committee reports or opinions and/or clinical experiences of respected authorities

Table A.9 Grades of recommendation.

A Requires at least one randomized controlled trial as part of a body of literature of overall good quality and consistency addressing the specific recommendation (evidence levels Ia, Ib)
B Requires the availability of well-conducted clinical studies but no randomized clinical trials on the topic of recommendation (evidence levels IIa, IIb, III)
C Requires evidence obtained from expert committee reports or opinions and/or clinical experiences of respected authorities. Indicates an absence of directly applicable clinical studies of good quality (evidence level IV)

Appendix B: sources of information for blood management

Table B.1 Algorithms and summaries of methods for a multimodal concept for blood management found in the literature.

Algorithms for what?	Included facets	Source
Abnormal bleeding in cardiac surgery	Transfusions, coagulation monitoring	Nuttall *et al.* [1]
Cardiac surgery	Thrombelastography	Shore-Lesserson *et al.* [2]
Coronary artery bypass graft	A wide variety	Helm *et al.* [3]
Craniomaxillofacial surgery	Hemodilution, controlled hypotension, call saver, PAD, rHuEPO	Rohling *et al.* [4]
Epistaxis in hereditary hemorrhagic telangiectasia	Surgical and pharmaceutical approaches	Lund and Howard [5]
Glanzmann's thrombasthenia	Different	Bell and Savidge [6]
Hemoptysis	Surgical and others	Jougon *et al.* [7]
Hip and knee joint replacement	rHuEPO, transfusion	Pierson *et al.* [8]
Joint arthroplasty	A variety	Callaghan *et al.* [9]
Joint replacement	Flowchart for anemic patients	Muller *et al.* [10]
Liver transplant	rHuEPO, ANH, etc.	Jabbour *et al.* [11]
Major orthopedic surgery	Normothermia, PAD; iron, rHuEPO, cell salvage, preoperative assessment, ANH, aprotinin	Slappendel *et al.* [12]
Orthopedic surgery	RBC transfusion, fluids	Helm *et al.* [13]
Orthopedic surgery	PAD, hemodilution, intra- and postoperative cell salvage	Sculco [14]
Orthopedic surgery	A wide variety	Tobias [15]
Prosthetic hip and knee infections	rHuEPO, antifibrinolytics	Lee and Cushner [16]
Spine surgery	A wide variety	Szpalski *et al.* [17]
Surgical patients	Planning	Nelson *et al.* [18]
Total knee arthroplasty	rHuEPO, hematinics, ANH, tourniquet, postoperative cell salvage, adapted transfusion trigger	Kourtzis *et al.* [19]
Transfusion decision for RBC	Hemoglobin value and physical signs	Garrioch *et al.* [20]
Unexpected bleeding disorder	Pharmacologic and blood-derived agents	Teitel [21]

PAD, preoperative autologous donation; ANH, acute normovolemic hemodilution.

Table B.2 Examples of current transfusion guidelines.

Institution and recommendation	Year issued	Patients	Blood products
Guidelines for red blood cell and plasma transfusion for adults and children	1997	All	Red cells, FFP
ASA: Practice guidelines for blood component therapy	1996	All	Red cells, platelets, FFP, cryoppt
NIH Consensus Conference (National Institute of Health): Perioperative red blood cell transfusion	1988	Surgical patients	Red cells
NIH Consensus Conference: Fresh frozen plasma: Indications and risks	1985	All	FFP
NIH Consensus Conference: Platelet transfusion therapy	1987	All	Platelets
American College of Obstetricians and Gynecologists: Blood component therapy	1984	Women	All
ACP: Practice strategies for elective red blood cell transfusion	1992	All	Red cells
College of American Pathologists. Practice parameter for the use of fresh frozen plasma, cryoprecipitate, and platelets	1994	All	FFP, platelets
Practice parameter for the use of red blood cell transfusions	1998	All	Red cells
ASCO: Platelet transfusion for patients with cancer	2001	Oncologic	Platelets
BCSH Guidelines for the use of platelet transfusions	2003	All	Platelets
BCSH Guidelines on the clinical use of leukocyte-depleted blood components	1998	All	Leukocyte-depleted blood components
BCSH Transfusion guidelines for neonates and older children	2004 updated from 1994	Intrauterine, pediatric	Red cells, platelets, granulocytes, FFP
BCSH Guidelines for the Clinical use of red cell transfusions	2001	All	Red cells
National Blood Users Group (Ireland): A guideline for transfusion of red blood cells in surgical patients	2000	Surgical patients	Red cells
BCSH Guidelines for the use of fresh frozen plasma, cryoprecipitate and cryosupernatant	2004	All	FFP, cryoppt

NIH, National Institute of Health; BCSH, British Society for Haematology; ASCO, American Society of Clinical Oncology; ASA, American Society of Anesthesiologists; ACP, American College of Physicians; FFP, fresh frozen plasma; cryoppt, cryoprecipitate.

Table B.3 Examples of guidelines formulated for specific diseases. They include recommendations for blood management.

	Year issued	Patients/diseases
Myelodysplastic syndromes clinical practice guidelines in oncology	2006	Myelodysplastic syndrome
The ASH/ASCO clinical guidelines on the use of erythropoietin	2005	
Japanese Society for Dialysis Therapy. Japanese Society for Dialysis Therapy guidelines for renal anemia in chronic hemodialysis patients	2004	Renal anemia in hemodialysis patients
American Academy of Pediatrics Subcommittee on Hyperbilirubinemia Management of hyperbilirubinemia in the newborn infant 35 or more weeks of gestation	2004	Hyperbilirubinemia in the newborn
European Best Practice Guidelines Working Group. Revised European best practice guidelines for the management of anemia in patients with chronic renal failure	2004	Anemia in renal failure
Management of von Willebrand disease: a guideline from the UK Haemophilia Centre Doctors' Organization	2004	von Willebrand disease
British Committee for Standards in Haematology General Haematology Task Force by the Sickle Cell Working Party. Guidelines for the management of the acute painful crisis in sickle cell disease	2003	Sickle cell crisis
Clinical Practice Obstetrics Committee and Executive and Council, Society of Obstetricians and Gynaecologists of Canada	2002	Hemorrhagic shock
NKF-K/DOQI Clinical Practice Guidelines for Anemia of Chronic Kidney Disease	2000	Patients with renal failure
BCSH Guideline: The Investigation and Management of Neonatal Haemostasis and Thrombosis	2002	Neonates with hemostatic alterations
Nursing Guidelines Committee for Anemia in Patients with HIV Infection. Treatment of anemia in patients with HIV Infection—Part 2: guidelines for management of anemia	2002	HIV
AIEOP consensus guidelines Acute childhood idiopathic thrombocytopenic purpura	2000	Children with acute ITP

Table B.4 Books about blood management and related issues.

Title	Author	Information
Erythropoietins and erythropoiesis	Graham Molineux, Mary A. Foote, Steven Elliott	2005
No man's blood	Gene Church	1986, ISBN 0-8666-155-7
Perioperative transfusion medicine	Bruce D. Spiess, Aryeh Shander, Richard K. Spence	Lippincott Williams and Wilkins 2005, ISBN 0781737559
The clinical use of blood	World Health Organization	Information on WHO homepage
Transfusion medicine and alternatives to blood transfusion	NATA	2000 edition, information on NATA homepage
Transfusion-free medicine and surgery	Nicolas Jabbour	Blackwell Publishing 2005; ISBN 1405121599
Your body, your choice: The laymen's complete guide to bloodless medicine and surgery	Shannon Farmer, David Webb	Media Masters Singapore 2000, ISBN 981-04-1708-X

Table B.5 Organizations relevant for blood management.

Organization	Contact
Bloodless Healthcare International (BHI)	www.noblood.org
Bloodless Medicine Research of the University of Pisa, Italy	www.bloodless.it
Medical Society for Blood Management	www.bloodmanagement.org
Network for the Advancement of Transfusion Alternatives (NATA)	www.nataonline.com
Physicians and Nurses for Blood Conservation (PNBC)	www.pnbc.ca
Society for the Advancement of Blood Management (SABM)	www.sabm.org
Watchtower Society	http://www.watchtower.org/medical_care_and_blood.htm

References

1 Nuttall, G.A., *et al.* Efficacy of a simple intraoperative transfusion algorithm for nonerythrocyte component utilization after cardiopulmonary bypass. *Anesthesiology*, 2001. **94**(5): p. 773–781; discussion 5A–6A.

2 Shore-Lesserson, L., *et al.* Thromboelastography-guided transfusion algorithm reduces transfusions in complex cardiac surgery. *Anesth Analg*, 1999. **88**(2): p. 312–319.

3 Helm, R.E., *et al.* Comprehensive multimodality blood conservation: 100 consecutive CABG operations without transfusion. *Ann Thorac Surg*, 1998. **65**(1): p. 125–136.

4 Rohling, R.G., *et al.* Multimodal strategy for reduction of homologous transfusions in cranio-maxillofacial surgery. *Int J Oral Maxillofac Surg*, 1999. **28**(2): p. 137–142.

5 Lund, V.J. and D.J. Howard. A treatment algorithm for the management of epistaxis in hereditary hemorrhagic telangiectasia. *Am J Rhinol*, 1999. **13**(4): p. 319–322.

6 Bell, J.A. and G.F. Savidge. Glanzmann's thrombasthenia proposed optimal management during surgery and delivery. *Clin Appl Thromb Hemost*, 2003. **9**(2): p. 167–170.

7 Jougon, J., *et al.* Massive hemoptysis: what place for medical and surgical treatment. *Eur J Cardiothorac Surg*, 2002. **22**(3): p. 345–351.

8 Pierson, J.L., T.J. Hannon, and D.R. Earles. A blood-conservation algorithm to reduce blood transfusions after total hip and knee arthroplasty. *J Bone Joint Surg Am*, 2004. **86-A**(7): p. 1512–1518.

9 Callaghan, J.J., M.R. O'Rourke, and S.S. Liu. Blood management: issues and options. *J Arthroplasty*, 2005. **20**(4, Suppl 2): p. 51–54.

10 Muller, U., *et al.* Effect of a flow chart on use of blood transfusions in primary total hip and knee replacement: prospective before and after study. *BMJ*, 2004. **328**(7445): p. 934–938.

11 Jabbour, N., *et al.* Live donor liver transplantation without blood products: strategies developed for Jehovah's Witnesses offer broad application. *Ann Surg*, 2004. **240**(2): p. 350–357.

12 Slappendel, R., *et al.* An algorithm to reduce allogenic red blood cell transfusions for major orthopedic surgery. *Acta Orthop Scand*, 2003. **74**(5): p. 569–575.

13 Helm, A.T., *et al.* A strategy for reducing blood-transfusion requirements in elective orthopaedic surgery. Audit of an algorithm for arthroplasty of the lower limb. *J Bone Joint Surg Br*, 2003. **85**(4): p. 484–489.

14 Sculco, T.P. Global blood management in orthopaedic surgery. *Clin Orthop Relat Res*, 1998. (357): p. 43–49.

15 Tobias, J.D. Strategies for minimizing blood loss in orthopedic surgery. *Semin Hematol*, 2004. **41**(1, Suppl 1): p. 145–156.

16 Lee, G.C. and F.D. Cushner. Blood management in patients with deep prosthetic hip and knee infections. *Orthopedics*, 2004. **27**(6, Suppl): p. s669–s673.

17 Szpalski, M., R. Gunzburg, and B. Sztern. An overview of blood-sparing techniques used in spine surgery during the perioperative period. *Eur Spine J*, 2004. **13**(Suppl 1): p. S18–S27.

18 Nelson, C.L., *et al.* An algorithm to optimize perioperative blood management in surgery. *Clin Orthop Relat Res*, 1998. (357): p. 36–42.

19 Kourtzis, N., D. Pafilas, and G. Kasimatis. Blood saving protocol in elective total knee arthroplasty. *Am J Surg*, 2004. **187**(2): p. 261–267.

20 Garrioch, M., *et al.* Reducing red cell transfusion by audit, education and a new guideline in a large teaching hospital. *Transfus Med*, 2004. **14**(1): p. 25–31.

21 Teitel, J.M. Unexpected bleeding disorders: algorithm for approach to therapy. *Clin Lab Haematol*, 2000. **22**(Suppl 1): p. 26–29; discussion 30–32.

Appendix C: program tools and forms

Table C.1 Example of data collection in orthopedics (initial analysis).

Patient (sex/age)	Numbers of red cell units given	Procedure performed, reason for hospital stay	Length of stay	Hematocrit at first presentation	Intra-operative blood loss in mL	Pretransfusion hematocrit	Post-transfusion hematocrit	Emergency or planned admission	Units given outside accepted policies	Units given to patients who initially were anemic	Units given to patients who bled heavily intra-operatively	Comments
1												
2												
3												
4												
5												
6												

Have the blood bank provide you with the names of the patients who received red cells.

Data collection is easier if every single transfusion episode is recorded rather than the summarized transfusion history of every patient.

Table C.2 Patient history: clotting.

		Physician notes	How to proceed
Please answer the following questions		• History negative	Check kidney and liver panel, blood count, coagulation tests, drugs
		• No history taken	
		• History positive as follows	
Do you suffer from nose bleeds?	Yes/No	One or both sides? Drug-related? Without obvious reason (flu, dry nose, trauma)?	Labs
Do you easily get black spots?	Yes/No	Larger than 3 cm diameter? Extremities: medial or lateral? Trauma-related? Joint hemorrhage? Congenital or start during lifetime?	Labs
Do you bleed for prolonged times after minor injuries, e.g., after shaving?	Yes/No	How long? Amount of bleeding? How stopped?	Labs
Are you aware of any bleeding abnormality you suffer from?	Yes/No	Diagnosis? Who diagnosed? Last consultation of physician? Therapy? Description of historical bleeding episodes	Confirm diagnosis, consult hematologist
Does any of your relatives suffer from a bleeding abnormality?	Yes/No	Diagnosis? What relative?	Confirm diagnosis, labs
Do you have or have you had prolonged menstrual bleeding (>7 d)?	Yes/No	Primary or secondary? Did Gyn provide reason?	Labs, Gyn consult
Do you suffer from kidney disease?	Yes/No	Diagnosis or symptoms	Labs, consider DDAVP
Do you suffer from a liver disease?	Yes/No	Diagnosis or symptoms	Labs, consider vitamin K, DDAVP, estrogens, antifibrinolytics
Did you ever bleed for prolonged times after surgery or having a tooth pulled?	Yes/No	Intra- or postoperative? Surgical revision needed?, rebleeding after initial hemostasis?	Confirm event
Did you ever receive a blood transfusion?	Yes/No	Reason? Blood products? Who transfused?	Confirm event
Do you take drugs ("blood thinners"), e.g., coumadin, aspirin?	Yes/No	Drug name	Stop/change
During the last 2 weeks, did you take any medication for flu, pain, psychiatric disease, epilepsy, cramps, or infection?	Yes/No	Drug name	Stop/change/Treat/ antagonize (?)
Do you take nutritional supplements or herbal medicines?	Yes/No	Ginkgo, ginseng, garlic, ginger, green tea, Chinese preparations? St John's wort, vitamins C or E	Reduce dose, stop 14 d prior to surgery

Table C.3 Initial analysis.

	Transfusion statistics	Organization	Established blood management	Resources
Questions	What is the number of all transfusions given during the last year by departments (and associated costs)? What are the top 10 procedures using blood? Which procedures are performed with >10% of patients transfused?	What are the mode of transfusion use and methods of blood management already established? How is staff educated? What area and number of patients does the hospital serve per year? Who refers patients to hospital?	Who already uses which methods of blood management?	What equipment (type, storage place, responsible person for maintenance) and personnel (number of physicians, nurses, ancillary staff, specialties, knowledge about blood management, motivation) is available? Who is the staff responsible for transfusions, blood bank, autologous blood? Who is interested in blood management? Where are available funding opportunities?
Methods to obtain answers	Chart review, transfusion statistics, transfusion committee reports, billing department	Ask for staff education, black-board, hospital intranet, education coordinator, quality assurance files, review policies and procedures, visit blood bank, laboratory, ward, ICU	Talk to pharmacist, check policies and procedures	Survey, talk to medical technicians, surgical nurses, perfusionists, medical maintenance

What are the strong sides of the hospital? For example, a very good orthopedic program? A renowned sickle cell clinic etc?

Table C.4 Surgical continuum.

Preoperative	Intraoperative	Postoperative
Evaluation	Optimize hemostasis minimize blood loss (surgical techniques, equipment)	Minimize iatrogenic blood loss
Develop a plan of care and communicate it	Positioning	Positioning
Create lead time to optimize patients/postponing surgeries and procedures if indicated	Embolization	Bandages, pressure applied to wounds
Optimizing hemoglobin levels (EPO, iron, vitamins, androgens)	Acute normovolemic hemodilution	Postoperative cell salvage
Treat coagulation abnormalities	Acute hypervolemic hemodilution	Optimizing anticoagulation
Optimize cardiopulmonary, renal, hepatic condition of the patient (referral to specialist)	Augmented acute normovolemic hemodilution	EPO, hematinics
Embolization	Plasmapheresis	Oxygen therapy
Informed consent	Plateletpheresis	Maintaining normothermia
Ensure availability of equipment and personnel	Synthetic and autologous tissue adhesives	Avoid hypertension
Minimize iatrogenic blood loss	Antifibrinolytics, desmopressin	Monitoring of the patient and his blood loss
Stop or adapt anticoagulation	Monitoring of coagulation and anticoagulation (TEG, Hepcon)	Prompt intervention in case of postoperative bleeding
	Controlled hypotension	Nutrition
	Regional anesthesia	Judicious use of anticoagulation
	Tourniquets	Antifibrinolytics
	Cell salvage	
	Staging	
	Packing	
	Maintaining normothermia	
	Induced hypothermia	
	Ultrafiltration	
	Retrograde priming of extracorporeal circulation circuits	
	Oxygen therapy	

Table C.5 Job description: coordinator blood management program.

The coordinator plays an important role in the blood management of patients. The coordinator is responsible to establish and run the blood management program, making (your hospital) a "Center of Excellence" in blood management.

Requirements
- Thorough knowledge in the organization of a blood management program
- Basic knowledge in clinical blood management
- Understanding for patients for whom allogeneic transfusion is no option
- Computer skills, e.g., Word, Excel, e-mail, Medline
- Preferably speaking English
- Leadership and management skills
- Excellency in communication, presentation, and conflict resolution

Work environment
- Office
- Clinical area of hospital

Contacts and communication
- Within the hospital: Communicates with patients and their family/significant others; program and hospital management; medical, nursing, ancillary, and research staff
- Outside the hospital: Communicates with the media, public, national and international organizations relevant for blood management, industry, general business contacts

Accountability
- Program and hospital management

Details of responsibilities
Education and advertisement
- Together with PR department, establishes advertisement and media contact, interacts with the public to ensure progress of the blood management program
- Organizes blood management seminars for the public
- Remains up-to-date with blood management, is a source of information
- Conducts orientation sessions for new staff members regarding blood management program
- Organizes educational interventions for medical, nursing, and ancillary hospital staff

Clinical work
- Screens and interviews patients participating in the blood management program, educates patients in blood management
- Assists patients to formulate advance directives and document living wills regarding blood management
- Collects patient data, gives recommendation regarding the patient's blood management as outlined in established policies and procedures
- Liaises with patients, patient advocates, medical, nursing and ancillary staff, and the public
- Informs patients about blood management, develops information material for patients
- Coordinates inter-hospital patient transfers and physician–patient contacts
- Coordinates and supports travel and accommodation of patients coming from far to use the service of the program
- Daily visits patients participating in the blood management program; ensures that the patient is treated according to his stated will and that treatment is adequate; supports and informs the patient as needed
- Maintains a 24-hr-emergency contact

Data collection and research
- Assists with designing of research initiatives in blood management
- Collects data for program evaluation and blood management database
- Assists with analysis and presentation of data
- Evaluates new equipment for innovative blood management

(*cont.*)

Table C.5 (*Continued*)

Management
- Coordinates and supervises service of the blood management program, develops strategies to overcome weaknesses of the program
- Corresponds in a timely fashion
- Organizes regular meetings with blood management committee, hospital administration, the public, patients, and patient advocates
- Records requests and transfers of patients in the program
- Reports about program service and other relevant data
- Works in accordance with established policies and procedures for the program
- Maintains confidentiality
- Participates regularly in training and educational interventions
- Manages finances including preparation of realistic budgets and works within its limits

Interpersonal communication and skills
- Creates a warm, secure, harmonic, and comfortable atmosphere for patients and staff
- Is confident, competent, and professional
- Resolves conflicts
- Facilitates communication between patient and family
- Recognizes fear and anxiety, proactively provides comfort
- Is a role model for other staff members
- Addresses inappropriate behavior
- Treats patients, their family, staff members with respect; recognizes their opinion
- Encourages staff to communicate their proposals for process and service improvement and problem solving; takes corrective measures to solve problems
- As part of a team, is observant about the work load of co-workers, supports team members to reach the goals of the blood management program using the strong points of each staff member to make the program a success

Table C.6 Model policy format.

Step #	Step	Responsible person	Tools	Remarks
1.1	*Receive call*	*Coordinator on call*	*Mobile phone*	
1.2.	*Record essential information*	*,,*	*Flow chart "transfer" (Item No xxx)*	
1.3.	*Confirm you will call back*	*,,*		
1.4.	*Contact physician on all*	*,,*	*Physicians list (Item no xxx)*	
1.5.	*Call back*	*physician*		

Literature:

Date, Signatures (CEO, coordinator, medical director)

Italics are examples: # of policy/procedure//Name of policy/procedure *1.4.3: Transfer*. Purpose of the policy/procedure: *Describes how patients are transferred from outside hospitals to our hospital, based on their wish to participate in the blood management program.*

Table C.7 Administrative policies and procedures.

Blood bank notification	What is to be done if a physician orders a transfusion that is not to be given? Convey patient-related restrictions regarding blood use to the blood bank computer to prevent unauthorized release of blood products
Budget	Line out how the program receives its annual budget, how budgets can be increased, how the program is accountable for the use of the program and establish a book keeping mode; modes to buy
Charting and administration in the program	Develop a system to collect data, chart patient encounters, etc.; consider to obtain computerized data storage and use, develop forms and checklists for redundant procedures
Creation of lead time	Define who is doing it and how, open lines of communication
Daily work with patients on the ward	Define what the responsibilities of the coordinator are who daily visit patients on the ward. What information does he have to be gathered? Prepare a case with utensils needed during ward visits, e.g., forms, stickers, wrist bands, list with contact information, etc.
Educational interventions for the hospital staff	Plan initial and continuing education; define how new staff members are reported to the program so that they can receive their orientation and can be included in educational interventions; develop information material and hand-outs for staff orientation
Informed consent	List essential components for an informed consent, develop patient education materials used to explain the features of blood management so that patient is adequately; establish ways to document the informed consent process (advance directive, living will, consent forms, exclusion of liability) and to make the content of the patient directive known to all participants in patient care
Marketing	Define marketing strategies that support in reaching the goals of the program and plan how to do this
Patient contacts	Establish how patients can contact the program when they want to use its service; define ways how patients enter the program when they present as emergencies as well as when they are scheduled for elective procedures; establish a "patient career" (where the patient has to go, what he has to fill in, which services he has to receive, who has to see the patient, etc.)
Patient identification	Describe how patients in the program are identified, e.g., by wrist bands, chart stickers, note on patient identification stickers, forms in the chart, markers in the blood bank computer, identification in the admission computer, the laboratory, on the wards
Program measurement	Define goals or quality criteria (e.g., patient satisfaction, reduction of transfusions, reduction of transfusion-related morbidity and mortality, cost reduction, increase in patients) and ways how to measure whether these goals have been reached (e.g., patient surveys, staff surveys); establish how corrective measures are initiated when goal is not reached
Referrals	If the program is established where patients can chose a physician, there must be a procedure how a patient is referred to a physician who is willing to take his case in accordance with the patient's preferences; keep an updated lists of physicians and their willingness to take certain patient groups, establish communication of the fact that a patient is referred to the physician, provide information about the physician to the patient (phone, office, etc.)
Screening of patients	Define which patients need to be screened regarding their eligibility to participate in the program; develop a checklist
Transferrals	There needs to be a procedure how patients are transferred from another institution to the program or from the program to another program; depict the ways how to transport patients, with what medical or nursing care, cost coverage, what information needs to be gained; e.g., using a check list for transferrals; define who coordinates emergency transferrals and how this person communicates
Use of donations	Establish a way how donations can be directed to the program; make sure this is a legally accepted way

Table C.8 Clinical guidelines.

Acute normovolemic hemodilution	Include recommendations for indications, contraindications, preparations, tools, monitoring, and documentation
Antifibrinolytics and desmopressin	For each agent, list indications, contraindications, dosing, and monitoring recommendations
Cell salvage, intra- and postoperatively	Include recommendations for indications, contraindications, preparations, tools, monitoring, and documentation. Consider patient populations requiring adaption of the method (e.g., patients with heparin sensitivity, children, Jehovah's Witnesses)
Compassionate use procedure	Outline how a compassionate use procedure is initiated, e.g., for the use of artificial oxygen carriers. Record emergency contacts and file needed forms
Intraoperative platelet or plasma sequestration	Include recommendations for indications, contraindications, preparations, tools, monitoring, and documentation
Marking of autologous erythrocytes in Jehovah's Witness patients	If marking of autologous red cells is a standard diagnostic procedure in your hospital, define a way how this procedure is performed in patients who do not agree to take their own red cells back
Minimization of iatrogenic blood loss	Define parameters which warrant the start of efforts to minimize iatrogenic blood loss. Explain how the blood loss is reduced, e.g., using neonatal blood sample containers, etc.
Therapy of severely anemic who do not receive allogeneic blood	If necessary, define a minimum treatment standard for those patients
Transfusion-free care of obstetric and pediatric patients	Outline the legal and ethical implications of the transfusion-free care of the patients. Describe a decision making process for cases with conflict potential
Use of autologous blood in patients who do not consent to allogeneic transfusions	Define how specific requests of patients are accommodated, e.g., how a closed circuit is established and maintained
Use of hematinics and erythropoietins	Include recommendations for indications, contraindications, preparations, tools, monitoring, and documentation. Standards, e.g., for a preoperative improvement of the hemoglobin level, may be helpful for infusion center
Use of point-of-care testing	Describe the methods used, the patients who should be assessed by the methods and provide an algorithm which indicates appropriate therapy when the point of care tests are pathologic
Use of recombinant clotting factors	For each agent, list indications, contraindications, dosing, and monitoring recommendations
Use of tissue adhesives	Include recommendations for indications, contraindications, preparations, tools, monitoring, and documentation, e.g., for the preparation of autologous glue, etc.

Table C.9 Legal and ethical guidelines.

Minors or parents of minors who refuse transfusions	Outline a legal way how to differentiate between mature and immature minors, how to accept their wishes and explain if and when court orders are to be obtained
Patients who refuse blood transfusion	Outline how patients who refuse transfusions are legally treated. Organize ways how the patients signs a release of liability, an advance directive and/or a sheet to document detailed wishes pertinent to the planned care. Adapt the used consent forms
Physician participation	Define a way how to ensure that physicians keep their promise to take care of patients according to present patient values and in accordance with program policy and procedures, e.g., as a contract between the hospital and the physician. If necessary, set a minimum education level in blood management required for physicians
Pregnant women who refuse transfusions	Define the status of pregnant women who refuse transfusions. Consider also what will happen to the newborn when the mother refuses transfusions for the baby. Think about bioethical consultations and ways how to resolve conflicts without or with using the service of a court of justice

Table C.10 Media for marketing.

Print media:
- Newspapers: Which one serves the area I want to advertise in? What is their readership? Do they publish my advertisements?
- Brochures: Is there one to which I should add my service? Do I need a brochure for my program?
- Posters: Am I allowed to place posters in strategically important spots, e.g., in nursing homes, on the roadside, etc.?
- Newsletters: Do I have or can I create a mailing list? What will be the content? Is it interesting? Who will contribute to the content?
- Direct mail: With what purpose?

Electronic media:
- Website: Have your own or participate in an existing one?
- E-mail: Do you have a mailing list (current and potential patients), need permission to contact them by e-mail? What will you say?
- Radio: Is there a radio station? Reasonable rate? Help produce content for them. Send your ads.
- TV: Is there a TV station? Costs? Content?

Person to person:
- Seminars: Content? How to promote them? Who will be speakers? Costs? Handout?
- Giveaways, gimmicks: The key ring theory—is useful? Will it last? Is it supposed to last?
- Word of mouth: Ambassadors, physicians, staff, religious, and community groups

Table C.11 Target groups for marketing.

Target group: Referring physicians
- Information letters about the initiation of the program sent to physicians in the vicinity and in the area the hospital serves or the area the program will serve (may be greater than the usual area the hospital serves)
- Occasional information letters about the ongoing development of the program and news regarding the program, e.g., once a year
- Information and recommendation letters to physicians who have referred patient previously, thanking for the good cooperation
- Seminars, information sessions
- Homepage, patient-oriented

Target group: Potential patients who already wish to avoid transfusions
- Regularly send information about blood management
- Sell key chains for emergencies, etc.
- Information sessions regarding blood management, seminars, use questionnaires and follow up
- Homepage, patient-oriented
- Register program in program lists, hit lists, etc.
- Gadgets as presents, e.g., pens
- Clubs for patient groups that continually require blood management (e.g., sickle cell patients)

Target group: Media, the public
- Report about the program and spectacular cases in the media
- Invite media to report
- Provide press releases, compile information material designed for media representatives
- Homepage

Target group: Colleagues
- Participation in meetings
- Publications
- Invite speakers
- Organize sessions for mutual exchange of experiences

Table C.12 Structures for business plans [1, 2].

Proposal 1
Introduction
    (history of blood management, no proven efficacy of transfusions, current trends and data)
Business purpose
    (feasibility and desirability of the program, benefits for patient care and revenue; continued reinforcement, that administrative
    support is essential)
Operations plan
    (structure of the program, roles of the key players—physician director and coordinator; short- and long-term goals)
Financial analysis
    (cite historical trends in blood use of the hospital, relate them to costs, project into the future, integrate the costs of the program,
    calculate return on investment)
Market assessment
    (2 basic markets for blood management: bloodless medicine for Jehovah's Witnesses or blood safety for the general public; mention
    existence or nonexistence of competing programs in the area)
Risk–benefit analysis
    Very few risks associated (nonperformance of program staff, failure to reach goals), many benefits
Recommendations
    Establish follow-up contact and time frame; recommend a contract for at least 3 years

Proposal 2
Background
    Description of the current situation of blood management in general and in the hospital, reasons to change current situation
Purpose and objectives
    State that the implementation of a formal blood management program is planned, cite its objectives
Strategies
    Describe in general what will be done to fulfil the purpose of the program (e.g., optimize blood use, introduce methods that reduce
    use of allogeneic blood transfusions, participate in research)
Benefits
    For the patient, for the hospital, for the staff, for the society
Structure
    Shortly explain the implementation of a physician director, a coordinator and possible, committees
Financial
    Project savings, calculate costs of the program, approximate the expected return on investment
Next steps and time frame
    Immediate next steps, short-, median-, and long-term goals
Appendix
    Job description of the coordinator; sources and references; tables and model calculations of key numbers using hospital data

Proposal 3: The four "P's" of program development:
    Purpose: a general statement of the program
    Philosophy: assumptions and beliefs about the blood management program. Who is served? How? With what intention?
    Policy: precise statements of the do's and don't's. Responsibilities are shortly stated
    Procedures: precise definitions of the policies
Followed by goals and objectives:
• Goals are overall statements which direct the program into a certain direction. Goals may be classified as immediate, intermediate,
and long-term
• Objectives are the specific statements, which touch on the patient care and the part all participants in the program play. They are
designed based on the above-formulated objectives. They define the behavioral changes that are intended to be achieved

Table C.13 An example of an outline for a formal one-to-one educational intervention.

Goals of the visit
- Introduce yourself as blood management coordinator
- Inform the visited persons about the goals, objectives, and structure of the planned blood management program
- Identify the benefits the program brings for the hospital in general and the visited individual in particular
- Define the role of the visited individual in the blood management program
- Encourage the visited individual to assume an active share in the program
- Provide information about the next steps that are planned to bring the program into existence
- Provide contact information

Materials/Visual aids to be used:

Summary of the accepted business proposal for the blood management program

Chart of the structure of the blood management program

Information sheet for visited individual with take home messages

Business card of the coordinator

Outline of the presentation

Allow for questions

Leave information sheet

Table C.14 Form: transfer of patients from outside hospitals into the program.

Transfer patient

    Transfer

    Date . . . . time . . . . coordinator . . . .

    Name of patient . . . . date of birth: . . . .

    Reason for transfer: . . . .

    Baseline disease: . . . .

    Medical history: . . . .

    . . . .

Clinical data:

    Last Hb/Hkt: . . . . g/dL/mmol/dL/% of . . . . coags? . . . .

    Active bleeding: yes/no? where? . . . . how much? . . . . therapy initiated? . . . .

Medication

Drug/mode of application	Dose	Remarks

Transport

Continuous intravenous therapy? . . . .

Monitoring? EKG, intravenous line?, arterial line?, central line? PAC? Others?

Is patient stable for transport? yes/no

Transferring hospital

Name of hospital . . . . ward . . . . cooperative yes/no?

Treating physician: . . . . phone: . . . .

Insurance? . . . .

Name of person who wishes transfer . . . . phone: . . . .

Bedanke Dich für Anruf, versichere Rückruf in ca. 15 Minuten

Table C.14 (*Continued*)

Performing the transfer

Contact in-hospital physician

Contacted physician . . . . time . . . .

Inform about patient, transfer possible yes/no

☐ stabile (no monitoring); ☐ not critical (constant monitoring); ☐ critical

If transfer, ask physician to   (a) contact transferring physician in 15 minutes time

                                   (b) book a bed for patient

Contact person, who asks for transfer

☐ call person who asked for transfer (time . . . .)

Ask to:

– inform treating physician about transfer

– tell treating physician, that out in-hospital physician will contact him shortly

– issue transport certificate

– organize transfer

– ask nursing to make copy of patient file

– provide information about trip to our hospital

– ask for return-call

Cave: when transport not cooperative, then transfer still possible (against will of treating physician)

Cave: transport costs, no insurance during transport, no liability

Notes:

☐ patient travels by himself, takes care of his own travel arrangements (give hints regarding travel)

☐ patient cannot travel alone

Stabil, without monitoring	Not critical, need for monitoring	Critically ill
Organize patient transport	Organize ambulance, possibly with emergency physician	Organize ambulance with intensivist, mobile intensive care unit, helicopter

☐ help required, do we have transport certificate/payment certificate?

☐ call emergency transport coordination center (Phone: XXXXX)

☐ call person who asks for transfer and inform about organized transfer

☐ call treating physician

☐ inform in-hospital physician about transfer time

Patient arrived: Date . . . . Time . . . .

Remarks . . . .

References

1 Gagliardi, K. Inservice education: a commitment to excellence. *Can J Med Technol*, 1991. **53**(1): p. 18–23.

2 Derderian, G.P. Establishing a business plan for blood conservation. *J Cardiothorac Vasc Anesth*, 2004. **18**(4 Suppl): p. 12S–14S.

Appendix D. Teaching aids: research and projects

Appendix D provides a number of model projects and a teaching story. These are meant to help to teach blood management.

Student projects

Project 1

Aim: Familiarize the student with methods to reduce blood loss and manage anemia and bleeding without the use of donor blood. Provide an overview over the possibilities available at the student's hospital.

Task: List all specialties and subspecialties offered in the hospital. Then approach each of them and ask for methods how to manage patients without donor blood or how to reduce the probability of allogeneic blood encounter. List all drugs and methods available, and describe the rationale for their use. Note whether the methods are used routinely, occasionally, or never.

Project 2

Aim: Encourage the students to reflect on current patient's rights and ethics.

Task:

1 Find out about the right patients have to determine whether they want to have a transfusion or not. Please, give the paragraphs of your current law, not your personal opinion.

• Can patients express their wishes concerning blood products?

• Are patients allowed to have a valid advance directive?

• Are you as physician bound to accept the refusal of a treatment, even if it seems to be contrary to what you think is good for them?

• Can minors express their wishes and do you have to accept it?

• Can parents say what they want for their baby and can you overrate them in an ethical manner?

• Do you have to call for a court order in case of a mature person/a minor?

• What happens if you accept the wish of a patient and what happens if you do not accept it?

2 Give your personal view of the questions mentioned under (1)

Survey your fellow workers about their opinion about the following questions. Analyze their answers in the light of what you learned during your study of current law and ethics.

1 Would you accept blood transfusion if you were patient?

2 At which hemoglobin level would you like to be transfused?

3 Would you transfuse a mature patient, if he refuses transfusion?

4 Would you use therapies that can reduce the likelihood of transfusions even if they were more expensive than blood transfusions?

5 What is the most important reason for you to reduce patient's exposure to donor blood?

Project 3

Aim: Students get to know available blood products.

Task: List all ways how blood is used for therapy in the hospital. (Do not include diagnostic procedures.) List all means of donor-blood-use and all possible ways how to use patient's own blood. Describe each product, its production, indication, contraindication, risks, costs for one unit/one vial, and how often it is used in the hospital (e.g., 10,000 units of erythrocyte concentrates per year), and how much of the produced products have to be discarded.

Project 4

Aim: Broaden the horizon of your students.

Task: Research traditional medicine of the country. Find out which methods are used in traditional medicine to treat anemia, coagulation disorders, reduce blood loss, etc. List as many possibilities as you can find (herbs, venoms, acupuncture, diet, etc.), describe them, and relate how it is explained to work. Note whether the method is accepted in hospital treatment or only used by traditional healers.

Project 5

Aim: Practice to integrate newly gained knowledge into a plan of care.

Task: Develop a plan of care for a severely anemic patient heavily bleeding from the upper gastrointestinal tract and for whom no donor blood is available. Please, follow the algorithms you have learned and develop a systematic plan. Explain every step you plan and discuss therapeutic options, if available. Write the management plan for 1 week, one day after another. Provide the rationale for every step.

The following questions are meant to be a guide only.

What information would you obtain by history taking and physical examination?

What diagnostic procedures do you order?

What laboratory diagnostics do you order?

What therapeutic measures do you take? (immediately and tomorrow and next week)

Which treatments are urgent and which ones can wait?

Prescribe with timing and dose regimen.

What do you do if the patient is allergic to the prescribed drugs? (give a hint for every prescribed drug)

Whom do you would involve in the care of the patient?

Teaching with stories

While reading the hospital fairy tale, think about your own hospital and its potentials to use existing features for a blood management program. Analyze the story and answer the questions below. Think about how you would answer the same questions using the hospital you work in.

How is the patient identified?

What is done to comply with legal requirements?

Which steps are taken to ensure the patient's wishes are heeded?

What direct support does the patient receive?

A Hospital Fairy Tale

Once upon a time, in a distant land, there was a smart medical student named Tony. One day, he got a bad cough, so he went to see a doctor. Happily, it was not pneumonia. But there was something about his heartbeat that made his family doctor listen a little longer than normal. After he had completed his examination, the doctor explained that there is a heart murmur that needed further evaluation and Tony was sent to a heart specialist. The specialist concluded that Tony's heart needed surgery. This came to him quite unexpectedly. He never had been seriously sick, and now he suddenly had to undergo surgery. A million things went through his mind. What now?

Tony was a smart student and he thought about what could happen to him during surgery. What bothered him was not so much the surgery. He would be fast asleep. But what about afterwards? During his studies he had joined physicians when they explained heart surgery to other patients. No problem! Everything was routine. But now he was the patient, and he had a strange feeling in his belly. No, of course he wasn't afraid. But time and again he thought about the blood he would receive. Would it be safe enough? Deep inside he had some doubts.

Tony had heard about many successful heart surgeries performed without the use of donor blood. After a night of discussing the pros and cons with his parents, he decided to give it a try. There was a blood management program in a nearby town. Without further delay, he called to make an appointment. A friendly voice on the telephone invited him for the next day and asked him to bring along a copy of his medical records.

The next morning, Tony got up early to be at the hospital on time. He had never been there before. While on the bus Tony tried to imagine the kind of hospital would be. Most probably it would be one of the huge glass buildings he had seen on TV. High-Tech equipment was what he expected and much more. Then again, maybe not. He just knew this hospital must be something very special.

To his surprise, he found that the hospital was not the shining glass building he had expected. Rather, he found himself standing in front of one of those hospitals built years ago. The building was made of red bricks. Flowers were planted along the pavement toward the main hospital entrance.

Hesitantly, Tony followed the path to the hospital reception. A poster right in the hallway caught his attention. Big letters said: "No Blood? No Problem." Never before had Tony seen anything like this. It was so different from the posters he was used to seeing: "Give blood, save lives." Tony looked around. Nothing was as he had imagined. The atmosphere in the hospital was rather familiar, almost cosy. Tony relaxed. The smile of the old lady at the reception was contagious. He smiled back and followed the signs to the blood management coordinator's office.

Another smiling face welcomed Tony. A young lady offered him a seat. Mr Dam, the lady said, was still with another patient but he would be with him soon. The lady brought him a cup of jasmine tea and chocolate chip cookies and left him alone in Mr Dam's office. Tony let his eyes wander. His attention was caught by a huge pin board full of cards and photos. Obviously, many patients had expressed their thanks by dropping a line.

It was not before long that the door opened and a man entered the room. The coordinator introduced himself: "Laban Dam," and gave Tony's hand a good shake. Taking some papers from a shelf, Mr Dam took a seat.

Tony told him about his heart murmur and his concerns about receiving someone else's blood. The coordinator listened carefully, nodding occasionally. When Tony had finished, Mr Dam said: "No problem! I will refer you to a heart surgeon who is experienced in doing the procedure without the use of donor blood. Let's discuss some details. Here I have a form for an advance directive. We will go over every point and I will explain all you need to know." The coordinator took the patient education material and went over it with Tony. Tony had so many questions. Using the pictures and charts in the education material, Mr Dam patiently explained everything. By the end, Tony knew all about the use of his own blood in a cell saver, about hemodilution, the heart-lung-machine, plasma expanders, human and recombinant clotting factors, and even about artificial oxygen carriers. Tony was relieved. He could easily fill in his advance directive and the consent form, allowing the physician to use the methods he chose. He felt that he was in competent hands.

What followed seemed to be mere routine for the coordinator. He had a look in his computer and gave Tony the name and the telephone number of his surgeon, Dr Lucas. A short message informed Dr Lucas about Tony's upcoming visit, and an e-mail to the blood bank ensured that the blood bank would be informed about Tony's decision regarding the use of his own and donor blood. Mr Dam asked to see the copies of Tony's medical records. A short glimpse at Tony's blood count told him that everything was all right. Otherwise, the coordinator would have alerted Dr Lucas right from the start. Tony was amazed. So much professionalism!

A few days later, Tony met with Dr Lucas. He was a tall man in his fifties. His calm personality was really reassuring. After reading through Tony's documents, taking his history and a physical examination, the surgeon explained the procedure. Tony's curiosity was satisfied by Dr Lucas friendly explanations. Dr Lucas had especially emphasized what measures he would take to reduce any unnecessary blood loss. As a future physician, Tony was fascinated and for a while he nearly forgot that he was the patient and not the physician. Since Tony's condition and especially his blood count were excellent, there was no reason to wait with the surgery. Had that not been the case, his surgery would have been postponed until erythropoietin and hematinics had done their part. Tony was scheduled for next Monday at 2 p.m.

On Monday morning, Tony traveled alone to the hospital again. His parents couldn't make it, since both had caught a cold. Admittedly, Tony was nervous. But as soon as he entered the corridor and saw the smiling lady at the reception again he felt an inner calm. He was convinced Dr Lucas and his team would know what to do.

Tony went to the admissions office. The clerk entered Tony's personal data into the computer. She asked if he is a participant of the blood management program and entered Tony's positive response into the computer. Now, every print-out on any form would not only state Tony's name and date of birth but also his status in the blood management program. When all required papers were printed, Tony was handed a folder with his new medical documents. The clerk took him to the office of the coordinator again. When he entered he felt quite at home. The same friendly faces welcomed him. Mr Dam checked Tony's folder. Everything was all right. A sticker was attached to his folder indicating his participation in the program. Copies of his advance directive and his signed consent form were also put into the folder. Now every physician—no matter what specialty—would be informed about his decision regarding the use of blood. After a little small-talk, Mr Dam took Tony to the ward and introduced him to Ms Florence Shiphrah, one of the nurses in the pre-op holding area.

Right away, Florence started with her work. She attached a wrist band to Tony's arm. The bracelet had a distinct color that indicated his blood management status. Florence was well informed. She didn't take as much blood as Tony was used to from his home hospital. Also, the nurses seemed to participate in saving every drop of blood. It was real team work!

As Tony was wheeled to the operating room he had the impression that everything was ready for him. He saw the cell saver already set up. And while he wondered why a weighing scale was needed in an operating room, he drifted off to sleep.

Tony tried to remember what had happened. His mind was so cloudy that it took quite a while until he realized that he was in a bed. The surroundings didn't look familiar at all. He felt drowsy. Didn't he have surgery? Yes, he remembered remotely. His eyes scanned his surrounding. Suddenly he shuddered. Blood! Three bags were hanging on a pole over his head. Tony felt a flush of adrenaline working through his body. It nearly made him sit up! But then he felt a warm hand resting reassuringly on his shoulder. Tony turned his head and saw the brown eyes of Florence. She seemed to have noticed his startled glance at the blood above his head and said: "It is your own." Phew! Tony relaxed. Mr Dam had told him before that there might be blood remaining from cell salvage and hemodilution. This would be given back to him after surgery. Tony again felt his drowsiness. Calmly he gave in to his medication.

Tony didn't know how long he had been asleep. He heard a noise as if someone was turning pages and opened his eyes. This time, his mind was much clearer. Mr Dam was about to check his chart. Tony's hoarse "hello" made Mr Dam turn his attention towards him. "Everything went well. There was some blood loss during surgery but not too much. And the blood coming from your drains is only minimal. You can rest assured. It's all right." Tony nodded and leaned back in his pillow. Florence approached Mr Dam and reported her findings about Tony. There was no reason to assume complications would develop. Even if they did—there would be several pairs of eyes ready to register any change in his condition. Help would be available immediately to prevent further blood loss. Before Mr Dam left the room he offered to keep Tony's parents informed about the progress he was making.

Three days had passed since Tony's surgery. He had recovered well and was ready to go home. Florence came in the room to give him last instructions. He was told what to do to speed up his recovery, which food to eat, how to take his iron tablets, and when to come back. Tony's parents had sent friends to give him a ride home. Before he finally went home, he stopped by Mr Dam's office to thank him for his extraordinary service. Tony's eyes again rested on the pin board with the many cards and pictures. Tony was sure the card he would send would soon join the collection on the board.

Appendix E: address book

Medications

Acetylstarch
Check: o normally available in hospital o available with special order o not available
Supplier/company:
Name: ....
Phone .... Fax ....
Address: ....
e-mail: .... Homepage: ....
Remarks: ....
Responsible sales representative
Name: ....
Phone .... Fax ....
Address: ....
e-mail: .... Homepage: ....
Remarks: ....

Androgens
Check: o normally available in hospital o available with special order o not available
Supplier/company:
Name: ....
Phone .... Fax ....
Address: ....
e-mail: .... Homepage: ....
Remarks: ....
Responsible sales representative
Name: ....
Phone .... Fax ....
Address: ....
e-mail: .... Homepage: ....
Remarks: ....

Aprotinin
Check: o normally available in hospital o available with special order o not available
Supplier/company:
Name: ....
Phone .... Fax ....
Address: ....
e-mail: .... Homepage: ....
Remarks: ....

Responsible sales representative
Name: ....
Phone .... Fax ....
Address: ....
e-mail: .... Homepage: ....
Remarks: ....

Bone wax
Check: o normally available in hospital o available with special order o not available
Supplier/company:
Name: ....
Phone .... Fax ....
Address: ....
e-mail: .... Homepage: ....
Remarks: ....

Responsible sales representative
Name: ....
Phone .... Fax ....
Address: ....
e-mail: .... Homepage: ....
Remarks: ....

Carnitine
Check: o normally available in hospital o available with special order o not available
Supplier/company:
Name: ....
Phone .... Fax ....
Address: ....
e-mail: .... Homepage: ....
Remarks: ....

Responsible sales representative
Name: ....
Phone .... Fax ....
Address: ....
e-mail: .... Homepage: ....
Remarks: ....

Cellulose
Check: o normally available in hospital o available with special order o not available
Supplier/company:
Name: ....
Phone .... Fax ....
Address: ....
e-mail: .... Homepage: ....
Remarks: ....

Responsible sales representative
Name: ....
Phone .... Fax ....
Address: ....
e-mail: .... Homepage: ....
Remarks: ....

Collagen mesh
Check: o normally available in hospital o available with special order o not available
Supplier/company:
Name: ....
Phone .... Fax ....
Address: ....
e-mail: .... Homepage: ....
Remarks: ....

Responsible sales representative
Name: ....
Phone .... Fax ....
Address: ....
e-mail: .... Homepage: ....
Remarks: ....

Conjugated estrogens
Check: o normally available in hospital o available with special order o not available
Supplier/company:
Name: ....
Phone .... Fax ....
Address: ....
e-mail: .... Homepage: ....
Remarks: ....

Responsible sales representative
Name: ....
Phone .... Fax ....
Address: ....
e-mail: .... Homepage: ....
Remarks: ....

Cyanoacrylate
Check: o normally available in hospital o available with special order o not available
Supplier/company:
Name: ....
Phone .... Fax ....
Address: ....
e-mail: .... Homepage: ....
Remarks: ....

Responsible sales representative
Name: ....
Phone .... Fax ....
Address: ....
e-mail: .... Homepage: ....
Remarks: ....

Danazol
Check: o normally available in hospital o available with special order o not available
Supplier/company:
Name: ....
Phone .... Fax ....
Address: ....
e-mail: .... Homepage: ....
Remarks: ....

Responsible sales representative
Name: ....
Phone .... Fax ....
Address: ....
e-mail: .... Homepage: ....
Remarks: ....

Darbepoetin (NESP)
Check: o normally available in hospital o available with special order o not available
Supplier/company:
Name: ....
Phone .... Fax ....
Address: ....
e-mail: .... Homepage: ....
Remarks: ....

Responsible sales representative
Name: ....
Phone .... Fax ....
Address: ....
e-mail: .... Homepage: ....
Remarks: ....

Desmopressin
Check: o normally available in hospital o available with special order o not available
Supplier/company:
Name: ....
Phone .... Fax ....
Address: ....
e-mail: .... Homepage: ....
Remarks: ....

Responsible sales representative
Name: ....
Phone .... Fax ....
Address: ....
e-mail: .... Homepage: ....
Remarks: ....

Dextran
Check: o normally available in hospital o available with special order o not available
Supplier/company:
Name: ....
Phone .... Fax ....
Address: ....
e-mail: .... Homepage: ....
Remarks: ....

Responsible sales representative
Name: ....
Phone .... Fax ....
Address: ....
e-mail: .... Homepage: ....
Remarks: ....

Epsilon aminocaproic acid
Check: o normally available in hospital o available with special order o not available
Supplier/company:
Name: ....
Phone .... Fax ....
Address: ....
e-mail: .... Homepage: ....
Remarks: ....

Responsible sales representative
Name: ....
Phone .... Fax ....
Address: ....
e-mail: .... Homepage: ....
Remarks: ....

Erythropoietin
Check: o normally available in hospital o available with special order o not available
Supplier/company:
Name: ....
Phone .... Fax ....
Address: ....
e-mail: .... Homepage: ....
Remarks: ....

Responsible sales representative
Name: ....
Phone .... Fax ....
Address: ....
e-mail: .... Homepage: ....
Remarks: ....

Ethamsylate
Check: o normally available in hospital o available with special order o not available
Supplier/company:
Name: ....
Phone .... Fax ....
Address: ....
e-mail: .... Homepage: ....
Remarks: ....

Responsible sales representative
Name: ....
Phone .... Fax ....
Address: ....
e-mail: .... Homepage: ....
Remarks: ....

Fibrin sealant
Check: o normally available in hospital o available with special order o not available
Supplier/company:
Name: ....
Phone .... Fax ....
Address: ....
e-mail: .... Homepage: ....
Remarks: ....

Responsible sales representative
Name: ....
Phone .... Fax ....
Address: ....
e-mail: .... Homepage: ....
Remarks: ....

Filgrastim (G-CSF)
Check: o normally available in hospital o available with special order o not available
Supplier/company:
Name: ....
Phone .... Fax ....
Address: ....
e-mail: .... Homepage: ....
Remarks: ....

Responsible sales representative
Name: ....
Phone .... Fax ....
Address: ....
e-mail: .... Homepage: ....
Remarks: ....

Folate
Check: o normally available in hospital o available with special order o not available
Supplier/company:
Name: ....
Phone .... Fax ....
Address: ....
e-mail: .... Homepage: ....
Remarks: ....

Responsible sales representative
Name: ....
Phone .... Fax ....
Address: ....
e-mail: .... Homepage: ....
Remarks: ....

Gelatin
Check: o normally available in hospital o available with special order o not available
Supplier/company:
Name: ....
Phone .... Fax ....
Address: ....
e-mail: .... Homepage: ....
Remarks: ....

Responsible sales representative
Name: ....
Phone .... Fax ....
Address: ....
e-mail: .... Homepage: ....
Remarks: ....

Hemoglobin-based oxygen carrier
Check: o normally available in hospital o available with special order o not available
Supplier/company:
Name: ....
Phone .... Fax ....
Address: ....
e-mail: .... Homepage: ....
Remarks: ....

Responsible sales representative
Name: ....
Phone .... Fax ....
Address: ....
e-mail: .... Homepage: ....
Remarks: ....

Hydroxyethylstarch
Check: o normally available in hospital o available with special order o not available
Supplier/company:
Name: ....
Phone .... Fax ....
Address: ....
e-mail: .... Homepage: ....
Remarks: ....

Responsible sales representative
Name: ....
Phone .... Fax ....
Address: ....
e-mail: .... Homepage: ....
Remarks: ....

Hypertonic volume expander, e.g., saline
Check: o normally available in hospital o available with special order o not available
Supplier/company:
Name: ....
Phone .... Fax ....
Address: ....
e-mail: .... Homepage: ....
Remarks: ....

Responsible sales representative
Name: ....
Phone .... Fax ....
Address: ....
e-mail: .... Homepage: ....
Remarks: ....

Interleukin 11 (Oprelvekin)
Check: o normally available in hospital o available with special order o not available
Supplier/company:
Name: ....
Phone .... Fax ....
Address: ....
e-mail: .... Homepage: ....
Remarks: ....

Responsible sales representative
Name: ....
Phone .... Fax ....
Address: ....
e-mail: .... Homepage: ....
Remarks: ....

Iron dextran
Check: o normally available in hospital o available with special order o not available
Supplier/company:
Name: ....
Phone .... Fax ....
Address: ....
e-mail: .... Homepage: ....
Remarks: ....

Responsible sales representative
Name: ....
Phone .... Fax ....
Address: ....
e-mail: .... Homepage: ....
Remarks: ....

Iron gluconate
Check: o normally available in hospital o available with special order o not available
Supplier/company:
Name: ....
Phone .... Fax ....
Address: ....
e-mail: .... Homepage: ....
Remarks: ....

Responsible sales representative
Name: ....
Phone .... Fax ....
Address: ....
e-mail: .... Homepage: ....
Remarks: ....

Iron polymaltose
Check: o normally available in hospital o available with special order o not available
Supplier/company:
Name: ....
Phone .... Fax ....
Address: ....
e-mail: .... Homepage: ....
Remarks: ....

Responsible sales representative
Name: ....
Phone .... Fax ....
Address: ....
e-mail: .... Homepage: ....
Remarks: ....

Iron sucrose
Check: o normally available in hospital o available with special order o not available
Supplier/company:
Name: ....
Phone .... Fax ....
Address: ....
e-mail: .... Homepage: ....
Remarks: ....

Responsible sales representative
Name: ....
Phone .... Fax ....
Address: ....
e-mail: .... Homepage: ....
Remarks: ....

Iron sulfate
Check: o normally available in hospital o available with special order o not available
Supplier/company:
Name: ....
Phone .... Fax ....
Address: ....
e-mail: .... Homepage: ....
Remarks: ....

Responsible sales representative
Name: ....
Phone .... Fax ....
Address: ....
e-mail: .... Homepage: ....
Remarks: ....

Lenograstim (G-CSF)
Check: o normally available in hospital o available with special order o not available
Supplier/company:
Name: ....
Phone .... Fax ....
Address: ....
e-mail: .... Homepage: ....
Remarks: ....

Responsible sales representative
Name: ....
Phone .... Fax ....
Address: ....
e-mail: .... Homepage: ....
Remarks: ....

M-CSF
Check: o normally available in hospital o available with special order o not available
Supplier/company:
Name: ....
Phone .... Fax ....
Address: ....
e-mail: .... Homepage: ....
Remarks: ....

Responsible sales representative
Name: ....
Phone .... Fax ....
Address: ....
e-mail: .... Homepage: ....
Remarks: ....

Metoclopramide
Check: o normally available in hospital o available with special order o not available
Supplier/company:
Name: ....
Phone .... Fax ....
Address: ....
e-mail: .... Homepage: ....
Remarks: ....

Responsible sales representative
Name: ....
Phone .... Fax ....
Address: ....
e-mail: .... Homepage: ....
Remarks: ....

Molgramostim (GM-CSF)
Check: o normally available in hospital o available with special order o not available
Supplier/company:
Name: ....
Phone .... Fax ....
Address: ....
e-mail: .... Homepage: ....
Remarks: ....

Responsible sales representative
Name: ....
Phone .... Fax ....
Address: ....
e-mail: .... Homepage: ....
Remarks: ....

Nandrolone
Check: o normally available in hospital o available with special order o not available
Supplier/company:
Name: ....
Phone .... Fax ....
Address: ....
e-mail: .... Homepage: ....
Remarks: ....

Responsible sales representative
Name: ....
Phone .... Fax ....
Address: ....
e-mail: .... Homepage: ....
Remarks: ....

Nartograstim (G-CSF)
Check: o normally available in hospital o available with special order o not available
Supplier/company:
Name: ....
Phone .... Fax ....
Address: ....
e-mail: .... Homepage: ....
Remarks: ....

Responsible sales representative
Name: ....
Phone .... Fax ....
Address: ....
e-mail: .... Homepage: ....
Remarks: ....

Oxidized cellulose
Check: o normally available in hospital o available with special order o not available
Supplier/company:
Name: ....
Phone .... Fax ....
Address: ....
e-mail: .... Homepage: ....
Remarks: ....
Responsible sales representative
Name: ....
Phone .... Fax ....
Address: ....
e-mail: .... Homepage: ....
Remarks: ....

Oxygen
Check: o normally available in hospital o available with special order o not available
Supplier/company:
Name: ....
Phone .... Fax ....
Address: ....
e-mail: .... Homepage: ....
Remarks: ....
Responsible sales representative
Name: ....
Phone .... Fax ....
Address: ....
e-mail: .... Homepage: ....
Remarks: ....

Oxygen, hyperbaric
Check: o normally available in hospital o available with special order o not available
Supplier/company:
Name: ....
Phone .... Fax ....
Address: ....
e-mail: .... Homepage: ....
Remarks: ....

Responsible sales representative
Name: ....
Phone .... Fax ....
Address: ....
e-mail: .... Homepage: ....
Remarks: ....

Paraaminobenzoic acid (PAMBA)
Check: o normally available in hospital o available with special order o not available
Supplier/company:
Name: ....
Phone .... Fax ....
Address: ....
e-mail: .... Homepage: ....
Remarks: ....

Responsible sales representative
Name: ....
Phone .... Fax ....
Address: ....
e-mail: .... Homepage: ....
Remarks: ....

Peg-filgrastim (G-CSF)
Check: o normally available in hospital o available with special order o not available
Supplier/company:
Name: ....
Phone .... Fax ....
Address: ....
e-mail: .... Homepage: ....
Remarks: ....

Responsible sales representative
Name: ....
Phone .... Fax ....
Address: ....
e-mail: .... Homepage: ....
Remarks: ....

Perfluorocarbon
Check: o normally available in hospital o available with special order o not available
Supplier/company:
Name: ....
Phone .... Fax ....
Address: ....
e-mail: .... Homepage: ....
Remarks: ....

Responsible sales representative
Name: ....
Phone .... Fax ....
Address: ....
e-mail: .... Homepage: ....
Remarks: ....

Recombinant factor Antithrombin
Check: o normally available in hospital o available with special order o not available
Supplier/company:
Name: ....
Phone .... Fax ....
Address: ....
e-mail: .... Homepage: ....
Remarks: ....

Responsible sales representative
Name: ....
Phone .... Fax ....
Address: ....
e-mail: .... Homepage: ....
Remarks: ....

Recombinant factor IX
Check: o normally available in hospital o available with special order o not available
Supplier/company:
Name: ....
Phone .... Fax ....
Address: ....
e-mail: .... Homepage: ....
Remarks: ....

Responsible sales representative
Name: ....
Phone .... Fax ....
Address: ....
e-mail: .... Homepage: ....
Remarks: ....

Recombinant factor VIIa (Eptacog)
Check: o normally available in hospital o available with special order o not available
Supplier/company:
Name: ....
Phone .... Fax ....
Address: ....
e-mail: .... Homepage: ....
Remarks: ....

Responsible sales representative
Name: ....
Phone .... Fax ....
Address: ....
e-mail: .... Homepage: ....
Remarks: ....

Recombinant factor VIII (Octacog)
Check: o normally available in hospital o available with special order o not available
Supplier/company:
Name: ....
Phone .... Fax ....
Address: ....
e-mail: .... Homepage: ....
Remarks: ....

Responsible sales representative
Name: ....
Phone .... Fax ....
Address: ....
e-mail: .... Homepage: ....
Remarks: ....

Recombinant factor XIII
Check: o normally available in hospital o available with special order o not available
Supplier/company:
Name: ....
Phone .... Fax ....
Address: ....
e-mail: .... Homepage: ....
Remarks: ....
Responsible sales representative
Name: ....
Phone .... Fax ....
Address: ....
e-mail: .... Homepage: ....
Remarks: ....

Recombinant human prolactin
Check: o normally available in hospital o available with special order o not available
Supplier/company:
Name: ....
Phone .... Fax ....
Address: ....
e-mail: .... Homepage: ....
Remarks: ....
Responsible sales representative
Name: ....
Phone .... Fax ....
Address: ....
e-mail: .... Homepage: ....
Remarks: ....

Recombinant human thrombopoietin
Check: o normally available in hospital o available with special order o not available
Supplier/company:
Name: ....
Phone .... Fax ....
Address: ....
e-mail: .... Homepage: ....
Remarks: ....
Responsible sales representative
Name: ....
Phone .... Fax ....
Address: ....
e-mail: .... Homepage: ....
Remarks: ....

Regramostim (GM-CSF)
Check: o normally available in hospital o available with special order o not available
Supplier/company:
Name: ....
Phone .... Fax ....
Address: ....
e-mail: .... Homepage: ....
Remarks: ....

Responsible sales representative
Name: ....
Phone .... Fax ....
Address: ....
e-mail: .... Homepage: ....
Remarks: ....

Sargramostim (GM-CSF)
Check: o normally available in hospital o available with special order o not available
Supplier/company:
Name: ....
Phone .... Fax ....
Address: ....
e-mail: .... Homepage: ....
Remarks: ....

Responsible sales representative
Name: ....
Phone .... Fax ....
Address: ....
e-mail: .... Homepage: ....
Remarks: ....

Somatostatin
Check: o normally available in hospital o available with special order o not available
Supplier/company:
Name: ....
Phone .... Fax ....
Address: ....
e-mail: .... Homepage: ....
Remarks: ....

Responsible sales representative
Name: ....
Phone .... Fax ....
Address: ....
e-mail: .... Homepage: ....
Remarks: ....

Tranexamic acid
Check: o normally available in hospital o available with special order o not available
Supplier/company:
Name: ....
Phone .... Fax ....
Address: ....
e-mail: .... Homepage: ....
Remarks: ....

Responsible sales representative
Name: ....
Phone .... Fax ....
Address: ....
e-mail: .... Homepage: ....
Remarks: ....

Vasopressin
Check: o normally available in hospital o available with special order o not available
Supplier/company:
Name: ....
Phone .... Fax ....
Address: ....
e-mail: .... Homepage: ....
Remarks: ....

Responsible sales representative
Name: ....
Phone .... Fax ....
Address: ....
e-mail: .... Homepage: ....
Remarks: ....

Vitamin A
Check: o normally available in hospital o available with special order o not available
Supplier/company:
Name: ....
Phone .... Fax ....
Address: ....
e-mail: .... Homepage: ....
Remarks: ....

Responsible sales representative
Name: ....
Phone .... Fax ....
Address: ....
e-mail: .... Homepage: ....
Remarks: ....

Vitamin B1
Check: o normally available in hospital o available with special order o not available
Supplier/company:
Name: ....
Phone .... Fax ....
Address: ....
e-mail: .... Homepage: ....
Remarks: ....

Responsible sales representative
Name: ....
Phone .... Fax ....
Address: ....
e-mail: .... Homepage: ....
Remarks: ....

Vitamin B2 (Riboflavin)
Check: o normally available in hospital o available with special order o not available
Supplier/company:
Name: ....
Phone .... Fax ....
Address: ....
e-mail: .... Homepage: ....
Remarks: ....

Responsible sales representative
Name: ....
Phone .... Fax ....
Address: ....
e-mail: .... Homepage: ....
Remarks: ....

Vitamin B6
Check: o normally available in hospital o available with special order o not available
Supplier/company:
Name: ....
Phone .... Fax ....
Address: ....
e-mail: .... Homepage: ....
Remarks: ....

Responsible sales representative
Name: ....
Phone .... Fax ....
Address: ....
e-mail: .... Homepage: ....
Remarks: ....

Vitamin B12
Check: o normally available in hospital o available with special order o not available
Supplier/company:
Name: ....
Phone .... Fax ....
Address: ....
e-mail: .... Homepage: ....
Remarks: ....

Responsible sales representative
Name: ....
Phone .... Fax ....
Address: ....
e-mail: .... Homepage: ....
Remarks: ....

Vitamin C
Check: o normally available in hospital o available with special order o not available
Supplier/company:
Name: ....
Phone .... Fax ....
Address: ....
e-mail: .... Homepage: ....
Remarks: ....

Responsible sales representative
Name: ....
Phone .... Fax ....
Address: ....
e-mail: .... Homepage: ....

Remarks: ....

Vitamin E
Check: o normally available in hospital o available with special order o not available
Supplier/company:
Name: ....
Phone .... Fax ....
Address: ....
e-mail: .... Homepage: ....
Remarks: ....

Responsible sales representative
Name: ....
Phone .... Fax ....
Address: ....
e-mail: .... Homepage: ....
Remarks: ....

Vitamin K group
Check: o normally available in hospital o available with special order o not available
Supplier/company: Name: ....
Phone .... Fax ....
Address: ....
e-mail: .... Homepage: ....
Remarks: ....

Responsible sales representative
Name: ....
Phone .... Fax ....
Address: ....
e-mail: .... Homepage: ....
Remarks: ....

Sources of equipment

Argon beam coagulation
Supplier/company:
Name: ....
Phone .... Fax ....
Address: ....
e-mail: .... Homepage: ....
Remarks: ....

Responsible sales representative
Name: ....
Phone .... Fax ....
Address: ....

e-mail: .... Homepage: ....

Remarks: ....

Bags for ANH
Supplier/company:
Name: ....
Phone .... Fax ....
Address: ....
e-mail: .... Homepage: ....
Remarks: ....

Responsible sales representative
Name: ....
Phone .... Fax ....
Address: ....
e-mail: .... Homepage: ....
Remarks: ....

Blood tubes, neonatal
Supplier/company:
Name: ....
Phone .... Fax ....
Address: ....
e-mail: .... Homepage: ....
Remarks: ....

Responsible sales representative
Name: ....
Phone .... Fax ....
Address: ....
e-mail: .... Homepage: ....
Remarks: ....

Cavitron ultrasonic surgical aspirator (CUSA)
Supplier/company:
Name: ....
Phone .... Fax ....
Address: ....
e-mail: .... Homepage: ....
Remarks: ....

Responsible sales representative
Name: ....
Phone .... Fax ....
Address: ....
e-mail: .... Homepage: ....
Remarks: ....

Cell salvage device with washing
Supplier/company:
Name: ....
Phone .... Fax ....
Address: ....
e-mail: .... Homepage: ....
Remarks: ....

Responsible sales representative
Name: ....
Phone .... Fax ....
Address: ....
e-mail: .... Homepage: ....
Remarks: ....

Electrocautery (Hemostatic scalpel)
Supplier/company:
Name: ....
Phone .... Fax ....
Address: ....
e-mail: .... Homepage: ....
Remarks: ....

Responsible sales representative
Name: ....
Phone .... Fax ....
Address: ....
e-mail: .... Homepage: ....
Remarks: ....

Electrosurgery (monopolar/bipolar, Bovie)
Supplier/company:
Name: ....
Phone .... Fax ....
Address: ....
e-mail: .... Homepage: ....
Remarks: ....

Responsible sales representative
Name: ....
Phone .... Fax ....
Address: ....
e-mail: .... Homepage: ....
Remarks: ....

Electrothermal bipolar vessel sealer
Supplier/company:
Name: ....
Phone .... Fax ....
Address: ....
e-mail: .... Homepage: ....
Remarks: ....

Responsible sales representative
Name: ....
Phone .... Fax ....
Address: ....
e-mail: .... Homepage: ....
Remarks: ....

Fluid warmer
Supplier/company:
Name: ....
Phone .... Fax ....

Address: ....
e-mail: .... Homepage: ....
Remarks: ....

Responsible sales representative
Name: ....
Phone .... Fax ....
Address: ....
e-mail: .... Homepage: ....
Remarks: ....

Harmonic scalpel (Ultrasonic scalpel)
Supplier/company:
Name: ....
Phone .... Fax ....
Address: ....
e-mail: .... Homepage: ....
Remarks: ....

Responsible sales representative
Name: ....
Phone .... Fax ....
Address: ....
e-mail: .... Homepage: ....
Remarks: ....

Hepcon monitor
Supplier/company:
Name: ....
Phone .... Fax ....
Address: ....
e-mail: .... Homepage: ....
Remarks: ....

Responsible sales representative
Name: ....
Phone .... Fax ....
Address: ....
e-mail: .... Homepage: ....
Remarks: ....

Infrared contact coagulator
Supplier/company:
Name: ....
Phone .... Fax ....
Address: ....
e-mail: .... Homepage: ....
Remarks: ....

Responsible sales representative
Name: ....
Phone .... Fax ....
Address: ....
e-mail: .... Homepage: ....
Remarks: ....

Laser
Supplier/company:
Name: ....
Phone .... Fax ....
Address: ....
e-mail: .... Homepage: ....
Remarks: ....

Responsible sales representative
Name: ....
Phone .... Fax ....
Address: ....
e-mail: .... Homepage: ....
Remarks: ....

Linton-Nachlas tube
Supplier/company:
Name: ....
Phone .... Fax ....
Address: ....
e-mail: .... Homepage: ....
Remarks: ....

Responsible sales representative
Name: ....
Phone .... Fax ....
Address: ....
e-mail: .... Homepage: ....
Remarks: ....

Microwave coagulator
Supplier/company:
Name: ....
Phone .... Fax ....
Address: ....
e-mail: .... Homepage: ....
Remarks: ....

Responsible sales representative
Name: ....
Phone .... Fax ....
Address: ....
e-mail: .... Homepage: ....
Remarks: ....

Plasma scalpel
Supplier/company:
Name: ....
Phone .... Fax ....
Address: ....
e-mail: .... Homepage: ....
Remarks: ....

Responsible sales representative
Name: ....
Phone .... Fax ....

Address: ....
e-mail: .... Homepage: ....
Remarks: ....

Pneumatic tourniquet
Supplier/company:
Name: ....
Phone .... Fax ....
Address: ....
e-mail: .... Homepage: ....
Remarks: ....

Responsible sales representative
Name: ....
Phone .... Fax ....
Address: ....
e-mail: .... Homepage: ....
Remarks: ....

Positioning materials
Supplier/company:
Name: ....
Phone .... Fax ....
Address: ....
e-mail: .... Homepage: ....
Remarks: ....

Responsible sales representative
Name: ....
Phone .... Fax ....
Address: ....
e-mail: .... Homepage: ....
Remarks: ....

Postoperative cell salvage device (wound drains) with washing step
Supplier/company:
Name: ....
Phone .... Fax ....
Address: ....
e-mail: .... Homepage: ....
Remarks: ....

Responsible sales representative
Name: ....
Phone .... Fax ....
Address: ....
e-mail: .... Homepage: ....
Remarks: ....

Postoperative cell salvage device without washing step
Supplier/company:
Name: ....
Phone .... Fax ....
Address: ....
e-mail: .... Homepage: ....
Remarks: ....

Responsible sales representative
Name: ....
Phone .... Fax ....
Address: ....
e-mail: .... Homepage: ....
Remarks: ....

Saline-enhanced thermal sealing
Supplier/company:
Name: ....
Phone .... Fax ....
Address: ....
e-mail: .... Homepage: ....
Remarks: ....

Responsible sales representative
Name: ....
Phone .... Fax ....
Address: ....
e-mail: .... Homepage: ....
Remarks: ....

Sengstaken-Blakemore tube
Supplier/company:
Name: ....
Phone .... Fax ....
Address: ....
e-mail: .... Homepage: ....
Remarks: ....

Responsible sales representative
Name: ....
Phone .... Fax ....
Address: ....
e-mail: .... Homepage: ....
Remarks: ....

Shortened cardiopulmonary bypass equipment
Supplier/company:
Name: ....
Phone .... Fax ....
Address: ....
e-mail: .... Homepage: ....
Remarks: ....

Responsible sales representative
Name: ....
Phone .... Fax ....
Address: ....
e-mail: .... Homepage: ....
Remarks: ....

Thermocoagulator
Supplier/company:
Name: ....
Phone .... Fax ....

Address: ....
e-mail: .... Homepage: ....
Remarks: ....

Responsible sales representative
Name: ....
Phone .... Fax ....
Address: ....
e-mail: .... Homepage: ....
Remarks: ....

Thrombelastograph
Supplier/company:
Name: ....
Phone .... Fax ....
Address: ....
e-mail: .... Homepage: ....
Remarks: ....

Responsible sales representative
Name: ....
Phone .... Fax ....
Address: ....
e-mail: .... Homepage: ....
Remarks: ....

Ultrafiltration for cardiopulmonary bypass
Supplier/company:
Name: ....
Phone .... Fax ....
Address: ....
e-mail: .... Homepage: ....
Remarks: ....

Responsible sales representative
Name: ....
Phone .... Fax ....
Address: ....
e-mail: .... Homepage: ....
Remarks: ....

Warming device for patient
Supplier/company:
Name: ....
Phone .... Fax ....
Address: ....
e-mail: .... Homepage: ....
Remarks: ....

Responsible sales representative
Name: ....
Phone .... Fax ....
Address: ....
e-mail: .... Homepage: ....
Remarks: ....

Water jet
Supplier/company:
Name: ....
Phone .... Fax ....
Address: ....
e-mail: .... Homepage: ....
Remarks: ....

Responsible sales representative
Name: ....
Phone .... Fax ....
Address: ....
e-mail: .... Homepage: ....
Remarks: ....

Sources of information

Compassionate Use Protocol
Name: ....
Phone .... Fax ....
Address: ....
e-mail: .... Homepage: ....
Remarks: ....

Embolization
Name: ....
Phone .... Fax ....
Address: ....
e-mail: .... Homepage: ....
Remarks: ....

Hospital Information Services of Jehovah's Witnesses
Name: ....
Phone .... Fax ....
Address: ....
e-mail: .... Homepage: ....
Remarks: ....

Program for Blood Management/Bloodless Medicine
Name: ....
Phone .... Fax ....
Address: ....
e-mail: .... Homepage: ....
Remarks: ....

Index

Page numbers in **bold** represent tables; those in *italics* represent figures.

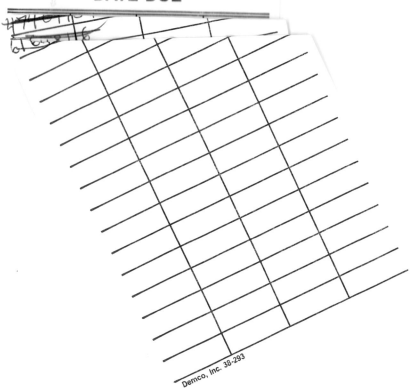

DATE DUE

Demco, Inc. 38-293